ACSM'S RESOURCES FOR CLINICAL EXERCISE PHYSIOLOGY:

MUSCULOSKELETAL, NEUROMUSCULAR, NEOPLASTIC, IMMUNOLOGIC, AND HEMATOLOGIC CONDITIONS

EDITORS

Jonathan N. Myers, PhD
Clinical Associate Professor
Department of Veterans Affairs Medical Center
Stanford University School of Medicine
Palo Alto, California

William G. Herbert, PhD
Human Nutrition, Foods and Exercise
Virginia Tech
Blacksburg, Virginia

Reed Humphrey, PhD, PT, FACSM
Physical Therapy
Medical College of Virginia
Virginia Commonwealth University
Richmond, Virginia

SECTION EDITORS

Stephen F. Figoni, PhD, RKT, FACSM
Research Health Scientist
Spinal Cord Injury Center
Veterans Administration Palo Alto Health Care System
Palo Alto, California

David C. Nieman, DrPH, FACSM
Professor
Department of Health, Leisure, and Exercise Science
Appalachian State University
Boone, North Carolina

Kenneth H. Pitetti, PhD, FACSM
Professor
College of Health Professions
Wichita State University
Wichita, Kansas

ACSM'S RESOURCES FOR CLINICAL EXERCISE PHYSIOLOGY:

Musculoskeletal, Neuromuscular, Neoplastic, Immunologic, and Hematologic Conditions

AMERICAN COLLEGE OF SPORTS MEDICINE

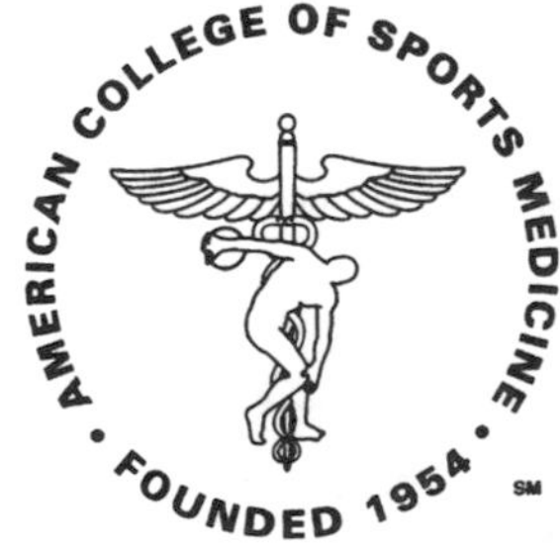

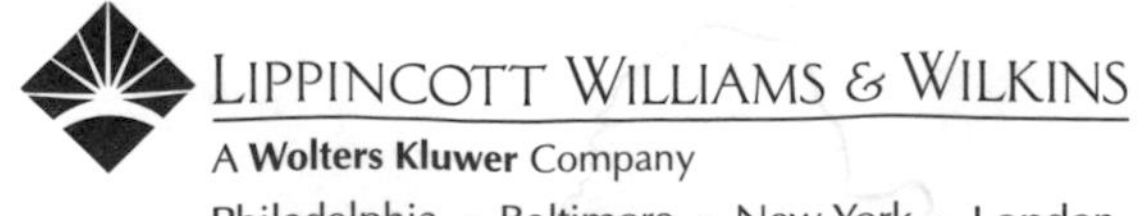

Philadelphia • Baltimore • New York • London
Buenos Aires • Hong Kong • Sydney • Tokyo

Editor: Peter J. Darcy
Managing Editor: Linda N. Napora
Marketing Manager: Christen DeMarco
Production Editor: Christina Remsberg
Compositor: Peirce Graphic Services, Inc.
Printer: Vicks Lithograph & Printing

351 West Camden Street
Baltimore, Maryland 21201-2436 USA

530 Walnut Street
Philadelphia, Pennsylvania 19106 USA

Printed in the United States of America

Library of Congress Cataloging-in-Publication Data

ACSM's guidelines and resources for clinical exercise physiology : musculoskeletal, neuromuscular, neoplastic, immunologic, and hematologic conditions / American College of Sports Medicine ; [editors, Jonathan Myers, William Herbert, Reed Humphrey].
p. cm.
Includes index.
ISBN 0-7817-3502-5
1. Exercise therapy. I. Myers, Jonathan, 1957– . II. Herbert, William. II. Humphrey, Reed H. IV. American College of Sports Medicine. V. Title: Guidelines and resources for clinical exercise physiology.
[DNLM: 1. Exercise—physiology. WE 103 A184 2002]
RM725.A34 2002
615.8'2—dc21 2001050354

The publishers have made every effort to trace the copyright holders for borrowed material. If they have inadvertently overlooked any, they will be pleased to make the necessary arrangements at the first opportunity.

To purchase additional copies of this book, call our customer service department at **(800) 638–3030** or fax orders to **(301) 824–7390.** International customers should call **(301) 714–2324.**

To purchase additional copies of this book or for information concerning American College of Sports Medicine certification and suggested preparatory materials, call **(800) 486–5643.**

02 03 04 05
1 2 3 4 5 6 7 8 9 10

Foreword

"... all parts of the body which have a function, if used in *moderation* and exercised in labours in which each is accustomed, become thereby healthy, well-developed, and age more slowly, but if unused and left idle they become liable to disease, defective in growth, and age quickly."

—Hippocrates

"We doctors can now state from our experience with people, both sick and well, and from a growing series of scientific researches that 'keeping fit' does pay richly in dividends of health and longevity."

—Paul Dudley White, MD

"From a public health perspective, the emphasis on getting sedentary adults to become moderately active is highly appropriate; the evidence shows that on a population-wide basis, this is where the majority of the health benefits are to be obtained."

—Steven N. Blair, PEd

"Smoking, body-mass index, and exercise patterns in midlife and late adulthood are predictors of subsequent disability. Not only do persons with better health habits survive longer, but in such persons, disability is postponed and compressed into fewer years at the end of life."

—James F. Fries, MD

Interest in the essential medical role of exercise testing, training, and prescription has continued to escalate in the primary, secondary, and tertiary prevention of disease. Endurance and resistance training and, more recently, complementary lifestyle activity, serve as self-improvement techniques, especially when combined with dietary alterations and effective pharmacotherapies. Moreover, physicians and allied health professionals have embraced the use of exercise in the prevention, diagnosis, and treatment of a variety of clinical conditions and chronic health problems.

Multistage exercise-tolerance testing provides invaluable information in assessing the patient's functional capacity, safety of physical exertion, and effect of various interventions. The corresponding electrocardiographic, hemodynamic, and cardiorespiratory responses also have long-term prognostic significance with regard to morbidity and mortality. Appropriately prescribed exercise training programs are associated with extremely low complication rates and numerous salutary effects. These include increases in aerobic capacity and the anaerobic or ventilatory threshold; reductions in body weight and fat stores; decreases in blood pressure (particularly among hypertensives), serum triglycerides, and low-density lipoprotein cholesterol; enhanced muscular strength and endurance; and improved bone mineral density, glucose tolerance, and insulin sensitivity.

Recently, increased attention has been directed toward the role of exercise for improving the health, physical fitness, and rehabilitation potential of patients who are challenged by varied chronic diseases and disabilities. Common medical conditions such as stroke, multiple sclerosis, muscular dystrophy, and traumatic injury to the central nervous system can elicit muscle paralysis, paresis, or spasticity. Special deficits or defects resulting from congenital deformities or musculoskeletal, neoplastic, immunological, or hematological anomalies, and the needs and contraindications imposed by these conditions, must also be taken into account. A superimposed sedentary lifestyle can exacerbate the associated disease-specific sequelae, causing these patient subsets to experience secondary conditions such as reduced cardiorespiratory fitness, muscle atrophy, osteoporosis, and impaired circulation to the lower extremities, leading to eventual thrombus formation and pressure ulcers. In addition, a diminished self-efficacy, greater dependence on others for daily living, depression, and a reduced ability for normal societal interactions can have a debilitating psychological impact.

Although there are numerous books on exercise testing and training for presumably healthy adults and patients with cardiovascular or pulmonary disease, the American College of Sports Medicine (ACSM) recognized the need for, and value of, an evidence-based resource that would comprehensively address a myriad of special patient populations. Accordingly, it is an honor and a privilege for me to introduce you to this unique text, *ACSM's Resources for Clinical Exercise Physiology: Musculoskeletal, Neuromuscular, Neo-*

plastic, Immunologic, and Hematologic Conditions, which was written to cover the critical knowledge, skills, and abilities (KSAs) in evaluating and exercising patients with varied comorbid conditions, alone or in combination. This text extends the scope of coverage for chronic disease conditions provided in *ACSM's Guidelines for Exercise Testing and Prescription* (6th edition) and *ACSM's Resource Manual* (4th edition).

This virtual pharmacopoeia of exercise physiology applications, which includes three sections, Neuromuscular Disorders, Musculoskeletal Conditions, and Neoplastic, Immunologic, and Hematologic Conditions, as well as appendices on KSAs and scope of practice, a plethora of tables and figures to highlight key or salient points, and 19 clinically germane chapters, provides an overview of the fundamentals and additional competencies that must be mastered by candidates applying for ACSM's Registered Clinical Exercise Physiologist (RCEP) credential. The content represents a contemporary distillation of the science and clinical applications that will assist any qualified clinician to provide safe and effective exercise programming for patients with the diseases and disorders presented. Accordingly, this text should become a standard reference for all practitioners, including RCEPs, as well as physicians and their assistants, nurses, physical and occupational therapists, geriatricians, and rehabilitation specialists in all areas of medicine.

ACSM's Resources for Clinical Exercise Physiology was conceived to more clearly define the benefits and limitations of exercise testing and training in the clinical evaluation and management of a broad spectrum of patients, including those with stroke, cerebral palsy, multiple sclerosis, Parkinson's disease, spinal cord injury, postpolio and Guillain-Barré syndrome, muscular dystrophy and other myopathies, peripheral neuropathy and chronic neurogenic pain, head injury, osteoarthritis and rheumatoid arthritis, fibromyalgia, chronic back pain, osteoporosis, vertebral disorders, amputation, neoplasms, immune system and hematological disorders, as well as HIV infection and chronic fatigue syndrome. The editors have recruited a prestigious group of scientists, clinicians, researchers, and extraordinary teachers who have painstakingly worked to summarize, in a clear and concise manner, pertinent information relative to the KSAs with specific reference to pathophysiology, epidemiology, risk factors, associated signs and symptoms, screening and diagnosis, medical and surgical treatments, benefits of exercise testing and training, special precautions, and motivational and adherence strategies.

Since 1975, ACSM workshops and certifications have served as the "gold standard" in professional development and continuing education, helping physicians and allied health professionals counsel their patients and clients with and without cardiopulmonary disease regarding the benefits of a physically active lifestyle. This extraordinary book extends these applications in two distinct ways. First, it serves as a pivotal resource in the preparation of individuals for credentialing by ACSM, filling a current void. Second, it broadens the scope of established principles and recommendations of exercise evaluation and programming to virtually all segments of the population. Perhaps most importantly, it provides scientific evidence that exercise offers an "equal opportunity" intervention to selected populations that have been previously underserved.

Barry A. Franklin, PhD
Director, Cardiac Rehabilitation
and Exercise Laboratories
William Beaumont Hospital
Royal Oak, Michigan
Past President, ACSM

Preface

ACSM's Resources for Clinical Exercise Physiology: Musculoskeletal, Neuromuscular, Neoplastic, Immunologic, and Hematologic Conditions has been written in response to the need for guidance among exercise clinicians working with patients who have a wide variety of chronic diseases and disabilities that extend beyond cardiovascular and pulmonary disease, areas for which there are ample resources. Indeed, this publication should be viewed as an extension of two existing ACSM publications, *ACSM's Guidelines for Exercise Testing and Prescription* and *ACSM's Resource Manual for Exercise Testing and Prescription.* It is written for post-baccalaureate-level clinicians, primarily those with training in the exercise sciences.

The text is unique in that a variety of diseases and disabilities are addressed under the common theme of exercise assessment and intervention. That the chapter authors represent a cross-section of allied health practitioners is no accident. Clinicians with varied professional training frequently play a role in the treatment of the patients addressed in this text, depending on a variety of factors that include the nature and severity of functional impairment, exercise risk, comorbidities, institutional staffing philosophy, and regulatory definition. Physicians and physician assistants, nurses and nurse practitioners, respiratory, occupational and physical therapists, kinesiotherapists, and clinical exercise physiologists often work in cooperation to meet the specific needs of these patient populations. The authorship of this text reflects the multidisciplinary nature of rehabilitation, and as such, it was the intent of the editors and contributors to produce a text that would be of benefit to all exercise clinicians.

Included in this text are the knowledge, skills, and abilities (KSAs) that have been developed to address the role of the clinical exercise physiologist in the exercise management of patients with chronic diseases and disabilities. Since the scopes of practice are well-defined for other allied health professionals, the organization of KSAs for clinical exercise physiologists is certainly appropriate. The most recent edition is included in this text in an effort to better clarify the role of the clinical exercise physiologist, and to assist in preparation for inclusion in ACSM's registry of clinical exercise physiologists. This is done with two caveats. First, the KSAs in the Appendix reflect patient populations beyond those described in this text, in particular patients with cardiovascular, pulmonary, and/or metabolic disease. The guidelines for these patients have been covered in prior publications, *ACSM's Guidelines for Exercise Testing and Prescription* and *ACSM's Resource Manual for Exercise Testing and Prescription*. Second, since the principal intent of this text was to address the overall exercise management of a wide variety of patients with chronic disease for exercise clinicians of all backgrounds, this text does not address all the KSAs in the Appendix. The clinical exercise physiologist preparing for the ACSM registry program may need supplemental resources to obtain complete coverage for all the KSAs.

The editors and contributors to this wide-ranging text hope that all exercise clinicians will find benefit from the content. In a competitive healthcare environment, scopes of practice inevitably overlap. Specific roles in practice may vary by institution and region; clarification of specific roles is essential. Such clarifications will hopefully be made with the combined and collegial wisdom of academic institutions, professional associations, and their constituents, to ensure that the perceived boundaries between health and fitness providers of different professional training are, at best, artificial. With this approach, our goals will be met.

Jonathan N. Myers
William G. Herbert
Reed Humphrey

Acknowledgments

The editors thank these individuals who contributed to this book by reviewing manuscripts and providing editorial assistance.

Yagesh Bhambhani, Ph.D.
J. Mark Davis, Ph.D.
Randy Eichner, MD
William Jay Gillespie, Ph.D.
Carol Harnett
Louis J. Jankowski, Ph.D.
Laurel T. Mackinnon, Ph.D.
Brian J. McKiernan, Ph.D., PT
Patrick J. O'Connor, Ph.D.
Carol Pitetti, BA
Robert J. Rinaldi, MD
Robert D. Rondinelli, MD, Ph.D.
Roy J. Shephard, MD
Jeffrey Woods, Ph.D.

Contributors

Mark A. Anderson, PhD, PT, ATC
Department of Physical Therapy
University of Oklahoma Health Sciences Center
Oklahoma City, Oklahoma

Thomas J. Birk, PT, PhD
Associate Professor
Department of Physical Therapy, Physical Medicine and Rehabilitation
Wayne State University
Detroit, Michigan

Louise Burke, MD
Head, Department of Sports Nutrition
Australian Institute of Sport
Belconnen, Canberra, Australia

Kerry S. Courneya, PhD
Professor
Department of Physical Education
University of Alberta
Edmonton, Alberta, Canada

Timothy J. Doherty, MD, PhD, FRCPc
Assistant Professor
Department of Physical Medicine and Rehabilitation
The University of Western Ontario
London, Ontario, Canada

Stephen F. Figoni, PhD, RKT, FACSM
Research Health Scientist
Spinal Cord Injury Center
Veterans Administration Palo Alto Health Care System
Palo Alto, California

Nadine M. Fisher, EdD
Assistant Professor
Department of Occupational Therapy
State University of New York at Buffalo
Buffalo, New York

Kenton C. Freeman, MD, DABPM&R
Director in Physical Medicine and Rehabilitation
Private practice
St. Joseph, Missouri

William Jay Gillespie, EdD
Associate Professor and Chair
Department of Cardiopulmonology and Exercise Sciences
School of Health Professions
Bouve College of Health Sciences
Northeastern University
Boston, Massachusetts

Kimberly Harbst, PhD, PT
Associate Professor
Department of Physical Therapy
University of Wisconsin—La Crosse
La Crosse, Wisconsin

Timothy Harbst, MD
Physical Medicine and Rehabilitation
Gundersen Lutheran Medical Center
La Crosse, Wisconsin

William G. Herbert, PhD
Human Nutrition, Foods and Exercise
Virginia Tech
Blacksburg, Virginia

Marianna Horea, MS
Graduate Research Associate
School of Physical Therapy
Texas Woman's University
Denton, Texas

Reed Humphrey, PhD, PT, FACSM
Physical Therapy
Medical College of Virginia
Virginia Commonwealth University
Richmond, Virginia

Leonard A. Kaminsky, PhD, FACSM
Professor
School of Physical Education
Division of Exercise Science
Ball State University
Muncie, Indiana

B. Jenny Kiratli, PhD
Research Health Scientist
Spinal Cord Injury Center
Veterans Administration Palo Alto Health Care System
Palo Alto, California

John J. LaManca, PhD
Research Coordinator/Exercise Physiologist
Heart Failure and Cardiac Transplantation
New York Presbyterian Hospital
New York, New York

James J. Laskin, PT, PhD
Department of Physical Therapy
University of Montana
Missoula, Montana

Jennifer E. Layne, MS
Jean Mayer USDA Human Nutrition Research Center on Aging
Tufts University
Boston, Massachusetts

John R. Mackey, MD
Department of Oncology
Faculty of Medicine
University of Alberta
Edmonton, Alberta, Canada

Laurel T. Mackinnon, PhD
Associate Professor
School of Human Movement Studies
The University of Queensland
Brisbane, Queensland, Australia

Robert C. Manske, MPT, CSCS
Assistant Professor
Department of Physical Therapy
Wichita State University
Wichita, Kansas

Karen Palmer McLean, PhD, PT
Associate Professor
Department of Physical Therapy
University of Wisconsin—La Crosse
La Crosse, Wisconsin

Janet A. Mulcare, PhD, FACSM
Associate Professor
Department of Physical Therapy
Andrews University—MPT Program
Dayton, Ohio

David L. Nichols, PhD
Assistant Research Professor
Institute for Women's Health
Texas Woman's University
Denton, Texas

Terry L. Nicola, MD, MS
Assistant Professor of Clinical Rehabilitation Medicine
Director of Sports Medicine Rehabilitation
Department of Orthopedics
University of Illinois Medical Center
Chicago, Illinois

Robin Parisotto, BAppSci
Laboratory Manager
Sports Haematology and Biochemistry Laboratory
Australian Institute of Sport
Leverrier Crescent
Bruce, Australian Capital Territory, Australia

Jack H. Petajan, MD
University of Utah MS Clinic
Salt Lake City, Utah

Mark T. Pfefer, RN, MS, DC
Director of Research
Department of Research
Cleveland Chiropractic College
Kansas City, Missouri

Kenneth H. Pitetti, PhD, FACSM
Professor
College of Health Professions
Wichita State University
Wichita, Kansas

Elizabeth J. Protas, PhD, PT
School of Physical Therapy
Texas Woman's University
Houston, Texas

H. Arthur Quinney, PhD
Faculty of Physical Education
University of Alberta
Edmonton, Alberta, Canada

James Rimmer, PhD, FACSM
Associate Professor
Institute for Disability and Human Development
University of Illinois
Chicago, Illinois

Jessica C. Roberts, MA
Department of Clinical Psychology
University of Kansas
Wichita, Kansas

Ronenn Roubenoff, MD, MHS
Associate Professor of Medicine
Jean Mayer USDA Human Nutrition Research Center on Aging
Tufts University
Boston, Massachusetts

Roy Sasaki, MD
Spinal Cord Injury Center
Veterans Administration Palo Alto Health Care System
Palo Alto, California

Heather R. Schmitz, BS
Department of Nutrition, Exercise Physiology and Sarcopenia Laboratory
Jean Mayer USDA Human Nutrition Research Center on Aging
Tufts University
Boston, Massachusetts

Maureen J. Simmonds, PT, PhD
Associate Professor
School of Physical Therapy
Texas Woman's University
Houston, Texas

Sue Ann Sisto, PT, MA, PhD
Director, Human Performance and Movement Analysis Laboratory
Kessler Medical Rehabilitation Research and Education Corporation (KMRREC)
West Orange, New Jersey
Assistant Professor of Physical Medicine and Rehabilitation
Clinical Assistant Professor of Physical Therapy
University of Medicine and Dentistry of New Jersey/ New Jersey Medical School and School of Health Related Professions
Newark, New Jersey
Assistant Professor of Clinical Physical Therapy
Columbia University
New York, New York

Sue Smith, PT, PhD
Associate Professor
School of Physical Therapy
Texas Woman's University
Dallas, Texas

Rhonda K. Stanley, PhD, PT
Assistant Professor
Department of Physical Therapy
University of Maryland School of Medicine
Baltimore, Maryland

Mark Tarnopolsky, MD, PhD, FRCPc
Neuromuscular Disease Unit
Chedoke/McMaster University Medical Center
Hamilton, Ontario, Canada

Elaine Trudelle-Jackson, MS, PT
School of Physical Therapy
Texas Woman's University
Dallas, Texas

Contents

SECTION ONE

Neuromuscular Disorders

SECTION EDITOR: *Stephen F. Figoni*

CHAPTER **1**

STROKE

James H. Rimmer and Terry Nicola

EPIDEMIOLOGY AND PATHOPHYSIOLOGY

Definition and Prevalence

Stroke has been defined by the World Health Organization (WHO) as rapidly developing clinical signs of focal (or global) disturbance of cerebral function, with signs lasting 24 hours or longer or leading to death with no apparent cause other than of vascular origin (1). This definition does not include transient ischemic attack (TIA) and hemorrhage or infarction related to infection or tumor (2). Stroke is the third leading cause of death and disability in the United States (3). It is considered the most common life-threatening neurological disorder and accounts for 1 of every 15 deaths in the United States (4). The health and economic consequences of stroke impose a substantial economic burden on the individual, family, and society at large (5, 6).

Current estimates are that there are 4 million stroke survivors living in the United States and that 731,000 new strokes occur each year (7). While all segments of the population are affected by stroke, African-Americans have a much greater risk than Caucasians or Hispanics and are more likely to be disabled from a stroke (8). The incidence of first stroke increases exponentially with age (1). In the 55–59-year-old age group, the risk of stroke increases approximately 5 percent per year. In the 80–84-year-old age group, the increased risk is closer to 25 percent a year (9). Men have a 30 percent greater risk of stroke than women in earlier life, while women have a greater risk in later life. Despite advances in medical treatment for stroke, it remains the leading cause of disability in adults (1). While the incidence of stroke has remained constant over the last 3 decades, the mortality rate from stroke and stroke severity has declined (10).

Classification

Strokes are often referred to as cerebrovascular accidents (CVAs) or brain attacks. They are considered a heterogeneous disorder that can involve the rupturing of a large blood vessel in the brain, or the occlusion of a tiny blood vessel that may affect a certain area of the brain (11). Strokes are classified as "hemorrhagic" or "ischemic." Hemorrhagic strokes constitute approximately 10 percent of all strokes, while the ischemic type make up the vast majority and remainder of strokes (1). Risk factors for stroke are listed in Table 1.1.

Pathophysiology

Stroke occurs from cell damage and impaired neurological function resulting from a restricted blood supply (ischemia) or by bleeding (hemorrhage) into the brain tissue. The injury to the brain affects multiple systems depending on the site of injury and the amount of damage sustained during the event. These include motor and sensory impairments and language, perception, affective, and cognitive dysfunction (1). Strokes can cause severe limitations in mobility and cognition or can be very mild with only short-term consequences that are often not permanent.

A hemorrhagic stroke results in blood leaking into the extravascular space within the cranium or into the brain tissue itself. Hemorrhagic strokes are classified as intracerebral (bleeding directly into the brain) or subarachnoid (bleeding into the spaces and spinal fluid around the brain), depending on where the injury occurs. This bleeding damages the brain by cutting off connecting pathways and by causing localized or generalized pressure injury to brain tissue. Biochemical substances released before and after the hemorrhage may also adversely affect vascular and brain tissues (11).

Ischemic strokes result from an infarction of some kind and are usually divided into two types: "thrombotic" and "embolic." "Thrombosis" refers to an obstruction of blood flow due to a localized occlusion within one or more blood vessels (11). "Thrombotic infarction" occurs when a thrombus or clot forms on an atherosclerotic plaque. "Embolic infarction" results when a material (embolus) formed elsewhere in the vascular system occludes an artery or arteriole (12). Infarcts resulting from occlusion of the carotid artery or proximal middle artery have the worst prognosis (12).

Clinical features of stroke depend on the location and severity of the injury. Signs of a hemorrhagic stroke include altered level of consciousness, severe headache, and

Table 1.1. Risk Factors for Stroke

Ischemic Stroke

- Atherosclerosis—associated with the following risk factors: hypertension, cigarette smoking, hyperlipidemia, diabetes, sedentary lifestyle
- Hypothyroidism
- Use of oral contraceptives
- Sickle cell disease
- Coagulation disorders
- Polycythemia vera
- Arteritis
- Dehydration combined with any of the previous conditions

Hemorrhagic Stroke

- Hypertension
- Arteriovenous malformation
- Anticoagulant therapy
- Drug abuse with cocaine, amphetamines, or alcohol

usually elevated blood pressure (1). Cerebellar hemorrhage usually occurs unilaterally and is associated with dysequilibrium, nausea, and vomiting. Hemorrhage into the brain stem is often fatal (12).

Cerebral blood flow (CBF) is the primary marker for assessing ischemic strokes. When CBF drops below 18 mL/100 g/min (normal CBF is 50–55 mL/100 g/min), synaptic transmission failure occurs. When CBF drops below 8 mL/100 g/min, cell death results. The "ischemic cascade" refers to a complex series of biochemical events that result from ischemic stroke (1). Acidosis, altered calcium homeostasis, transmitter dysfunction, free radical production, cerebral edema, and microcirculatory obstruction are all involved in the injury phase. Diagnostic tests used to assess stroke include computed tomography (CT) and magnetic resonance imaging (MRI) (1).

FUNCTIONAL CONSEQUENCES OF STROKE

Comorbidities and Secondary Conditions[1]

The loss in function that often accompanies a stroke affects both physical and psychological systems (13, 14). The magnitude of disablement will vary depending on the severity of stroke (15). More than 50 percent of people who have a stroke will develop major depression (16). The likelihood of a second stroke is also increased as a result of continuing to lead an unhealthy lifestyle (17).

Many stroke survivors require extensive care (18). "Comorbidities" that are common in this group include coronary heart disease, obesity, hypertension, type 2 diabetes, and hyperlipidemia (19).

"Secondary conditions" include a higher incidence of injury from falls, spasticity, memory loss, aphasia, sleep apnea, back pain, stress, depression, and social isolation (1). Symptoms of stroke include weakness (hemiparesis, quadriparesis) or paralysis (hemiplegia, tetraplegia) and impaired balance.

The synergy between the loss of physical function and an exacerbation of one or more comorbidities severely compromises the functional independence and quality of life of many stroke survivors (20). These conditions add complexity to the design of the exercise prescription for this population. A list of comorbidities and secondary conditions can be found in Table 1.2.

CLINICAL EXERCISE PHYSIOLOGY

Acute Responses to Exercise

The major physiological consequence of stroke is loss of functional muscle mass (21). Most stroke survivors show some residual loss of function on either the right or left side of the body, referred to as hemiplegia or hemiparesis. Because the majority of strokes are caused by vascular disease, physiological responses to acute exercise may be limited by CAD (21, 22). Few studies have assessed the peak oxygen uptake ($\dot{V}O_2$) of stroke survivors, but those that have been completed have reported low peak $\dot{V}O_2$ levels in this cohort. In two of the largest studies to date (23, 24), investigators reported that in male and female stroke survivors (Potempa et al.: age range 43–72 yr; Rimmer et al.: *M* age = 53.2 ± 8.3), peak $\dot{V}O_2$ ranged from 13.3 $mL \cdot kg^{-1} \cdot min^{-1}$ (23) to 16.6 $mL \cdot kg^{-1} \cdot min^{-1}$ (24). Both studies involved an exercise intervention aimed at improving peak $\dot{V}O_2$. Potempa et al. (23) reported peak $\dot{V}O_2$ values after 10 weeks of training ranging from 0% to 35.7%. Rimmer et al. (24) used a more severely disabled stroke population and reported a mean improvement of 8.2% after a 12-week intervention. The relatively low baseline aerobic capacity is associated with a number of factors, including multiple comorbidities (i.e., CAD, obesity) and lifestyle-related behaviors (i.e., lack of regular physical activity).

Table 1.2. Common Sequelae and Comorbidities in Stroke Survivors

Physical Sequelae	Psychological Sequelae	Comorbidities
Spasticity	Depression	Coronary artery disease
Muscle weakness	Social isolation	Hypertension
Balance impairments	Cognitive impairment	Hyperlipidemia
Obesity	Memory loss	Diabetes mellitus
Paralysis	Low self esteem	Obesity
Paresis	Low self efficacy	Peripheral vascular disease
Fatigue	Emotional ability	
Falls		
Aphasia		
Visual Impairments		

[1]A comorbidity exists prior to having a stroke (i.e., obesity, hypertension). A secondary condition is the direct result of having a stroke (i.e., hemiplegia, impaired balance).

Peak heart rate during acute exercise will vary for persons with stroke depending on their age, level of disability (extent of muscle atrophy on hemiparetic side), number and severity of comorbidities (i.e., hypertension, CAD) and secondary conditions (i.e., degree of spasticity, cognitive impairment), and medication use (i.e., beta-blockers). Potempa et al. (21) noted that some stroke survivors may reach near-normal peak heart rates, while others may attain significantly lower peak heart rates for a similar bout of exercise. While this will vary for each individual, in general peak heart rates for stroke survivors during acute exercise will be lower than those for persons of the same age and gender who do not have a disability. The relatively low aerobic capacity reported in stroke survivors is likely attributed to a reduction in the number of motor units capable of being recruited during dynamic exercise, the reduced oxidative capacity of paretic muscle (21), and the sedentary lifestyle of most stroke survivors (25).

Muscular strength and endurance are also deficient in stroke survivors. Rimmer et al. (24) evaluated the strength levels of a relatively young group of male and female stroke survivors (*M* age = 53 yr). Mean strength scores (10-RM) on two LifeFitness machines were 26 lb on the bench press and 147 lb on the leg press. Grip strength on the nonaffected side was 30.7 lb, and on the affected side, 20.4 lb. Considering the average weight of the subjects (*M* = 200 lb), scores on both of these measures would be less than the 10th percentile according to data reported on nondisabled individuals of the same age and gender (26). Other studies have confirmed low strength scores in this population (27–29).

Physical Examination

The extent of damage occurring from a stroke can be both physical and cognitive. Left-hemisphere lesions are typically associated with expressive and receptive language deficits compared to right-hemisphere lesions (30). The motor impairment from stroke usually results in hemiplegia (paralysis) or hemiparesis (weakness). When damage occurs to the descending neural pathways, there is an abnormal regulation of spinal motor neurons resulting in adverse changes in postural and stretch reflexes and difficulty with voluntary movement. Deficits in motor control may involve muscle weakness, abnormal synergistic organization of movements, impaired regulation of force, decreased reaction times, abnormal muscle tone, and loss of active range of motion (31).

EXERCISE TESTING AND SCREENING CRITERIA

Screening Protocol

Before conducting a graded exercise test, persons with stroke should be screened by their primary care physician. The screening should include a fasting blood draw, resting ECG, resting heart rate, resting blood pressure (standing, seated, supine), and basal temperature. In order to be approved for peak $\dot{V}O_2$ testing, participants' blood screening tests (i.e., CBC, enzymes, protein levels) should be within normal limits. If the preliminary blood work is acceptable, the participant can be scheduled for testing. Participants who successfully complete the graded exercise test can be recommended for an exercise program. Individuals who have adverse cardiovascular changes during exercise testing should be advised for further follow-up and may need to begin an exercise program in a closely supervised setting such as cardiac rehabilitation.

Exercise Testing

Peak Oxygen Uptake (Cardiovascular Fitness)

Because of a significant loss of muscle function resulting from hemiparesis or hemiplegia, stroke survivors have a severely reduced maximal or peak oxygen uptake (23, 24). Since many stroke survivors also have cardiovascular comorbidities (e.g., hypertension, CAD), graded exercise tests are often symptom-limited, thus not allowing the person to achieve high peak capacities.

A symptom-limited graded exercise test (peak $\dot{V}O_2$) can be performed on a stationary bike or treadmill, or in persons with severe hemiplegia, with an arm ergometer. While it may be necessary to perform the exercise test with an arm ergometer, performance will be limited because of the limited amount of muscle recruitment and a greater strain on the cardiac system per unit of peripheral muscle mass recruited. Goodman (32) notes that arm cranking yields a peak $\dot{V}O_2$ 30–35 percent less than treadmill performance. The preferred exercise mode is the stationary cycle since most stroke survivors have difficulty with gait and balance (21). The stationary cycle makes it easier to quantify external workload, because the energy requirements of treadmill walking will vary as individuals change stride length, shift center of gravity, swing arms, or hold onto railings. Additionally, it is easier to record blood pressure measurements on the cycle ergometer and likely results in less artifact in ECG monitoring of stroke survivors.

Ramp Cycle Protocol

Rimmer et al. (24) measured peak $\dot{V}O_2$ in 35 stroke survivors using a ramp cycle ergometer testing protocol. Participants began cycling at a workload of 20 W and increased by 10 W every minute until maximal effort was achieved. They were instructed to pedal at 60 revolutions per minute (rpm). Heart rate and blood pressure were recorded every 2 min. Tests were terminated if one of the following criteria was observed: (a) respiratory exchange ratio (RER) ≥ 1.1, (b) peak heart rate within ± 10 beat $\cdot$ min^{-1} of age-predicted maximal value, (c) abnormal blood pressure or ECG response, or (d) unable to continue pedaling above 50 rpm. Potempa et al. (23) used a similar ramp cycle ergometer protocol with stroke survivors. Testing began at 10 W and increased 10 W each minute until maximal effort was attained. During testing, blood pressure should be measured on the unaffected arm. Testing time in both studies ranged from 4 to 12 minutes.

Strength

Strength can be assessed in a number of ways using standard exercise machines, free weights, or dynamometers (33). Instruction on proper lifting technique must be conducted prior to testing. Persons with cognitive impairments or severe mobility limitations may require more time to perform the test correctly. Adaptive gloves or Velcro may be necessary to secure a hand to the weight or bar.

Rimmer et al. (24) used the 10-RM method on two exercise machines, one measuring upper body strength and one measuring lower body strength in stroke survivors. A handgrip dynamometer was also used to measure grip strength on the affected and nonaffected sides. During the strength assessment, it is important to evaluate each limb separately to determine the disparity in strength between the hemiparetic and nonhemiparetic side. The clinical exercise physiologist should also evaluate if the affected side has enough residual innervation to allow strength gains.

Flexibility

Hamstring and low back flexibility are important muscle groups to evaluate in stroke participants because of the increased spasticity on the hemiparetic side. These muscle groups can be assessed using a modified version of the sit-and-reach test. If sitting on the floor is difficult, a modified version can be performed using a bench. The client is asked to sit on a bench with legs fully extended and feet placed against the sit-and-reach box. Participants extend their arms and reach in the direction of their feet. The distance from the middle finger to the center of the box is recorded.

A good measure of functional shoulder flexibility is to have the person put one hand over the shoulder (slide the hand down the back) and the other hand behind the back (slide the back of the hand up the middle of the back). The participant is asked to bring the fingers as close as possible to each other. The distance between the two middle fingers of each hand is recorded. Record scores on both sides of the body by reversing the position of the arms. A more comprehensive evaluation of flexibility can be performed with a goniometer.

Body Composition

Body composition measurements should include height, weight, skinfold measures, body mass index (BMI) and waist-to-hip ratio (WHR). The sum of skinfold measurements can be used in place of an estimated percent body fat if the skinfold calipers do not open wide enough to obtain the entire skinfold. Many stroke survivors are severely obese and it may not be possible to obtain an accurate skinfold measure at certain sites (i.e., thigh). Because it is sometimes difficult to distinguish between subcutaneous fat and muscle tissue on the hemiparetic side, it is recommended that skinfold measurements be taken on the noninvolved side.

EXERCISE PRESCRIPTION AND PROGRAMMING

The emphasis in working with stroke survivors has been traditionally directed at rehabilitation during the first six months of recovery (31, 34, 35). Few studies have been conducted on improving the functional capacity of stroke survivors after rehabilitation (36, 37). The small number of training studies that have been completed, however, have supported the use of exercise in improving mobility and functional independence and in preventing or reducing further disease and functional impairment in persons with stroke (10, 37, 38).

Most persons with stroke go through a significant recovery period during the first 6 months after having a stroke, while others will see significant recovery for up to a year or longer (33). The goal of resistance training is to maximize recovery and sustain and improve fitness throughout the lifespan. The clinical exercise physiologist should work closely with the client's physician or therapist in developing a safe and effective program. Stroke survivors who return home from a hospital or rehabilitation facility shortly after their injury will need greater attention to ensure that cardiovascular adaptations are conducted in a safe environment with timely and appropriate emergency medical equipment and care available.

Endurance Training

Endurance (aerobic) training for stroke survivors requires adequate supervision. Stroke survivors often vary widely in age; severity of disability; motivational level; and number and severity of comorbidities, secondary conditions, and associated conditions (see Table 1.2). While strength and gait training have been the hallmark components of stroke rehabilitation, researchers are suggesting that recovery from stroke should include the reduction of cardiovascular, pulmonary, and metabolic sequelae (21, 24, 29). Appropriate cardiovascular exercise may reduce these comorbidities and improve functional capacity. Aerobic exercise training can result in improved tolerance to activities of daily living and allow more physical activity to occur at a lower submaximal threshold, thus reducing myocardial oxygen demand (21).

Frequency and Duration

The goal of the exercise program should be to have each stroke participant engage in an hour of physical activity, a *minimum* of three days a week, in a clinical (i.e., hospital wellness program) or community-based setting (i.e., fitness center, university-based program or clinic). Self-initiated exercise should occur on the days that the client does not attend the program (i.e., riding a stationary bike in the home at a low perceived exertion level). The exercise intervention should consist of the following components: cardiovascular endurance, muscle strength and endurance, and flexibility. After the comprehensive screening has been completed according to ACSM guidelines (26), the first 2 to 4 weeks of the program should be used to train participants in using the equipment. Individual goals should be established for each participant to ensure that they are exercising within their comfort zone and are achieving the desired training effect.

Intensity Level

The intensity level of the cardiovascular exercise should be established for each participant from the graded exercise test. In the few studies that have been conducted on stroke survivors, intensity was set at different levels. Rimmer et al. (24) based the intensity level on the participants' peak $\dot{V}O_2$ measure. The heart rate that the participant reached at a respiratory quotient (RQ) of 1.00 was used to set the target heart rate range (THRR). Five beats per minute was subtracted from this value, and the THRR for the participant was then set from this heart rate to 10 bpm below this heart rate. For example, if a participant's heart rate was 130 $b \cdot min^{-1}$ at an RQ = 1.00, subtracting five beats per minute from this value would put the ceiling heart rate at 125 $b \cdot min^{-1}$. The THRR would be 115 to 125 bpm.

In the work by Potempa et al. (21, 23), initial training for stroke survivors was set at 40–60% of measured peak $\dot{V}O_2$ for a duration of 30 minutes of continuous or discontinuous exercise. The emphasis during the early stages of the program was on duration as opposed to intensity. Once the person was able to exercise for 30 minutes, training intensity was progressively increased to the highest workload tolerance without cardiac symptoms. It is important to note that the investigators used telemetry monitoring with their subjects and were thus able to be more aggressive in their training intensity (23).

Smith and coworkers (39) developed a conditioning program for 14 individuals with mild-to-moderate stroke using a motorized treadmill 3 $days \cdot wk^{-1}$ for three months. The training intensity was limited at the beginning of the study to 40% of the calculated heart rate reserve (HRR) and increased to 60–70% of HRR over the course of the training program. Teixeira-Salmela et al. (29) used an intensity of 70% of the maximal heart rate attained from an exercise test with a higher functioning group of stroke survivors. However, subjects underwent a dobutamine stress echocardiogram prior to exercise to rule out evidence of cardiac risk.

In the study by Rimmer et al. (24), participants who had an abnormal blood pressure response during the exercise test (systolic ≥220 mm Hg, diastolic ≥110 mm Hg) had a modification to their exercise prescription. They were instructed not to exceed a rate pressure product (RPP) of 200. The RPP was calculated by multiplying heart rate times systolic blood pressure, divided by 100. For example, if a participant's blood pressure response during an exercise session was 180 mm Hg at a heart rate of 130 bpm^{-1}, the RPP would be 180 × 130/100 or 234. Because the value is more than 200, the participant would not be allowed to exercise on that day or should wait until RPP dropped below 200.

Resting diastolic blood pressure (DBP) should be less than 100 mm Hg to begin exercising. If resting diastolic pressure is greater than 100 mm Hg, range-of-motion exercises should be performed until DBP drops below 100. Exercise should be terminated if blood pressure is elevated to 220/110 mm Hg or higher and should only be resumed when blood pressure drops below this value.

Participants should begin with intermittent exercise during the first 4 weeks of the program. At the end of four weeks, most participants should be able to complete 30 minutes of continuous exercise in their THRR.

Training Modalities

Examples of cardiovascular training modalities for stroke survivors include stationary cycling (recumbent and upright), over-ground walking or walking on a treadmill (provided the clients have adequate balance, are closely supervised, and do not experience joint pain), elliptical cross-training, and recumbent stepping (especially useful for clients with severe hemiplegia). Stair stepping in a vertical position was found to elicit high heart rates and spikes in blood pressure and may be contraindicated for certain stroke survivors (24). Participants should be given the opportunity to select their own equipment as long as it is considered safe and does not cause adverse cardiovascular (i.e., excessive rise in blood pressure or heart rate) or musculoskeletal complications (i.e., pain, injury).

Strength Training

Muscle weakness has been recognized as a major symptom resulting from stroke (29). Research has demonstrated that the torque generated by the knee extensors, ankle plantar flexors, and hip flexors is correlated to gait performance in stroke survivors (40, 41, 42). Low strength levels have also been reported to increase the risk of falls (43).

Training Intensity

Rimmer et al. (24) initiated a strength training protocol for stroke survivors at 70% of each participant's 10-RM for one set of 15–20 repetitions. When participants were able to complete 25 repetitions for 2 consecutive sessions with proper lifting technique (i.e., proper biomechanical motion, without Valsalva maneuver), the weight was increased by 10% of their 10-RM. Participants trained using a variety of exercises, including the bench press, leg press, leg curl, triceps push-down, seated shoulder press, seated row, lat pull-down, and biceps curl. Blood pressure and rating of perceived exertion (RPE) should be recorded at the completion of each set.

Training Volume

A major determinant of training volume is the amount of muscle mass that is still *functional*. Persons with paralysis, hemiplegia, impaired motor control, or limited joint mobility have less functional muscle mass and will therefore only tolerate a lower training volume. For individuals who cannot lift the minimal weight on certain resistance machines, resistance bands or cuff weights are recommended. If bands and cuff weights are too difficult, use the person's own limb weight as the initial resistance. For example, lifting an arm or leg against gravity for 5–10 seconds may be the initial starting point for clients with very low strength levels. Also, use gravity-eliminated exercises if manual muscle test grade is <3/5 (i.e., horizontal movements, aquatic exercises, manual resistance, isometrics).

Training volume will also depend on the client's health status. Many individuals with stroke have been inactive for much of their lives and will need only a small amount of resistance exercise during the *initial* stage of the program to obtain a training effect. How responsive clients with stroke will be to resistance exercise during the *conditioning* stage will depend on their current health status and the severity of their stroke. For individuals who start out at very low levels of strength, significant improvements can be made with very light resistance.

Training Modalities

Modes of resistance exercise fall into three general categories: free weights, portable equipment (i.e., elastic bands, tubing), and machines. Any of these modalities is acceptable for improving strength levels in stroke survivors, provided the client is not at risk for injury. When an instructor feels that the resistance mode presents a danger to the client, the exercise routine should be either adapted (i.e., securing the weight to the hand, changing the movement) or substituted with a safer piece of equipment.

Some experts argue that free-weight exercises have greater value for persons with physical disabilities because the resistance can be tailored to resemble a *functional* daily activity (29). Lifting free weights requires *stabilizing* muscles around the torso and joints while lifting and lowering the resistance. These muscle groups need strengthening in persons with physical disabilities (including stroke survivors) to maintain the ability to perform Activities of Daily Living (ADL—i.e., dressing and undressing) and Instrumental Activities of Daily Living (IADL—i.e., lifting and carrying items). However, lifting free weights requires good trunk stability and may be difficult to perform in individuals who have severe limitations in motor control and coordination.

In clients with very low strength levels, *gravity-resistance* exercise (lifting limbs against gravity) may be all that the person is capable of performing. Abducting an arm or extending a leg for several repetitions may be a good entry point. These exercises can be used for persons who are extremely weak after a stroke, while other modes of resistance exercise can be used with stronger clients. Once an individual is able to complete 8–12 reps of a gravity-resistance exercise, the person could progress to free weight, bands, or machines. If a client is unable to move a limb against gravity because of extreme weakness, the instructor could place the limb in a certain position (i.e., shoulder abduction) and have the client hold the position isometrically for a few seconds, gradually increasing the time. Horizontal movements and aquatic exercises can be performed with gravity eliminated, thus allowing the limb to move more freely.

Active-assistive exercise may be required for certain individuals who do not have enough strength to overcome the force of gravity. The instructor can assist the client in performing the movement by providing as much physical assistance as necessary. At various points in the concentric phase, the instructor may have to assist the client in overcoming the force of gravity. During the eccentric phase, the instructor may need to control the movement so that the weight or limb is not lowered too quickly. In many instances, active-assistive exercise can be used with severely weak musculature while *active* exercise can be used with stronger muscle groups.

Flexibility Training

Participants should be taught a variety of stretching exercises targeting both upper and lower body muscle groups. Participants should stretch at the beginning of each exercise session, at the end of the cardiovascular exercise session, between strength exercises, and at the end of the exercise session. Stretches should held for 15 to 30 seconds. A particular emphasis should be made to stretch the tight (spastic) muscle groups on the hemiparetic side, which include the finger and wrist flexors, elbow flexors, shoulder adductors, hip flexors, knee flexors, and ankle plantar flexors.

GENERAL PROGRAM GUIDELINES

Exercise sessions should be supervised by a clinical exercise physiologist along with several assistants. Assistants should be trained in monitoring blood pressure, heart rate, and vital signs. A good staff-to-client ratio would be one to three participants per staff member, particularly during the early stages of the program when more assistance is needed. Participants should wear a heart rate monitor for the entire session to ensure that they are exercising in the appropriate target heart rate zone.

Participants should be taught how to measure their own RPE, use the equipment safely, and understand the warning signs for when to stop exercising. A sample checklist of safety guidelines for self-regulating exercise is shown in Table 1.3.

Blood pressure and heart rate should be recorded prior to exercise and several times during the exercise session. If possible, participants should wear heart rate monitors

Table 1.3. Sample Checklist for Teaching Clients to Perform Exercise Safely

Client Name: ______________________ Staff Name: ______________________ Date: ______________

Before participation in an exercise program, you must be able to competently execute the tasks listed below. If you have difficulty performing any of these tasks, you will receive additional training before participating in the program.

Task	
Able to monitor target heart rate.	
Able to use the rating of perceived exertion (RPE) scale.	
Knows the warning signs to stop exercising.	
Able to safely operate the treadmill.	
Able to program the treadmill.	
Able to safely operate the upright bike.	
Able to program the upright bike.	
Can record aerobic and strength activities on assigned log sheet.	
Display knowledge of the goals of strength training.	
Know what a set is.	
Know what a repetition is.	
Can adjust the bench press to fit him or her.	
Can display proper form when using the bench press.	
Can display proper breathing (lack of Valsalva maneuver) when using the bench press.	
Can adjust the leg press to fit him or her.	
Can display proper form when using the leg press.	
Can display proper breathing (lack of Valsalva maneuver) when using the leg press.	
Can adjust the shoulder press to fit him or her.	
Can display proper form when using the shoulder press.	
Can display proper breathing (lack of Valsalva maneuver) when using the shoulder press.	
Can adjust the triceps push-down to fit him or her.	
Can display proper form when using the triceps push-down.	
Can display proper breathing (lack of Valsalva maneuver) when using the triceps push-down.	
Can adjust the biceps curl to fit him or her.	
Can display proper form when using the biceps curl.	
Can display proper breathing (lack of Valsalva maneuver) when using the biceps curl.	
Can adjust the front row to fit him or her.	
Can display proper form when using the front row.	
Can display proper breathing (lack of Valsalva maneuver) when using the front row.	
Can adjust the lat pull-down to fit him or her.	
Can display proper form when using the lat pull-down.	
Can display proper breathing (lack of Valsalva maneuver) when using the lat pull-down.	
Can adjust the hamstring curl to fit him or her.	
Can display proper form when using the hamstring curl.	
Can display proper breathing (lack of Valsalva maneuver) when using the hamstring curl.	

that indicate when the exercise intensity exceeds the target heart rate range. Persons with type 1 diabetes should bring their own portable glucometer to the fitness center and take a blood glucose measurement before and after each exercise session. Orange juice and other high carbohydrate snacks should be available for those subjects who become hypoglycemic (<50 mg $\cdot$ dL^{-1}).

Each exercise session should be recorded on a SOAP form. This is a standard form that has been used widely in cardiac rehabilitation programs. "S" stands for Subjective, which is a client self-report of their current state (i.e., how much sleep they had, do they feel well, did they eat breakfast, did they take their medication(s), symptoms). "O" stands for Objective, which is the exercise instructor's evaluation of the participant's current state and quantitative performance during the exercise session (i.e., modality, workload, blood pressure response, physiologic signs). "A" stands for Assessment, which is how the clinician interprets *S* and *O*. "P" stands for *Plan*, which refers to prescribed/recommended treatment plan, including modifications that need to be made to the exercise prescription in the next session (i.e., trying a new piece of cardiovascular equipment, increasing resistance to 70% of 10-RM). At the end of each session, blood pressure and heart rate should be recorded to ensure that they return to resting values before departure from the fitness center. Participants should be encouraged to drink plenty of water during the exercise session to avoid dehydration.

The instructor should make every effort to avoid prolonged or unusual *fatigue* and *delayed-onset muscle soreness*. Although this is a common side effect of any new resistance training program, it could present a problem for persons with physical disabilities if the soreness prevents them from conducting their normal ADLs. Even though a client with stroke may aspire to make rapid gains in strength and can train at a moderate-to-high intensity level, the instructor should be cautious not to overwork the muscle groups. Use light resistance for at least the first month of the program (30–50% of 1-RM), and only proceed to higher training loads if muscle soreness and fatigue are not present.

If soreness in certain muscle groups prevents the person from performing routine daily activities, the exercise should be stopped until the pain subsides. If it continues after the program resumes, the instructor may need to reduce the training volume or avoid certain exercises that induce pain or fatigue. If there are prolonged bouts of pain or soreness 24–48 hours after exercise, the client should consult with his or her physician to determine the cause.

Many individuals with stroke have *hand dysfunction* on the hemiparetic side. This may make it difficult to grasp barbells or the railings or handles on aerobic training equipment. There are several versions of specially designed gloves that are available commercially that will allow the person's hand to maintain contact with the equipment. Gloves will also protect the hand from injury while performing resistance training routines. Participants who do not have good grip strength can use wrist cuffs or leather mitts with Velcro and buckles to secure their hands to dumbbells or weight equipment.

Many individuals with stroke will exhibit *asymmetrical weakness* or will have a disproportionately greater amount of weakness to the flexor or extensor muscle groups. It is important to evaluate individual muscle groups on both sides of the body, including both agonists and antagonists, to isolate the degree of weakness in key muscle groups. Individuals with asymmetrical weakness will often "hike" their body toward the weaker side in order to compensate for this weakness while performing resistance training. This could impose mild or moderate muscle strain. Make sure that the client is performing the activity with proper form. If there is a tendency to "hike" the body, lower the resistance and emphasize good form.

Blood pressure must be monitored closely in persons with stroke. Since hypertension is a common comorbidity, follow the guidelines in *ACSM's Guidelines for Exercise Testing and Prescription* for working with persons with hypertension (26). It is especially important for the person's blood pressure to be under control before initiating the program. A group of experts recently noted that persons with recent stroke and hypertension should not participate in exercise until resting mean arterial pressure (MAP = diastolic pressure + 1/3 [systolic − diastolic]) is <130 mm Hg (19).

During the first 4 weeks of the program, monitor blood pressure frequently to ensure that complications or adverse changes are not occurring. If blood pressure continually fluctuates, contact the client's physician to determine how to proceed with a safe program. Under no circumstances should a person who has had a stroke and continues to have difficulty maintaining a stable blood pressure be allowed to exercise.

An emergency contact number should be posted in the exercise facility. Physician pager numbers of clients with stroke should be readily available. A portable automated external defibrillator is a good safety device to keep in the fitness center. An infectious waste container for blood specimens should be available for clients who must check their blood glucose level. Blood specimens should be performed in a sterile setting away from equipment and high-volume traffic areas.

Stroke survivors should also be taught the warning signs for when they should stop exercising. Table 1.4 provides a list of items that should be reviewed with each client. Once the persons understands these warning signs and can repeat them back to the instructor, both parties should sign the form. This assures the instructor that the client has a basic understanding of how to exercise safely.

Education and Counseling

The clinical exercise physiologist has an important responsibility to teach stroke participants the importance of good health promotion practices (mind/body relationship) in a structured classroom setting where clients can learn about various strategies to enhance their health. Many stroke survivors do not understand the importance of good health maintenance (e.g., diet, exercise, health behavior) in preventing a second stroke or further comorbidity (4). The perception is that they have already had a major life event and therefore exercise and good nutritional habits are of little benefit to them. Structured lectures that address questions and misconceptions should be an integral part of the educational component.

Rimmer et al. (25) have developed an exercise, nutrition, and health behavior intervention for stroke survivors. The health behavior curriculum uses a wellness model that re-

Table 1.4. Guidelines for Self-Regulating Exercise in Stroke Participants

You understand that you are being asked to exercise within your own comfort level. During exercise, your body may give you signs that you should stop exercising.

These signs include:

- Lightheadedness or dizzyness
- Chest heaviness, pain, or tightness; angina
- Palpitations or irregular heart beat
- Sudden shortness of breath **not due to increased activity**
- Discomfort or stiffness in muscles and joints persisting for several days after exercise

Call your doctor if you experience any of these sensations.

Please call your exercise instructor at (111-1111) if you experience any of the following signs:

- A change in your medication.
- A change in your health, such as:
  - An increase or change in blood pressure, resting heart rate (just sitting around), or other symptoms related to your heart
  - Hospitalization for any reason
  - Cold/flu
  - Emotional stress or upset at work or at home
  - Any other change that you feel is important
  - Your doctor advises you to stop exercising for any reason

I realize that it is my responsibility to report any of these signs/symptoms to my **DOCTOR.** Once the situation is resolved, I must contact **MY INSTRUCTOR, Clinical Exercise Physiologist, at 111-1111.**

____________________ ____________
Signature of Participant Date

____________________ ____________
Signature of Instructor Date

inforces what is being taught in the exercise and nutrition components of the program (44). It offers participants new ways to think about changes in their lives following a stroke and thus facilitate healthier living. The model provides a positive framework for change and promotes active involvement of the participants.

Information about causes and risk factors for stroke as related to secondary conditions (i.e., overweight, social isolation, physical inactivity) established the basis for the intervention. A presentation of Prochaska's stage of change model provided the background for making and maintaining change and led to goal setting by individual participants (45). Group discussions about stressful events related to stroke (i.e., change in family roles) were an important part of the health behavior classes and were used to facilitate development of peer support relationships. Through these peer relations, participants helped each other develop new ways to think about coping and adapting following their stroke. Participants identified ways to incorporate exercise, healthier cooking and eating habits, and new approaches to coping with their disability into their daily lives.

Barriers to Exercise

Rimmer et al. (46) examined barriers to exercise in persons with stroke and other physical disabilities. Data were collected through an in-depth telephone interview using an instrument that addressed issues related to physical activity and the subjects' disability (Barriers to Physical Activity and Disability Survey–B-PADS). Subjects were asked questions pertaining to their participation or interest level in structured exercise. The four major barriers were: *cost of the exercise program* (84.2%), *lack of energy* (65.8%), *transportation* (60.5%), and *did not know where to exercise* (57.9%). Barriers commonly reported in nondisabled persons (e.g., lack of time, boredom, too lazy) were not observed in this cohort. Interestingly, only 11% of the subjects reported that they were not interested in starting an exercise program. The majority of subjects (81.5%) wanted to join an exercise program but were restricted by the number of barriers reported. The investigators noted that African-American women with stroke and other physical disabilities were interested in joining exercise programs but were limited in doing so because of their inability to overcome several barriers to increased physical activity participation.

To increase exercise adherence among stroke survivors, the clinical exercise physiologist must consider the actual (i.e., transportation) and perceived (i.e., exercise will not improve condition) barriers that are evident in each client. To achieve successful adherence to the exercise program, the identified barriers to exercise must first be eliminated.

CASE STUDIES

In all cases, physical, occupational, and speech therapists had completed treatment programs in these allied health care disciplines. Physician care included primary management by an internist and neurologist, with other specialty consults as needed. A psychiatrist and/or neuropsychologist were also involved in patient care where needed, for depression and deficits in task processing where noted.

CASE 1

RM: 55-year-old married gentleman, businessman, retired due to cerebrovascular accident, which left him with partial left hemiplegia (hemiparesis). Chief complaint at time of visit was tightness of the left shoulder and reduced grip strength, especially notable when golfing. There was also a long-standing history of recurrent low back pain. *Medications:* Plavix, Bayer ASA, Procardia, Zocor, MVI, vitamins B6, B12, and folic acid. His stance showed a slightly lower posture on the left side. Romberg sign was negative. Gait up to 2 miles per hour was normal. He was unable to walk on a narrow straight line for 10 feet without making a side balance error. He was able to do a partial squat. Spine range of motion showed blocking of movement with side tilt to the right side. The shoulder range of motion was limited to 90 degrees for abduction and 100 degrees for forward flexion, 50 degrees of 90-degree abducted-external rotation. There were no one-sided sensory, position sense, or one-sided sensory neglect deficits detected. Babinski sign was absent, and muscle stretch reflexes were normal. Cranial nerves showed a mild left facial paresis. A program with the clinical exercise physiologist was conducted for 20 sessions over a 9-month period. Initially, he was able to walk 2 mph for 10 minutes and reached a heart rate of 130 b·min^{-1}. He could hold a 2 lb weight in his left hand but was unable to use the thumb. He could not control a full cup of coffee without spilling it. Exercises to establish a neutral spine posture were initiated. An isometric program for the left scapular muscles was initiated with feedback from a take-home electrical muscle stimulation device. He was able to progress to diagonal-pattern upper-extremity exercises and some grip movements of the left thumb. His endurance improved to 4 mph for 20 minutes at a heart rate of 140 b·min^{-1}. Low back pain became more evident as the patient became more active and played 18 holes of golf three times a week using a golf cart. X-rays showed osteophytes and degenerative joint changes in the facets, sacroiliac, symphysis pubis, and hip joints, with no change since x-rays taken 5 months earlier. Fluoroscopically guided injection was done to the left sacroiliac joint, which reduced pain and interference from guarding of that area during sessions with the clinical exercise physiologist.

Problems to Consider

Left hemiparesis primarily involved the left upper extremity, the most common form of hemiparesis. Usually, some muscles are spared; it is rare to see complete sensorimotor hemiplegia of every muscle group on the left side.

Deficits on the left side are sometimes more obvious with fatigue after a period of ambulation at a given speed, or after an increased challenge to coordination such as line-walking. Low back pain may lateralize to side of poorest function (hemiparetic side). Presence of pain alerts the health practitioner to the fact that he or she should check for biomechanical deficits. X-rays show a long history of low back cumulative wear that probably extends prior to the onset of the stroke. It is important to address motor control of the low back and avoid fatigue to those muscles. Isometric exercises should be performed while maintaining the neutral spine (the most relaxed midposition between lumbar flexion and extension). It is important to see if exercises should be emphasized for either weakness or flexibility for increased tone of the hemiplegic side.

Patient was able to continue playing golf by swinging the golf club with his right arm. Assistive devices, such as the tube device hooked to a glove for the left hand, may minimize the grip deficits and optimize the patient's ability to coordinate the movements of the upper extremity. He was also able to golf sometimes in the 90s score range, because of focus on ball direction instead of distance. The emphasis in this program was to first establish normal trunk control and then head position with retraining of the scapular movement with the golf swing.

CASE 2

DK: 46-year-old female with juvenile onset diabetes mellitus (type 1), smoker, suffered a cerebrovascular accident at age 17 with history of seizures. This left her with spastic hemiparesis of the right upper and lower extremities and expressive aphasia. Her chief complaint was difficulty with sustained daily activities (including exercise) because of the hemiparesis. In addition, she had complaints of tender points in the left hand over the thenar eminence, the left tensor fasciae latae, and the left heel. She was functionally independent in the community and had a long-term relationship with a boyfriend. She finished high school but never developed a career. *Medications:* Tegretol, Dilantin, Provera, Valium, and insulin pump (implantable device for infusion of insulin instead of injection needles). On physical exam, she was alert and oriented and understood simple and multistep instructions. Speech was markedly limited by nonfluent use of single words and phrases, and she often corrected herself. Naming of simple objects like a pen or watch resulted in mispronunciations and nonwords. She could communicate most routine conversation if allowed to correct herself. Sensation was decreased but present for the right side; no neglect or sensory extinction was noted. The presence of the trigger points in the areas of tenderness supported the absence of neglect on the right side. Increased tone was noted in the right lower extremity with a knee-extended gait. Posturing of the foot was partially masked by previous ankle/tendon surgery for equinovarus ankle posturing. Increased tone was noted in the right hand in the form of a grip posture. Range of motion was otherwise normal. Pressure over any of the trigger points caused a sudden spastic response. Reflexes were increased for the right upper and lower extremities. Babinski sign was positive on the right side and negative on the left side. Volitional movements tended to follow flexion/extension synergy patterns on the right side. Movement could be isolated for the scapulothoracic and hip musculature. Patient could assume upright posture with cueing.

The patient entered a clinical exercise physiology program for a period of 6 months. The first 3 months involved biweekly visits for endurance and a home exercise program. She was independent and safe in the community at time of initial visit. However, her speed of gait was approximately 1.5 mph and inefficient with aerobic-level heart rates greater than 130 bpm. Initially, she was unable to progress in the program due to the painful trigger points. Phenol blocks were performed twice over the treatment period, which provided marked relief of symptoms and reduction in spasticity. The second 3 months of the program were in an exercise class setting. She made marked progress in her ability to control the right lower extremity during the swing phase of gait. She was also prescribed a polypropylene ankle-foot orthosis. Her right upper extremity function improved with the combined effect of improved scapular control using electrical muscle stimulation and a neutral hand splint to prevent wrist and finger flexion contractures from spasticity and help in positioning for gross grip of objects for daily activity and weight training. She initially avoided use of her right upper extremity. By the end of the treatment session, she was able to use it as an assist in two-handed activities with the left upper extremity. Throughout the program, blood glucose levels were monitored, and low blood sugars less than 60 mg·dL^{-1} would be treated with a high glucose content beverage. High blood glucose (hyperglycemia) was addressed with increased water ingestion.

Dietary adjustments and insulin pump (physician/nurse adjusted) dosage changes were made in response to increased physical activity and blood glucose and glucometer readings and patient symptoms. Education and counseling were instituted toward the end of treatment.

Problems to Consider

In insulin-dependent diabetes, even with an implantable device, wide fluctuations of blood sugar can occur, resulting in loss of consciousness or lethargy. Lethargic mood can be mistakenly misinterpreted as fatigue, lack of enthusiasm, or poor ability to follow instructions. *Aphasia* is a broad family of classifications used to describe communication deficits in relationship to organic brain disorders. They are primarily disorders of comprehension and/or expression. This patient was primarily in the expressive disorders category. Aphasias should not be confused with *apraxias,* which involve difficulty in formulating words. Also, *paralysis* of facial muscles or tongue, such as an injury to a nerve, is not an aphasia. If a patient has an aphasia, communication through a few written words and pictures can improve exercise comprehension and compliance.

Spasticity and *increased tone* in spine and extremities must be addressed by first working with muscles that have near-normal function. Progression should then extend to the next group of muscles, usually spine-related muscles first, followed by more distal muscles, with the intention of spreading sequential motor control. Spasticity usually responds by an undesirable increase in response to fast movements or sudden large loads during resistance training. Slow and controlled submaximal contractions may be better than fast repetitions. *Proprioceptive neuromuscular facilitation* is used to describe various forms of feedback, either the caretaker tapping or applying light pressure during use of a muscle desired. Positioning the patient in a lying or sitting position will avoid excessive spasticity response. Electrical muscle stimulation may have a facilitative biofeedback effect in combination with a voluntary contraction of a given muscle.

Tender points and *trigger points* are specific areas where tenderness can be greatest in a muscle. The tenderness can cause a noxious (painful) response that may cause muscle guarding and spasticity. Phenol blocks either to a trigger point or to the actual nerve or its junction in the muscle may reduce spasticity and pain.

CASE 3

JP: 72-year-old male suffered a cerebrovascular accident 2 years prior to visit. He was a depressed gentleman, a retired successful businessman, and had a history of participation in competitive sports. His chief complaints were lack of improvement from a left hemiparesis after the stroke and lack of energy. Extensive medical workup did uncover sleep apnea, and a home airway (CPAP) device was implemented through an affiliated sleep lab. He needed help in bathing, dressing, and for community walks greater than household distances (i.e., 50 feet). He could eat but not cut his own food. A wheelchair was used for community mobility and was usually pushed by his wife. His wife noted that he had several falls at home while ambulating, although none caused injury. *Medications:* Dilantin, Coumadin, Synthroid, Prozac, Zocor, MVI, Digoxin. The physical exam noted a tall, slender gentleman with clear speech and communication but with wandering thoughts during his responses and slowed response. He showed a left facial hemiparesis. He could repeat 5 of 7 numbers verbally given to him in forward order, but was unable to repeat the numbers in reverse order. He had a tendency to avoid looking at his left side and did not attend to his left arm hanging off the wheelchair. He displayed minimal movement of the proximal scapular muscles and had no voluntary motor control in the more distal upper extremity. The lower extremity had only fair-grade strength in the proximal muscles of the hip and knee and poor-grade strength in the more distal muscles of the ankle and foot. Sensation was partially decreased on the left side, with sensory extinction on simultaneous (left and right tested at the same time) light touch. Graphesthesia (the ability to describe an object that is drawn on the skin such as the number 8) was also impaired but present on the left side. Reflexes were decreased on the left side, and there was a positive Babinski sign on the left and right sides. Cranial deficits were noted in facial muscles on the left side. No aphasia was present. He needed several attempts to rise from a sitting to a standing position. However, with a quad cane he did ambulate at less than 1 mph with no deviations at that speed on a noncarpeted surface. As a result of foot drop, he had difficulty clearing his toe during swing phase of gait.

He entered the clinical exercise physiology program to improve safety in ambulation and improve focus on details as they related to a home exercise program. The goal was to facilitate maximum use of the left upper extremity and attention to his left side. Throughout the program, he displayed interruption in ambulation, reaching tasks, and therapeutic exercises. He would periodically bump his left side in the doorway or into other obstacles. The program was tailored to raise his awareness of objects by developing various obstacle courses that he would navigate to reach a specific destination point. He was taught to avoid bumping into the contrived obstacles by navigating around them. He also gradually responded to verbal cues to the left side. Resistance exercise for the right side involved lifting the left extremities. Electrical muscle stimulation, pulsed to turn on every 5 seconds' for 5 seconds duration, was used to cue muscles of the left shoulder and left hip and knee related muscles. No gait training was done on the treadmill, since his speed of ambulation was initially 0.6 mph and never faster than 1.5 mph. He did not report any additional falls at home. His speed of ambulation increased, and he could discontinue his left ankle foot orthosis without foot drop at the end of 6 months of the program on a semimonthly (once every 2 weeks) basis. His left upper extremity became functional for arm swing during ambulation. He and his wife were successfully connected with psychological support care.

Problems to Consider

One-sided neglect is a problem most common to people who have had a stroke to the right (or dominant) hemisphere with left hemiplegia. They will often ignore the left side of their body as if it did not exist. Setting up safe challenges that require the person to become aware of that side, such as an obstacle course, is one technique that helps to cue that side. Other strategies are to use the recognized extremities to find and use the neglected side in bilateral two-extremity exercises. *Biofeedback* such as electrical stimulation with activities can be useful.

Sensory extinction is the absence of recognition of a sensory stimulus to one extremity when both are touched. For example, if both extremities recognize a sensory stimulus when touched or pin-pricked one at a time, one side will not be recognized if both are simultaneously touched. This sensory extinction is considered a sign of a one-side brain injury or disease. *Graphesthesia,* or the recognition of numeric signs gently traced (without marker or inks), is another organic brain function test.

Depression and distractibility appear the same, but are different in the underlying cause. Depression is a mental disorder, with feelings of helplessness and hopelessness. Some individuals with stroke may not be very *arousable* and will appear distractible. Organic brain diseases will often have distractibility without depression because of lack of arousal. In this patient's case, depression played a significant role.

Flaccid hemiparesis is distinct from *spastic hemiparesis* in that the muscles show flaccid (flaccid = no reflexes; no spasticity) paralysis and decreased activity both with voluntary and sudden involuntary movement. The hemiparesis described above was of the flaccid type. For muscles that do function, repetitive movement exercises are not a problem as with the spastic form.

Domestic falls are considered a functional concern, even if the patient is noted to have strength and coordination adequate for ambulation and arising from a sitting position. The problem may be distractibility, fatigue, or desire to move to another location faster than is safe to move with a hemiparesis. Challenges in the clinic such as fast ambulation and obstacle courses help prevent further falls. Other causes, such as vertigo, heart failure, medication side effects, and an unsafe household with throw rugs, uneven surfaces, and slippery bathrooms, must also be addressed.

References

1. Stewart DG. Stroke rehabilitation. 1. Epidemiological aspects and acute management. Arch Phys Med Rehabil 1999; 80: S4–S7.
2. Groer MW, Shekleton ME. Basic Pathophysiology. A Holistic Approach. 3rd ed. St. Louis, MO: C. V. Mosby Company, 1989: 356–358.
3. Kohl HW III, McKenzie JD. Physical activity, fitness, and stroke. In: Bouchard C, Shephard RJ, Stephens T, eds. Physical Activity, Fitness, and Health. International Proceedings and Consensus Statement. Champaign, IL: Human Kinetics, 1994: 609–621.
4. Wolf GE, D'Agnostino RB. Epidemiology of stroke. In: Barnett HJM, Mohr JP, Stein BM, Yatsu FM, eds. Stroke. Pathophysiology, Diagnosis and Management. 3rd ed. New York: Churchill Livingstone, 1998: 3–28.
5. Holloway RG, Benesch CG, Rahilly CR, et al. A systematic review of cost-effectiveness research of stroke evaluation and treatment. Stroke 1999;30: 1340–1349.
6. Taylor TN, Davis PH, Torner JC, et al. Lifetime cost of stroke in the United States. Stroke 1996;27: 1459–1466.
7. Gorelick PB, Sacco RL, Smith DB. Prevention of a first stroke. A review of guidelines and a multidisciplinary consensus statement from the National Stroke Association. JAMA 1999;281: 1112–1120.
8. Broderick JT, Brott R, Kothari R, et al. The greater Cincinnati/northern Kentucky stroke study. Preliminary first-ever and total incidence rates of stroke among blacks. Stroke 1998;29: 415–421.
9. Thompson DW, Furlan AJ. Clinical epidemiology of stroke. Neurol Clin 1996;14:309–315.
10. Duncan P, Richards L, Wallace D, et al. A randomized, controlled pilot study of a home-based exercise program for individuals with mild and moderate stroke. Stroke 1998;29: 2055–2060.
11. Caplan LR. Stroke. A Clinical Approach. 2nd ed. Boston, MA: Butterworth-Heinemann, 1993: 24–25.
12. Whisnant JP, Basford JR, Bernstein EF, et al. Classification of cerebrovascular disease. III. Special report from the National Institute of Neurological Disorders and Stroke. Stroke 1990; 21: 637–676.
13. Wolf PA, Claggett GP, Easton JD, et al. Preventing ischemic stroke in patients with prior stroke and transient ischemic attack. A statement for healthcare professionals from the Stroke Council of the American Heart Association. Stroke 1999;30:1991–1994.
14. Ramasubbu R, Robinson RG, Flint AJ, et al. Functional impairment associated with acute poststroke depression: The Stroke Data Bank study. J Neuropsych Clin Neurosci 1998; 10: 26–33.
15. Ebrahim S. Clinical Epidemiology of Stroke. New York: Oxford University Press, 1990: 164–183.
16. Kelly JF. Stroke rehabilitation for elderly patients. In: Kemp B, Brummel-Smith K, Ramsdell JW, eds. Geriatric Rehabilitation. Boston, MA: Little, Brown and Company, 1990: 61–89.
17. Hoenig H, Nusbaum N, Brummel-Smith, K. Geriatric rehabilitation: state of the art. J Am Geriatr Soc 1997;45:1371–1381.
18. Abrams WB, Beers MH, Berkow R, eds. The Merck Manual of Geriatrics. Whitehouse Station, NJ: Merck Research Laboratories, 1995: 1162–1188.
19. Black-Schaffer RM, Kirsteins AE, Harvey RL. Stroke rehabilitation. 2. Co-morbidities and complications. Arch Phys Med Rehab 1999;80: S8–S16.
20. Gordon NF. Stroke. Your Complete Exercise Guide. The Cooper Clinic and Research Institute Fitness Series. Champaign, IL: Human Kinetics, 1993: 14–16.
21. Potempa K, Braun LT, Tinknell T, Popovich J. Benefits of aerobic exercise after stroke. Sports Med 1996;21: 337–346.
22. Macko RF, DeSouza CA, Tretter LD, et al. Treadmill aerobic exercise training reduces the energy expenditure and cardiovascular demands of hemiparetic gait in chronic stroke patients. A preliminary report. Stroke 1997;28: 326–330.
23. Potempa K, Lopez M, Braun LT, et al. Physiological outcomes of aerobic exercise training in hemiparetic stroke patients. Stroke 1995;26: 101–105.

24. Rimmer JH, Riley B, Creviston T, et al. Exercise training in a predominantly African-American group of stroke survivors. Med Sci Sports Exerc 2000;32: 1990–1996.
25. Rimmer JH, Braunschweig C, Silverman K, et al. Effects of a short-term health promotion intervention for a predominantly African-American group of stroke survivors. Am J Prev Med 2000;18: 332–338.
26. American College of Sports Medicine. ACSM's Guidelines for Exercise Testing and Prescription. 6th ed. Baltimore: Lippincott Williams & Wilkins, 2000.
27. Sharp SA, Brouwer BJ. Isokinetic strength training of the hemiparetic knee: effects of function and spasticity. Arch Phys Med Rehab 1997;78: 1231–1236.
28. Stein J. Stroke. In: Frontera WR, Dawson DM, Slovik DM, eds. Exercise in Rehabilitation Medicine. Champaign, IL: Human Kinetics, 1999: 293–312.
29. Teixeira-Salmela LF, Olney SJ, Nadeau S, et al. Muscle strengthening and physical conditioning to reduce impairment and disability in chronic stroke survivors. Arch Phys Med Rehab 1999;80: 1211–1218.
30. Richards JS, Jackson WT, Novack TN. Central nervous system conditions. In: Fuhrer MJ, ed. Assessing Medical Rehabilitation Practices. The Promise of Outcomes Research. Baltimore, MD: Paul H. Brookes, 1997: 319–346.
31. Duncan PW. Synthesis of intervention trials to improve motor recovery following stroke. Top Stroke Rehab 1997;3: 1–20.
32. Goodman JM. Assessment of exercise capacity and principles of exercise prescription. In: Shephard RJ, Miller HS, eds. Exercise and the Heart in Health and Disease. New York: Marcel Dekker, 1996: 59–98.
33. Lockette KF, Keys AM. Conditioning with Physical Disabilities. Champaign, IL: Human Kinetics, 1994: 3–21.
34. Boult C, Brummel-Smith K. Post-stroke rehabilitation guidelines. J Am Geriatr Soc 1997;45: 881–883.
35. Reutter-Bernays D, Rentsch HP. Rehabilitation of the elderly patient with stroke: an analysis of short-term and long-term results. Dis Rehab 1993;15: 90–95.
36. Rimmer JH, Hedman G. A health promotion program for stroke survivors. Top Stroke Rehab 1998;5: 30–44.
37. Fujitani J, Ishikawa T, Masami A, et al. Influence of daily activity on changes in physical fitness for people with post-stroke hemiplegia. Am J Phys Med Rehab 1999;78:540–544.
38. Monga TN, Deforge DA, Williams J, et al. Cardiovascular responses to acute exercise in patients with cerebrovascular accidents. Arch Phys Med Rehab 1988;69: 937–940.
39. Smith GV, Silver K, Goldberg AP, et al. "Task-oriented" exercise improves hamstring strength and spastic reflexes in chronic stroke patients. Stroke 1999;30: 2112–2118.
40. Bohannon R, Walsh S. Nature, reliability, and predictive value of muscle performance measures in patients with hemiparesis following stroke. Arch Phys Med Rehab 1992; 73: 721–725.
41. Nakamura R, Watanabe S, Handa T, et al. The relationship between walking speed and muscle strength for knee extension in hemiparetic stroke patients: a follow-up study. Tohoku J Exp Med 1988;154: 111–113.
42. Olney S, Griffin M, Monga TN, et al. Work and power in gain of stroke patients. Arch Phys Med Rehab 1991;67: 92–98.
43. Luukinen H, Koski K, Paippala P, et al. Risk factors for recurrent falls in the elderly in long-term institutional care. Public Health 1995;109: 57–65.
44. Benson H, Stuart EM. The Wellness Book: The Comprehensive Guide to Maintaining Health and Treating Stress-related Illness. New York, NY: Fireside, 1993.
45. Prochaska JO, Velicer WF, Rossi JS, et al. Stages of change and decisional balance for 12 problem behaviors. Health Psych 1994;13: 39–46.
46. Rimmer JH, Rubin SS, Braddock D. Barriers to exercise in African-American women with physical disabilities. Arch Phys Med Rehab 2000;81: 182–188.

CHAPTER 2
CEREBRAL PALSY

James J. Laskin and Mark Anderson

EPIDEMIOLOGY AND PATHOPHYSIOLOGY

Cerebral palsy (CP) was defined in 1959 as "a persistent though not unchanging disorder of movement and posture, appearing early in life and due to a non-progressive lesion of the developing brain" (1). More recently, Mutch et al. (2) defined CP as "an umbrella term covering a group of non-progressive, but often changing, motor impairment syndromes secondary to lesions or anomalies of the brain arising in the early stages of its development." It is important to note that while the brain lesion is static, the resultant movement disorder many times is not, with changes occurring for either the better or the worse (3). Nelson and Ellenberg (4) found that half of all children diagnosed with "cerebral palsy" and two-thirds of those diagnosed with spastic diplegia by their first birthdays had "outgrown" the motor signs of CP by age 7. Other studies have shown that the motor skills of children diagnosed with dystonic and athetoid CP can continue to worsen for years (5, 6).

The overall incidence of CP in the United States is 1.5–2.5 per 1000 live births (3). However, the incidence is higher among African-American children (7) and among ethnic minority children in other parts of the world (8, 9). For example, Sinha et al. (10) report incidences of CP among Asian families in the Yorkshire region of Britain of between 5.48 and 6.42 per 1000 live births.

The most readily identified cause of CP is the combination of prematurity and low birth weight (11). The diagnosis of CP has been associated with several prenatal factors, including viral infections, maternal substance abuse, multiple births, congenital brain malformations, and certain genetic conditions. In addition, certain perinatal factors such as anoxia from traumatic delivery, hemorrhage with direct brain damage from birth trauma, and kernicterus may all result in CP. Postnatal factors occurring before the age of two such as viral and bacterial meningitis, traumatic head injury, anoxia, and toxin-induced encephalopathy are also considered risk factors for CP (11). However, according to Stanley et al. (12), CP is the result of a causal pathway rather than a single event. This pathway identifies multiple causal factors, which lead to the child developing CP. For example, multiple births may lead to preterm delivery that may lead to neonatal cerebral damage in CP. These factors increase the child's vulnerability to later causal factors such as intrauterine growth restriction that may decrease the child's capacity to cope with intrapartum stress.

Classification of CP may be done using physiological (Table 2.1) or anatomical (Table 2.2) categorization, or by predominant movement disorder (Table 2.3). Classification allows one to categorize CP into subtypes that display certain specific characteristics. However, for each child with CP, the type and degree of motor impairment combined with other effects of diffuse brain damage ultimately determine the child's functional level and the need for a variety of intervention services, regardless of how that child is classified.

The prevalence of other conditions related to CP has also been noted in the literature. Saito et al. (13) reported an incidence of scoliosis of 68% in those patients diagnosed with spastic CP. Scoliosis usually started before the age of 10 and progressed rapidly during the growth period. Risk factors for progression of scoliosis in this population included having a spinal curve of 40° before the age of 15 years, having spasticity that involved the total body, being bedridden, and having a thoracolumbar curve.

Several gastrointestinal (GI) manifestations are prevalent in children with CP (14). In this report, 92% of children with CP had clinically significant GI symptoms; these included swallowing disorders, regurgitation and/or vomiting, abdominal pain, chronic pulmonary aspiration, and chronic constipation. They concluded that most of these GI clinical manifestations were the result of disorders of GI motility and not related to any specific computed tomography or magnetic resonance imaging finding of the brain.

CLINICAL EXERCISE PHYSIOLOGY

There is limited research as to the exercise response of individuals with CP. This may be related to the fact that

Table 2.1. Physiological Classification of Cerebral Palsy (11)

Type	Site of injury	Presentation
Pyramidal	Cortical system	Spastic, hyperreflexia, "clasp-knife" hypertonia, prone to contractures
Extrapyramidal	Basal ganglia and cerebellum	Athetosis, ataxia, "lead-pipe" rigidity, chorea
Mixed	Combination of above	Combination of above

Table 2.2. Anatomical Classification of Cerebral Palsy (11)

Type	Presentation
Hemiplegia	Unilateral involvement; upper extremity generally more involved than lower extremity
Diplegia	Bilateral involvement; legs generally more involved than arms
Tetraplegia	Total body involvement, including cranial nerves; frequently seen with mental retardation
Monoplegia	Single limb involvement
Paraplegia	Legs only involved; arms normal
Triplegia	One limb unaffected

participation in exercise programs has been limited in this population. This lack of participation should not be construed as a lack of desire to participate. In many instances, lack of participation is related to a paucity of programs designed for or accessible to persons with disabilities.

In some individuals with CP, impaired motor function may cause a decrease in daily activity and diminished function associated with physical activity (15, 16). Persons with CP have also been reported to have increased adiposity (15), low muscle force (17), lower aerobic and anaerobic power (16, 18), decreased mechanical efficiency (18), and decreased respiratory function (19). All of these factors are signs of poor overall fitness. This may be related to poor exercise habits, difficulty in performing skilled movements, muscle imbalances, or overall poor functional strength. It has also been reported that fatigue and stress associated with a strenuous exercise program may cause a transient increase in spasticity and incoordination in the person with CP (20).

Exercise testing of individuals with CP may be difficult due to their spasticity and dyskinesia, and the inefficient nature of their mobility often leads to higher than expected exercise response values. Studies examining heart rate, blood pressure, expired air, and blood lactate have shown that individuals with CP respond with higher heart and respiratory rates as well as elevated blood pressures and blood lactate levels for a given submaximal work rate than those without CP. Peak physiological responses are also lowered (10–20%) in persons with CP. Physical work capacity has been shown to be 50% that of able-bodied subjects (20). However, Bowen et al. (21) reported no statistically significant differences in the percentage of variability of oxygen cost, oxygen consumption, or physiological cost index between subjects with and without CP at free-walking velocity.

PHARMACOLOGY

Pharmacotherapy for the movement disorders of CP has focused on the dyskinesia that most affects the person's functional level. Several drugs are used to treat the types of involuntary movements found in CP. These may be broken down by type of involuntary movement: dystonia, myoclonus, chorea and athetosis, and spasticity (22).

The main categories of drugs used to treat dystonia, myoclonus, chorea/athetosis, and spasticity are listed in Table 2.4. Up to 50% of patients with dystonia respond positively to anti-Parkinsonian drugs, and less than 25% respond positively to antispasticity, dopaminergic, or anticonvulsant

Table 2.3. Classification of Cerebral Palsy based on Movement Disorder (3,37)

Classification	Presentation
Spastic cerebral palsy (CP) (diplegia, hemiplegia, tetraplegia, paraplegia, monoplegia, triplegia)	Present in ~65% of those with CP; diplegia most common; typically greater lower extremity involvement than upper extremity; involves flexors, adductors, and internal rotators greater than their antagonists; hypotonia at birth progressing to spasticity after infancy; increased deep tendon reflexes (DTRs); clonus; abnormal postural reflexes.
Dyskinetic CP (athetosis; dystonia, chorea, ataxia)	*Athetosis*—slow, writhing motions of the appendicular musculature; present in ~25% of those with CP; impairment of postural reflexes; nonrhythmical involuntary movement; dysarthria; dysphagia; signs increase with anxiety, absent during sleep. *Dystonia*—sustained muscle contractions that result in twisting and repetitive movement or abnormal posture; present in 15–25% of those with CP; persists throughout life, but no joint contractures or deformities due to continuous movement. *Chorea*—state of excessive, spontaneous movements, irregularly timed; nonrepetitive and abrupt; unable to maintain voluntary muscle contraction; present in ~25% of those with CP. *Ataxia*—uncoordinated, voluntary movements; wide-based gait with genurecurvatum; mild intention tremors; in the infant, generalized hypotonia; normal DTR; in its mildest form, called *apraxia,* which is an inability to perform coordinated voluntary gross and fine motor skills.
Mixed	Present in ~20% of those with CP; both spastic and dyskinetic components

Table 2.4. Pharmacological Management of Cerebral Palsy (22)

MOVEMENT DISORDER	CATEGORY OF DRUG	EXAMPLES	POSSIBLE SIDE EFFECTS
Dystonia	Anti-Parkinsonian drugs, anticholinergic medications and dopaminergic drugs, anticonvulsants, antispasticity drugs, antidopaminergic drugs, and antidepressants	baclofen, carbamazepine, clonazepam, levadopa/carbidopa, lorazepam, reserbine, tetrabenazine, and trihexyphenidyl	Drowsiness, dizziness, weakness, fatigue, skin rash, bone marrow suppression, hepatotoxicity, ataxia, nausea, psychosis, depression, dry mouth, blurred vision, nervousness
Myoclonus	Anticonvulsants	clonazepam, valproate, phenobarbital, baclofen, piracetam, lorazepam	Drowsiness, dizziness, weakness, fatigue, ataxia, sedation, dry mouth, hyperactivity
Chorea/Athetosis	Anticonvulsants, neuroleptics	baclofen, clonazepam, fluphenazine, haloperidol, pimozide, reserbine, tetrabenazine, valproate	Drowsiness, dizziness, weakness, fatigue, skin rash, bone marrow suppression, hepatotoxicity, ataxia, sedation, extrapyramidal reactions, depression
Spasticity	Muscle relaxants, antispasticity drugs	baclofen, dantrolene, diazepam	Drowsiness, dizziness, weakness, fatigue, hepatotoxicity, ataxia, diarrhea

drugs. Anticholinergic drugs may be helpful in controlling the drooling in CP and may be delivered via transdermal patch. Drugs used for myoclonus typically are anticonvulsants, which facilitate the action of gamma-aminobutyric acid (GABA), the principal inhibitory neurotransmitter in the brain. Benzodiazepines are often used to treat chorea and athetosis but are subject to development of tolerance. Neuroleptics, which block dopamine receptors, are effective drugs for chorea and athetosis, but they are also associated with the most permanent side effects and are the most problematic with chronic use. Spasticity may be of either cerebral or spinal origin, and each requires a specific drug therapy. However, baclofen has been shown to be effective in controlling both cerebral and spinal spasticity (22).

Continuous intrathecal baclofen (CIB) is perhaps the first highly effective medical treatment of spasticity in persons with CP (23). It has been used to treat the movement disorders associated with CP for more than 15 years (24). The first double-blind study on the use of intrathecal baclofen for spinal spasticity was published by Penn and colleagues (25) in 1989. They found that lower-extremity spasticity was significantly reduced and that muscle tone on the Ashworth scale (Table 2.5) was decreased from 4.0 before treatment to 1.2 after baclofen use.

General indications for CIB infusion are to improve function, to facilitate care, and to retard or prevent the development of contractures. Another uncommon indication is to decrease pain associated with involuntary muscle spasms. According to Albright (23) and Bodensteiner (26), CIB is indicated for treating spasticity in four distinct groups: (1) those whose gait and lower-extremity movements are impeded by spasticity, but whose underlying strength is poor; (2) individuals older than age 16 with spasticity of the lower or both the upper and lower extremities that is interfering with gait or lower-extremity function; (3) nonambulatory persons with spastic tetraparesis whose spasticity interferes with their activities of daily living, comfort, and endurance; and (4) nonfunctional persons in whom the goal is to enable their care.

Almeida et al. (27) described a case study in which the reflex status, range of motion (ROM), strength, and motor performance of an 11-year-old boy with spastic diplegia were assessed prior to and following implantation of an intrathecal baclofen pump. They showed that spasticity, Babinski reflexes, clonus, strength, and coactivation of antagonist muscles during voluntary movement were decreased following baclofen administration. They also reported an increase in hip and ankle ROM and upper-extremity movement speed, as well as improved independence in dressing and transfers and elimination of orthoses. Gerszten et al. (28) reported that CIB for the treatment of spastic CP reduces the need for subsequent orthopedic surgery for the effects of lower-extremity spasticity. They further recommended that for patients with spastic CP, spasticity should be treated before orthopedic procedures are performed.

Continuous intrathecal baclofen has no affect on athetosis, ataxia, and chorea and is contraindicated for choreoathetoid CP, ataxic CP, and for individuals with severe contractures. However, it may be effective in treating extensor rigidity that occurs after anoxic episodes and appears to

Table 2.5. Ashworth Scale of Muscle Tone (23)

ASHWORTH SCORE	DEGREE OF MUSCLE TONE
1	No increase in tone
2	Slight increase in tone, giving a "catch" when affected part is moved in flexion or extension
3	More marked increase in tone; passive movements difficult
4	Considerable increase in tone; passive movements difficult
5	Affected part rigid in flexion and extension

improve generalized dystonia in CP. An insignificant increase in plasma baclofen level also occurs in children receiving CIB (29). Excessive dosages of baclofen result in listlessness, apathy, urinary hesitancy, or leg weakness. However, these symptoms respond readily to lowering the dosage (23). Complications relating to the intrathecal catheter occur in approximately 20% of patients, and infection requiring the removal of the pump occurs in approximately 5% of patients (30).

Physicians have used neuromuscular blocking agents such as 45% ethyl alcohol, 4–6% phenol, local anesthetics, or botulinum A toxin (Botox) to treat the muscle imbalance, spasticity, and joint deformities associated with CP for more than 30 years. The neuromuscular blockade may be used to interrupt the function of the nerve, the neuromuscular junction, or the muscle. The blockade is used to balance agonist-antagonist muscle forces by (a) diminishing stretch reflexes through neural destruction and blocking of nerve transmission (phenol, alcohol, local anesthetic), (b) preventing or decreasing muscle fiber contraction by direct muscle fiber destruction (alcohol or phenol), or (c) blocking neuromuscular junction activity (Botox). The goal is complete or partial paralysis of the agonist muscle while leaving antagonist muscles unaffected. All neuromuscular blockade procedures are contraindicated in the presence of fixed contractures (31).

Local anesthetics may be used diagnostically to differentiate between dynamic deformity and fixed contracture or to evaluate the performance of antagonist muscles and to determine the potential functional effects of longer-acting agents. Injection of the drugs within the target muscle in the vicinity of the myoneural junction produces the maximum blockade effect. There are no well-controlled studies documenting the effectiveness of alcohol injection in modifying spasticity in those with CP. There are reports in peer-reviewed literature that the clinical effects of alcohol vary in duration and that there are occasional complications, including the need for anesthetic due to the pain. Phenol, which produces a functional and clinical effect for 3–18 months, depending on the concentration and duration of exposure, may also be extremely painful if injected in the vicinity of a sensory nerve. However, phenol has been reported as safe, simple, and economically advantageous in pediatric patients with CP (31).

The use of Botox, while widely used as a neuromuscular blockade, is a bit more controversial. Botulinum A toxin was first introduced to treat strabismus and blepharospasm and is now being used in an increasing number of conditions, including involuntary tremor, focal dystonias such as spasmodic torticollis, and autonomic disorders such as focal hyperhidrosis of the palms (32). However, its widest use is probably in treating spasticity or athetosis associated with CP.

Botulinum A toxin has been used in persons with CP to diminish paravertebral spasticity, to facilitate positioning and hygiene, to improve ambulation, as an alternative to serial casting, diagnostically to determine the efficacy of surgery, as an adjunct to further therapy, to facilitate or replace bracing, to delay surgery, and to improve upper-extremity function (31–34). Following injection, the onset of weakness is usually detectable in 2 or 3 days. Generally, weakness wears off by 3 months, but functional improvement may last considerably longer (34). Treatment may be given at periodic intervals, as long as continued efficacy is documented. A positive response rate of 70% has been reported in appropriately selected ambulatory patients (31).

Massin and Allington (35) demonstrated that Botox was effective in reducing the energy cost of movement and in improving the endurance of spastic muscles in children with CP. Few adverse effects have been reported. The most common complaints were excessive muscle weakness in the injected muscle or unwanted weakness in adjacent muscles (34). Contraindications for the use of Botox include fixed contracture, the presence of certain neuromuscular diseases (e.g., myasthenia gravis), patients being treated with medications that may exaggerate the neuromuscular blockade response, muscles that failed to respond to alcohol or phenol injections, the presence of Botox antibodies, or the absence of objective benefit to the patient (31).

Disadvantages of this treatment include the requirement of repeated treatment at regular intervals and the cost of the treatment (32). The controversy that exists regarding the use of Botox relates to a perceived lack of scientifically rigorous studies on the efficacy of the treatment. Forssberg and Tedroff (36) reviewed the literature on Botox and found scientific rigor lacking in the published studies. While they conceded that Botox studies are justified and needed, they called for studies that conform in every way to scientific research protocols, including the use of proper design and statistical analysis as well as objective and valid measures with which to evaluate functional improvement in clients with CP.

PHYSICAL EXAMINATION AND DIAGNOSIS

In children with CP, movement disorders become apparent as the nervous system matures and new motor skills are learned. This produces what appears to be a progressive rather than a static disorder. The extent of the disorder may not be recognized until the child reaches age 2 or 3 or even later. A definitive diagnosis of CP is rarely made before age 6 months and many times occurs much later. However, certain clinical findings should arouse suspicion of the diagnosis (37).

Children with CP commonly exhibit tonal abnormalities such as hypotonia, hypertonia, or a combination of both. Hypotonia may be identified by increased range of motion of the shoulders and hips. Hypertonicity of the lower extremities may be present if the infant displays a scissoring posture of the legs. Asymmetry of movement or posture between the right and left sides of the body should be evaluated for possible dysfunction (37). Prechtl (38) reports that, even at very early infancy, distinct movement patterns called general movements are predictive of neurological outcome over 2 years, in particular CP. The Early Motor Pattern Profile (EMPP) has been shown to be an effective instrument to identify children in their first year of life who are at greatest risk for the development of CP. This profile, consisting of 15 items related to variations in muscle tone, reflexes, and movement and organized into a standardized format, may be incorporated into a routine health screening. The format only adds minutes to the routine screening and has high sensitivity and specificity (39).

Persistence of primitive reflexes and the delayed appearance of postural reflexes are consistent with a diagnosis of CP. Asymmetry of reflex response should also be regarded as significant. Hyperreflexia of the deep tendon reflexes and ankle clonus both should signal further evaluation. Abnormal behavioral characteristics are more subtle. However, irritability, irregular sleep patterns, continuous gross motor activity, delayed speech, and diminished attention span are behaviors that may signify central nervous system dysfunction. Additional behavioral signs include delayed achievement of motor milestones, which is often the first recognized sign and primary complaint (37).

There are also a number of tests and measures that are useful in documenting and quantifying the outcomes of intervention for children with CP. These tests may be categorized in a variety of ways, including tests for assessing disability in daily activity (Table 2.6); tests of functional limitations (Table 2.7); and measures of impairment (Table 2.8) (40).

CONSERVATIVE AND SURGICAL INTERVENTION

Conservative management of people with CP is directed at improving overall function and facilitating care. Besides traditional physical and occupational therapy, a number of different approaches have been used. Traditional therapy has focused on improving strength and range of motion to promote improved function, through a combination of therapeutic exercise, neurodevelopmental treatment (NDT), and motor learning approaches (41).

Table 2.6. Tests for Assessing Disability in Daily Activity (40)

Test	Use
Canadian Occupational Performance Measure	Assist client/family to choose therapeutic goals and rate performance and satisfaction
Pediatric Evaluation of Disability Inventory	Assess needs for caregiving assistance and equipment modifications
Functional Independence Measure for Children (WeeFIM)	Assess independence in mobility, self-care, and cognition

Table 2.7. Tests of Functional Limitations (40)

Test	Use
Pediatric Evaluation of Disability Inventory	Assess skills in mobility, self-care, and social function
Gross Motor Function Measure	Assess gross motor skills
Peabody Developmental Motor Scales	Assess gross and fine motor skills
Bruininks-Oseretsky Test of Motor Proficiency	Assess gross motor and eye-hand coordination, strength, balance, and agility
The Test of Infant Motor Performance	Assess head and trunk postural control needed for functional movement in early infancy
Alberta Infant Motor Scale	Identify children with delayed gross motor development or with abnormal posture and coordination

The efficacy of such treatments alone has been questioned. Law et al. (42) found no significant differences in upper-extremity function, quality of movement, or parent's perception of functional performance in children with CP between a group receiving intensive NDT and casting or a group receiving regular occupational therapy programs. Weindling et al. (43) conducted a study to determine if infants at high risk of CP would benefit from early physical therapy utilizing NDT. There was no difference in functional outcomes between the group receiving NDT and the group whose therapy was delayed until abnormal signs were present. Bower et al. (44) reported that in children with CP, the use of specific measurable goals directed at motor skill acquisition was more strongly associated with the actual skill acquisition than either conventional amounts or intensive amounts of physical therapy alone.

Several studies have demonstrated the positive effects of various conservative interventions. Normal movement with emphasis on weight bearing in children with spastic CP has been shown to significantly increase femoral neck bone mineral content and volumetric bone mineral density (45). Carlson et al. (46) showed that using an ankle-foot orthosis during gait training provided biomechanical benefits with more efficient gait in children with spastic diplegia, whereas using supramalleolar orthoses appeared to have little measurable effect. It has also been shown that there are no differences between walking speed, energy cost, and perceived exertion between the use of anterior and posterior walkers in children with CP who were familiar with both walkers and that most children preferred the posterior walker (47).

Damiano and Abel (48) showed that children with spastic diplegia and spastic hemiplegia could have significant strength gains in targeted muscles following a 6-week strength training program. In addition, they demonstrated that with increased strength, these children had higher gait velocities with increased cadence as well as an increase in the Gross Motor Function Measure with no in-

Table 2.8. Measurements of Impairment (40)

IMPAIRMENT	HOW MEASURED	USE
Involuntary movement	Motion analysis—position and orientation of multiple joints and body segments	Biofeedback training to reduce unwanted movements or to measure changes following intervention
Speed/progression of movement	Motion analysis—position and orientation of multiple joints and body segments	Measure changes following intervention
Spasticity	Ashworth scale	Measure resistance to passive movement following intervention
Postural control and alignment	*Gross Motor Performance Measure*	Quantifying impairment in postural alignment, weight-shifting, coordination, and select activation of specific joints/segments during gross motor skill performance
	Assessment of Behavioral Components	Capture disordered postural alignment in children with CP using illustrated criterion referenced postures in children
	Sitting Assessment Scale	Ratings of postural control of the head, trunk, and feet during performance of reaching and various functional tasks in addition to functional performance measures of these skills
	Melbourne Assessment of Unilateral Upper Limb Function	Quality-of-movement scale addressing trunk control and alignment, fluence and range of movement, and quality of grasp and release during 12 fine motor and reaching activities
	Examination of a Child with Mild Neurological Dysfunction	Measures balance, coordination, posture, and motor function
Force	Hand-held dynamometry or isokinetic dynamometry	Useful measures of outcomes of strength training programs for children with CP
Range of motion	Goniometry or electrogoniometry	Goniometry lacks satisfactory reliability in the presence of spasticity; electrogoniometry shown to be more reliable than traditional approaches
Balance	Functional Reach Test	Assess ability to reach forward in standing without losing one's balance—simple, fast, and reliable
Energy cost	Physiological Cost Index	Indicates biological cost of ambulation using heart rate (bpm) during walking minus resting heart rate divided by speed of walking; due to inefficient gait of persons with CP, this measure is only an estimate of energy cost

crease in energy expenditure. Swimming has been shown to improve baseline vital capacity in children with CP (19). Van den Berg-Emons et al. (16) looked at the effects of two 9-month sports programs on level of daily physical activity, fat mass, and physical fitness in children with spastic CP. They found that the children involved in the training had no change in fat mass compared to the control group who showed an increase. There was also a favorable increase in muscle strength and peak aerobic power in those students involved in the training program.

Surgical intervention in persons with CP is designed to improve function by relieving spasticity or by correcting deformity. Selective dorsal (posterior) rhizotomy (SDR) is the surgery used to treat spastic diplegia and tetraplegia in children with spastic CP. Numerous studies have demonstrated the effectiveness of this procedure (49). Wright et al. (50), Steinbok et al. (51), and Steinbok, Reiner, and Kestle (52) found that SDR in combination with physical and/or occupational therapy leads to significantly greater functional improvement at 1 year following surgery than either PT or OT alone. The functional improvement was achieved through reduced knee and ankle tone, increased ankle dorsiflexion ROM, and more normal foot-floor contact during gait. Subramanian et al. (53) reported SDR alleviated spasticity, resulting in lasting functional benefits as measured by improved gait in children with spastic CP.

Several authors have reported postoperative weakness following SDR (54). However, this does not agree with the studies of Engsberg et al. (55, 56) who found no loss of hamstring or ankle plantar flexor strength following SDR. In Abbot's review (54) of the literature on SDR, he reports various complications, either immediately postoperatively or at long-term follow-up. Besides postoperative hypotonia, other complications reported include a persisting sensory loss, postoperative urological dysfunction, cerebral spinal fluid leakage around the wound, subdural hematomas, and headache. Long-term complications include changes in postural spinal alignment, low back pain, spondylolisthesis, soft-tissue contractures, hip dislocation, and persisting neurogenic bladder. Buckon et al. (57) reported no significant decrease in upper-extremity muscle tone at 1 year following SDR in ambulatory children with spastic CP.

Stereotactic surgery of the basal ganglia for the improvement of rigidity, choreoathetosis, and tremor in persons with CP is another option (58). The surgery involves placing a well-planned lesion either in the ventrolateral nucleus of the thalamus or ventroposterior pallidum. The site is chosen based on the predominance of the symptoms of a given patient. Speelman and van Manen (59) reported a 21-year follow-up on patients receiving stereotactic surgery for CP. They reported a subjective improvement in function in 44% of patients with 64% of patients reporting side effects such as hemiparesis and speech impairments. For patients with unilateral dystonia, tremor, and choreoathetoid symptoms, it is the consensus that this surgery is very successful (58).

Surgery to correct upper- and lower-extremity deformity in persons with CP generally falls into one of three categories: (1) soft-tissue releases, (2) tendon transfers, or (3) bone/joint stabilization. Table 2.9 describes these procedures with specific examples of how each is used in the upper and lower extremity (60, 61).

Van Heest (60) reported significant improvement with regards to upper limb function following surgical intervention for upper-extremity dysfunction in patients with CP over a 25-year period. Patients were rated pre- and post-surgery on a Classification of Upper Extremity Functional Use scale from 0 (does not use) to 8 (spontaneous use, complete) by House et al. (62). The average functional use score was 2.3 before surgery (range 0–7) and 5.0 after surgery (range 2–8). The average change in functional use scores, 2.7 levels of improvement, was statistically significant.

Persons with CP commonly develop deformities of the spine such as scoliosis, kyphosis, and lordosis. Kyphosis and lordosis are usually treated conservatively unless tendon lengthenings of the hip flexors or extensors are required to correct the deformity. Conservative management of scoliosis in persons with CP is usually ineffective in stopping the progression of the deformity. Surgical intervention is indicated if the scoliosis curve exceeds 40–50° and the spine will not be severely shortened by arrest of its further growth. Spinal arthrodesis with internal fixation is the definitive treatment of progressive scoliosis in persons with CP. This procedure should produce a balanced spine over a level pelvis to facilitate sitting balance, improve sitting endurance, facilitate care and personal hygiene, and improve patient outlook (61).

EXERCISE/FITNESS/FUNCTIONAL TESTING

Given the varied presentations of CP in terms of an individual's physical attributes, cognitive abilities, communication abilities, visual/hearing deficits, and chronological age, it not possible to provide a simple recipe for exercise testing in this population. In addition, there is limited research available to support the use of the able-bodied exercise adaptation model, testing protocols, principles, and techniques in the CP population (20, 63). Therefore, it is up to clinicians to use their experience, common sense, the details provided in this chapter, and the basic principles of exercise testing as published by the ACSM (64, 65) to devise the most appropriate exercise testing protocols for a given client. To assist in the assessment of the client's needs, goals, and objectives, it is suggested that the clinician utilize the Cerebral Palsy—International Sports and Recreation Association's Functional Classification System (see Table 2.10) (66). This classification system, though developed for sport, can be used as a tool to help the clinician gain insight into the client's functional abilities. With this information, the clinician will be better prepared to recommend specific exercise test protocols and recognize the need for adaptations that will help ensure the success of the testing session.

Cardiovascular

Evaluating cardiovascular fitness using some form of wheelchair ergometer (preferably the individual's own chair on wheelchair rollers) provides the most functional assessment for the wheelchair users with CP. However, various forms of arm crank ergometers are frequently used in the research literature (63). One of the disadvantages of the wheelchair roller ergometer is the difficulty in accu-

Table 2.9. Common Surgical Procedures to Correct Deformities Associated with Cerebral Palsy (60, 61)

PROCEDURE	TYPE	EXAMPLES SEEN IN UPPER EXTREMITY	EXAMPLES SEEN IN LOWER EXTREMITY
Soft-tissue releases	Tendon lengthening; tendon release; aponeurosis release	Biceps lengthening for elbow flexion contracture; Biceps aponeurosis release for pronation contracture; Adductor pollicis and 1st dorsal interosseous release for thumb in palm	Achilles tendon lengthening for equinus deformity; Fasciectomy of medial and lateral hamstrings for knee flexion contracture; Long head of the rectus femoris release for hip flexion contracture
Tendon transfers	Tendon rerouting; tendon transfer for muscle substitution	Pronator teres rerouting for pronation contracture; Flexor carpi ulnaris transfer to extensor digitorum communis for finger deformity	Distal rectus femoris tendon transfer to sartorius to assist knee flexion during gait; Posterior tibial tendon rerouting for supination/varus deformity of forefoot
Bone/joint stabilization	Rotational osteotomies; arthrodesis; capsulodesis	Rotational osteotomy of the radius for pronation contracture; Wrist arthrodesis with proximal row carpectomy for wrist flexion/ulnar deviation deformity; Palmar plate capsulodesis for finger deformity	External rotation osteotomy of the femur for femoral anteversion; Extra-articular subtalar arthrodesis for valgus deformity of the foot; Palmar plate capsulodesis for hammer toe deformity

Table 2.10. Overview of the Cerebral Palsy—International Sports and Recreation Association's Functional Profiles for Athletes with Nonprogressive Brain Injuries(66)

	Functional Profile
1	Moderate to severe spasticity—severe involvement of all four limbs. Poor trunk control and functional strength in upper extremities (UE).
2 (Lower)	Moderate to severe spasticity—severe involvement of upper extremities and trunk. Poor functional strength and control of UE. Propels wheelchair with legs.
2 (Upper)	Moderate to severe spasticity—severe involvement of lower extremities and trunk. Poor functional strength and control of lower extremities. Propels wheelchair poorly with arms.
3	Fair functional strength and moderate control in UE. Almost full functional strength in dominant UE. Propels wheelchair slowly with one or both arms.
4	Moderate to severe involvement of lower limbs. Functional strength and minimal control problems in UE.
5	Good functional strength; minimal control problems in UE. Usually ambulates with an assistive device.
6	Moderate to minimal involvement of all four limbs and trunk (typically athetoid); competes without an assistive device.
7	Moderate to minimal hemiplegia. Good functional ability on nonaffected side. Ambulates well.
8	Minimally affected or monoplegic. Good coordination and balance.

rately calculating, controlling, and progressing the rolling resistance. Often, the clients are asked to wheel at progressively faster cadences during each stage of the test protocol. Unfortunately, spasticity and athetosis may be aggravated by the increased speed of movement. Ultimately, coordination and therefore performance may be limited.

The literature has documented starting power outputs ranging from 0 to 15 W at 30–50 rpm and increasing in 5–10-W increments every 2 minutes during a typical arm crank ergometry test to volitional exhaustion (63). The client should be positioned so that during the pedaling action their forearms do not rise above the horizontal plane and their elbows do not fully extend. Stability of the client in the seated position is critical. An axiom in rehabilitation is that one cannot achieve distal mobility without proximal stability. Participants with CP typically present with increased muscle tone in the extremities and decreased tone in the trunk. Using the client's own wheelchair and/or some other stable seating system with or with out strapping of the trunk, pelvis, and lower extremities (LEs) may be necessary. Be very cautious if you choose to strap the client's hand to the handle. This type of strapping is most commonly done for those with hemiplegia or marked weakness of the hands. With the person with hemiplegia, if the limb that is strapped does not have sufficient range of motion to complete the same pedal stroke as the sound side, serious injury could result to the wrist, elbow, or shoulder. The specific resistance/cadence will depend on the client's functional abilities and the presence of any concomitant secondary conditions. The clinician must also consider the handle position of the ergometer. It is preferable to use handles that are in the vertical versus the horizontal plane. If the handles are grasped in the horizontal plane, the shoulder is forced into marked internal rotation, thereby increasing the risk for impingement and/or rotator cuff overuse syndromes (20). A final consideration is the distance between the client and the ergometer. The typical setup described above works primarily the upper-extremity (UE) musculature with the trunk muscles cocontracting for proximal stability. The clinician may choose to increase the distance between the ergometer and the client. This adaptation forces the trunk to move through a greater range of motion and therefore a more dynamic role.

Many wheelchair users, though not functional for ambulation, will have some level of LE use. Exercise modalities such as the Schwinn Air-Dyne™ and the NuStep™ Recumbent Stepper both allow for the use of all four extremities. The utilization of all four limbs in a dynamic rhythmic movement pattern will help control the spasticity and/or athetosis experienced by the client. This form of exercise will also maximize the number of muscle groups involved in the exercise. The clinician may choose to perform a graded exercise test on a Schwinn Air-Dyne™; however, the only way to increase the resistance is to increase the cadence. Increasing the cadence often increases the spasticity in the participant with moderate to severe resting spasticity, thus significantly increasing both their perceived effort and absolute energy expenditure at any given workload. The NuStep™ Recumbent Stepper allows the client to maintain a constant cadence while resistance is increased, therefore minimizing the velocity of movement-related increased spasticity.

The treadmill will optimize the exercise test response for those with CP who are ambulatory (20, 67). However, limitations in balance and coordination may force the clinician to choose a cycle ergometer or some other form of ergometry. The clinician should note that, as the client fatigues, the spasticity of the hip adductors might increase (20, 67). As the client's hip abductors fatigue and become less able to offset the increasing hip adductor spasticity, an increase in the genu valgus (knocked knees) will result. The risk on the treadmill is that the client will hit his or her knees together and fall, or on a cycle ergometer that his or her knees may start to hit against the frame of the ergometer. Using a treadmill protocol that allows the client to choose a self-selected pace and increase only the inclination has been demonstrated to be the most appropriate for clients with mild to moderate spasticity/athetosis. Due to the increased risk of falls in this population (even those experienced with treadmill use), a spotter should always be in place. For persons with minimal motor deficits, any of the typical able-bodied treadmill protocols would be appropriate.

In the literature, the power outputs used with cycle ergometry varied from an initial 25–50 W at 50–60 rpm and increased by 15–25 W for each 2-minute increment until volitional fatigue (20, 63). The clinician will find that cage-type toe clips will prove to be invaluable for keeping the client's feet on the pedals of a cycle ergometer, especially with moderate to high resistances and cadences.

The literature available has documented high test-retest reliability coefficients for testing maximal aerobic capacity using wheelchair, arm crank, and cycle ergometry (68, 69). The determination of anaerobic threshold in wheelchair athletes with CP using a discontinuous protocol, however, has been found to demonstrate poor reliability. Bhambhani et al. (69) suggested that the poor reliability may have been a result of the protocol used and/or inconsistencies related to the effect of spasticity and lactate diffusion from the working muscles into the blood.

Clinicians who elect to collect metabolic data should be aware that the mouth often develops abnormally in a person with CP. The long-term effects of increased tone of the facial muscles and tongue results in a very acute mandibular angle. This results in oral deformities that may make the use of the typical mouthpiece difficult in terms of fit, comfort, and the assurance of an airtight seal. Also, a spastic tongue typically trusts outward, thus making it difficult for the client to keep the mouthpiece in place (20). Clinicians who resort to using a mask must be careful to ensure that the seal remains unbroken at rest and during exercise.

Muscular Strength and Endurance

Muscular strength and endurance testing in individuals with spasticity and/or athetosis has often been considered inappropriate and invalid (70, 71). Bohannon has reported from his own work and others that in fact these measures are appropriate (71–74). Strength testing is a measurement of the capacity of the person to activate a specific muscle or group while inhibiting the antagonist. Bohannon presents a body of evidence that not only highlights the appropriateness of muscular strength and endurance testing in this population, but also demonstrates the predictive traits between the initial and final clinical evaluations (71, 73–75). Other research has documented high test-retest reliability coefficients for both upper and lower extremity one repetition maximal (1-RM) strength testing (63). The clinician must remember that as a result of spasticity, the involuntary contraction of the opposing muscle group during a manual muscle test may result in a situation of co-contraction. The co-contracting muscle groups may both be "strong," but net little functional muscle strength during the manual muscle testing procedure.

Prior to muscular strength and endurance testing, the appropriate range-of-motion (ROM) measurements should be performed. These measurements will help the clinician determine if there are substantial side-to-side differences and if contractures exist. With substantial side to side differences, the case can be made to test muscle strength and endurance unilaterally versus bilaterally. Both active and passive measurements should be made. If the passive ROM is substantially greater than the active ROM, then the difference is likely caused by increased tone/spasticity of the antagonist or weakness of the agonist. If the both the passive and active ROM are equally clinically less than the expected normal limits, then the loss is most likely due to a permanent contracture (76, 77).

The main considerations for muscular strength and endurance testing are stability, coordination, range of motion, and timing (76). The forms and protocols for testing do not necessarily need to be modified from the able-bodied model. Typically, an 8-RM muscular strength testing protocol can be used. This protocol will adequately estimate approximately 80–85% of the individual's 1-RM. Using a protocol that utilizes moderate resistances will help to minimize the risk of increased spasticity resulting in decreased coordination and functional movement. The goal for this protocol is to reach volitional fatigue (6–10 repetitions) in no more than three sets. When assessing muscular endurance, a resistance in the order of 50–60% of the predicted 1-RM should be used (63).

The clinician must pay particular attention to the client's technique. Any deviation from the prescribed technique and/or cadence would be reason to discontinue the test even if the client does not reach volitional fatigue. Fatigue-related increases in spasticity and incoordination should be expected (20, 76).

As mentioned previously, proximal (trunk) stability is critical for the optimal performance of the extremity movements. Wide benches, low seats (so the client's feet can rest on the floor), and trunk and pelvic strapping are potentially necessary adaptations for the client with CP. Given the potential for altered coordination and balance, it would be preferable to use selectorized weight machines for this population. With the movements guided, the client can focus on muscular effort, the learning curve of the task is diminished, and ultimately the client's performance is optimized. Clients with athetosis can especially benefit from the guided movement that the weight machines offer. Free weights, although more functional, may pose a safety threat to all but the most experienced client.

Using a metronome or other timing system to ensure slow, controlled movements will help optimize the client's performance. Slow, controlled movements will facilitate coordination of movement and lessen the impact of spasticity.

Another consideration when testing for muscular strength and endurance is the use of large, nonslip hand grips. This adaptation helps those clients with weak and/or dysfunctional handgrip. The clinician may also consider the use of gloves, tension wraps, or other hand-strapping systems to augment the client's grip.

When testing participants with CP, it is not uncommon for the participant to report short-term increases in spasticity, athetosis, and/or incoordination (76, 77). After the testing session, provide clients with plenty of time to recover, and be prepared to assist the client if his or her function has been significantly impaired. Clients often express that one of the most profound changes that they observe when performing a regular exercise program is a decrease in their long-term neurological symptoms (63). When documenting the testing session, be sure to record this and other behavioral observations such as changes in gait pattern and function/independence.

Regardless of the exercise mode and test protocol used when testing a participant with CP, provide adequate practice and make the necessary adaptations to the equipment to help ensure a successful testing session. At the very least, the clinician must provide clients with an adequate period of time to familiarize themselves with the equipment and testing protocol. This learning period may be substantially longer than the time needed for the able-bodied population due to differences in cognitive ability, previous experience, and the amount of spasticity/athetosis and incoordination.

EXERCISE PRESCRIPTION AND PROGRAMMING

Although limited, the literature available has clearly documented the positive adaptations of people with CP to both muscular strength and cardiovascular exercise programs (20, 63, 67, 78). The literature has also demonstrated the overall low levels of physical fitness of this population and their extremely high risk for secondary chronic disease (63, 78–80). These low levels of physical fitness also relate to perceptions of poor quality of life, difficulties with activities of daily living, and limited abilities to gain and retain employment.

Two valuable resources for information regarding the prescription of exercise are *ACSM's Exercise Management for Persons with Chronic Diseases and Disabilities* (65) and *ACSM's Resource Manual for Guidelines for Exercise Testing and Prescription* (64). These resources will help guide the clinician when developing an individual's exercise program. For each client, the specific exercise modes, frequency, intensity, duration, and progressions are completely individual and will require the clinician to be observant and request feedback from the client on a regular basis. As discussed in the Exercise Testing section, a comprehensive initial evaluation will help identify the needs/goals of clients, their activity preferences, specific precautions, and potential barriers to the exercise program. This section also addressed the considerations for modification of equipment and its setup.

In general, the exercise program should be simple and easy to follow. Initially, it is better to underestimate the capabilities to the client. The clinician must remember that the exercise program is just one component of the client's day and that, if they are unable to complete their daily activities because of an exercise program that was too demanding, they might discontinue their participation in the program.

The detrained ambulatory client will be used as an example of an initial exercise program. This initial exercise program may consist of 10–15 minutes on the treadmill or cycle ergometer at a self-selected pace. *ACSM's Guidelines* (64, 65) suggest that the activity should be at a conversational pace (50–65% of the maximal age-predicted heart rate) and that the desired health benefits may be gained by continuous and/or discontinuous exercise. Because many ambulatory clients with CP have limited dorsiflexion due to spasticity of the plantar flexors, it is best to keep the inclination of the treadmill relatively flat. Following their cardiovascular exercise, clients should do a few generalized stretches (3–5 repetitions for 15–20 seconds each) for the upper and lower extremities. Due to potential balance and coordination problems, clients should be advised to stretch in a seated or supine position. Typically, 1–2 sets of 10–12 repetitions are sufficient for each of the strength training exercises. To help the client's technique and to maximize the functional nature of strength exercises, an emphasis is placed on slow, controlled eccentric phase (count of two concentrically and a count of four eccentrically) (64). As suggested in the Exercise Testing section, the clinician's first choice would be motion-controlled strength training equipment. Initial strength exercises could include the following: chest press, seated row, lat pull-down, seated leg press, seated leg curl, and abdominals. Progression of these exercises and the addition of new exercises would be at the discretion of the clinician and the desire of the client. Another consideration when trying to determine the appropriate resistance for a given strengthening exercise is whether or not the antagonistic muscle presents with increased muscle tone. If this is the case, then the working muscle must not only overcome the resistance provided by the exercise, but also the resistance to movement being created by the spastic antagonist. To minimize this effect, ensure that the client is well supported and the exercise is being performed in a relatively slow controlled manner.

In general, the clinician must be aware that spastic muscles respond best to slow, controlled movements. Therefore, stretching is best performed once the client has completed a warm-up and is in a stable, safe position. Many people with CP present with altered and/or non-functional movement patterns. These movement patterns have developed because of the neurological involvement of the condition or due to the client developing substitution strategies. When using strapping, avoid direct contact with the skin and watch for reddened areas. Since CP is a condition that must be addressed across the life span, the clinician must take into account the client's chronological age; the activities should be age-appropriate and related to the client's needs and goals. In addition, the authors have found that these clients often have limited opportunities for social engagement; therefore, group-oriented programs that facilitate social interaction have proven to help maintain adherence to the program. The authors have also found that frequent positive feedback and routine supervision can help maintain adherence.

EDUCATION AND COUNSELING

Clinicians can educate people with CP by developing a rapport with each client and facilitating adherence to a program. The congenital nature of CP results in a population that often has a long history of contact with the medical and allied health professions. They may also have lived very sheltered, protected lives. For many, instead of a childhood of play-related recreation and sport, their experience with exercise is one of regimented stretching, positioning, and rehabilitation. This scenario has dramatically changed with the advent of early intervention programs and the IDEA legislation (67). However, the adult population with which the clinician may work may have a very jaded and negative opinion of exercise and health professionals, hence the need for client education and participant-driven, goal-oriented programming. The participant may need to be educated in areas such as exercise as it related to prevention of secondary chronic disease, the effects of exercise on depression, exercise as a component of weight management, and the ways in which exercise may facilitate improvements in ADL and quality of life. Table 2.11 summarizes some of the primary reasons why a person with CP might be motivated to exercise. Due to communication disorders, this information may have to be provided in a variety of formats, repeated numerous times, as well as including the participants in an appropriate support network. The role of education must also include the other health professionals involved with the client.

The primary educational objective of the clinician is to educate the participant about the benefits of a lifelong health-oriented exercise program. However, given an appropriate client, the clinician could also present information regarding the recreational and sporting opportunities that are available to the individual with CP. Besides the obvious easily integrated recreational activities of walking, cycling, and swimming, numerous sporting opportunities are available to the person with CP. Clinicians should familiarize themselves with the variety of local, regional, statewide, national, and international organizations that provide sporting opportunities for people with CP. DePauw and Gavron (66) is an excellent resource that provides an overview of the variety of options and the appropriate contact organizations. Rehabilitation centers, school districts, community fitness facilities, and city parks and recreation departments are also potential sources for information regarding recreation and sporting opportunities for people with disabilities.

A variety of barriers, including communication, physical limitations, medications, and limited prior exposure to participating in an exercise program, have already been presented in the earlier sections of this chapter. Common barriers to exercise in the general population are also addressed in the *ACSM's Resource Manual for Guidelines for Exercise Testing and Prescription* (65). However, other barriers may exist for those with CP as well as for anyone with a physical disability. Social and environmental isolation, embarrassment to be in public, difficulty with accessing and using public transportation, unsupportive caregivers, and financial considerations must all be taken into consideration when working with participants with CP. Do not underestimate the importance of attendance. Just showing up for the initial evaluation may be a significant step for your client. Take advantage of this opportunity to use your knowledge, experience, and creativity to encourage and motivate the participant.

Table 2.11. Primary Benefits of an Exercise Program for People with Cerebral Palsy (20, 87)

1	Risk reduction for secondary chronic diseases
2	Maintain and/or improve bone health
3	Maintain and/or improve muscular strength
4	Maintain and/or improve cardiovascular fitness
5	Maintain and/or improve flexibility and mobility
6	Maintain and/or improve balance and coordination
7	May facilitate a decrease in spasticity/athetosis
8	Facilitate weight management
9	Reduce anxiety and stress
10	Provide a sense of well-being
11	Increased participation in individual pursuits and community engagement

References

1. Little Club. Memorandum on terminology and classification of 'cerebral palsy.' Cereb Palsy Bull 1959;1:27–35.
2. Mutch L, Alberman E, Hagberg B, et al. Cerebral palsy epidemiology: where are we now and where are we going? Dev Med Child Neurol 1992;34:574–551.
3. Albright AL. Spasticity and movement disorders in cerebral palsy. J Child Neurol 1996;11(Suppl 1):S1–S4.
4. Nelson KB, Ellenberg JH. Children who "outgrew" cerebral palsy. Pediatrics 1982;69:529–536.
5. Arvidsson J, Hagberg B. Delayed onset dyskinetic 'cerebral palsy': a late effect of perinatal asphyxia? Acta Pediatr Scand 1990;79:1121–1123.
6. Lesny I. The development of athetosis. Dev Med Child Neurol 1968;10:441–446.
7. Murphy CC, Yeargin-Allsopp M, Decoufle P, et al. Prevalence of cerebral palsy among ten year old children in metropolitan Atlanta, 1985 through 1987. J Pediatr 1993;123: S13–S19.
8. Arens LJ, Molteno CD. A comparative study of postnatally-acquired cerebral palsy in Cape Town. Dev Med Child Neurol 1989;31:246–254.
9. Al-Rajah S, Bademosi O, Awada A, et al. Cerebral palsy in Saudi Arabia: a case-control study of risk factors. Dev Med Child Neurol 1991;33:1048–1052.
10. Sinha G, Corry P, Subesinghe D, et al. Prevalence and type of cerebral palsy in a British ethnic community: the role of consanguinity. Dev Med Child Neurol 1997;39:259–262.
11. DeLuca PA. The musculoskeletal management of children with cerebral palsy. Pediatr Clin North Amer 1996;43(5): 1135–1150.

12. Stanley F, Blair E, Alberman E. Cerebral Palsies: Epidemiology and Causal Pathways. Clinics in Developmental Medicine. London: Mac Keith Press, 1999:51.
13. Saito N, Ebara S, Ohotsuka K, et al. Natural history of scoliosis in spastic cerebral palsy. Lancet 1998;351:1687–1692.
14. Del Giudice E, Staiano A, Capano G, et al. Gastrointestinal manifestations in children with cerebral palsy. Brain Dev 1999;21:307–311.
15. Bandini LG, Schoeller DA, Fukagawa NK, et al. Body composition and energy expenditure in adolescents with cerebral palsy or myelodysplasia. Pediatr Res 1991;29:70–77.
16. van den Berg-Emons RJ, van Baak MA, Speth L, et al. Physical training of school children with spastic cerebral palsy: effects on daily activity, fat mass and fitness. Int J Rehab 1998; 21:179–194.
17. Damiano DL, Kelly LE, Vaughn CL. Effects of quadriceps femoris muscle strengthening on crouch gait in children with spastic cerebral palsy. Phys Ther 1995;75:658–671.
18. Bar-Or O, Inbar O, Spira R. Physiological effects of a sports rehabilitation program on cerebral palsied and post-poliomyelitic adolescents. Med Sci Sports Exerc 1976;8: 157–161.
19. Hutzler Y, Chacham A, Bergman U, et al. Effects of a movement and swimming program on vital capacity and water orientation skills of children with cerebral palsy. Dev Med Child Neurol 1998;40:176–181.
20. Ferrara M, Laskin J. Cerebral palsy. In: ACSM's Exercise Management for Persons with Chronic Diseases and Disabilities. Champaign, IL: Human Kinetics, 1997: 206–211.
21. Bowen TR, Lennon N, Castagno P, et al. Variability of energy-consumption measures in children with cerebral palsy. J Pediatr Orthop 1998;18:738–742.
22. Pranzatelli MR. Oral pharmacotherapy for the movement disorders of cerebral palsy. J Child Neurol 1996;11(Suppl 1):S13–S22.
23. Albright AL. Intrathecal baclofen in cerebral palsy movement disorders. J Child Neurol 1996;11(Suppl 1):S29–S35.
24. Penn RD, Kroin JS. Intrathecal baclofen alleviates spinal cord spasticity. Lancet 1984;1:1078.
25. Penn RD, Savoy SM, Corcos D, et al. Intrathecal baclofen for severe spinal spasticity. N Engl J Med 1989;320:1517–1521.
26. Bodensteiner JB. The management of cerebral palsy: subjectivity and conundrum. J Child Neurol 1996;11(2): 75–76.
27. Almeida GL, Campbell SK, Girolami GL, et al. Multidimensional assessment of motor function in a child with cerebral palsy following intrathecal administration of baclofen. Phys Ther 1997;77(7):751–764.
28. Gerszten PC, Albright AL, Johnstone GF. Intrathecal baclofen infusion and subsequent orthopedic surgery in patients with spastic cerebral palsy. J Neurosurg 1998;88:1009–1013.
29. Albright AL, Shultz BL. Plasma baclofen levels in children receiving continuous intrathecal baclofen infusion. J Child Neurol 1999;14:408–409.
30. Albright AL. Baclofen in the treatment of cerebral palsy. J Child Neurol 1996;11:77–83.
31. Koman LA, Mooney JF, and Smith BP. Neuromuscular blockade in the management of cerebral palsy. J Child Neurol 1996;11(Suppl 1):S23–S28.
32. Gordon N. The role of botulinus toxin type A in treatment—with special reference to children. Brain Dev 1999;21:147–151.
33. Gouch JL, Sandell TV. Botulinum toxin for spasticity and athetosis in children with cerebral palsy. Arch Phys Med Rehabil 1996;77:508–511.
34. Carr LJ, Cosgrove AP, Gringras P, et al. Position paper on the use of botulinum toxin in cerebral palsy. Arch Dis Child 1998;79:271–73.
35. Massin M, Allington N. Role of exercise testing in the functional assessment of cerebral palsy children after botulinum A toxin injection. J Pediatr Orthop 1999;19:362–365.
36. Forssberg H, Tedroff KB. Botulinum toxin treatment in cerebral palsy: intervention with poor evaluation? Dev Med Child Neurol 1997;39:635–640.
37. Davis DW. Review of cerebral palsy, part II: identification and intervention. 1997;16(4):19–25.
38. Prechtl HFR. State of the art of a new functional assessment of the young nervous system. An early predictor of cerebral palsy. Early Hum Dev 1997;50:1–11.
39. Morgan AM, Aldag JC. Early identification of cerebral palsy using a profile of abnormal motor patterns. Pediatrics 1996;98:692–697.
40. Campbell SK. Quantifying the effects of interventions for movement disorders resulting from cerebral palsy. J Child Neurol 1996;11(Suppl 1):S61–S70.
41. Barry MJ. Physical therapy interventions for patients with movement disorders from cerebral palsy. J Child Neurol 1996;11(Suppl 1):S51–S60.
42. Law M, Pollock N, Rosenbaum P, et al. A comparison of intensive neurodevelopmental therapy plus casting and a regular occupational therapy program for children with cerebral palsy. Dev Med Child Neurol 1997;39:664–670.
43. Weindling AM, Hallam P, Gregg J, et al. A randomized controlled trial of early physiotherapy for high-risk infants. Acta Paediatr 1996;85:1107–1111.
44. Bower E, McLellan DL, Arney J, et al. A randomised controlled trial of different intensities of physiotherapy and different goal-setting procedures in 44 children with cerebral palsy. Dev Med Child Neurol 1996;38:226–237.
45. Chad KE, Bailey DA, McKay HA, et al. The effect of a weight-bearing physical activity program on bone mineral content and estimated volumetric density in children with spastic cerebral palsy. J Pediatr 1999;135:115–117.
46. Carlson WE, Vaughan CL, Damiano DL, et al. Orthotic management of gait in spastic diplegia. Am J Phys Med Rehabil 1997;76:219–225.
47. Mattsson E, Andersson C. Oxygen cost, walking speed, and perceived exertion in children with cerebral palsy when walking with anterior and posterior walkers. Dev Med Child Neurol 1997;39:671–676.
48. Damiano DL, Abel MF. Functional outcomes of strength training in spastic cerebral palsy. Arch Phys Med Rehabil 1998;79:119–25.
49. Morton R. New surgical interventions for cerebral palsy and the place of gait analysis. Dev Med Child Neurol 1999;41: 424–428.
50. Wright FV, Sheil EM, Drake JM, et al. Evaluation of selective dorsal rhizotomy for the reduction of spasticity in cerebral palsy: a randomized controlled trial. Dev Med Child Neurol 1998;40:239–247.
51. Steinbok P, Reiner AM, Beauchamp R, et al. A randomized clinical trial to compare selective posterior rhizotomy plus physiotherapy with physiotherapy alone in children with

spastic diplegic cerebral palsy. Dev Med Child Neurol 1997; 39: 178–184.
52. Steinbok P, Reiner A, Kestle JRW. Therapeutic electri-cal stimulation following selective posterior rhizotomy in children with spastic diplegic cerebral palsy: a randomized clinical trial. Dev Med Child Neurol 1997;39: 515–520.
53. Subramanian N, Vaughan CL, Peter JC, et al. Gait before and 10 years after rhizotomy in children with cerebral palsy spasticity. J Neurosurg 1998;88:1014–1019.
54. Abbott R. Sensory rhizotomy for the treatment of childhood spasticity. J Child Neurol 1996;11(Suppl 1):S36–S42.
55. Engsberg JR, Olree KS, Ross SA, et al. Spasticity and strength changes as a function of selective dorsal rhizotomy. J Neurosurg 1998;88:1020–1026.
56. Engsberg JR, Ross SA, Park TS. Changes in ankle spasticity and strength following selective dorsal rhizotomy and physical therapy for spastic cerebral palsy. J Neurosurg 1999;91: 727–732.
57. Buckon CE, Thomas SS, Aiona MD, et al. Assessment of upper extremity function in children with spastic diplegia before and after selective dorsal rhizotomy. Dev Med Child Neurol 1995;38:967–975.
58. DeSalles AAF. Role of stereotaxis in the treatment of cerebral palsy. J Child Neurol 1996;11(Suppl 1):S43–S50.
59. Speelman JD, van Manen J. Cerebral palsy and stereotatic neurosurgery: long term results. J Neurol Neurosurg Psychiatry 1989;52:23–30.
60. Van Heest AE, House JH, Cariello C. Upper extremity surgical treatment of cerebral palsy. J Hand Surg 1999;24A: 323–330.
61. Renshaw TS, Green NE, Griffin PP, et al. Cerebral palsy: orthopaedic management. Instruct Course Lect 1996;45:475–490.
62. House JH, Gwaathmey FW, Fidler MO. A dynamic approach to the thumb-in-palm deformity in cerebral palsy. J Bone Joint Surg 1981;63A:216–225.
63. Laskin JJ. Physiological adaptations to concurrent muscular strength and aerobic endurance training in functionally active people with a physical disability. Unpublished doctoral dissertation, University of Alberta, 2001.
64. American College of Sports Medicine. ACSM's Guidelines for Exercise Testing and Prescription. 6th ed. Baltimore, Lippincott Williams & Wilkins, 2000.
65. American College of Sports Medicine. ACSM's Resource Manual for Guidelines for Exercise Testing and Prescription. 3rd ed. Philadelphia, PA: Lippincott Williams & Wilkins, 1998.
66. DePauw KP, Gavron SJ. Disability and Sport. Champaign, IL: Human Kinetics, 1995, 122.
67. DePauw KP, Gavron SJ. Disability and Sport. Champaign, IL: Human Kinetics, 1995.
68. Bhambhani YN, Holland LJ, Steaward RD. Maximal aerobic power in cerebral palsied wheelchair athletes: validity and reliability. Arch Phys Med Rehabil 1992;73(3): 246–252.
69. Bhambhani YN, Holland LJ, Steaward RD. Anaerobic threshold in wheelchair athletes with cerebral palsy: validity and reliability. Arch Phys Med Rehabil 1993;74(3): 305-311.
70. Bohannon RW. Is the measurement of muscle strength appropriate in patients with brain lesions? A special communication. Phys Ther 1989;69(3):225–229.
71. Bohannon RW, Walsh S. Nature, reliability, and predictive value of muscle performance measures in patients with hemiparesis following stroke. Arch Phys Med Rehabil 1992; 73: 721–725.
72. Bohannon RW. Relative decreases in knee extension torque with increased knee extension velocities in stroke patients with hemiparesis. Phys Ther 1987;67(7): 1218–1220.
73. Bohannon RW, Larkin PA, Smith MB, et al. Relationship between static muscle strength deficits and spasticity in stroke patients with hemiparesis. Phys Ther 1987;67(7): 1068–1071.
74. Bohannon RW, Smith MB. Assessment of strength deficits in eight paretic upper extremity muscle groups of stroke patients with hemiplegia. Phys Ther 1987;67(4): 522–525.
75. Bohannon RW, Smith MB. Upper extremity strength deficits in hemiplegic stroke patients: relationship between admission and discharge assessment and time since onset. Arch Phys Med Rehabil 1987;68: 155–157.
76. Bennett SE, Karnes JL. Neurological Disabilities: Assessment and Treatment. Philadelphia, PA: Lippincott Williams & Wilkins, 1998.
77. Tecklin JS. Pediatric Physical Therapy. 3rd ed. Philadelphia: Lippincott Williams & Wilkins, 1999.
78. Fernandez JE, Pitetti KH, Betzen MT. Physiological capacities of individuals with cerebral palsy. Hum Factors 1990; 32(4): 457–466.
79. Parker DF, Carriere L, Hebestreit H, et al. Muscle performance and gross motor function of children with spastic cerebral palsy. Dev Med Child Neurol 1993;35(1): 17–23.
80. Parker DF, Carriere L, Hebestreit H, et al. Anaerobic endurance and peak muscle power in children with spastic cerebral palsy. Am J Dis Child 1992;146(9):1069–1073.

CHAPTER 3

Multiple Sclerosis

Janet A. Mulcare and Jack H. Petajan

EPIDEMIOLOGY

Multiple sclerosis (MS) is a very common disease with a prevalence ranging from 50–100/100,000 people (1, 2). Studies of migrating populations have indicated that where one resides in relation to the equator before the age of 15 appears to determine the likelihood of developing MS (3). The incidence of MS is nearly 3/100,000 in temperate zones, and below 1/100,000 in tropical areas (4). Women are more affected than men in a ratio of approximately 2:1 (4). The initiation of MS, either propensity for the disease or the disease itself, begins in childhood. A variety of infections, including exanthemata such as measles and upper-respiratory infections, may be etiological (4). There is a threefold increase in the incidence of exacerbations of MS following an upper-respiratory infection(5, 6). Exacerbation rate is reduced during pregnancy and is increased threefold in the postpartum period up to approximately 3 months (7). MS usually makes its onset between the ages of 20 and 40. However, it is often possible to obtain a history of transient neurological deficits, such as numbness of an extremity, weakness, blurring of vision, and diplopia, in childhood or adolescence prior to the development of more persistent neurological deficits, which lead to the definitive diagnosis (8, 9). It is possible that viruses causing upper-respiratory infections may be responsible for sensitizing the brain to subsequent autoimmune insult, producing inflammatory demyelination.

Patients who have a definite diagnosis of MS are more likely to have a variety of other illnesses of an autoimmune nature such as systemic lupus erythematosus, rheumatoid arthritis, polymyositis, myasthenia gravis, etc. (10). If a first-degree relative has MS, there is a 12–20-fold increase in the likelihood of having MS (11). In monozygotic twins there is a 33% increase in the incidence of MS, whereas in dizygotic twins the incidence is about 8%, or that found in the normal population (12, 13).

Pathophysiology

MS is a disease of the central nervous system in which there are multiple areas of inflammatory demyelination with a predilection for distribution around the ventricles and vascular spaces. Multiple mechanisms are involved in producing damage to central nervous system myelin, as well as axons (14–18). An immune reaction to myelin (myelin basic protein, or MBP) and myelin oligodendrocyte glycoprotein (MOG) occurs. Activated T cells attach to the endothelium of capillaries within the brain and migrate into the brain parenchyma, where activated macrophages attack and digest myelin. A number of cytokines, including tumor necrosis factor (TNR), and interferons, as well as IgG, are involved in the immune attack. B cells produce IgG directed at MOG. There is increased production of IgG and an increased prevalence of specific IgG moieties, some of which represent antiviral IgG. Antigenic specificity of most of the IgG is unknown, "nonsense antibody" (19–22). Recent studies of total brain NAA/creatine ratios have provided evidence for loss of axons, as well as evidence for membrane damage (demyelination) as an increase in choline/creatine ratio (23).

Lesions representing focal areas of inflammatory demyelination can be present in the cerebral hemispheres, brain stem, and spinal cord. For a definite diagnosis to be established, two or more areas of demyelination (white matter lesions) must be established. Furthermore, there must be two or more remissions of neurological deficits. This must be accompanied by paraclinical evidence of disease seen as the presence of MRI T2 weighted lesions in white matter, as well as evidence of increased IgG synthesis with positive oligoclonal bands (OCBs) in the spinal fluid (26). OCBs result from a reduction in the number of different migrating species of IgG obtained on electrophoresis. Other conditions, such as bacterial or viral infection, autoimmune diseases such as systemic lupus erythematosus and vasculitis, may also produce increased IgG or oligoclonal bands.

Clinical Features

Long-fiber pathways or tracts are more likely to be involved in the process of demyelination. For example, it is very common for patients to have posterior column signs, such as loss of vibration sense, and pyramidal signs early in the course of the disease when the disease is virtually asymptomatic. A common feature of MS is profound fatigue often with a diurnal pattern. This is characterized as malaise or a lack of motivation for the performance of any physical activity, as well as motor fatigue, which develops with continued physical activity (24, 25). Another extremely interesting phenomenon is a marked decrease in heat tolerance with the development of neurological signs when the individual is passively heated or during physical exercise (26). Blurring of vision in one or both eyes may occur with physical exercise (Uhthoff's phenomenon). Demyelination reduces the efficiency of axonal conduction so that less current is available for depolarization at nodes of Ranvier. With demyelination and reduction of current density, the safety factor for conduction can be exceeded. In an animal model, increasing brain temperature by less than 0.5°C may be sufficient to produce conduction block (18).

Common signs and symptoms of MS include painful blurring or loss of vision in one eye with evidence of deafferentation (the Marcus-Gunn pupil) occurring as the result of optic neuritis. Eventually, there will be marked loss of visual acuity. Most patients will begin to recover vision within 6 weeks. Recovery is more rapid, pain is reduced, and MS less likely to occur over time when treated with methylprednisolone (28, 29). Various visual complaints include blurring of vision with rapid eye movements, difficulty with visual fixation, diplopia (double vision), decreased night vision, and an inability to ascertain contrast. The patient may complain of facial numbness or pain typical of trigeminal neuralgia. Numbness of the tongue and loss of taste may occur. Patients rarely complain of difficulty swallowing, though the prevalence of dysphagia is higher than commonly appreciated. Often, weakness and loss of coordination affect first the lower extremities and then the upper extremities, sometimes in a typical hemiparetic pattern. Spastic paraparesis along with ataxia is a common combination referred to as the "spastic ataxic syndrome." Early in the illness, neurogenic bladder manifests itself as an inability of the bladder to hold an adequate volume of urine. Consequently, urinary frequency and urgency exceeds six times per day, often with incontinence. Nocturia is common. There is a high incidence of urinary tract infections. Greater than 50% of early diagnosed patients complain of urinary urgency and frequency (30–34).

Sexual dysfunction is common with loss of sensation, lack of the ability to have an orgasm, and impotence being very common (35, 36). Adynamia of the colon is also common with most patients experiencing severe constipation. Some patients require partial colectomy secondary to obstipation (intractable constipation). In view of the prevalence of bowel complaints, development of effective therapies is essential. A variety of skin sensations and loss of sensation occur, most commonly vibration sense loss in both feet with position sense preserved until vibration sense loss is severe. Dysesthesias, characterized as abnormal sensations produced by touching or stroking the skin, are also very common. These sensory disturbances do not occur in a distribution characteristic of involvement of a peripheral nerve. Abnormal sensation over the trunk, particularly a band-like sensation around the abdomen or chest, is also characteristic. Fortunately, allodynia is uncommon and most patients do not complain of severe pain in the extremities, but this does sometimes occur.

Cognitive difficulties develop along with cranial, motor, and sensory symptoms (37–42). The patient may complain of an inability to function in the workplace when he or she is required to monitor two or more activities at the same time. Attentiveness is decreased so that the patient may be unable to register information accurately in memory. Emotional lability is also common in association with subfrontal demyelination, which produces a pseudobulbar palsy. Studies have shown that cognitive deficit is greater in individuals with prominent signs of pseudobulbar palsy or excessive emotional lability.

There are several different clinical courses for MS. The disease usually begins as a relapsing-remitting (RR) form of disease, with exacerbations occurring two to three times per year at the beginning of the disease. Gradually, the exacerbations decrease to less than one per year approximately beyond year five (8, 9). As the disease progresses, neurological deficits accumulate. Finally, the disease can be characterized as secondary progressive or progressive relapsing disease with periods of accelerated progression or exacerbation with the development of new deficits superimposed on those that are preexisting. Finally, the illness may be primary progressive (the Marburg variant). In this form of MS, the disease does not manifest any ability to remit, but progresses immediately from the outset. This form of MS has been characterized as being more benign than the usual expression of the illness but in some cases, particularly when male patients are involved, the illness may be extremely severe, as well as being progressive.

Medical and Surgical Treatments

Exacerbations of MS are usually treated with high-dose adrenocortical steroids customarily administered intravenously at a dose of 1000 mg per day for 3 to 5 days, followed by a prednisone taper over approximately 6 weeks (28, 29). It has been demonstrated that patients with monosymptomatic MS initially treated with methylprednisolone defer the development of more typical MS when they are treated with methylprednisolone (29). Development of two or more deficits, marked weakness and incoordination, and/or loss of sensation in both lower extremities are indications for treatment with adrenocortical steroids.

Prophylactic treatments include interferon beta-1a and -1b, which reduce lymphocytic invasion of the brain, induce a suppressor immune reaction provide an antiviral action, reduce the number of exacerbations over time, and preserve brain mass (43–45). Glatiramer (copolymer I or Copaxone), a peptide consisting of four amino acids—glycine, alanine, lycine, and tyrosine—act by inducing immune tolerance to myelin basic protein (46). This is also effective in reducing the number of exacerbations and preserving brain mass over time. Chemotherapy such as methotrexate and Novantrone (mitoxantrone) are also recommended for patients with chronic progressive disease (47, 48).

Symptomatic management includes the treatment of neurogenic bladder with anticholinergic medications such as oxybutynin for urinary frequency and urgency. Regimens for treating obstipation include psyllium preparations, laxatives, suppositories, and physical activity. Spasticity, particularly flexor and extensor spasms, is treated with either GABA-b-ergic compound (baclofen), which increases spinal inhibition, or Tizanidine, which increases supra-spinal inhibitors of spinal reflex activities (49, 50).

Diagnostic Techniques

If the patient's history is highly suggestive of MS, then an MRI of the brain often combined with imaging of the spinal cord are obtained. Sometimes in order to establish the existence of another lesion characteristic of MS, evoked potentials of the visual systems (visual evoked potential, VEP), the brain stem, or somatosensory (SSEP) systems are obtained. In MS, there is a marked delay in conduction of the action potential. Evaluation of the spinal fluid during an exacerbation early in the disease may reveal a mild pleocytosis of usually less than 100 cells consisting predominantly of lymphocytes and a mild elevation of protein, usually less than 100 mg %. An increase in IgG synthesis and decreased variability of the different moieties of IgG is also characteristic. In the first few months of the disease, spinal fluid findings may be normal, but repeat examination a year or so later may reveal increased IgG synthesis and OCBs. Early definitive diagnosis is important so that prophylactic treatment can be instituted to prevent injury to the central nervous system (51).

CLINICAL EXERCISE PHYSIOLOGY

Acute Exercise Response

Most studies have shown that persons with MS will not respond to an acute bout of exercise as would the average age- and gender-matched, nondisabled adult without MS (52–54). Furthermore, variability in the type and magnitude of symptoms manifested with this disease often results in a wide range of responses to exercise (55). Despite the variability, one common effect of acute exercise in individuals with MS is an overwhelming sense of fatigue during postexercise recovery.

To understand basic physiological responses to an acute bout of exercise, it is helpful to use the two directions commonly taken in the literature: (1) as it relates to muscle performance (i.e., strength and endurance) and (2) cardiovascular responses (i.e., heart rate, blood pressure, oxygen utilization).

Muscle Performance

In the absence of documented spasticity or use of antispasmodic drugs, muscle endurance for persons with MS during a sustained isometric contraction at 30% of maximal voluntary contraction (MVC) is similar to that of a nondisabled, healthy adult (57). Although these findings are in direct conflict with earlier studies of acute muscle response (58–61), it is important to consider that in none of the earlier studies was the presence of spasticity and/or the use of antispasmodic drugs controlled in the design. Engardt and colleagues (62) have shown that in the presence of an upper motor neuron lesion, antagonist muscles are also activated during concentric contraction of an agonist. This would support Chen et al. (60) and Ponichtera et al. (58) in their hypothesis that spasticity was one of the factors that resulted in a reduction in agonist force production of their MS subjects. In contrast, antagonists are not stretched during the eccentric contraction, while the agonist receives additional stretch to facilitate its contraction (75, 76). This supports the results from Ponichtera and associates (65) who hypothesized that, while spasticity in 44% of their sample may have contributed to a significantly lower force production during concentric knee extension, force production during eccentric knee extension for the MS patients was normal. Therefore, the common MS symptom of spasticity may be one factor that can reduce concentric muscle performance in this population. There is ample evidence from other patient populations with spasticity that these individuals would have difficulty producing force, as well as experience trouble in controlling forces that modulate movement speed and direction (66–68).

However, to believe that spasticity is the sole contributor to differences in isometric muscle endurance observed between MS and non-MS persons would be naïve. Other contributors to observed differences have been attributed to conduction block of demyelinated fibers (69–71), reduced muscle metabolic responses to voluntary exercise (72–74), muscle weakness related to fiber atrophy of exercising muscles (72), as well as sensory deficits.

Maximal muscle force during sustained dynamic exercise has also been shown to be consistently lower for persons with MS. Commonly, this has been observed during tests of maximal aerobic power using leg cycling or combination leg/arm cycling protocols (54, 56, 75, 76). During maximal upright and recumbent leg cycling, patients with MS were able to exercise at loads that were 20–68% (54, 75, 76) less than matched controls. Performance during arm cranking and combined arm/leg cycling shows similar findings: 31% lower during arm cranking and 24%

lower during combined arm/leg cycling (54). Once again, the source of this reduced muscle strength during dynamic exercise is thought to be related to reduced muscle metabolic responses (73, 74), muscle weakness secondary to muscle fiber atrophy (72), and muscle weakness secondary to spasticity, sensory loss, and behavioral disuse.

Acute Cardiorespiratory Responses

Physiological responses to an acute bout of submaximal aerobic exercise appear to be normal for many persons with MS. Heart rate (HR), blood pressure (BP), and oxygen uptake ($\dot{V}O_2$) have been shown to increase in a linear fashion to increments in workload (52, 65, 75). This is also true of ventilatory responses such as respiratory rate and minute ventilation (52). Furthermore, these responses are consistent over a wide range of impairment levels. However, there is some evidence that HR response, while linear, may be blunted (i.e., less increase per absolute workload increment) in some persons with MS (52). However, this may not be true of all persons with MS. Use of the standard practice of calculating HR_{max} as 220 − age and subsequently establishing a target HR range between 60–70% of HR_{max} is a safe method for this population.

Maximal aerobic power ($\dot{V}O2_{max}$) varies greatly based on the degree of physical impairment and neurological symptoms present (64, 68). When compared with that of healthy adults, even minimally impaired MS clients will perform more poorly (i.e., lower $\dot{V}O_{2max}$), regardless of whether the test is performed using leg, arm, or combined arm/leg exercise (66). Comparison of $\dot{V}O_{2max}$ (mL/kg/min) of 20 minimally to moderately impaired sedentary persons with MS against normative fitness standards showed that 75% fell into the "low fitness" range, whereas 15% and 10% were "fair" and "average," respectively (88). In these same studies, HR_{max} at test termination has often not been at a level that would be termed "maximum," (i.e., 220 − age) (64, 66). The inability to reach a predicted HR_{max} before test termination is believed to be related to a need to terminate the exercise test due to local muscle fatigue rather than cardiovascular limitations. When queried using the Category-Ratio Rating of Perceived Exertion Scale (77), subjects consistently rated "peripheral" stress than "central" (i.e., cardiovascular) both during submaximal and maximal levels of exercise (52, 78).

Aerobic exercise endurance (i.e., time to fatigue) also varies greatly among clients with MS. Furthermore, endurance time does not appear to be directly related to the level of physical impairment. At a moderate level of exercise (i.e., 50% $\dot{V}O_{2max}$) patients have been able to exercise for as little as 15 minutes to as long as 60 minutes (78). Again, the correlational analysis found no relationship between endurance time and the level of physical impairment.

Chronic Exercise Response

There is very little research regarding the effects of training on muscle performance in persons with MS. However, from the available research, we can conclude that MS patients have the capacity to improve muscle strength following a supervised program of aerobic exercise training (56, 79). Petajan and colleagues reported a mean improvement of 17% in upper-extremity isometric strength (sum of four different muscle groups) and an 11% improvement in lower-extremity isometric strength (sum of five different muscle groups) in a sample of 21 MS subjects (79). Ponichtera-Mulcare et al. observed a 29% improvement in power output during leg cycling following 24 weeks of supervised aerobic exercise training (80). Certainly, these findings are very encouraging, but more research is needed to completely understand the benefits of training on muscle performance in this population.

A supervised program of aerobic exercise for as little as 15 weeks can improve aerobic fitness level (i.e., $\dot{V}O_{2max}$) in some persons with MS. Petajan and colleagues reported a 22% increase in $\dot{V}O_{2max}$ and a 48% increase in physical work capacity (79). Ponichtera-Mulcare and colleagues (68) found similar improvements in persons with equivalent impairment level (+19%), but less dramatic for those more severely impaired (+7%) after a 24-week supervised program (80). This raises an important issue regarding the development of realistic expectations based on the baseline impairment level of the individual. Subtle neurological changes may not be observable to the clinician. However, small unnoticeable changes may affect exercise training outcomes. It is important to carefully monitor neurological changes by periodically interviewing the client regarding subjective impressions of their disease status. Consideration must also be given to the fact that training outcomes observed under strict supervision may not be similar outside the supervised, controlled program environment, as would be the case of a home exercise program.

Exercise/Fitness/Functional Testing

General principles of fitness testing as outlined by the American College of Sports Medicine (81) can be appropriately applied to many persons in this population. However, when evaluating fitness in the person with MS, it is important to consider special needs related to the specific symptoms experienced by the client.

Flexibility

Because many MS patients experience lower-extremity spasticity, flexibility may be restricted in the hip, knee, and ankle joints. Hip flexor, hamstring, and gastrocsoleus tightness is particularly problematic and should be evaluated in the sitting position (e.g., Sit-and-Reach Test). Use of this particular test will serve to eliminate any problem with balance during testing. Lateral trunk flexibility should also be evaluated from a sitting position or, if standing, the clinician may place his/her hands on the client's waist to prevent loss of balance.

Balance

To truly appreciate how balance deficits might affect the MS client's ability to perform exercise safely, balance should be evaluated under both static and dynamic conditions. A fairly short and easy battery of tests can be found using the Berg Balance Scale (82). This test is valid for neurological conditions such as MS and takes approximately 15 minutes to administer. The results of this test will provide a better understanding of the client's ability to exercise safely using standard equipment.

Aerobic Fitness

As previously noted, many persons with MS experience problems with balance. In addition, foot drop associated with dorsiflexor weakness can be present prior to exercise, or it may appear shortly after the onset of weight-bearing exercise. Therefore, for safety purposes, aerobic fitness is best evaluated using a bicycle ergometer. Even so, this mode of exercise testing can also present challenges. Ankle clonus (i.e., spasmodic alternation of contraction and relaxation of muscles) and sensory abnormalities (e.g., numbness, tingling, deficits in joint proprioception) can make it difficult for the client to keep his or her feet on the pedals. The use of standard toe clips and Velcro™-secured heel straps can reduce or eliminate this problem.

The general procedures for submaximal testing of cardiorespiratory endurance using a cycle ergometer published by the American College of Sports Medicine can be applied to this population; however, workloads suggested in standard tests such as the YMCA Cycle Ergometry Protocol (83) or the Astrand-Rhyming test may need to be reduced. Modification of these protocols can be accomplished simply by beginning with a warm-up phase of no-load pedaling, followed by a fixed rate pedaling at 50 W for 6 minutes (84) or by proceeding with increments of 0.25 kp at 50 rpm until the appropriate HR response is achieved (83). Of these two protocols, the latter may be more appropriate with extremely sedentary MS clients (male and female), who may have maximal workload capacities less than 50 W.

Muscular Strength and Endurance

The general procedures for measuring muscle strength and endurance suggested by the American College of Sports Medicine can be applied to this population. Again, to proceed safely, any reduction in joint range of motion, sensory loss (upper and lower extremity), coordination deficits, ataxia, and spasticity need to be considered prior to testing. Suggestions for activities and special considerations during testing, training, and counseling are summarized in Tables 3.1 and 3.2, respectively.

EDUCATION AND COUNSELING

Many people with disabilities (87) and persons with MS, in particular (88), *believe* that they do not possess the

Table 3.1. General Guidelines for Prescribing Physical Activity and Exercise Programming

Mode of Exercise/Activity	General Goals	Intensity/Frequency/Duration	Special Consideration
Physical Activity • Activities of Daily Living • Built-in Inconveniences • Leisure Activities and Hobbies	• Increase daily activity energy expenditure	• 30 minutes of accumulated physical activity each day on most days	• Strategies for energy conservation may be necessary.
Aerobic and Endurance Exercise • Cycling • Walking • Water aerobics • Chair exercise	• Increase cardiovascular function	• 60–75% HR_{peak} /50–65% $\dot{V}O_{2peak}$ • 3 sessions/week • 1 30-min session or 3 10-min sessions/day	• Air temperature should be kept cool; fans may be helpful; therapeutic swimming pool water temperature is too warm.

Strength Training
• Resistance training
  • Elastic bands
  • Free weight
  • Weight machines
  • Pulley weights
	• Increase general muscle strength
	• Improve muscle tone
	• Equalize agonist/antagonist strength
		• Perform on nonendurance training days.	• With any upper-extremity sensory deficit, free weights should not be used.
			• Exercises should be performed in a seated position when possible.

Flexibility (Stretching) • Passive range of motion (ROM) • Active ROM • Yoga • Tai Chi	• Increase joint range of motion • Counteract effects of spasticity • Improve balance	• Perform daily for short periods, preferably more than once per day if fatigue occurs.	• Should be performed from a seated or lying position.

Table 3.2. Special Considerations When Prescribing Physical Activity Exercise

Heat Sensitivity: There is ample research documenting the presence of heat sensitivity in most persons with MS. The exact mechanism of how either external (e.g., environmental) or internal (e.g., metabolic) heat affects these individuals remains unknown. However, the resulting sequelae can include any one or all of the following: general or severe fatigue, loss of balance, foot drop, visual changes (e.g., blurred vision), speech changes (e.g., slurred speech), and muscle weakness and/or paralysis. Sweating has also been shown as being abnormal in as much as 50% of the population (76). The absence of sweating may contribute to a perception of being overheated as capillary skin blood flow increases in an effort to dissipate heat generated from exercising muscles. As such, the perception of overheating coupled with heat-related fatigue may preempt the exercise session before the desired time. Use of fans, wet neck wraps, and spray bottles may help reduce the perception of overheating. Surface cooling has been shown to improve aerobic endurance slightly (85). Others have shown that precooling before exercise also has a beneficial effect on performance (86). Exercise is also recommended to occur early in the day. This is when circadian body temperature is at its lowest. Subjective reports from most individuals with MS indicate that there is a decline in energy level during the afternoon hours, with the occurrence of fatigue and other MS-related symptoms.

Bladder Dysfunction: Bladder dysfunction is an MS symptom that can indirectly affect exercise performance. Because of symptoms such as bladder urgency and exertional incontinence, MS clients may limit their daily intake of liquids. This is also a common practice observed during exercise. Recommendations for proper hydration prior to exercise and rehydration following should be addressed when working with this population.

Sensory Deficits: Subtle losses in tactile and proprioceptive sensation may make using some equipment difficult and even dangerous. Deficits may be reflected in an inability to grasp and control free weights, as well as to perceive muscle and joint position. Visual feedback by training in front of a mirror or performing rhythmic counting during repetitions can provide alternate forms of input to ensure proper performance. When possible, the use of machines such as the LifeCycle Series™ is recommended since it reduces the amount of control and coordination needed by the client and provides visual feedback regarding range of motion and force produced for each repetition.

Incoordination: Safety is also an issue for persons who have coordination deficits. The presence of spasticity, ataxia, and/or tremor may result in uncoordinated movement patterns in the affected extremities. Therefore, use of equipment that requires coordinated movement (i.e., free weights) is contraindicated. Use of synchronized arm/leg ergometers may improve exercise performance by allowing the arms to assist the less-coordinated legs.

Cognitive and Memory Deficits: Subtle cognitive changes and memory deficits may require a modified approach to instructing the MS client. This might include providing information in both written and diagrammatic format, and reminders of proper form, repetitions, and use of equipment. In addition, providing an easy form of recording exercises will eliminate the need for accurate recall.

Neurological Impairment Level: Depending on the level of neurological impairment, it may take longer for some persons with MS to experience notable improvements in muscle strength, endurance, and/or aerobic fitness. In more extensively impaired clients, this may be related to any or all of the following: the need to (1) begin with very low levels of resistance, (2) reduce the number of weekly sessions due to a protracted recovery time, and (3) disperse the daily exercise time into 2–3 smaller bouts.

knowledge and skills needed to exercise safely. Because of these beliefs, it is not surprising to find that preliminary evidence shows that persons with MS are less active than the average, nondisabled American (89). However, before one can counsel the person with MS regarding exercise and physical activity, it is important to understand the perceived barriers that may be present.

In nondisabled populations, the four major barriers to participation in an exercise program have been reported as financial cost, lack of energy, transportation, and not knowing where to exercise (90). Other barriers that have been cited include not having someone to exercise with, childcare responsibilities, and lack of confidence (91). These factors, some more than others (e.g., lack of energy, lack of confidence), are more than likely real issues for the person with MS also. Such barriers need to be overcome before we can facilitate successful participation in a program of regular exercise.

At the foundation, counseling should focus on the basic principles of training (i.e., frequency, intensity, duration, and mode). Special emphasis on how to modify each principle specific to the client's lifestyle and physical impairments is very important. Advice related to dealing with spasticity, tremor, incoordination, balance deficits, and general fatigue, when appropriate, will set a tone of "understanding" that will help to promote a level of confidence for these individuals. These issues have been outlined in the section "Special Considerations."

While evidence related to the efficacy of surface cooling for improving exercise performance is equivocal, previous research has shown that persons with MS perceive exercise to be less stressful when surface cooling is present (64, 88). As such, strategies to promote surface cooling may improve exercise tolerance and adherence. These include (1) selecting water exercise instead of land, (2) using a bicycle ergometer with a fan-style flywheel, (3) wearing a presoaked neck scarf, (4) ingesting ice chips prior to exercise, and (5) skin surface misting with cool water. Prehydration and drinking during exercise should also be discussed.

Providing information to the client regarding cost, accessibility, and scheduling of local exercise opportunities sponsored by community recreational facilities, senior citizen centers, universities, and hospital outreach programs can reduce or eliminate several other barriers. However, if the clients feel sufficiently confident in their general knowledge base, they may prefer to exercise at home. This will require the clinician to provide basic information regarding appropriate choices of home equipment, particularly as it relates to safety, cost, and ease of use.

Finally, an important key to successful counseling and education with the person with MS, or any other disability, is the building of confidence to practice self-advocacy. A candid and comprehensive discussion of basic exercise responses, training principles, modifications related to symptomatology, safety issues, and programming can provide a solid foundation for this to occur.

REFERENCES

1. Anderson DW, Ellenburg JH, Leventhal M, et al. Revised estimate of the prevalence of MS in the United States. Ann Neurol 1992;31:333–336.
2. Dean G. How many people in the world have MS? Neuroepidemiology 1994;13:1–7.
3. Rosati G. Descriptive epidemiology of MS in Europe in the 1980's: a critical overview. Ann Neurol 1994;36:5164–5174.
4. Weinshenker BG. Epidemiology of MS. Neurol Clin 1996; 14:291–308.
5. Sibley WA, Bamford CR, Clark K. Clinical viral infections and MS. Lancet 1985;1:1313–1315.
6. Panitch HS. Influence of infection on exacerbation of MS. Ann Neurol 1994;36:525–528.
7. Korn-Labetzki I, Khana E, Cooper G, et al. Activity of MS during pregnancy and puerperium. Ann Neurol 1984; 16:229–231.
8. Weinshenker BG, Rice GPA, Noseworthy JH, et al. The natural history of MS: a geographically based study. 3. Multivariate analysis of predictive factors and models of outcome. Brain 1991;114:1045–1056.
9. Kurtzke JF, Beebe GW, Nagler B, et al. Studies on the natural history of MS. VIII: Early prognostic features of the later course of the illness. J Chron Dis 1997; 30:819–830.
10. Wynn DR, Rodriguez M, O'Fallon M, et al. A reappraisal of the epidemiology of MS in Olmstead County, Minnesota. Neurology 1990;40:780–786.
11. Haegert DG, Marrosu MG. Genetic susceptibility to MS. Ann Neurol 1994;36:2S04–S210.
12. Mumford CJ, Wood NW, Kellar-Wood H, et al. The British Isles survey of MS in twins. Neurology 1994;44:11–15.
13. Sadovnick AD, Armstrong H, Rice GP, et al. A population-based study of MS in twins: update. Ann Neurol 1993; 33:281–285.
14. Prineas JW. Pathology of MS. In: Cook SD, ed. Handbook of MS. New York: Marcel Dekker. 1990:187–218.
15. Sobel RA. The pathology of MS. Neurol Clin 1995;13:1–21.
16. Giovannoni G, Hartung HP. The immunopathogenesis of MS and Guillain-Barre syndrome. Curr Opin Neurol 1996; 9:165–177.
17. Waxman SG. Pathophysiology of MS. In: Coo DS, ed. Handbook of MS. New York: Marcel Dekker, 1990:219–249.
18. Prineas JW, Barnard RD, Revesz T, et al. MS: pathology of recurrent lesions. Brain 1993;116:681–693.
19. Genain CP, Cannella B, Hauser SL, et al. Identification of autoantibodies associated with myelin damage in MS. Nat Med 1999;5:170–175.
20. Linington C, Bradl M, Lassmann H, et al. Augmentation of demyelination in rat acute allergic encephalomyelitis by circulating mouse monoclonal antibodies directed against myelin/oligodendrocyte glycoprotein. Am J Pathol 1988; 130:443–454.
21. Morris MM, Piddlesden S, Groome N, et al. Anti-myelin antibodies modulate experimental allergic encephalomyelitis in Biozzi ABH mice. Biochem Soc Trans 1997;24:168S.
22. Gerritse K, Deen C, Fasbender M, et al. The involvement of specific anti-myelin basic protein antibody-forming cells in MS immunopathology. J Neuroimmunol 1994;49:153–159.
23. Gonen O, Patalace I, Babb JS, et al. Total brain N-acetylaspartate, a new measure of disease load in MS. Neurology 2000;54:15–19.
24. Poser CM, Paty DW, Scheinberg L, et al. New diagnostic criteria for MS: guidelines for research protocols. Ann Neurol 1983;13:227–231.
25. Krupp LB, Alvarez LA, LaRocca NG, et al. Fatigue in MS. Arch Neurol 1988;45:435–437.
26. Freal JE, Kraft GH, Coryell JK. Symptomatic fatigue in MS. Arch Phys Med Rehabil 1984;65:165–168.
27. Weinshenker BG, Bass B, Rice GPA, et al. The natural history of MS: a geographically based study. I. Clinical course and disability. Brain 1989;112:133–146.
28. Thompson AJ, Kennard C, Swash M, et al. Relative efficacy of intravenous methylprednisolone and ACTH in the treatment of acute relapse in MS. Neurology 1989;39:696–971.
29. Beck RW, Cleary PA, Anderson MM, et al. A randomized controlled trial of corticosteroids in the treatment of acute optic neuritis. N Engl J Med 1992;326:581–588.
30. Miller H, Simpson CA, Yeates WK. Bladder dysfunction in MS. Br Med J 1965;1:1265–1269.
31. Blaivas JG. Management of bladder dysfunction in MS. Neurology 1980;30:12–18.
32. Bradley WE, Logothetis JL, Timm GW. Cystometric and sphincter abnormalities in MS. Neurology 1973;23:1131–1139.
33. Schoenberg HW, Gutrich J, Banno J. Urodynamic patterns in MS. J Urol 1979;122:648–650.
34. Blaivas JG, Bhimani G, Labib KB. Vesicourethral dysfunction in MS. U Urol 1979;122:324–327.
35. Stenager E, Stenager EN, Jensen K. Sexual aspects of MS. Semin Neurol 1992;2:120–124.
36. Valleroy ML, Kraft G. Sexual dysfunction in MS. Arch Phys Med Rehabil 1984;65:125–128.
37. Rao SM, Leo GJ, Bernadin L, et al. Cognitive dysfunction in MS: frequency, patterns, and prediction. Neurology 1991; 41:685–691.
38. Krupp LB, Sliwinski M, Masur DM, et al. Cognitive functioning and depression in patients with chronic fatigue syndrome and MS. Arch Neurol 1994;51:705–710.
39. Rao SM, Leo GJ, Ellington L, et al. Cognitive dysfunction in MS. II. Impact on employment and social functioning. Neurology 1991;41:692–696.
40. Peyer JM, Edwards KR, Poser CM, et al. Cognitive functioning in patients with MS. Arch Neurol 1980;37:577–579.
41. Rao SM, Hammeke TA, McQuillen MP, et al. Memory disturbance in chronic progressive MS. Arch Neurol 1984;41: 625–631.
42. Heaton RK, Nelson LM, Thompson DS, et al. Neuropsychological findings in relapsing-remitting and chronic-progressive MS. J Consult Clin Psychol 1985; 53:103–110.
43. The IFNB MS study group and the University of British Columbia MS/MRI analysis group. Interferon beta-1b in the treatment of MS: final outcome of the randomized controlled trial. Neurology 1995;45:1277–1285.
44. Jacobs LD, Cookfair DL, Rudick RA, et al. Intramuscular interferon beta-la for disease progression in relapsing MS. Ann Neurol 1996;39:285–294.
45. Lublin FD, Whitaker JN, Eidelman BH, et al. Management of patients receiving interferon beta-1b for MS: report of a consensus conference. Neurology 1996;46:12–18.
46. Johnson KP, Brooks BR, Cohen JA, et al. Copolymer-1 reduces relapse rate and improves disability in relapsing-

remitting MS: results of a phase III multicenter double-blind placebo-controlled trial. Neurology 1995;45:1268–1276.

47. Thompson AJ, Noseworthy JH. New treatments for MS: a clinical perspective. Curr Opin Neurol 1996;9:187–198.
48. Fidler JM, DeJoy SQ, Smith FR, et al. Selective immunomodulation by the antineoplastic agent mitoxantrone. Nonspecific adherent suppressor cells derived from mitoxantrone-treated mice. J Immunol 1986;136:2747–2754.
49. Katz R. Management of spasticity. Am J Phys Med Rehabil 1988;67:108–116.
50. Nance DW, Sheremata WA, Lynch SG, et al. Relationships of the antispasticity effect of Tizanidine to plasma concentration in patients with MS. Arch Neurol 1997;54:731–736.
51. Rudick RA, Goodman A, Herndon RM, et al. Selecting relapsing-remitting MS patients for treatment: the care for early treatment. J Neuroimmunol 1999;98:22–28.
52. Ponichtera-Mulcare JA, Glaser RM, Mathews T, et al. Maximal aerobic exercise in persons with MS. Clin Kinesiol 1983;46(4):12–21.
53. Pepin EB, Hicks RW, Spender MK, et al. Pressor response to isometric exercise in patients with MS. Med Sci Sport Exerc 1996;28(6):656–660.
54. Ponichtera-Mulcare JA, Mathews T, Glaser RM, et al. Maximal aerobic exercise of individuals with MS using three modes of ergometery. Clin Kinesiol 1995;49:4–13.
55. Schwid SR, Thornton CA, Pandya S, et al. Quantitative assessment of motor fatigue and strength in MS. Neurology 1999;53:743–750.
56. Ponichtera-Mulcare JA, Mathews T, Barrett PJ, et al. Change in aerobic fitness of patients with MS during a 6-month training program. Sport Med Training Rehab 1997;7:265–272.
57. Ng AV, Dao HT, Miller RG, et al. Blunted pressor and intramuscular metabolic responses to voluntary isometric exercise in MS. J Appl Physiol 2000;88:871–880.
58. Ponichtera JA, Rodgers MM, Glaser RM, et al. Concentric and eccentric isokinetic lower extremity strength in persons with MS. J Orthop Sport Phys Ther 1988;16(3):114–122.
59. Armstrong LE, Winant DM, Swasey PR, et al. Using isokinetic dynamometry to test ambulatory patients with MS. Phys Ther 1983;63:1274–1279.
60. Chen W-Y, Peirson FM, Burnett CN. Force-time measurements of knee muscle function in MS. Phys Ther 1987;67:934–940.
61. Rice CL, Volmer TL, Bigland-Ritchie B. Neuromuscular responses of patients with MS. Muscle Nerve 1992;15:1123–1132.
62. Engardt M, Knutsson E, Johsson M, et al. Dynamic muscle strength training in stroke patients: effects on knee extension torque, electromyographic activity and motor function. Arch Phys Med Rehabil 1995;76:419–425.
63. Knutsson E, Matensoon A. Dynamic motor capacity in spastic paresis and its relation to prime mover dysfunction, spastic reflexes and antagonistic co-activation. Scand J Rehabil Med 1982;12:93–106.
64. Knutsson E. Analysis of spastic paresis. Proceedings, 10th International Congress of the World Confederation for Physical Therapy. Sydney, Australia; 1987;626–633.
65. Ponichtera JA. Cardiorespiratory responses in persons with MS. (Contract No. CDFA 84.133). Washington, DC: Department of Education, 1991.
66. Kramer JF, McPhail HE. Relationship among measures of walking efficiency, gross motor ability, and isokinetic strength in adolescents with cerebral palsy. Pediatr Phys Ther 1994;3:3–8.
67. Olney SJ, MacPhail HE, Hedden DM, et al. Work and power in hemiplegic cerebral palsy gait. Phys Ther 1990;70(7):431–438.
68. Olney SJ, Costigan PA, Hedden DM. Mechanical energy patterns in gait of cerebral palsied children with hemiplegia. Phys Ther 1987;67(9):1348–1354.
69. McDonald WI, Sears TA. Effect of a demyelinating lesion on conduction in the central nervous system studied in single nerve fibers. J Physiol (London), 1970;207:53–54P.
70. Schauf CL, Davis FA. Impulse conduction in MS: a theoretical basis for modification by temperature and pharmacological agents. J Neurol Neuosurg Psychiatry 1974;37:152–161.
71. Schauf CL, Pencek TL, Davis FA, et al. Physiological basis for neuroelectric blocking activity in multiple sclerosis. Neurology 1981;31:1338–1341.
72. Kent-Braun JA, Ng AV, Castro M, et al. Strength, skeletal muscle composition, and enzyme activity in MS. Muscle Nerve 1994;17:835–841.
73. Kent-Braun JA, Sharma KR, Weiner MW, et al. Effects of exercise on muscle activation and metabolism in MS. Muscle Nerve 1994;17:1162–1169.
74. Sharma KR, Kent-Braun J, Mynhier MA, et al. Evidence of an abnormal intramuscular component of fatigue in MS. Muscle Nerve 1995;18(12):1403–1411.
75. Tantucci C, Massucci M, Piperno R, et al. Energy cost of exercise in MS patients with low degree of disability. Mult Scler 1996;2(3):161–167.
76. Mulcare JA, Webb P, Mathews T, et al. Sweat response in persons with MS during exercise. (*Unpublished manuscript*).
77. Noble BJ, Borg GAV, Jacobs I, et al. A category-ratio perceived exertion scale: relationship to blood and muscle lactates and heart rate. Med Sci Sports Exerc 1983;15:523–528.
78. Mulcare JA, Mathews T. Exercise testing and training of MS patients. (*Final Report, Merit Review B940714-A—unpublished manuscript*), 1998.
79. Petajan JH, Gappmaier E, White AT, et al. Impact of aerobic training on fitness and quality of life in MS. Ann Neurol 1996;34:432–441.
80. Ponichtera-Mulcare JA, Mathews T, Barrett PJ, et al. Maximal aerobic exercise of persons with multiple sclerosis following a 6-month endurance training program. Med Sci Sports Exerc 1995;27(5):S81.
81. American College of Sports Medicine. ACSM's guidelines for exercise testing and prescription. 5th ed. Lippincott William & Wilkins, 1995.
82. Berg KO, Wood-Dauphine SL, Williams JI, Maki B. Measuring balance in the elderly: validation of an instrument. Can J Public Health 1992;83(Suppl 2):S7–S11.
83. Golding LA, Myers CR, Sinning WE, eds. Y's way to physical fitness. 3rd ed. Champaign, IL: Human Kinetics Publishers, 1989.
84. Astrand P-O, Ryhming I. A nomogram for calculation of aerobic capacity (physical fitness) from pulse rate during submaximal work. J Appl Physiol 1954;7:218.
85. Mulcare JA, Webb P, Mathews T, et al. The effect of body cooling on the aerobic endurance of persons with MS following a 3-month aerobic training program. Med Sci Sports Exerc 1997;29(5,Suppl):S83.

86. White AT, Wilson TE, Petajan JH. Effect of pre-exercise cooling on physical function and fatigue in MS patients. Med Sci Sports Exerc 1997;29(5):S83.
87. Stuifbergen A, Becker H. Predictors of health promoting lifestyles in persons with disabilities. Res Nurs Health 1994; 17:3–13.
88. Stuifbergen A. Health promoting behaviors and quality of life among individuals with MS. Schol Inq Nurs Pract 1995; 9:31–50.
89. Ng AV, Kent-Braun J. Quantification of lower physical activity in persons with MS. Med Sci Sports Exerc 1997;29(4):517–523.
90. Rimmer JH, Rubin SS, Braddock D. Barriers to exercise in African American women with physical disabilities. Arch Phys Med Rehabil 2000;81(2):182–188.
91. Abramson S, Stein J, Schaufele M, et al. Personal exercise habits and counseling practices of primary care physicians: a national survey. Clin J Sport Med, 2000;10(1):40–48.

Suggested Reading

Petajan JH, White AT. Recommendations for physical activity in patients with MS. Sports Med 1999;27(3):179–191.

CHAPTER 4

Parkinson's Disease

Rhonda K. Stanley and Elizabeth J. Protas

EPIDEMIOLOGY

Parkinsonism is a progressive, degenerative neurological disorder. The pathology of PD is associated with the dysfunction of the central nervous system resulting in the decrease, or abnormal activity, of neurotransmitter systems. The resulting neurotransmitter imbalance is exhibited by abnormal movements of the body.

Parkinsonism is ranked as one of the most common neurological syndromes affecting individuals over the age of 50 and includes a variety of disorders that consist of varying degrees of resting tremor, bradykinesia (slowness of movement), rigidity, and impaired postural reflexes (1–4). Primary or idiopathic Parkinson's disease (IPD) is the most common type of Parkinsonism and most often presents itself between the ages of 50 and 79 years (5, 6).

Idiopathic Parkinson's disease is thought to occur worldwide, and to date, no population has been found immune to the disease (4, 7). Although this may be the case, races are affected differently by the disease. Crude prevalence ratios in the white population vary from 84 to 270 per 100,000 population (7). African blacks and Asians appear to have lower prevalence rates ranging from 4 to 85.7 per 100,000, depending on race (1). The ratio of blacks to whites is reported to be 1:4 (7). In the United States alone, based on a population of 250 million, and using an average prevalence ratio of 160 per 100,000, the number of persons affected by IPD would be approximately 400,000 (6).

Incidence has been studied less often than prevalence with varying rates from 5 to 24 per 100,000 population (7). Because incidence of PD increases with age, after the age of 50, age-specific incidence is said to sharply increase varying from 53 to 229 per 100,000 (1, 8).

Because prevalence and incidence are closely related, changes in one can affect the other. Prevalence is "the proportion of individuals in a population who have the disease at a specific instant" (9), whereas "incidence quantifies the number of new events or cases of disease that develop in a population of individuals at risk during a specified time interval" (9). Since the advent of levodopa (L-dopa) therapy in the late 1960s, incidence of PD has remained relatively constant, although the prevalence has increased. This increase in prevalence has been attributed to an increase in the age at time of death, which has resulted due to the success of L-dopa therapy (1, 6). Consequently, individuals with IPD are living longer with the disease.

Prevalence and/or incidence rates between males and females vary depending on whether crude or sex-specific calculations are determined. In studies performed by Marttila and Rinne and Rajput et al., where sex-specific prevalence and incidence calculations were used, results indicated no differences between the sexes in being affected by PD (10, 11). Other studies have found that prevalence and incidence are lower in females versus males (12,13,14).

As with prevalence and incidence, mortality rates associated with PD vary between studies. Prior to L-dopa therapy, mortality related to PD was reported by Hoehn and Yahr to be 2.9 times higher than in the general population (15). Since the advent of L-dopa therapy, this rate has decreased to 1.3 to 1.9 times higher than that in the general population (1, 16–19). Because coding and reporting of diseases on death certificates can be inconsistent and often times inaccurate, the underlying cause of death due to complications related to the PD is thought to be underestimated (10). Respiratory and urinary infections are the leading causes of death in individuals having PD (15, 20, 21).

CLASSIFICATION

Parkinsonism is a complex of neurological syndromes characterized by clinical symptoms consisting of varying degrees of tremor, bradykinesia, rigidity, and impaired postural reflexes (2). Idiopathic Parkinson's disease (IPD) is classified as such because the damage to the dopaminergic nigrostriatal pathway is unknown and because there is the distinct presence of Lewy body inclusions found in the substantia nigra and locus ceruleus (6, 22, 23). In contrast, secondary parkinsonism is a neurological syndrome displaying similar motor symptoms as IPD, but the cause of damage to the nigrostriatal system has been identified (24).

This secondary classification includes postencephalitic, drug-induced, toxic, traumatic, metabolic, and neoplastic causes (22, 24). A third classification includes Parkinsonism due to multiple system degenerations or atrophies and has also been labeled Parkinsonism-plus syndromes (22). This classification includes striatonigral and pallidonigral degenerations, olivopontocerebellar atrophy, progressive supranuclear palsy, and Shy-Drager syndrome (2, 24). This category also includes various degenerative diseases and disorders of the nervous system that are inherited, all of which can present with or cause parkinsonian-like symptoms (22). According to Jankovic, approximately 10% of all patients with Parkinsonism have "secondary" parkinsonism, and 15% of all patients seen in specialized clinics are diagnosed with multiple system degenerations (22).

For purposes of this chapter, emphasis will be placed on IPD. As much as 75 to 90 percent of the parkinsonian syndromes are thought to be IPD (22). Within this classification, distinct clinical pictures occur with the descriptive subgroups labeled depending on which authority one reads (2, 22, 24).

A possible classification schema for IPD is that presented by Koller and Hubble (2). Clinical symptoms are categorized within three subgroups: (1) tremor predominant; (2) postural instability-gait difficulty (PIGD) and that group that is; and (3) akinetic-rigidity predominant. In addition, there are differentiating features dependent upon age of onset, mental status, and clinical course of the disease (2). Age of onset is broken down into juvenile, less than 40 years, between 40 and 75 years, or greater than 75 years. Classification of mental status is dependent upon dementia being present or absent. The clinical course of the disease can be classified as benign, progressive, or malignant.

As a means to classify the severity of the disease, one of the historical scales, which continues to be used by neurologists today, is the Hoehn and Yahr Staging Scale (15). The original scale simply stages the progression or severity of the disease on a I to V scale based on symptoms being unilateral or bilateral, impairment of balance, functional capability in relation to normal activities, and/or employment status, and level of independence. In the original version, the descriptives under each stage lack congruity and allow for extreme subjectivity when trying to rate an individual (Table 4.1).

Although a modified version of this scale has been developed that is more congruent and less ambiguous and wordy, it still allows for extreme subjectivity when rating an individual (Table 4.2) (25). This scale is frequently used in the clinic and in research as a means of classifying patients according to the severity of their disease. Despite its measurement limitations, after many years of its use by specialists in PD, when reference is made to a particular stage there is immediately some concept of where an individual is in the possible progression of the disease.

Table 4.1. Original Hoehn and Yahr Classification of Disability

STAGE	DESCRIPTION OF DISABILITY
I	Unilateral involvement only, usually with minimal or no functional impairment.
II	Bilateral or midline involvement, without impairment of balance.
III	First sign of impaired righting reflexes. This is evident by unsteadiness as the patient turns or is demonstrated when he is pushed from standing equilibrium with the feet together and eyes closed. Functionally, the patient is somewhat restricted in his activities but may have some work potential depending upon the type of employment. Patients are physically capable of leading independent lives, and their disability is mild to moderate.
IV	Fully developed, severely disabling disease; the patient is still able to walk and stand unassisted but is markedly incapacitated.
V	Confinement to bed or wheelchair unless aided.

CLINICAL SYMPTOMS

As stated above, clinical symptoms can be classified within three subgroups: (1) tremor predominant; (2) PIGD predominant; or (3) akinetic-rigidity predominant. The tremor-predominant group has been characterized as having more severe tremor, an earlier age of onset, less cognitive impairment, and a more favorable prognosis as compared to the PIGD group (26, 27). The PIGD-predominant group is characterized as having greater gait and postural instability, increased episodes of falling and/or freezing, and greater difficulties walking than those individuals within the tremor-predominant group (28). The akinetic-rigidity predominant group has a significant decrease or a complete lack of movement (akinesia) along with rigidity. Because the akinesia and rigidity can be significant, these individuals have major problems with all movements. Tremor may or may not be present.

In a study performed by Jankovic et al., tremor-predominant patients were found to have more severe resting tremor as well as greater action-postural tremor in comparison to the PIGD group (28). In the same study,

Table 4.2. Modified Hoehn and Yahr Classification of Disability

STAGE	DESCRIPTION OF DISABILITY
0.0	No signs of disease
1.0	Unilateral disease
1.5	Unilateral plus axial involvement
2.0	Bilateral disease, without impairment of balance
2.5	Mild bilateral disease, with recovery on pull test
3.0	Mild to moderate bilateral disease; some postural instability; physically independent
4.0	Severe disability; still able to walk or stand unassisted
5.0	Wheelchair bound or bedridden unless aided

the PIGD patients were found to have more severe bradykinesia, increased difficulty rising from a chair, and more postural dysfunction than the tremor-predominant patients. In addition, the PIGD patients had greater occupational disability, more intellectual impairment and depression, decreased motivation, and increased impairment in activities of daily living (ADLS) as measured by the Unified Parkinson's Disease Rating Scale (UPDRS) (28).

Many individuals having IPD also have autonomic nervous system (ANS) dysfunction. These problems can include cardiovascular abnormalities, gastrointestinal motility disorders, bowel and bladder dysfunction, thermoregulatory abnormalities, pupillary abnormalities, and sexual dysfunction. Some of the most common problems include disorders of motility, drooling, difficulty in voiding, detrusor hyperactivity, and impaired sweating response (29).

Other problems that may be encountered by those with Parkinson's disease are listed in Table 4.3.

PATHOPHYSIOLOGY

As stated previously, IPD is a neurodegenerative process that can result in movement disorders. In addition, these symptoms of dysfunctional movement are often accompanied by cognitive changes and mood disturbances. The anatomical structure within the central nervous system known to be a primary area affected by the disease is the basal ganglia. Collectively, the basal ganglia are thought to control the more complex aspects of motor planning. In addition, parts of the thalamus and reticular formation work in close association with the above structures and are therefore considered to be part of the basal ganglia system for motor control. Furthermore, the basal ganglia is anatomically linked to other parts of the brain that control not only motor and sensory programs, but cognitive and motivational aspects of the human body and psyche as well. Therefore, any disease of the basal ganglia can result in various movement disorders, as well as cognitive changes and mood disturbances.

Although it is not the only area affected by the disease, the structure within the basal ganglia most vulnerable to the pathological process of IPD is the substantia nigra. Widespread destruction of the pigmented neurons in the substantia nigra pars compacta is associated with IPD, and as a result of this destruction, the nigrostriatal tract degenerates. The degeneration of the dopaminergic nigrostriatal pathway has been recognized as the primary pathological event resulting in parkinsonian syndromes (24, 30, 31). This degeneration results in the loss of dopamine normally secreted in the caudate nucleus and putamen, resulting in the classic motor symptoms. The cause of the destruction within the substantia nigra in IPD remains to be answered.

The pathogenesis of ANS abnormalities in PD are not well understood. There have been lesions found/indicated within the hypothalamus and the locus ceruleus that are both involved in the central control of the ANS (32). In addition, abnormalities within the dorsal nucleus of the vagus nerve, a disturbed metabolism of catecholamines, as well as Lewy bodies found within the enteric system have been implicated in ANS dysfunction (29, 33–37).

Table 4.3. Possible Secondary Problems Encountered by Those with Parkinson's Disease

Incoordination
Gait deficits
Balance deficits
Masked facies
Dysphagia
Dysarthria
Sialorrhea
Scoliosis
Kyphosis
Pain and sensory symptoms
Seborrhea
Constipation
Dementia
Urinary incontinence
Impotence
Depression
Fall risk
Muscle atrophy and weakness

ETIOLOGY

Although the cause of IPD is currently unknown, there are two theories that have been frequently studied and debated. These are the theories of genetic predisposition and of environmental etiology. In addition, there are factors that must be considered as mechanisms that may contribute to the pathogenesis of the disease.

Early twin studies lead researchers to believe that genetics do not provide a significant contribution in the cause of IPD (38–43). Reexamination of some of the old studies as well as design of newer studies have brought investigators back to reconsidering IPD as a genetically inherited disease.

As support for an environmental cause, a bizarre outbreak in 1983 of Parkinsonism in northern California led to the theory that environmental factors play a role in the etiology of IPD. These individuals were drug abusers and had been inadvertently exposed to 1-methyl-4-phenyl-1,2,3,6-tetrahydropyridine (MPTP). MPTP can result as a by-product during the synthesis of the narcotic, 1-methyl-r-phenyl-r-proprionorypiperidine (MPPP), which is a synthetic form of heroine. The drug abusers were exposed to the MPTP as a result of injecting contaminated MPPP and later developed rapid and severe parkinsonian symptoms that included bradykinesia, rigidity, weakness, severe speech difficulties, tremor, masked facies, seborrhea, festinating gait, drooling, flexed posture, as well as fixed stare and decreased blinking (44). L-dopa/carbidopa treatment was initiated with all patients and improved symptoms, but within a few weeks, drug-related side effects of dyskinesias and clinical fluctuations ensued. Thus began the earnest endeavor in the search for an environmental cause of IPD.

As of yet, there are no definitive data clearly supporting a genetic or environmental cause. Some believe that it is probably a combination of both. Consequently, the search goes on.

Two newer theories that have been introduced as possible mechanisms that may contribute to the pathogenesis of the disease include mitochondrial dysfunction and free-radical toxicity. Several studies currently suggest that nigral mitochondrial Complex I is abnormal in those with IPD (45–48). This abnormality appears to be specific to the brain because other studies looking at tissues such as platelets and muscle, as well as other components of the electron transport chain, have been less consistent in their results. Consequently, more research is needed in this area.

Another body of evidence is growing that suggests that free-radical toxicity causes nigral cell degeneration in those with IPD (49–52). This theory suggests that free radicals are produced in the basal ganglia and lead to the progressive degeneration and eventual cell death of neurons in the substantia nigra. Here, too, more research is needed.

There are no definitive risk factors for the development of IPD.

FUNCTIONAL IMPACT

The functional problems that a person with PD displays will be dependent upon the symptoms with which they present. Some of the common problems related to function in those with Parkinson's disease include gait and balance deficits and difficulty getting out of bed, out of a car, and arising from a chair. Other problems include difficulties with getting dressed, especially fastening buttons, writing, and speech and swallowing problems. In general, the person with PD has trouble with doing more than one task at a time. As the disease progresses, these problems will usually become more pronounced and the person will eventually lose the ability to perform activities of daily living (ADLS). In the last stage of the disease, the person is usually wheelchair- and/or bed-bound.

The classic gait pattern displayed by the person with PD is a decrease in step length and foot clearance. The heel-toe pattern is lost, and there is a tendency to shuffle the feet. Posture is flexed forward out of the base of support, which causes the person to take quicker and quicker steps with an inability to stop. This propulsion forward with quick steps is called festination. The person often has difficulty stopping and may eventually fall. In addition, the natural arm swing with gait is greatly decreased or absent.

Balance deficits are also common in those with PD. Because postural reflexes are absent, if the person is perturbed outside the base of support, he or she is often unable to recover and will fall. Falls are a major concern in those with Parkinson's disease and should be kept in mind when prescribing any kind of exercise program.

In addition to gait and balance deficits, segmental movements in the joints, especially in the vertebrae, are greatly decreased if rigidity is present. As a result, the person will have difficulty isolating movements such as rolling from side-to-side as is required when getting out of bed, or being able to rotate the trunk when getting out of a car. In general, movement can be very difficult due to the rigidity and bradykinesia.

Another phenomenon that can greatly impact function is called "freezing." This most typically occurs during gait. The person will be unable to initiate gait or while walking will suddenly become "frozen" in place. It is as if the person's feet become glued to the floor. Various techniques such as taking a step backward, marching in place, or visualizing stepping over a line on the floor can bring the person out of the "freeze."

It is important to remember that the functional problems experienced by those with PD are extremely variable from person to person. This requires that an individualized approach be taken with each person.

CLINICAL EXERCISE PHYSIOLOGY

Research that has studied the effects of exercise for individuals having PD has been directed toward interventions that would most likely impact the motor control problems associated with the disease. Typical treatment protocols that might be used include range of motion (ROM) and flexibility exercises, balance and gait training, mobility, and/or coordination exercises (53–60). Little research has been conducted assessing the aerobic capacity of, or the impact that aerobic exercise might have on, those having the disease. Likewise, there have been few studies assessing strength or using strength training as the intervention.

As far as aerobic capacity is concerned, most studies have found no difference in those with IPD and healthy normals in maximum or peak oxygen consumption ($\dot{V}O_2$). In a study conducted by Stanley and colleagues, a one-time exercise bout using a stationary bicycle was performed with 20 men and women having IPD and 23 healthy men and women (61). It was determined that peak $\dot{V}O_2$ levels for males and females did not differ between those with PD and the healthy group. The only significant difference found was in time to maximum exercise in the male subjects. Those with IPD reached $\dot{V}O_{2peak}$ sooner than the healthy group. The other difference between groups in the study was the response to submaximal exercise. Males and females with IPD appeared to have higher submaximal $\dot{V}O_2$ levels for each stage of exercise. These authors concluded that those with IPD might be less efficient during exercise.

In a study by Canning et al., exercise capacity of those with PD was assessed during cycle ergometry to determine if exercise capacity is affected by abnormalities in respiratory function and gait (62). These researchers did not compare subjects to healthy individuals, but compared actual values to predicted values. No differences were found in peak work or $\dot{V}O_{2peak}$ during exercise. These researchers also found certain respiratory abnormalities at rest and during exercise.

Another study finding differences in certain respiratory measures with exercise is a study by Koseoglu et al. (63). They also found impairment in maximum voluntary ventilation and exercise tolerance when compared to the healthy group. Following a 5-week exercise program involving "unsupported upper-extremity exercises" (specifics not explained), they found improvement in some of the respiratory measures, as well as in exercise tolerance and decreases in rating of perceived exertion for those with PD.

In a study by Reuter et al., patients with PD and age-matched health controls were tested using a ramped, cycle ergometer protocol (64). Heart rate variability and lactate levels were measured during exercise with the assumption that these would be impaired if a deficit in the respiratory chain was present. Other variables measured included systolic and diastolic blood pressures and heart rate. Heart rate variability was significantly abnormal in those with PD for all tests. Heart rate increase during exercise was not significantly different between groups nor was diastolic blood pressure. Systolic blood pressure was lower in those with PD at submaximal and maximal levels of exercise, and lactate levels tended to be lower at higher rates of exercise for those with PD, but were not statistically significant. Researchers concluded that those with PD can be tested for aerobic capacity and would be expected to condition aerobically with appropriate exercise intervention.

As with studies looking at aerobic capacity, research looking at strength issues in those with PD is also limited. In a study by Kakinuma et al., it was found that lower-extremity strength was less on the affected side versus the unaffected side and this difference increased as the speed of movement increased (65). Another study by Nogaki et al. also found that muscle weakness increases as performance velocity increases (66). Other studies comparing strength when on and off anti-parkinsonian medications found strength to be significantly less when off medications (67, 68, 69).

PHARMACOLOGY

Pharmacological treatment is the primary therapeutic intervention for the problems associated with idiopathic Parkinson's disease. This treatment is based on what is currently known about the neurochemical imbalances that exist in the neurotransmitter concentrations within the basal ganglia of individuals having IPD. Treatment modes have been classified into two general categories by Berg et al. (70): (1) reduction of the functional excess of acetylcholine with anticholinergics, and (2) alleviation of the pathological deficiency of dopamine with drugs that act on the dopaminergic system. In more recent years, protective therapy aimed at slowing the progression of the disease has been introduced (71).

The most frequent drug classifications used for treatment include dopaminergics, anticholinergics, monoamine oxidase type "B" (MAO-B) inhibitors, and catechol-O-methyltransferase (COMT) inhibitors. In addition, there are various other drugs that are often prescribed depending on signs and symptoms of the disease (i.e., baclofen, clozapine). The most common medications for each of the above classifications are:

Dopaminergics (levodopa, levodopa/carbidopa, amantadine, pergolide, bromocriptine)
Anticholinergics (benztropine, trihexyphenidyl)
MAO-B inhibitors (selegiline)
COMT inhibitors (entacapone, tolcapone)

Acute and long-term side effects can be considerable for all the medications taken for PD. Peripheral side effects include gastrointestinal upset, orthostatic hypotension, bradycardia, tachycardia, arrhythmia, dry mouth, blurred vision, and headaches. Central side effects include motor disturbances, insomnia, ataxia, vivid dreams, cognitive/psychiatric disturbances, and edema.

Some of the most debilitating side effects are those that occur after long-term use of L-dopa. These side effects are motor disturbances that include dyskinesias, dystonias, and clinical fluctuation. These frequently appear approximately 5 to 7 years after L-dopa therapy was initiated. Consideration should be taken when exercising an individual who exhibits any of these side effects. The abnormal movements may interfere in any activity that the person tries to perform.

For considerations to be taken during exercise testing and training, please refer to *ACSM's Exercise Management for Persons with Chronic Diseases and Disabilities* (72).

PHYSICAL EXAMINATION

When examining an individual with Parkinson's disease, it is important to take a thorough history, as well as perform a complete neurological exam and an orthopedic screen. It is also important to determine how the individual is responding to the anti-parkinsonian medications, especially whether they are beginning to experience any of the long-term side effects.

During the neurological exam, rigidity, tremor, bradykinesia, and postural reflexes must be examined. To illicit rigidity, the examiner can grasp one or both wrists and shake the hand(s) up and down. Looseness and ease of the movement is observed. Flexing and extending the forearm repetitively while feeling the ease of movement can also be done to assess rigidity. The same can be done with the lower extremities (LES) at the hip, knee, and ankle. The neck and trunk must also be examined by moving the part through all planes of movement. Ease of movement and the amount of range will determine the extent of the rigidity. When assessing for rigidity, the movement should be passive with the individual relaxed.

To assess for resting tremor, have the individual sit with his/her hands resting in the lap. Have the individual recite a specific sentence or count backwards by 2s or 7s. The stress of this activity will allow the tremor to become obvious. Action tremor can be elicited by having the individual reach for a cup of water on a table, pick it up, and bring it to the mouth to take a drink, then return the cup to the table. Watch for tremor during the course of the movement.

Assess bradykinesia by having the individual sit with both hands in his/her lap. Ask the person to supinate and pronate the forearm as fast as possible for at least 30 seconds. If bradykinesia is present, the quality of the movement will begin to break down after a few seconds. There may be a slowing of the movement, a decrease in ROM, or decreased coordination of the movement.

Postural reflexes can be examined by having the individual stand with his/her back to the examiner. The individual keeps the eyes open while the examiner reaches around to the front of the shoulders and pulls quickly and firmly posteriorly. The examiner is observing for recovery from the pull test. Does the individual stay in place, step or stagger backwards but recover independently, step or stagger backwards requiring assistance from the examiner to recover, or does the individual fall straight back without any attempt to recover? It is important that the examiner be behind the individual during this test in order to guard the individual from falling.

In addition to these tests, a general coordination, sensory, and cognitive examination should be performed. The Unified Parkinson's Disease Rating Scale (UPDRS) is a comprehensive examination administered by a health professional (25). The UPDRS examines cognition, ADL, motor behaviors, complications of therapy, and assesses a disability rating.

Since the person with PD can have significant postural changes, a postural screen should be performed. This should be done in sitting and in standing. The examiner is observing for forward head, rounded shoulders, kyphosis and scoliosis, decreased lordosis, and excessive hip and knee flexion.

To determine responsiveness to the anti-parkinsonian medications, certain questions should be asked. To determine whether the individual is having dyskinesias or dystonias, the examiner should ask whether the person is having any abnormal involuntary movements or postures. If yes, when do these movements occur in relation to taking his/her dose of medication? Are there times after taking his/her dose that the medication does not seem to work and their parkinsonian symptoms are worse? If this is the case, the individual may be having clinical fluctuations, also known as "on/off" phenomenon. All of this information can be important in determining the best time for the person to exercise.

MEDICAL AND SURGICAL TREATMENTS

As stated previously, drug therapy is the primary means of medical management for IPD. Secondary lines of treatment include sophisticated surgeries to the brain. Surgical procedures include thalamotomy, pallidotomy, and deep brain stimulation (73, 74). For the thalamotomy and pallidotomy, neuroablation procedures, lesions are made to specific areas in the thalamus or globus pallidus. This procedure is an irreversible disruption of the abnormal functioning structure that gets rid of the undesired movement disorder such as tremor, leaving other volitional movement intact. Thalamotomy is done to correct drug-resistant tremor, and pallidotomy, which is the most widely used, can decrease rigidity, bradykinesia, tremor, muscular spasms, and off-state dystonias.

Another surgical procedure is deep brain stimulation. In this procedure, a programmable pulse-generating device is implanted in the brain. The advantages over lesioning are that it is safer and it is reversible and adaptable. Disadvantages include cost and maintenance of the device. These devices are usually implanted in the thalamus or globus pallidus. Although clinical effects will vary depending on where the device is implanted, results are similar to those mentioned above for the thalamotomy and pallidotomy.

A third type of surgery is the fetal mesencephalon graft transplantation. These surgeries are currently only investigational and are also controversial because of the use of fetal tissue. To address this issue, researchers are investigating the use of genetically engineered cells, encapsulated cells, and gene therapy, as well as xenografts.

DIAGNOSTIC TECHNIQUES

There are no definitive diagnostic tests for the detection of Parkinson's disease.

EXERCISE/FITNESS/FUNCTIONAL TESTING

Before exercise testing is performed, it is recommended that balance, gait, general mobility, range of motion and flexibility, and manual muscle testing be performed. Results of these tests will give guidance in how to safely exercise test the individual.

Both static and dynamic balance while in sitting and standing should be performed. Clinical balance tests that can be used with those having PD include the Functional Reach (75), the Berg Balance Scale (76), or sensory organization testing (77).

Gait can be observed while the individual walks a 20- to 50-foot pathway. The examiner observes step length, stride width, and heel strike. Because those with PD have trouble turning, the examiner should observe the individual changing directions. Continuity of steps and coordination during the transition are noted. It is also important to observe the person having to come to a sudden stop while walking, looking for ease of stopping the momentum. Does the individual stop easily, have to take several steps, stagger or stutter step, or possibly fall? Also have the individual step over an object in the path. The examiner should also take note of any freezing episodes that occur. If balance and gait are compromised, it is not recommended that the treadmill be used when exercise testing an individual with PD.

General mobility can be tested by using a tool like the Duke Mobility test (78). Although the scoring of this test uses an ordinal scale, it incorporates several of the above tasks such as walking, turning, and stepping over an object, as well as reaching, bending down, chair transfers, stairs, and static sitting and standing. It only takes about 10 minutes to administer. Even though mobility may appear to be greatly compromised, the person may still be able to perform an exercise test using a stationary bicycle or arm ergometry protocol. Try the activity before assuming the individual cannot do something.

For the rehabilitation specialist, the standard way of testing muscle strength is by manual muscle testing specific muscles or muscle groups. More objective measures include using devices such as cable tensiometers, handgrip dynamometers, and isokinetic equipment. Because this area has not been well researched, there are no recommendations as to which strength testing protocols should be used. Therefore, recommendations as outlined by the ACSM should be followed for testing muscle strength and endurance (79).

When deciding to test for aerobic endurance, the absolute and relative contraindications for exercise testing outlined by the ACSM should be followed (79). In addition, precautions should be taken if the individual is experiencing severe dyskinesias or dystonias. As with strength testing, little research has been done trying different exercise testing protocols with those having PD. The results of the physical and functional exam should guide the examiner in what exercise protocol is safe to use.

EXERCISE PRESCRIPTION AND PROGRAMMING

When prescribing exercise for the person with IPD, an overall, individualized program should be the goal. Because the disease is chronic and progressive, an exercise program should begin early when the disease is first diagnosed and be maintained on a regular long-term basis. The program should be updated and revised as the disease progresses and the needs of the individual change. Each of the following areas should be addressed: flexibility, aerobic conditioning, strengthening, functional training, and motor control.

To address flexibility, slow static stretches should be performed for all major muscle groups. In addition, ROM exercises should be prescribed for all joints. The upper quadrant and trunk should be emphasized early on because the disease affects these areas first and because frozen shoulders and loss of segmental movements in the spine are common as the disease progresses.

Although the optimal frequency for flexibility and ROM exercises for IPD is not established, suggestions range from once a week to daily. Schenkman et al. conducted a randomized, clinical trial with 51 people with PD (80). Twenty-three people participated in a 10-week, 3 times per week program focused on spinal flexibility. This program resulted in improvements in trunk flexibility and functional reach, a measure of balance, but no improvements in the time to move from supine to standing. Even though moving from supine to standing may be limited due to reduced trunk flexibility, increased trunk movement did not result in improved function in this study.

Since few studies conducted have used aerobic conditioning or strength training for those with IPD, specifics for prescribing exercise are lacking. Guidelines as outlined by the ACSM should be followed for frequency, intensity, duration, and progression (79). The mode of exercise should depend on the problems the individual exhibits. As mentioned previously, caution should be taken in placing someone on a treadmill if he/she has gait or balance problems or a history of falls. A stationary bicycle, recumbent bicycle, or arm ergometer may be safer. If walking is used, recommend an environment with a level surface with minimal obstacles such as a walking track. Mall walking might be possible if the person goes when pedestrian traffic is at a minimum. Anecdotal reports from those with IPD indicate that swimming can be a good mode of exercise. Some report that the water enables them to move more easily. If prescribing a strengthening program, exercise machines may be safer than the use of free weights because the movement can be more controlled. If a person has severe intention tremor or dyskinesias, free weights may not be as safe as strengthening machines.

Functional training often includes gait and balance training, as well as fall prevention and specific training in activities of daily living. Again, little research supports the efficacy of these interventions. Training the patient to use visual and auditory cues demonstrates improvements in gait and a reduction in freezing (81).

Motor control strategies emphasize slow, controlled movement for specific tasks, through various ranges of motion while lying, sitting, standing, and walking. Dietz et al. reported that using a body-weight support system while individuals with IPD walked on a treadmill improved some gait parameters (82).

This strategy has not been used as a long-term training approach. In a study by Viliani and colleagues, physical training was given to those with PD that included active mobilization for the lower and upper extremities, spinal mobility exercises, limb coordination exercises, and postural and gait exercises (83). Specific motor tasks were measured that included supine to sitting, sitting to supine, rolling to supine, and standing from a chair. All the variables showed significant improvement following the intervention. These researchers conclude that specific motor task training can improve movements with which individuals with PD have problems.

Because of the potential demands of an exercise program, it is necessary that the participant be able to understand and follow instructions in order to safely complete the requirements of the program. Cognitive changes for those with IPD can be mild to severe; consequently, it is important that the instructor determine whether the person is able to safely follow the program. Ways to ensure this include providing both verbal and written instructions, giving repetitive demonstrations, closely observing the individual while performing all tasks, and instructing the spouse, a friend, or other caregiver in the program so that support and direction can be given as needed when at home.

For the older person with IPD, comorbidity can be an issue. Cardiopulmonary disease as well as coexisting arthritis and related musculoskeletal abnormalities should be considered and included in patient screening. Some of the cardiac abnormalities that may be present include frequent preventricular contractions, ST-depression, blunted heart rate response similar to cardiac patients on beta-blockers, as well as tachycardia during peak-dose–related dyskinesias.

As mentioned previously, it is important to have a clear understanding of how the individual responds to his/her medications. Although timing the medication so that the individual is at his/her best during the exercise session is important, precautions should be taken if the person is having dose-related dyskinesias during his/her peak time. Depending on the severity of the dyskinesias, exercise during this time may be contraindicated. For those having "on/off" phenomenon, exercising during an "off" time may be difficult or impossible.

Depending on the severity of the disease, supervision during exercise may or may not be required. For those more involved or those having cognitive deficits, group exercise may be more beneficial in order to ensure safety, adherence, and socialization.

EDUCATION AND COUNSELING

Because the person with PD may decrease his/her activity level as it becomes more difficult to move or the tremor becomes an embarrassment, it is imperative that the individual and his/her family be educated about the importance of maintaining an active lifestyle. Parkinson's support groups are organized in larger cities. These groups can be very important in educating the individual and family about the disease as well as encouraging continued socialization. Exercise groups are often available through these organizations as well as educational presentations.

Barriers to exercise can be many for the person with Parkinson's disease, but the number one barrier may well be the inability to do the activity because of the movement difficulties. When prescribing exercise, careful consideration should be given to the ability of the person and the complexity of the program being prescribed. The more complex the program, the less likely the individual will adhere.

References

1. Marttila RJ. Diagnosis and epidemiology of Parkinson's disease. Auton Nerv Sys 1983;95(suppl):9–17.
2. Koller WC, Hubble JP. Classification of parkinsonism. In: Koller WC, ed. Handbook of Parkinson's disease. 2nd ed. New York: Marcel Dekker, Inc., 1992:59–103.
3. Yahr MD, Pang SWH. Movement disorders. In: Abrams WB, Berkow R, Fletcher AJ, et al., eds. The Merck manual of geriatrics. Rahway, NJ: Merck Sharp & Dohme Research Laboratories, 1990:973–994.
4. Caird FI. Parkinson's disease and its natural history. In: Caird FI, ed. Rehabilitation in Parkinson's disease. New York: Chapman & Hall, 1991:1–7.
5. Maguire GH. Occupational therapy. In: Abrams WB, Berkow R, Fletcher AJ, et al., eds. The Merck manual of geriatrics. Rathway, NJ: Merck Sharp and Dohme Research Laboratories, 1990:274–278.
6. Rajput AH. Current concepts in the etiology of Parkinson's disease. In: Schneider JS, Gupta M, eds. Current concepts in Parkinson's disease research. Seattle: Hagrefe & Huber Publishers, 1993:11–19.
7. Marttila RJ. Epidemiology In: Koller WC, ed. Handbook of Parkinson's disease. 2nd ed. New York: Marcel Dekker, Inc., 1992:35–57.
8. Marttila RJ, Rinne UK. Epidemiology of Parkinson's disease—an overview. J Neural Transm 1981;51:135–148.
9. Hennekens CH, Buring JE. Epidemiology in medicine. Boston: Little, Brown and Co., 1987:57.
10. Marttila RJ, Rinne UK. Epidemiology of Parkinson's disease in Finland. Acta Neurol Scand 1976;53:80–102.
11. Rajput AH, Offord, Beard CM, et al. Epidemiology of parkinsonism: incidence classification and mortality. Ann Neurol 1984;16:278–282.
12. Kessler II. Epidemiologic studies of Parkinson's disease II. A hospital-based survey. Am J Epidemiol 1972;95(4):308–318.
13. Kessler II. Epidemiologic studies of Parkinson's disease III. A community-based survey. Am J Epidemiol 1972;96(4): 242–254.
14. Kessler II, Diamond EL. Epidemiologic studies of Parkinson's disease I. Smoking and Parkinson's disease: a survey and explanatory hypothesis. Am J Epidemiol 1972;94(1): 16–25.
15. Hoehn M, Yahr MD. Parkinsonism: onset, progression, and mortality. Neurology 1967;17(5):427–442.
16. Diamond SG, Markham ChC. Present mortality in Parkinson's disease: the ratio observed to expected deaths with a

method to calculate expected deaths. J Neural Transm 1976; 36: 259–269.
17. Sweet RD, McDowell FH. Five years' treatments of Parkinson's disease with levodopa. Ann Intern Med 1975;83: 456–463.
18. Yahr MD. Evaluation of long-term therapy in Parkinson's disease. Mortality and therapeutic efficacy. In: Birkmayer W, Hornykiewicz O, eds. Advances in parkinsonism. Basle: Editiones Roche 1976:435–443.
19. Marttila RJ, Rinne UK, Siirtola T, et al. Mortality of patients with Parkinson's disease treated with levodopa. J Neurol 1977;216:147–153.
20. Schenkman M, Butler RB. A model for multisystem evaluation treatment of individuals with Parkinson's disease. Phys Ther 1989;69(11):932–943.
21. Stefaniwsky L, Bilowit DS. Parkinsonism: facilitation of motion by sensory stimulation. Arch Phys Med Rehab 1973; 54(2): 75–77.
22. Jankovic J. Parkinsonism—plus syndromes. Mov Disord 1989;4(suppl 1):S95–S119.
23. Gershanik OS, Nygaard TG. Parkinson's disease beginning before age 40. In: Streifler MB, Korcqyn AD, Melamed E, et al., eds. Advances in neurology: Parkinson's disease: anatomy, pathology, and therapy. New York, NY: Raven Press, Ltd., 1990;53:251–258.
24. Gerstenbrand F, Poewe WH. The classification of Parkinson's disease. In: Stern G, ed. Parkinson's disease. Baltimore, MD: John Hopkins University Press, 1990:315–331.
25. Fahn S, Elton RL, Members of the UPDRS Development Committee. Unified Parkinson's disease rating scale. In: Stanley F, Marsden CD, Goldstein M, et al, eds. Recent developments in Parkinson's disease volume II. Florham Park, NJ: MacMillan Healthcare Information, 1987:153–303.
26. Jankovic J, Marsden CD. Therapeutic strategies in Parkinson's disease. In: Jankovic J, Tolosa E, eds. Parkinson's disease and movement disorders. 2nd ed. Baltimore, MD: Williams & Wilkins, 1993:115–144.
27. Marttila RJ, Rinne RK. Disability and progression of Parkinson's disease. Acta Neurol Scand 1977;56:159–169.
28. Jankovic J, McDermott M, Carter J, et al. Variable expression of Parkinson's disease: a base-line analysis of the DATATOP cohort. Neurology 1990;40:1529–1534.
29. Tanner CM, Goetz CG, Klawans HL. Autonomic nervous system disorders. In: Koller WC, ed. Handbook of Parkinson's disease. New York, NY: Marcel Dekker, Inc., 1992:185–215.
30. Gupta M. Parkinson's disease pathology: multineurotransmitter systems defects. In: Schneider JS, Gupta M, eds. Current concepts in Parkinson's disease research. Seattle, WA: Hogufe & Haber Publishers, 1993:21–40.
31. Wichmann T, DeLong MR. Pathophysiology of parkinsonian motor abnormalities. In: Narabayashi H, Nagatau T, Yanagisawa N, et al, eds. Advances in neurology. New York, NY: Raven Press, Ltd., 1993;60:53–61.
32. Ludin SM, Steiger MJ, Ludin. Autonomic disturbances and cardiovascular reflexes in idiopathic Parkinson's disease. J Neurol 1987;235:10–15.
33. Piha SJ, Rinne UK, Rinne RK, et al. Autonomic dysfunction in recent onset and advanced Parkinson's disease. Clin Neurol Neurosurg 1988;90(3):221–226.
34. Wakabayashi K, Takahashi H, Takeda S, et al. Parkinson's disease: the presence of Lewy bodies in Auerbach's and Meissner's plexuses. Acta Neuropathol 1988;76:217–221.
35. Wakabayashi R, Takahashi H, Ohama E, et al. Parkinson's disease: an immunohistochemical study of Lewy body-containing neurons in the enteric nervous system. Acta Neuropathol 1990;79:581–583.
36. Wakabayashi K, Takahashi H, Takeda S, et al. Louie bodies in the enteric nervous system in Parkinson's disease. Arch Histol Cytol 1989;52(suppl 1):191–194.
37. Martignoni E, Micieli G, Cavallini A, et al. Autonomic disorders in idiopathic parkinsonism. J Neural Transm 1986; 22(suppl):149–61.
38. Duvoisin RC, Eldridge R, Williams A, et al. Twin study of Parkinson's disease. Neurology 1981;31:77–80.
39. Ward CD, Duvoisin RC, Ince SE, et al. Parkinson's disease in 65 pairs of twins and in a set of quadruplets. Neurology 1983;33:815–824.
40. Kondo K, Kurland LT, Schull WJ. Parkinson's disease, genetic analysis and evidence of a multifactorial etiology. Mayo Clin Proc 1973;48:465–475.
41. Marsden CD. Parkinson's disease in twins. J Neurol Neurosurg Psychiatry 1987;50:105–106.
42. Martilla RJ, Kaprio J, Kistenvuo MD, et al. Parkinson's disease in a nationwide twin cohort. Neurology 1988;38:1217–1219.
43. Duvoisin RC. Genetics of Parkinson's disease. Adv Neurol 1986;45:307–312.
44. Sonsalla PK, Nicklas WJ. MPTP and animal models of Parkinson's disease. In: Koller WC, ed. Handbook of Parkinson's disease. 2nd edition. New York, NY: Marcel Dekker, Inc., 1992:319–340.
45. Bindoff LA, Birch-Machin MA, Cartlidge NEF, et al. Mitochondrial function in Parkinson's disease. Lancet 1989: 2:49.
46. Blin O, Desnuelle C, Rascol O, et al. Mitochondrial respiratory failure in skeletal muscle from patients with Parkinson's disease and multiple system atrophy. J Neurol Sci 1994;125: 95–101.
47. Taylor DJ, Krige D, Barnes PRJ, et al. A^{31} P magnetic resonance spectroscopy study of mitochondrial function in skeletal muscle of patients with Parkinson's disease. J Neurol Sci 1994;125:77–81.
48. Schapira AHV, Cooper JM, Dexter DT, et al. Mitochondrial complex I deficiency in Parkinson's disease. Lancet 1989; 1:1269.
49. Ebadi M, Srinivasan SK, Baxi MD. Oxidative stress and antioxidant therapy in Parkinson's disease. Prog Neurobiol 1996;48: 1–19.
50. Hirsch EC. Does oxidative stress participate in nerve cell death in Parkinson's disease? Eur Neurol 1993;33(suppl 1):52–59.
51. Jenner P, Olanow CW. Oxidative stress and the pathogenesis of Parkinson's disease. Neurology 1996;47(suppl 3): S161–S170.
52. Olanow CW. An introduction to the free radical hypothesis in Parkinson's disease. Ann Neurol 1992;32(suppl): S2–S9.
53. Hurwitz LJ. Improving mobility in severely disabled parkinsonian patients. Lancet 1964:953–955.
54. Stern PH, McDowell F, Miller JM, et al. Levodopa and phys-

ical therapy in treatment of patients with Parkinson's disease. Arch Phys Med Rehab 1970;(5):273–277.

55. Gibberd FB, Page NGR, Spencer KM, et al. A controlled trial of physiotherapy for Parkinson's disease. In: Rose FC, Capildeo R, eds. Research progress in Parkinson's disease. Kent: Pitman Medical 1981:401–403.
56. Flewitt B, Capildeo R, Rose FC. Physiotherapy and assessment in Parkinson's disease using the polarised light goniometer. In: Research progress in Parkinson's disease. Rose FC, Capildeo R, eds. Kent: Pitman Medical 1981:404–413.
57. Palmer SS, Mortimer JA, Webster DD, et al. Exercise therapy for Parkinson's disease. Arch Phys Med Rehabil 1986;67: 741–745.
58. Banks MA, Caird FI. Physiotherapy benefits patients with Parkinson's disease. Clin Rehabil 1989;3:11–16.
59. Pedersen SW, Oberg B, Insulander A, et al. Group training in parkinsonism: quantitative measurements of treatment. Scand J Rehab Med 1990;22:207–211.
60. Comella CL, Stebbins GT, Brown-Toms N, et al. Physical therapy and Parkinson's disease: a controlled clinical trail. Neurology 1994;44:376–378.
61. Stanley RK, Protas EJ, Jankovic J. Exercise performance in those having Parkinson's disease and healthy normals. Med Sci Sports Exerc 1999;31(6):761–766.
62. Canning CG, Alison JA, Allen NE, et al. Parkinson's disease: an investigation of exercise capacity, respiratory function, and gait. Arch Phys Med Rehabil 1997;78:199–207.
63. Koseoglu F, Inan L, Ozel S, et al. The effects of a pulmonary rehabilitation program on pulmonary function tests and exercise tolerance in patients with Parkinson's disease. Funct Neurol 1997;12:319–325.
64. Reuter I, Engelhardt M, Stecker K, et al. Therapeutic value of exercise training in Parkinson's disease. Med Sci Sports Exerc 1999;31(11):1544–1549.
65. Kakinuma S, Hiroshi N, Pramanik B, et al. Muscle weakness in Parkinson's disease: isokenetic study of the lower limbs. Eur Neurol 1998;39:218–222.
66. Nogaki H, Kakinuma S, Morimatsu M. Movement velocity dependent muscle strength in Parkinson's disease. Acta Neurol Scand 1999;99:152–157.
67. Pedersen SW, Oberg B. Dynamic strength in Parkinson's disease. Eur Neurol 1993;33:97–102.
68. LeWitt PA, Bharucha A, Chitrit I, et al. Perceived exertion and muscle efficiency in Parkinson's disease: L-dopa effects. Clin Neuropharmacol 1994;17(5):454–459.
69. Corcos DM, Chen CM, Quinn NP, et al. Strength in Parkinson's disease: relationship to rate of force generation and clinical status. Ann Neurol 1996;39:79–88.
70. Berg MJ, Ebert B, Willis DK, et al. Parkinsonism—drug treatment: part I. Drug Intell Clin Pharm 1987;21(1):10–21.
71. Montgomery EB, Lipsy RJ. Treatment of Parkinson's disease. In: Geriatric pharmacology. Bressler R, Kane MD, eds. New York, NY: McGraw Hill, Inc., 1993:309–328.
72. Protas EJ, Stanley RK, Jankovic J. Parkinson's disease. In: ACSM's exercise management for persons with chronic diseases and disabilities. Champaign, IL: Human Kinetics, 1997:212–218.
73. Honey C, Gross RE, Lozano AM. New developments in the surgery for Parkinson's disease. Can J Neurol Sci 1999; 26(Suppl 2):S45–S52.
74. Arle JE, Alterman RL. Surgical options in Parkinson's disease. Med Clin North Am 1999;83(2):483–498.
75. Duncan PW, Weiner DK, Chandler J, et al. Functional reach: a new clinical measure of balance. J Gerontol 1990;45: M192–197.
76. Berg K, Wood-Dauphinee S, Williams JI, et al. Measuring balance in the elderly: preliminary development of an instrument. Physiother Can 1989;41(6):304–311.
77. Liston RAL, Brouwer BJ. Reliability and validity of measures obtained from stroke patient using the balance master. Arch Phys Med Rehabil 1996;77:425–430.
78. Studenski S, Duncan PW, Hogue C, et al. Progressive mobility skills: a mobility scale with hierarchical properties. In: American Geriatrics Society Annual Meeting, Boston MA, 1989;41.
79. American College of Sports Medicine. ACSM's guidelines for exercise testing and prescription. 6th ed. Baltimore, Lippincott Williams & Wilkins, 2000.
80. Schenkman M, Cutson TM, Kuchihhatla M, et al. Exercise to improve spinal flexibility and function for people with Parkinson's disease: a randomized, controlled trial. J Am Geriatr Soc 1998;46:1207–1216.
81. Thaut MH, McIntosh GC, Rice RR, et al. Rhythmic auditory stimulation in gait training for Parkinson's disease patients. Mov Disord 1996;11(2):193–200.
82. Dietz V, Colombo G. Influence of body load on the gait pattern in Parkinson's disease. Mov Disord 1998;13(2): 255–261.
83. Viliani T, Pasquetti P, Magnolfi S, et al. Effects of physical training on straightening-up processes in patients with Parkinson's disease. Disabil Rehab 1999;21(2):68–73.

CHAPTER **5**

Spinal Cord Dysfunction

Stephen F. Figoni, B. Jenny Kiratli, and Roy Sasaki

INTRODUCTION

In this chapter, the term "spinal cord dysfunction" (SCD) will represent either acquired spinal cord injury (SCI) or spina bifida (SB), both of which involve lesions on the spinal cord. It will not include poliomyelitis, postpolio, or postpolio syndrome (see chapter 6). Also, due to the continuity of the spinal cord and cauda equina in the spine, SCD will include both injury to the spinal cord itself (part of the central nervous system) and/or the cauda equina (part of the peripheral nervous system). The resulting damage to the neural elements within the spinal canal results in impairment or loss of motor and/or sensory function in the trunk and/or extremities. Depending on the neurological level and severity of the lesion, SCI may result in (a) "tetraplegia/-paresis" (formerly "quadriplegia/-paresis"—paralysis/weakness of upper and lower extremities) or (b) "paraplegia/-paresis" (paralysis/weakness of the lower extremities).

SCI is acquired after birth by trauma to or disease in the spinal cord. The resulting compression, contusion, or severance of the spinal cord or the associated spinal arteries cause spinal cord necrosis and dysfunction. This is in contrast to SB, which is a congenital neural tube defect in which the posterior arch of the spine fails to close during the first month of pregnancy. The most severe type of SB with functional consequences is "myelomeningocele," (1) where the spinal meninges and nerves herniate through an opening in the lumbar or sacral vertebrae, damaging the spinal cord (Fig. 5.1).

EPIDEMIOLOGY

Spinal Cord Injury

Most SCIs are acquired from trauma, with approximately 10,000 new SCIs/yr in the U.S. The incidence of SCI is approximately 30–40/million people in the population, with another 20/million (5000/yr) not surviving the initial injury. The highest per capita rate of SCI occurs between ages 16 and 30. An estimated 250,000–400,000 people with SCI live in the U.S., with about 80% being male. Mean age at time of injury is 33 yr (median 26, mode 19). Causes of traumatic SCI in the U.S. include motor vehicle accidents (44%), violence (24%), falls (22%), and sports (8%). An undetermined number also acquire SCI from diseases such as tumor, infection, and thrombosis. Approximately 50% of SCIs involve the cervical spine, 25% thoracic, 20% lumbar, and 5% sacral. About 45% of SCIs are "complete" with total loss of sensorimotor and autonomic function below the injury level. The remaining 55% are "incomplete" with partial loss. This proportion is increasing with improved emergency medical treatment. Approximately half of all SCIs result in tetraplegia, and this proportion increases with the age at onset (2, 3).

Spina Bifida

In the U.S., SB occurs in about 0.6 per 1000 live births and is steadily declining. At least 2000 children with SB are born annually in the U.S. Incidence is greatest among Hispanic-Americans, lower among Caucasian-Americans, and lowest among African-Americans. About 80% of SB cases involve myelomeningocele (1).

PATHOPHYSIOLOGY

Spinal Cord Injury

SCI results in impairment or loss of motor and/or sensory function in the trunk and/or extremities due to damage to the neural elements within the spinal canal. Injury to the cervical segments (C1–C8) or the highest thoracic segment (T1) causes tetraplegia/-paresis, with impairment of the arms, trunk, legs, and pelvic organs (bladder, bowels, and sexual organs). Injury to the thoracic segments T2–T12 causes paraplegia/-paresis, with impairment to the trunk, legs, and/or pelvic organs. Injury to the lumbar or sacral segments of the cauda equina (L1–S4) impairs the legs and/or pelvic organs. The neurological level and completeness of injury determines the degree of impairment. See Figure 5.2 for an illustration of spinal cord segmental innervation of muscles and other organs

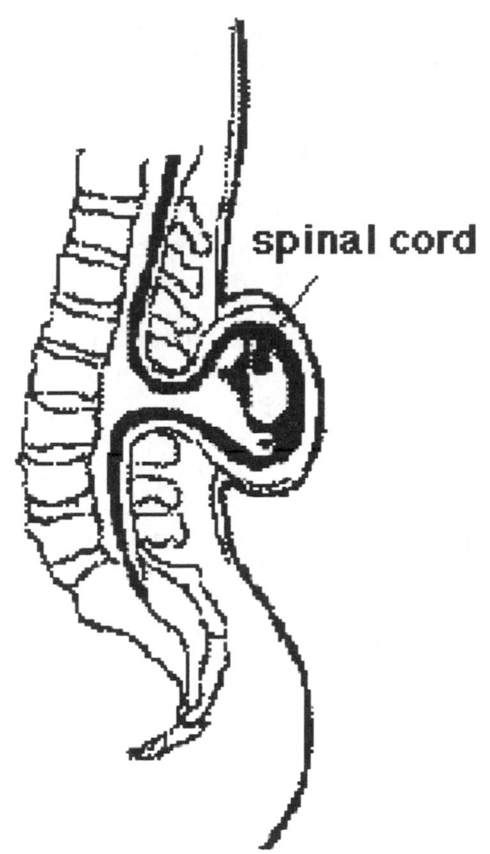

Figure 5.1. Lumbar myelomeingocele with spinal nerves and meninges protruding from the newborn's spine.

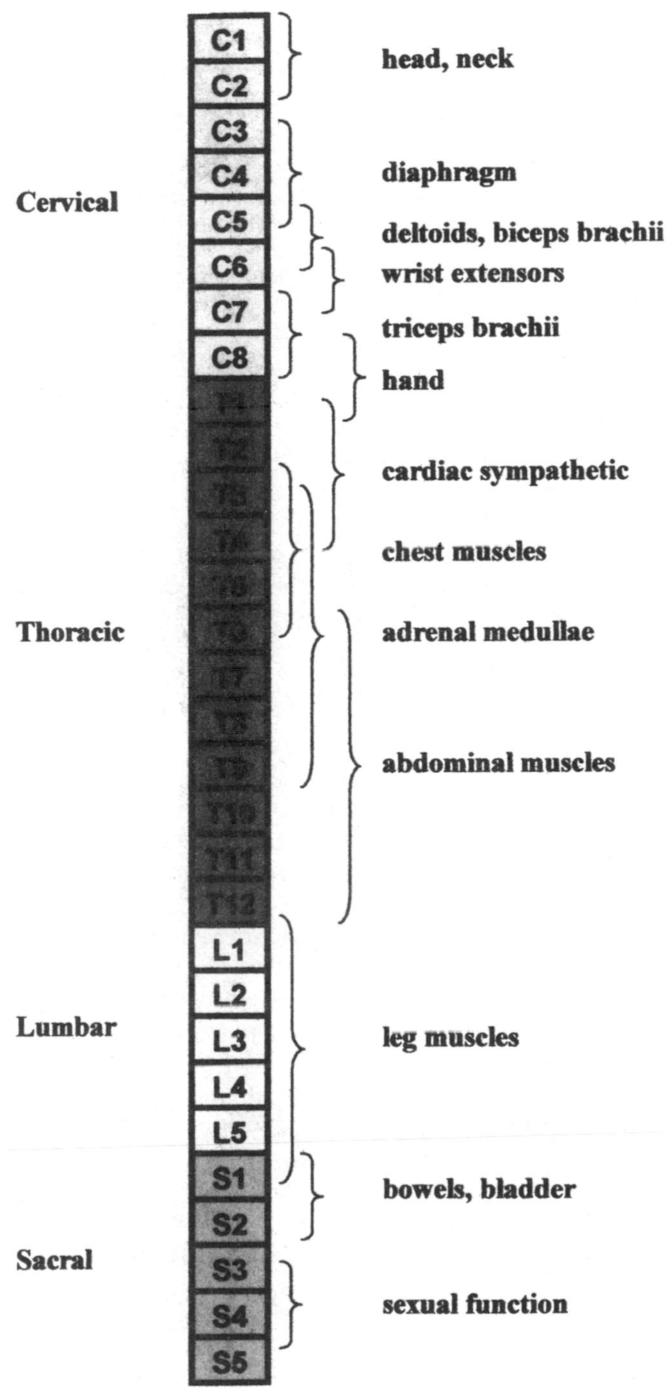

Figure 5.2. Segmental innervation of some key muscles and organs in spinal cord dysfunction.

(4, 5). The ASIA Impairment Scale in Table 5.1 is used to grade the degree of impairment or completeness at a given level (6, 7).

Physiological impairment from either acquired or congenital SCI may include sensory loss, muscular paralysis, and sympathetic nervous system impairment. These frequently impact the magnitude and quality of acute physiological responses to exercise and the ultimate trainability of the person with SCI. Basic anatomical and physiological impairments and residual functions are often summarized by physicians on the form shown in Figure 5.3 (6, 7).

Clinical SCI Syndromes

Six major SCI syndromes are recognized (7), usually associated with incomplete SCI or low-level paraplegia.

- **Brown-Sequard syndrome** results in relatively greater ipsilateral proprioceptive and motor loss and contralateral loss of sensitivity to pinprick and temperature.
- **Central cord syndrome** results from cervical cord lesion, spares sacral sensory function, and produces greater weakness in the upper limbs than in the lower limbs.
- **Posterior cord syndrome** produces loss of pinprick and temperature sensation, but largely preserves motor function and proprioception.
- **Anterior cord syndrome** results in profound motor loss, but may spare light touch and pressure sensation.
- **Conus medullaris syndrome** is an injury to the sacral cord (conus) and lumbar nerve roots within the spinal canal, usually resulting in an areflexic bladder, bowel, and lower limbs.

Table 5.1. ASIA Impairment Scale for Assessing the Severity of Spinal Cord Injury (6, 7)

CLASS	DESCRIPTION
A	Complete. No sensory or motor function is preserved in the sacral segments S4–5.
B	Incomplete. Sensory but no motor function is preserved below the neurological level and extends through the sacral segments S4–5.
C	Incomplete. Motor function is preserved below the neurological level, and the majority of key muscles below the neurological level have a muscle grade <3/5.
D	Incomplete. Motor function is preserved below the neurological level, and the majority of key muscles below the neurological level have a muscle grade ≥3/5.
E	Normal. Sensory and motor function is normal.

- **Cauda equina syndrome** is an injury to the lumbosacral nerve roots within the neural canal, resulting in an areflexic bladder, bowel, and lower limbs.

Immediate Neurological Consequences of SCI

1. Sensorimotor and autonomic function: (a) normal function above neurological level of lesion, (b) impaired function (flaccid paralysis) at the level of lesion, (c) impaired function (spastic paralysis) below the level of lesion (spasticity in skeletal and smooth muscles)—according to myotome and dermatome diagrams (see Figs. 5.2 and 5.3).
2. Expected levels of functional independence varies by level of lesion (8):
   - Tetraplegia: impaired lower and upper body, cardiac and adrenal sympathetic innervation, vasomotor paralysis, susceptibility to hypotension and autonomic dysreflexia, impaired cough.
   - Paraplegia: impaired lower body.
3. Spastic/flaccid bladder requires catheterization or urinary collection system for emptying and management, risk of urinary incontinence.
4. Bowel constipation, risk of bowel incontinence.
5. Bone demineralization/osteopenia, risk of fracture.

Secondary Conditions and SCI

Secondary medical conditions may further compromise the health and function of persons with SCI as they age. These conditions generally increase with time since SCI. The most prevalent secondary conditions are chronic pain, problematic spasticity, depression, obesity, urinary tract infections, and pressure sores (9–12). Many years of dependence on the upper extremities for daily activities (wheelchair and/or crutch use, and transfers) makes the shoulders, elbows, and wrists susceptible to overuse injury, tendon inflammation, joint degeneration, and pain. Severe spasticity can cause joint contractures and loss of range of motion. Paralysis of abdominal (expiratory) musculature impairs cough and increases susceptibility to respiratory infections. Frequent bladder infections and use of antibiotics can lead to kidney damage and systemic infection. Inactivity, hyperlipidemia, insulin resistance, and hypertension put long-surviving persons with SCD at risk for cardio- and cerebrovascular disease (13, 14).

Exercise-related Consequences of SCI

SCI can result in two major exercise-related problems: (a) reduced ability to perform large-muscle-group aerobic exercise voluntarily, i.e., without using functional electrical stimulation leg cycle ergometry (FES-LCE) with paralyzed leg muscles, and (b) the inability to stimulate the autonomic and cardiovascular systems to support higher rates of aerobic metabolism (15, 16). Therefore, catecholamine production by the adrenal medullae, skeletal muscle venous pump, and thermoregulation may be impaired, which restricts exercise cardiac output (CO) to subnormal levels. Hopman et al. (17) examined the properties of the venous vasculature in the lower extremities in persons with paraplegia. Compared with non-SCI subjects, they noted lower venous distensibility and capacity and higher venous flow resistance. They attributed these to vascular adaptations to inactivity and muscle atrophy rather than the effect of an inoperable leg muscle pump and sympathetic denervation.

Common secondary complications during exercise, especially in persons with tetraplegia, may include limited positive cardiac chronotropy and inotropy, excessive venous pooling, venous atrophy, orthostatic and exercise hypotension, exercise intolerance, and autonomic dysreflexia. This latter condition is a syndrome resulting from mass activation of autonomic reflexes causing extreme hypertension (arterial blood pressure ≥300/200 mm Hg), headache, bradycardia, flushing, gooseflesh, unusual sweating, shivering, and/or nasal congestion.

Tetraplegia usually results in a sedentary lifestyle with profound deconditioning of many physiological systems. This exacerbates mobility impairment, bone demineralization, skeletal muscle and myocardial atrophy, and changes in body composition such as decreased lean body mass, body water content, blood volume, and increased percentage of fat (18).

Spina Bifida

Immediate Neurological Consequences of SB

Infants with SB generally have surgery within 24 hours of birth to close the spinal malformation to minimize the risk of infection and prevent further neurological damage. About 80% of SB affects the lumbosacral nerve roots (1), resulting in damage to the lumbar and/or sacral segments of the cauda equina from L1 to S4. Like SCI at the same neurological level, SB usually results in sensorimotor and autonomic impairment to the legs and/or pelvic organs (bladder, bowels, and sexual organs). The exact neurological level and completeness of injury determines the degree of impairment (see Figures 5.2 and 5.3). Also like

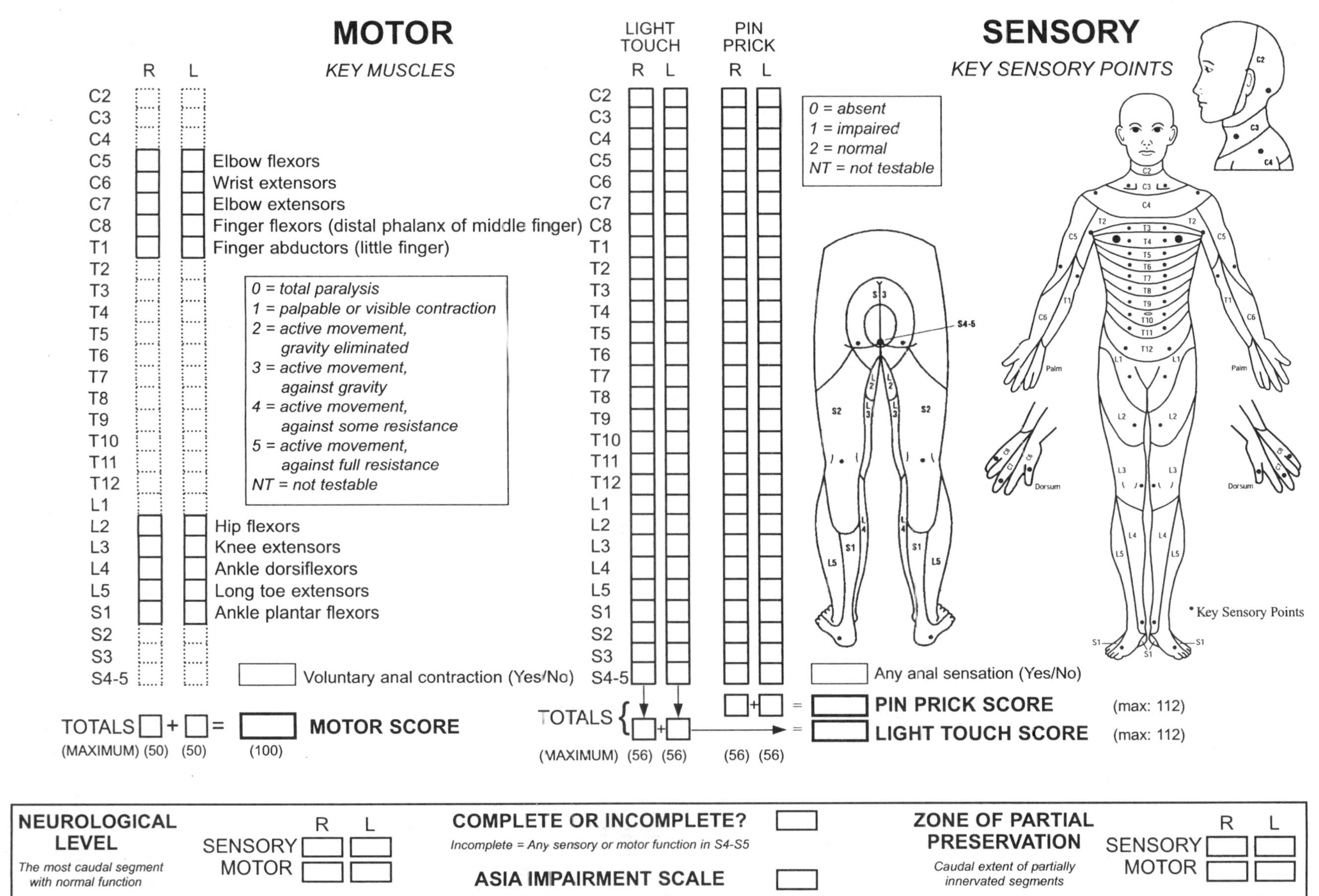

ASIA

STANDARD NEUROLOGICAL CLASSIFICATION OF SPINAL CORD INJURY

MOTOR

KEY MUSCLES

	R	L	
C2			
C3			
C4			
C5	☐	☐	Elbow flexors
C6	☐	☐	Wrist extensors
C7	☐	☐	Elbow extensors
C8	☐	☐	Finger flexors (distal phalanx of middle finger)
T1	☐	☐	Finger abductors (little finger)
T2			
T3			
T4			
T5			
T6			
T7			
T8			
T9			
T10			
T11			
T12			
L1			
L2	☐	☐	Hip flexors
L3	☐	☐	Knee extensors
L4	☐	☐	Ankle dorsiflexors
L5	☐	☐	Long toe extensors
S1	☐	☐	Ankle plantar flexors
S2			
S3			
S4-5			

0 = total paralysis
1 = palpable or visible contraction
2 = active movement, gravity eliminated
3 = active movement, against gravity
4 = active movement, against some resistance
5 = active movement, against full resistance
NT = not testable

☐ Voluntary anal contraction (Yes/No)

TOTALS ☐ + ☐ = ☐ **MOTOR SCORE**
(MAXIMUM) (50) (50) (100)

SENSORY

KEY SENSORY POINTS

	LIGHT TOUCH R	LIGHT TOUCH L	PIN PRICK R	PIN PRICK L
C2	☐	☐	☐	☐
C3	☐	☐	☐	☐
C4	☐	☐	☐	☐
C5	☐	☐	☐	☐
C6	☐	☐	☐	☐
C7	☐	☐	☐	☐
C8	☐	☐	☐	☐
T1	☐	☐	☐	☐
T2	☐	☐	☐	☐
T3	☐	☐	☐	☐
T4	☐	☐	☐	☐
T5	☐	☐	☐	☐
T6	☐	☐	☐	☐
T7	☐	☐	☐	☐
T8	☐	☐	☐	☐
T9	☐	☐	☐	☐
T10	☐	☐	☐	☐
T11	☐	☐	☐	☐
T12	☐	☐	☐	☐
L1	☐	☐	☐	☐
L2	☐	☐	☐	☐
L3	☐	☐	☐	☐
L4	☐	☐	☐	☐
L5	☐	☐	☐	☐
S1	☐	☐	☐	☐
S2	☐	☐	☐	☐
S3	☐	☐	☐	☐
S4-5	☐	☐	☐	☐

0 = absent
1 = impaired
2 = normal
NT = not testable

☐ Any anal sensation (Yes/No)

TOTALS ☐ + ☐ = ☐ **PIN PRICK SCORE** (max: 112)
☐ + ☐ = ☐ **LIGHT TOUCH SCORE** (max: 112)
(MAXIMUM) (56) (56) (56) (56)

NEUROLOGICAL LEVEL
The most caudal segment with normal function
SENSORY R ☐ L ☐
MOTOR R ☐ L ☐

COMPLETE OR INCOMPLETE? ☐
Incomplete = Any sensory or motor function in S4-S5

ASIA IMPAIRMENT SCALE ☐

ZONE OF PARTIAL PRESERVATION
Caudal extent of partially innervated segments
SENSORY R ☐ L ☐
MOTOR R ☐ L ☐

2000 Rev.

Figure 5.3. ASIA standard neurological classification of spinal cord injury (7).

SCI, the ASIA Impairment Scale in Table 1 can be used to grade the degree of impairment or completeness in SB at a given level (6, 7).

A frequent complication of SB is "hydrocephalus," occurring in about 90% of individuals with SB (1). SB impairs proper absorption and drainage of cerebrospinal fluid (CSF) and allows excessive accumulation of CSF in the ventricles of the brain. If ineffectively treated or left untreated, hydro-cephalus compresses the brain and causes brain damage and permanent cognitive impairment and learning disabilities. Most people with SB have a plastic shunt implanted to drain CSF from the ventricles of the brain under the skin into the chest or abdomen. Shunts will fail if they become obstructed; people with SB typically have their failed shunt replaced twice in their lifetime.

Presence of the Arnold-Chiari malformation may result in compression of the brain stem and cerebellum (1). Symptoms in children or adolescents may include neck pain, changes in sensorimotor function, or problems with swallowing, speech, or breathing. The only treatment is surgical decompression. Some may exhibit cerebellar dysfunction with dysmetria, fine motor incoordination, tremors, nystagmus, and ataxic gait. These individuals may experience difficulty with fine motor skills.

Spinal cord function must be closely monitored in people with SB. Changes in muscle tone or strength, rapidly progressing scoliosis, or changes in bowel or bladder function may indicate the presence of "hydromyelia" or "tethered cord" (1). In hydromyelia (or syringomyelia), a fluid cavity develops in the central canal of the spinal cord that further impairs neurological function. It could develop at any time or level, requiring surgical shunting of fluid. Spinal cord tethering is stretching of the spinal cord with longitudinal growth of the spine or with movement/exercise. When this occurs, surgical correction of tethering is necessary to prevent further spinal cord damage and loss of neurological function.

Secondary Conditions and SB

Unlike most people with SCI, SB survivors endure their condition over their entire life span. By the time children with SB reach adulthood, they usually have had multiple orthopedic and neurological surgeries that can compromise long-term functional status. If children with SB have walked with assistive devices for years, stress/strain on spinal and lower-extremity joints may require several orthopedic surgeries to correct deformities such as scoliosis, hip subluxation/dislocation, Achilles tendon contracture, and muscle imbalance (1). Scoliosis is reported to occur in 80% of people with SB and is treated often with spinal fusion. Similarly, lifelong wheelchair users may acquire upper-extremity overuse syndromes, such as carpel tunnel syndrome, tendinitis, and arthritis, further impairing their mobility. Osteoporosis is common in children and adults with flaccid paralysis of the lower extremities who use wheelchairs. Thus, they are vulnerable to painless fractures with symptoms such as local redness, deformity, or fever.

Like those with SCI, many people with SB need to pay close attention to skin care and hygiene. If the skin over the ischial tuberosities, greater trochanters, or sacrum is insensitive, then frequent weight shifts, pushups, seat cushioning, pressure relief, and cleanliness are necessary to prevent pressure sores on these areas. Also, chronic urinary tract infections over a lifetime may cause renal damage and failure, especially if bacteria become antibiotic-resistant.

Obesity is particularly prevalent as children with SB reach adolescence. Many children with SB are highly mobile with weight-bearing ambulation using braces and crutches. However, during adolescence, weight gain frequently interferes with and precludes efficient upright ambulation, forcing the person to use a manual wheelchair for mobility. This encourages further weight gain, inactivity, and the vicious cycle of deconditioning and declining health and functional independence. Wheelchair use also exposes the person to unusually high upper-extremity stresses, increasing his/her susceptibility to upper-extremity repetitive motion disorders. Special attention should be paid to weight management throughout adolescence and adulthood.

About 30% of persons with SB frequently have mild-to-moderate cognitive and/or learning disabilities necessitating special education (19). Many have low self-esteem, immature social skills, lack of initiative, and depression that make independent living difficult. Lifelong guidance, support, and medical/therapeutic follow-up may be necessary to maintain independence in the community.

Exercise-related Consequences of SB

If extensive lower-extremity paralysis is present, SB can result in reduced ability to perform large-muscle-group aerobic exercise voluntarily. Consequently, FES will not reactivate flaccidly paralyzed gluteal, hamstring, and quadriceps muscle groups; therefore, FES is not usually an option unless the neurological level of lesion is above L1. During aerobic exercise testing and training, ambulatory people with SB can probably walk/jog on a treadmill. On the other hand, people with SB who primarily use wheelchairs for mobility will require an exercise mode involving wheelchair treadmill exercise, wheelchair ergometry (WERG), arm-crank ergometry (ACE), or combined arm and leg ergometry to elicit maximal physiological responses.

Therapeutic exercises are recommended to maintain balanced strength and flexibility in the upper extremities. These are intended to help prevent upper-extremity overuse syndromes such as nerve entrapment syndromes and degenerative joint disease in lifelong wheelchair or crutch users (20).

About 70% of people with SB have an allergic hypersensitivity to latex (natural rubber) (1). Therefore, they should not touch exercise, clinical, or research equipment made of or covered with latex (e.g., elastic bands or tubing, rubber-coated dumbbells, latex gloves, blood pressure cuffs). If latex touches their skin or mucous membranes or enters their circulation, they react with watery eyes, wheezing, hives, rash, swelling, and in severe cases, life-threatening anaphylaxis.

Poor fitness and low physical activity have been documented among adults and youth with SCD (21, 22). Compared with peers with disability, adolescents with SCD have 27% lower handgrip strength, 47% greater skinfold thicknesses (i.e., higher body fatness), 65% lower VO_{2peak} (16 vs. 40 mL/kg/min), and very slow long-distance mobility times (23, 24).

CLINICAL EXERCISE PHYSIOLOGY

Acute Responses to Exercise

Spinal Cord Injury

Table 5.2 summarizes representative physiological responses during rest and peak arm ergometry (ACE or WERG) in two relatively large samples of adults with SCI. The data from Morrison et al. (25) are from subjects who were 6 mo after discharge from SCI rehabilitation. Notable differences among groups with different lesion levels are (a) blunted tachycardia in subjects with tetraplegia, (b) lack of pressor response and very low $\dot{V}O_{2peak}$ in subjects with tetraplegia and high-lesion paraplegia, (c) inverse relationship between lesion level and peak power output (PO), and (d) substantial variability of most responses. Also in Table 5.2, the data of Hjeltnes and Jansen (26) are from persons with long-standing SCI, i.e., 4–16 yr after SCI. Mean $\dot{V}O_{2peak}$ was substantially higher than in the Morrison et al. study (25). Higher $\dot{V}O_{2peak}$ was also strongly associated with higher functional mobility and lower incidence of secondary conditions such as chronic pain, spasticity, urinary tract infection, and osteoporosis.

Stewart et al. (27) factor-analyzed physiological and functional data on 102 subjects with SCI from the study by Morrison et al. (25). They concluded that the predominant fitness factor was "aerobic fitness and muscle strength/endurance" as indicated by high loadings on several peak physiological responses, followed by "blood pressure" (maintenance) and "general health."

Raymond et al. (28) compared cardiorespiratory responses during ACE to those during combined ACE and FES-leg cycle ergometry ("hybrid exercise") in seven subjects with T4–T12 paraplegia. FES-LCE involved 18% (35 vs. 30 W) higher PO than ACE alone. Compared with ACE

Table 5.2A. Mean ±SD Physiological Responses of 94 (ASIA class A-B) Adults with Spinal Cord Injury, 6 wk after Discharge from Rehabilitation, during Rest and Peak Arm Ergometry (25)

	HR (BPM)	SBP (MM HG)	DBP (MM HG)	$\dot{V}O_2$ (ML/KG/MIN)	$\dot{V}_E$ (L/MIN)	RPE (6–20)	PO (W)
REST							
Tetraplegia	83 ±16	98 ±16	66 ±13	—	—	—	—
High Paraplegia	92 ±19	104 ±12	72 ±11	—	—	—	—
Low Paraplegia	97 ±14	119 ±13	79 ±11	—	—	—	—
PEAK ARM ERGOMETRY							
Tetraplegia	117 ±16	95 ±22	65 ±14	8.3 ±2.9	30 ±12	17 ±2	34 ±11
High Paraplegia	152 ±29	107 ±30	67 ±13	8.9 ±2.6	36 ±11	17 ±2	51 ±15
Low Paraplegia	161 ±11	140 ±19	81 ±15	13.5 ±3.7	46 ±13	17 ±2	63 ±16

Mean age = 30 ±10 yr (range = 16–58): M = male, F = female.
Tetraplegia (C6–C8): n=24; 20 M, 4 F; mean ±SD body mass = 71 ±13 kg
High-lesion Paraplegia (T1–T5): n=15; 15 M, 13 F; mean ±SD body mass = 79 ±10 kg
Low-lesion Paraplegia (T6–L2): n=55; 42 M, 13 F; mean ±SD body mass = 71 ±18 kg

Table 5.2B. Mean ±SD VO_{2peak} (mL/kg/min) for 72 Women and Men with Long-standing SCI (26)

	TETRAPLEGIA (C5–C8)	HIGH PARAPLEGIA (T1–T6)	MID PARAPLEGIA (T7–T11)	LOW PARAPLEGIA (T12–L3)	VERY LOW PARAPLEGIA (L4–S2)	INCOMPLETE TETRAPLEGIA (C5–C8)	INCOMPLETE PARAPLEGIA (T1–L3)
FEMALES							
n	0	0	2	2	1	3	1
VO_{2peak}	—	—	23 ±1	23 ±2	40	20 ±5	12
MALES							
n	10	6	14	8	11	10	4
VO_{2peak}	14 ±5	17 ±6	26 ±8	28 ±7	24 ±7	23 ±11	23 ±7

alone, submaximal steady-state ACE + FES-LCE elicited 25% higher $\dot{V}O_2$ (1.58 vs. 1.26 L/min), 13% lower HR (132 vs. 149 bpm), and 42% higher O_2 pulse ($\dot{V}O_2$/HR, 12.2 vs. 8.6 L/b), with no differences in $\dot{V}_E$ or respiratory exchange ratio. These results demonstrate that during submaximal or maximal exercise, there was a greater metabolic stress elicited during combined arm and leg ergometry compared with arm ergometry. The higher cardiac stroke volume (SV) observed during submaximal combined arm and leg ergometry in the absence of any difference in HR implies reduced venous pooling and higher cardiac volume loading. These results suggest that training incorporating both arm and leg muscles may be more effective in improving aerobic fitness in people with paraplegia than ACE alone.

Paraplegia. In persons with paraplegia, the primary neuromuscular effect is paralysis of the lower body, precluding exercise modes such as walking, running, and voluntary leg cycling. Therefore, the upper body must be used for all voluntary activities of daily living (ADLs) and exercise: arm cranking, wheelchair propulsion, and/or ambulation with orthotic devices and crutches. The most common clinical exercise modes for exercise testing of persons with paraplegia are ACE and WERG. ACE is believed to be the more general exercise stressor and less likely to be influenced by the specific wheelchair skill of the user. It is the most available and standardized instrumentation for upper body exercise testing. WERG is specific to wheelchair propulsion, and if the person's own everyday or sports/racing wheelchair can be used for testing, it is also highly specific to the wheelchair task. WERGs are constructed by research laboratories and can take the form of a standardized wheelchair linked with a flywheel or rollers (29–31), or a wheelchair on a wide treadmill (32).

In paraplegia, the proportionally smaller active upper-body muscle mass typically restricts peak values of PO, $\dot{V}O_2$, and CO to approximately one-half of those expected for maximal leg exercise in individuals without SCI (16). Additionally, "circulatory hypokinesis," a reduced CO for any given $\dot{V}O_2$, has been reported by several investigators. Presumably, this condition is due to lack of the leg muscle pump to assist venous return during exercise, excessive venous pooling due to vasomotor paralysis, excessive skin perfusion to aid thermoregulation (33), and/or subnormal blood volume (34). The effect of this condition would be to impair delivery of O_2 and nutrients to and removal of metabolites and CO_2 from working muscles, facilitating muscle fatigue.

The most active people with SCI can achieve high upper body fitness levels. Veeger et al. (35) reported that the average peak PO, HR, and $\dot{V}O_2$ of 17 elite adult wheelchair athletes (basketball and track and field) were 93 W, 184 bpm, and 2.8 L/min (40 mL/kg/min) during maximal wheelchair treadmill exercise.

Tetraplegia. In persons with tetraplegia, the pathological effects on neuromuscular and autonomic function are more extensive than with paraplegia. The active upper body muscle mass will be partially paralyzed, and the sympathetic nervous system may be completely separated from control by the brain. Upper body PO, $\dot{V}O_2$, and CO are typically reduced to approximately one-half to one-third of those levels seen in individuals with paraplegia (36–38). In the upright sitting posture, peak HR, CO, SV, and arterial blood pressure (BP) are often subnormal for given levels of $\dot{V}O_2$ (39–41). Furthermore, strenuous exercise may not be tolerated due to orthostatic and exercise hypotension, which may produce overt symptoms of dizziness, nausea, etc. (42). Peak HRs for persons with tetraplegia typically do not exceed approximately 125 bpm due to small exercising muscle mass, impaired sympathetic adrenal and cardiac innervation, and vagal cardiac dominance (16).

Posture of subjects with tetraplegia affects peak hemodynamic and metabolic responses to ACE. Figoni et al. (43) compared peak physiological responses in supine vs. upright sitting postures in 11 subjects with tetraplegia. Supine posture produced higher PO by 39%, $\dot{V}O_2$ by 26%, CO by 20%, and SV by 14%, even though mean arterial pressure was lower (75 vs. 83 mm Hg). Pitetti et al. (32) observed higher peak $\dot{V}O_2$, pulmonary minute ventilation ($\dot{V}_E$), and PO during ACE and higher $\dot{V}O_{2peak}$ during treadmill wheelchair exercise in 10 men with tetraplegia using an anti-G suit to compress the abdomen and legs. Hopman et al. (44) also found 12% higher $\dot{V}O_{2peak}$ during supine ACE in five men with tetraplegia. These support the concept that excessive lower body venous pooling limits maximal arm exercise performance in this population with severe autonomic impairment.

Ready (45) studied acute responses of athletes with tetraplegia during prolonged ACE at 75% $\dot{V}O_{2peak}$ and found no changes in HR or skin/rectal temperatures across 10 exercise stages. They attributed the surprising lack of "cardiovascular drift" to lack of adequate muscle mass to increase body temperature and lack of skin vasodilation to compete with CO, thus maintaining a more stable SV.

Hooker et al. (46) compared acute physiological responses of eight subjects with tetraplegia performing moderate-intensity voluntary ACE, FES-LCE, and hybrid exercise. Although each mode elicited a $\dot{V}O_2$ of 0.66 L/min separately, the POs used to elicit this metabolic response were very different (arms 19 W vs. legs 2 W). This indicates markedly lower higher efficiency of over FES-LCE compared with voluntary ACE. Compared with ACE or FES-LCE, hybrid exercise elicited higher levels of $\dot{V}O_2$ (by 54%), $\dot{V}_E$ (by 33–53%), HR (by 19–33%), and CO (by 33–47%). Total peripheral vascular resistance during hybrid exercise was also lower (by 21–34%). Compared with ACE, FES-LCE and hybrid exercise produced higher SV by 41–56%.

Spina Bifida. Few investigators have reported physiological responses to exercise in children or adults with SB. Krebs et al. (47) observed the cardiorespiratory and perceptual/cognitive responses to a 6-min bout of moderate calisthenics in a small group of 9–12-yr-old children with SB. Besides normal increases in HR, $\dot{V}_E$, respiratory rate, and tidal volume, they noted acute improvements in peripheral vision, learning, and memory. Agre et al. (48) conducted aerobic and strength testing on 33 children and adolescents, ages 10–15, with SB of various functional levels. As shown in Table 5.3, peak $\dot{V}O_2$, HR, and $\dot{V}_E$ during walking or wheeling treadmill exercise varied inversely with functional level. Overall, the data suggest that people with SB respond similarly to people with SCI with comparable functional status.

Training Responses

Spinal Cord Injury

ADLs have been shown to require only 15–24% of their $HR_{reserve}$. This level of exertion is insufficient for developing physical fitness in people with SCD (49, 50). The exception was propulsion of a manual wheelchair up inclines or crutch walking, which elicited 50% $HR_{reserve}$, the equivalent to moderate exercise intensity. After acute inpatient SCI rehabilitation (mean of 76 days for paraplegia, 96 days for tetraplegia), the mean cardiovascular/ aerobic fitness ($\dot{V}O_{2peak}$) plateaus and remains stable for at least 8 wk (25).

Arm exercise training adaptations are believed to be primarily peripheral (muscular) in nature and may include increased muscular strength and endurance of the arm musculature in the exercise modes used. These may result in 10–60% improvements in peak PO and $\dot{V}O_2$ and an enhanced sense of well-being. However, central cardiovascular adaptations to exercise training, such as increased maximal SV or CO, have not yet been documented (51), suggesting that increases in $\dot{V}O_{2peak}$ are probably not due to central cardiovascular limitations, but increases in muscular strength and O_2 absorption/utilization by trained muscle tissue. People with paraplegia can expect increases in peak $\dot{V}O_2$ and PO approximately 20% through aerobic training with arm ergometry (51–55). Representative training studies are discussed below.

Arm Ergometry. Since 1973, several investigators have reported a variety of training effects of ACE or WERG in persons with SCI. Knutsson et al. (56) trained one group of SCI patients during initial rehabilitation with ACE 4–5 days/wk for 6 wk. A second similar group trained with calisthenics. Both groups increased peak ACE PO by about 40%.

Nilsson et al. (53) trained 12 people with paraplegia for 7 wk with both ACE and resistance training. Subjects increased their $\dot{V}O_{2peak}$ significantly by 0.20 L/min (10%), muscular strength by 16%, and muscular endurance (bench press) by 80%.

Davis et al. (51) compared training responses of nine men with SCI paraplegia to those of five controls without SCI. After 16 wk of arm ergometer exercise, heart rates of trained individuals were 9 bpm lower during isometric handgrip effort (30% of MVC for 3 min), with a substantial (20%) and decrease of rate-pressure product. Despite a significant increase of $\dot{V}O_{2peak}$ (19% and 31% after 8 and 16 wk, respectively), left ventricular mass and dimensions and indices of left ventricular performance at rest were unchanged by training. SVs were increased by 12–16% after training during submaximal and maximal ACE, with a trend toward higher peak CO. A short period of arm training was apparently insufficient to induce cardiac hypertrophy. An increase of SV with a decreased rate-pressure product, but no change in indices of left ventricular performance, implies improved myocardial efficiency. Possible explanations are a greater strength of the trained arms and increased cardiac preload.

Davis and Shephard (57) examined cardiorespiratory responses to four patterns of ACE training (@ 50/70% $\dot{V}O_{2peak}$, 20/40 min/session, 3 sessions/wk, 24 wk) in 24 initially inactive subjects with paraplegia. Training was associated with a significant increase of the $\dot{V}O_{2peak}$ during ACE tests except in control subjects and those combining a low intensity (50% peak) with short-duration training (20 min/ session). There were associated increases in SV during submaximal exercise. They suggest that the performance of inactive wheelchair users is limited by a pooling of blood in paralyzed regions, with a reduction of cardiac preloading.

Based upon the demonstrated hemodynamic advantages of arm exercise in the supine posture for people with tetraplegia (42), McLean and Skinner (58) conducted a 10-wk training study to compare training responses in each posture. Seven subjects with tetraplegia used ACE in the upright sitting posture, while another seven subjects used the supine posture. Both posture groups improved comparably: 0.08-L/min increase in $\dot{V}O_2$peak, 160% increase in arm exercise endurance, 7-mm decrease in the sum of four skinfolds, 5-bpm increase in resting HR, and nearly significant increase in peak HR.

Table 5.3. Mean ±SD Peak Physiological Responses and Usual Walking Speed of Children with Spina Bifida during Treadmill Walking or Wheeling (48)

Functional Level	$\dot{V}O_2$ (mL/kg/min)	HR (bpm)	$\dot{V}_E$ (L/min)	Usual Speed (km/hr)
L2 and above (n = 6)	17.7 ±3.8	167 ±9	32.6 ±6.7	1.9 (n = 1)
L3–L4 (n = 7)	20.2 ±3.8	172 ±9	36.4 ±6.7	3.5 ±0.6 (n = 5)
L5–S (n = 17)	29.6 ±2.2	186 ±5	49.1 ±3.8	3.9 ±0.3 (n = 16)
No motor deficit (n = 3)	41.6 ±5.3	202 ±12	63.6 ±9.4	4.8 ±0.7 (n = 3)

Lassau-Wray and Ward (59) compared the cardiorespiratory and metabolic responses to ACE in 25 men with cervical and thoracic SCIs and five controls without SCI. $\dot{V}O_{2peak}$ decreased progressively with increasing impairment (i.e., from subjects without SCI to paraplegia to tetraplegia). Great variability in maximum performance levels among groups were noted.

FES Leg Cycle Ergometry (FES-LCE). Several studies have documented physiological training effects of FES-LCE. Hooker et al. (60) trained 18 subjects with SCI for 12 wk with FES-LCE and noted higher posttraining peak PO (+45%), $\dot{V}O_2$ (+23%), $\dot{V}_E$ (+27%), HR (+11%), and CO (+13%) and lower total peripheral resistance (−14%). Nash et al. (61) trained eight subjects with tetraplegia using FES leg cycle ergometry for 6 mo and noted reversal of echocardiographically determined myocardial atrophy with the increased volume-load during exercise (62). Faghri et al. (63) reported FES-LCE training responses of seven subjects with tetraplegia and six subjects with paraplegia. Twelve weeks of LCE training resulted in a 270% increase in 30-min training PO (4.6 vs. 17.3 W). Resting HR, SBP, and SV increased in subjects with tetraplegia (suggesting more cardiovascular stability), whereas they decreased in subjects with paraplegia. SBP, DBP, and MAP responses decreased during submaximal exercise in both groups.

Janssen et al. (64) have summarized the training effects and clinical efficacy of training with FES-LCE. While many studies have documented physiological training effects, no randomized, controlled clinical trials have been conducted to determine efficacy or effectiveness of FES-LCE for improving health or functional status.

Combined Arm and Leg Ergometry. One group has trained SCI subjects using voluntary ACE combined with FES-LCE (hybrid exercise). Figoni et al. (65) trained 14 subjects with tetraplegia for 12 wk on an experimental hybrid ergometer and observed the following increases in peak responses: PO by 18% (40 vs. 47 W), $\dot{V}O_2$ by 18% (1.28 vs. 1.51 L/min), and $\dot{V}_E$ by 36% (49 vs. 66 L/min). No changes in peak cardiovascular responses (HR, SV, CO, or BP) were observed.

Resistance Training. Cooney and Walker (66) trained 10 SCI subjects (with tetra- or paraplegia) with hydraulic resistance exercise (3 sessions/wk, 9 wk @ 60–90 HR_{peak}). Mean peak PO and $\dot{V}O_2$ during ACE increased 28 and 37%, respectively. Also, Jacobs et al. (67) tested the effects of circuit resistance training on peak upperbody cardiorespiratory endurance and muscle strength in 10 men with T5–L1 SCI paraplegia. Subjects completed 12 wk of training, using isoinertial resistance exercises on a multistation gym and high-speed/low-resistance ACE. Peak arm ergometry tests, upper-extremity isoinertial strength testing, and testing of upper-extremity isokinetic strength were all performed before and after training. Subjects increased $\dot{V}O_{2peak}$ and peak PO by 30%. Increases in isoinertial muscular strength ranged from 12 to 30%. Increases in isokinetic strength were also observed for shoulder internal rotation, extension, abduction, adduction, and horizontal adduction.

Spina Bifida

Arm Ergometry. Ekblom and Lundberg (68) trained 10 adolescents (7 SB and 3 SCI, mean age 17 yr, 7 female and 4 male) with wheelchair exercise (30 min/session, 2–3 sessions/wk, 6 wk). Although $\dot{V}O_{2peak}$ (1.1 L/min) did not change, peak PO increased by 5.5 W (10%) to 60 W.

Resistance Training. Although no resistance exercise training studies are published that utilized adults with only SB, a few small-scale studies have documented training responses of children/adolescents with SB. Andrade et al. (24) found that a 10-wk exercise program significantly increased cardiovascular fitness, isometric muscle strength, and self-concept in eight children with spina bifida compared with control children. Also, O'Connell and Barnhart (69) resistance-trained three children (ages 4, 5, and 16) with thoracic SB. Training consisted of seven upperbody exercises using free weights: 30 min/session, 3 sets × 6-repetition maximum (RM), 3 sessions/wk for 9 wk. All children improved 6-RM muscular strength by 70–300%, 50-m dash time by 20%, and 12-min wheelchair propulsion distance by 29%. Thus, similar to youth without SCD, resistance training results in improved strength and general fitness.

PHYSICAL EXAMINATION

To adequately design a program for the participant with SCD, a systematic neurological examination of the sensory and motor function is required. A well-defined sequence is provided in the International Standards for Neurological and Functional Classification of Spinal Cord Injury (6). Beyond motor and sensory evaluation, attention must be paid to joint range of motion (ROM), spasticity status, and skin integrity. Programs will need to be tailored depending on contracture status, severe spasticity or flaccidity, and the presence of open pressure sores in weight-bearing areas. Some people with SCI require comprehensive pain management for chronic dysesthetic, spinal, or upper-extremity overuse syndromes. These and other functional tests (70, 71) may include joint flexibility/range of motion; manual muscle testing to determine muscle imbalance and risk of contracture; testing of reflexes, muscle tone, and spasticity; equipment evaluation (wheelchair and cushion, assistive/orthotic devices); home evaluation for accessibility and modification; and psychological evaluation to promote adjustment/coping and to assess/control depression and substance abuse. Due to susceptibility to pressure sores, people with SCD also need to perform frequent inspections of insensitive weight-bearing skin areas to assess skin integrity.

MEDICAL AND SURGICAL TREATMENTS

Multiple medical, nursing, and allied health professional services are utilized during SCD (re)habilitation (73). Shortly after injury, neurosurgery and/or orthopedic surgery are usually necessary to stabilize spinal fractures/dislocations. Internal fixation devices and fusion (rodding, plating, screws, bone grafts) are often necessary to accomplish this after traumatic SCI. The instrumentation and postsurgical healing must be adequate to withstand exercise demands. External spinal orthoses such as halo and other spinal orthoses are common for several weeks after surgery to stabilize the healing spine. Other orthopedic injuries often acquired during traumatic SCI include limb fracture and closed head injury.

Physiatrists coordinate the rehabilitation team (73). Typically, physical therapists, occupational therapists, and/or kinesiotherapists mobilize patients as soon as possible after SCI to restore tolerance of upright posture, joint flexibility/range of motion, muscular strength, and independence in ADLs (bed and mat mobility, transfers, wheelchair propulsion, ambulation, orthotic self-care activities such as dressing, eating, grooming). They also provide adapted driver education/training, home exercise programs, referral to community fitness programs, and prescribed self-care equipment and assistive technology, including a wheelchair with cushion. Nursing coordinates inpatient personal care, education, and follow-up, especially bowel, bladder, and hygienic concerns. Therapeutic recreation contributes to community reintegration through leisure counseling, social activities, and sports. Other rehab team members include the dietician for nutrition assessment and education and the social worker for planning about financial, discharge, placement, and family/social support issues. A vocational rehabilitation specialist will deal with reemployment training/education. Patients with orthostatic hypotension may use abdominal binders and compression stockings, which may affect exercise options.

A urologist will treat bladder dysfunction with medications and/or surgery to improve bladder filling/emptying and urinary drainage. Further, a careful history of adequate bowel and bladder management should be obtained. These programs should be well managed prior to initiation of exercise therapy. A detailed history of the patient's autonomic dysreflexia status should be investigated, including identification of known stimuli in order to prevent exacerbating the condition with exercise. Also, any implanted device, including cardiac pacemakers, intrathecal pumps, and FES devices, should be checked for adequate functional status and to be sure that the system/device does not preclude exercise interventions.

PHARMACOLOGY

Table 5.4 summarizes medications commonly used by people with SCD (72). These fall into three classes: spasmolytics (antispasticity, e.g., baclofen and Valium) and antithrombics (anticoagulation, e.g., warfarin), and antibiotics (e.g., Bactrim). Neurogenic bladder treatment may require alpha-blocking agents that induce hypotension, especially in persons with tetraplegia (73). Persons with a history of deep venous thrombosis may be taking warfarin, which leads to easy bruisability. Aging persons with SCD are at risk for cardiovascular disease and may take medications for hypertension, diabetes, dyslipidemia, dysrhythmia, and congestive heart failure.

DIAGNOSTIC PROCEDURES

The participant's file should include baseline radiographs (including plain x-rays, scans for osseous tissue, and MRIs for soft tissues) showing adequacy of spinal alignment and integrity of internal stabilization. Baseline pulmonary function tests are necessary for those with tetraplegia or tetraparesis. The nature and extent of the changes in ventilatory function and cough depend to a great extent on level of neurological injury/dysfunction. Electrocardiograms and myocardial perfusion tests should be obtained as baseline evaluations of the participant's cardiac status. Also, laboratory analysis of baseline hematological and metabolic status would be useful, including a complete blood count, electrolytes, renal indices, thyroid and liver function, lipid panel, fasting blood sugar, and glucose tolerance. Urodynamic evaluation is necessary to assess bladder responses to filling and emptying (e.g., voiding cystourethrogram). Finally, because osteoporosis is common below the level of injury in SCD and with immobilization in other conditions, one may consider evaluation of bone mineral status (bone densitometry) as part of the initial workup.

EXERCISE/FITNESS/FUNCTIONAL TESTING

Guidelines

During (re)habilitation of persons with SCD, functional testing takes priority over physiological testing to promote functional independence at the fastest rate possible. For example, (re)habilitation goals usually include independent mobility via weight-bearing or wheelchair ambulation, transfers, and self-care with or without assistive devices. The fitness requirements of these tasks are specific to the functional tasks themselves. The cardiovascular and metabolic demands of walking and wheelchair ambulation are the greatest of all functional tasks, hence, the importance of exercise tolerance and capacity during (re)habilitation. Aerobic fitness is necessary for long-distance mobility, some recreational activities, competitive sports, and long-term cardiovascular health. However, neuromuscular coordination/skill, balance/stability, and muscular strength/endurance are necessary to various degrees for safe standing, ambulation, transfers, driving, and other self-care activities.

Table 5.5 lists relative and absolute contraindications for cardiovascular exercise testing of persons with SCD. These are the same as for people without disabilities and include several disability-specific conditions.

When considering a cardiovascular exercise test for a person with SCD, consult a medical or allied health professional with experience in adapted exercise testing

Table 5.4. Common Medications in People with SCD (72)

Brand Name	Generic Name	Daily Dosage	Action	Therapeutic Purpose	Exercise Side Effects
			Spasmolytics		
Dibenzyline	phenoxybenzamine	20–40 mg, BID/TID	long-acting adrenergic alpha-receptor blocking agent	relax bladder smooth muscle, prevent autonomic dysreflexia	tachycardia, hypotension, palpitations
Ditropan	oxybutynin hydrochloride	5–15	direct spasmolytic and antimuscarinic (atropine-like) effect on bladder smooth muscle	facilitate bladder filling and emptying	tachycardia, hypotension
Lioresal	baclofen	20–80	centrally acting GABA agonist	decrease spasticity	CNS depression, hypotension
Valium	diazepam	15–30	centrally acting, facilitates postsynaptic effects of GABA	decrease spasticity	transient CV depression, sedation, dizziness, incoordination
Dantrium	dantolene sodium	50–400	decrease calcium release from sarcoplasmic reticulum at neuromuscular junction in spinal cord	decrease spasticity	sedation, dizziness, weakness
Catapres	clonidine hydrochloride	1–2 mg	centrally acting alpha-2 adrenergic antagonist	decrease spasticity	hypotension, bradycardia
Zanaflex	tizanidine hydrochloride	8 mg/8 hr	alpha-2 adrenergic antagonist	decrease spasticity	mild sedation
			Antithrombotic/coagulants		
Coumadin	warfarin	—	blood anticoagulation	prevent/treat blood clots	hemorrhage, bruisability
Heparin	heparin sodium	100 units/kg/ 4 hr via IV	blood anticoagulation	prevent/treat blood clots	hemorrhage, bruisability
			Antibiotics		
Bactrim	cotrioxazole (sulfamethoxazole-trimethoprim)	800 mg tablet PO q 12 hr × 14 days	Inhibits formation of dihydrofolic acid from PABA, bacteriocidal	prevent/treat urinary tract infections	none

techniques relevant to such persons. Use advice from the person with SCD concerning exercise modes and proper positioning/strapping. Adapt the exercise equipment as needed, and provide for the following special needs (74):

1. Trunk stabilization (straps)
2. Securing hands on crank handles (holding gloves)
3. Skin protection (seat cushion and padding)
4. Prevention of bladder overdistension (i.e., empty bladder or urinary collection device immediately before test)
5. Vascular support to help maintain low BP and improve exercise tolerance (elastic stockings and abdominal binder)
6. Use an environmentally controlled thermoneutral or cool laboratory or clinic to compensate for impaired sweating and thermoregulation. If necessary, use fans and water for compresses, misting, and hydration.
7. Design a discontinuous incremental testing protocol that allows monitoring of both HR, BP, RPE, and exercise tolerance at each stage. PO increments may range from 1 to 20 W, depending on exercise mode, level and completeness of injury, and training status.
8. Expect peak PO for persons with tetraplegia to range from 0 to 50 W and 50 to 150 W for persons with paraplegia.
9. Treat postexercise hypotension and exhaustion with rest, recumbency, leg elevation, and fluid ingestion.

Aerobic Exercise Test Protocols

A. Field Tests

1. University of Toronto Arm Crank Protocol (15, 75): This field test is a discontinuous submaximal protocol to predict $\dot{V}O_{2peak}$ from submaximal HR responses to arm-crank ergometry. Subjects performed three 5-min exercise stages at approximately 40, 60 and 80% of age-predicted HR_{peak} with 2-min rest periods between stages. HR was monitored continuously and recorded during the last 10 s of each stage. Based on laboratory assessment of $\dot{V}O_{2peak}$ in 49 subjects with lower-limb disabilities including tetraplegia and paraplegia, the

Table 5.5. Disability-specific Relative and Absolute Contraindications for Exercise Testing of Persons with Spinal Cord Injury (SCI) and Spina Bifida (SB)

	SCI		
RELATIVE	**T**	**P**	**SB**
Asymptomatic hypotension	X		
Muscle and joint discomfort	X	X	X
ABSOLUTE			
Autonomic dysreflexia	X		
Severe or infected skin pressure sore on weight-bearing skin areas	X	X	X
Symptomatic hypotension (dizziness, nausea, palor, extreme fatigue, visual disturbance, confusion)	X		
Illness due to acute urinary tract infection	X	X	X
Uncontrolled spasticity or pain	X	X	X
Unstable fracture	X	X	X
Uncontrolled hot humid environments	X		
Inability to safely seat and stabilize the person on well-cushioned/padded ergometers or equipment	X	X	X
Insufficient range of motion to perform exercise task	X	X	

T = tetraplegia; P = paraplegia; X = special relevance to SCI (T or P) or SB.

following regression equations were developed to predict $\dot{V}O_{2peak}$ in L/min; for males: $\dot{V}O_{2peak} = 0.018 \times$ (Arm-crank power output in watts) + 0.40 (r = 0.88, SEE = 0.20 L/min); for females: $\dot{V}O_{2peak} = 0.017 \times$ (Arm-crank power output in watts) + 0.37 (r = 0.85, SEE = 0.15 L/min). The coefficient of variation of individual differences between direct and predicted values was 12.5% for males and 14.5% for females.

2. Franklin et al. (76) developed a wheelchair field test to estimate $\dot{V}O_{2peak}$. Thirty male adult wheelchair users (mean age 34 yr) performed an arm-crank $\dot{V}O_{2peak}$ test in a laboratory and a 12-min maximal wheelchair propulsion test for distance using a standardized lightweight wheelchair (Quickie II) on a 0.1-mile indoor synthetic track. The mean peak PO, $\dot{V}O_2$ and wheelchair propulsion distance were 89 W, 22 mL/kg/min, and 1.11 miles, respectively. The following regression equation was developed to predict $\dot{V}O_{2peak}$ in mL/kg/min: $\dot{V}O_{2peak}$ = (Distance in miles − 0.37) ÷ 0.0337; r = 0.84.
3. Pare et al. (77) developed a regression equation to predict $\dot{V}O_{2peak}$ from submaximal wheelchair ergometry PO in 35 adults with SCI paraplegia: $\dot{V}O_{2peak}$ in L/min = (0.02 × Peak PO in watts) + 0.79; r = 0.80, SEE = 0.22 L/min). Prediction improved slightly when predicted $\dot{V}O_{2peak}$, %HR_{peak}, and body mass were included in the equation, but they admitted great variability among subjects.

B. Laboratory Tests

Generally, graded exercise testing for people with SCD involves discontinuous arm-crank ergometry protocols with 5–6 stages/test, 2–4 min/stage, and an initial stage of 0–20 W (warm-up). PO increments must be appropriate for the individual, depending upon his/her functional level of SCI, muscular strength, and conditioning level. Most persons with tetraplegia require very small PO increments (5–10 W/stage). People with paraplegia may require PO increments of 10–20 W/stage. If deconditioned, PO increments may be lower. Allow 2–3-min rest periods between stages to prevent premature fatigue and to allow monitoring of HR, ECG, BP, RPE, and symptoms. After the test, allow several minutes for cool-down and recovery, especially if the subject experienced symptoms of hypotension or severe exhaustion (74). Similar protocols have been utilized by Glaser et al. (78, 79), Kofsky et al. (75), Franklin et al. (76), and Morrison et al. (25).

Fitness Testing

Winnick and Short (23) have published detailed physical fitness assessment protocols and standards for youths with SCD, ages 10–17. The recommended test items include the "Target aerobic movement test" (80); triceps skinfold or triceps + subscapular skinfolds for body composition; reverse curl, seated push-up, and dominant handgrip; modified Apley and Thomas tests; and target stretch tests adapted for specific joint motions for musculoskeletal functioning. No such standardized tests exist for adults with SCD, but the above items could be adapted for adults. The field tests of Kofsky et al. (75) and Franklin et al. (76) can also be useful for estimating $\dot{V}O_{2peak}$ from arm-crank ergometry or wheelchair propulsion performance.

Functional Testing

During rehabilitation, the Functional Independence Measure (8, 81) is used most often to assess functional independence. Different versions exist for adults and children with SCD. A variety of other functional outcome measures in SCI rehabilitation are discussed by Cole et al. (82). HR responses and timed performances of various daily living functional tasks such as mobility and transfers are also used to reflect functional status (25, 47, 48).

EXERCISE PRESCRIPTION AND PROGRAMMING

General Guidelines

Little research is available to support specific training guidelines, but the following are offered largely out of clinical, recreational, and research experience of the authors, their professional colleagues, and people with SCD. It is hoped that these guidelines can contribute to the development of safe, effective, and standardized methods for (re)habilitative exercise evaluation/treatment and long-term fitness services and sports programming for people with SCD:

1. *Exercise modes:* Aerobic cardiopulmonary training modes may include ACE, WERG, wheelchair propulsion on extra-wide treadmill or rollers; free wheeling over ground; swimming and other aquatic exercises; vigorous sports such as wheelchair basketball, quad rugby, and wheelchair racing; arm-powered cycling; seated aerobic exercises; FES-LCE, with or without ACE; and vigorous ADLs, such as ambulation with assistive devices.
2. *Regulation of exercise:* In general, using HR to gauge exercise intensity for the SCD population is problematic due to the poor relationships between HR, $\dot{V}O_2$, and symptoms (83, 84). Discrepancies are attributable to varying amounts of active muscle mass, completeness of spinal cord lesion, levels of spinal neurological function, and autonomic control of HR and hemodynamics. However, within individuals, the relationship between HR and $\dot{V}O_2$ is likely to be more predictable and may be useful to guide exercise training intensity. Janssen et al. (49) and Dallmeijer et al. (50) have used percentage of HR reserve successfully to gauge the relative exercise intensity (physical strain) of various daily activities and exercise performance relative to individually determined HR_{peak} values. With continuous HR monitoring, $\%HR_{reserve}$ can be calculated as follows: $\%HR_{reserve} = (HR_{peak} - HR_{observed}) \div (HR_{peak} - HR_{rest}) \times 100$.

   If accurate HR monitoring is not possible, the Borg CR-11 rating of perceived exertion (RPE) scale (85) can be used to obtain a reliable estimate of relative exercise intensity. Therefore, "moderate"-intensity exercise would be perceived as RPE = 3, "strong" as RPE = 5, "very strong" as RPE = 7, "extremely strong" as RPE = 10, and "absolute maximum" as RPE = 11. As exercise tolerance and fitness improves through training, the exerciser performs at higher POs while reporting the same RPE values.
3. *Environment:* For training, use an environmentally controlled, thermoneutral or cool gym, lab, or clinic for persons with tetraplegia. Individuals with impaired thermoregulation can exercise outdoors if provisions are made for extreme conditions. If necessary, drink fluids before, during, and after exercise. Exercise only in thermally neutral environments such as in a laboratory or clinic with air-conditioning to control temperature and humidity, especially for persons with tetraplegia.
4. *Safety:*
   - Always supervise persons with SCD, especially those with SCI tetraplegia.
   - If they are not exercising in their wheelchairs, two people may be necessary for manual transfer of large individuals to/from exercise equipment.
   - A person with tetraplegia may need assistance to perform an exercise, to adjust machines and selected weights, and to perform flexibility exercises.
   - Follow all disability-specific precautions concerning skin, bones, stabilization, handgrip, bladder, bowels, illness, hypo-/hypertension, pain, orthopedic complications, and medications. For individuals with tetraplegia who are susceptible to orthostatic and exercise hypotension, monitor BP and symptoms regularly. Be prepared to reposition a symptomatic hypotensive person with tetraplegia to a more recumbent posture, and apply support stockings and abdominal binder to help maintain BP.
   - To prevent and treat upper-extremity overuse syndromes, vary exercise modes from week to week, strengthen muscles of the upper back and posterior shoulder (especially shoulder external rotators), and stretch muscles of anterior shoulder and chest.
   - Emptying the bladder or urinary collection device immediately beforehand may prevent dysreflexic symptoms during exercise. People with tetraplegia should *not* "boost" (i.e., self-induce "controlled" autonomic dysreflexia) during exercise to improve exercise tolerance (i.e., prevent hypotension) due to the danger of stroke and renal infection/damage.
5. *Follow-up:* Consult a physician and appropriate nursing/allied health personnel to answer specific questions concerning medical complications to which the persons with SCD may be susceptible.
6. *Training principles:* Following the universal training principles is necessary for achieving training outcomes.
   - Specificity: Focus exercise training activities on functional tasks to improve mobility and increase general lifestyle physical activity for health. Include all components of fitness: flexibility, muscular

strength/endurance, aerobic fitness, and coordination for high-skill functional or recreational tasks. For aerobic training, the greater the exercising muscle mass, the greater the expected improvements in all physiological and performance parameters. Arm training may prevent profound deconditioning, but will probably only induce peripheral training effects in the arm muscles. Combined arm and leg ergometry or exercise may induce both muscular and central cardiopulmonary training effects.

- Overload: Perform exercise at a higher intensity, duration, and/or frequency than that to which the person is accustomed. Fine-tune these according to feedback from the exerciser's subsequent soreness, etc.
- Progression: Expect small absolute (peak PO or $\dot{V}O_2$) improvements. Health maintenance and prevention of secondary conditions are essential for progressing to high levels of fitness for sports and optimal functional performance.
- Regularity: Exercise every week for at least 2–3 sessions/wk as per ACSM recommendations (86). Plan to continue the exercise training program indefinitely. Fulfill the ACSM-CDC recommendation of at least 30 min of daily, moderate, and varied physical activities.

Exercise Prescription

Useful exercise prescriptions specify the modes, frequency, intensity, and duration of exercises for an individual with known abilities and needs. Due to the diverse functional presentations of SCD and varying fitness goals, it is impossible specify these parameters. However, approximations for beginners and advanced exercisers with SCD are listed in Table 5.6.

EDUCATION AND COUNSELING

Coyle and Kinney (87) indicated that leisure satisfaction was the most important and significant predictor of life satisfaction among adults with disability. Edwards (88) noted that the leading two services desired but not received by individuals following SCI were planning an exercise program (43%) and providing a referral to a fitness center (26%). Moreover, the ability to meet the physical and psychosocial needs of the person affected by SCD is

Table 5.6. Components of the Beginning and Advanced Exercise Prescription for Persons with Spinal Cord Dysfunction

COMPONENT	BEGINNING (MINIMUM)	ADVANCED (MAXIMUM)
Flexibility		
Modes	Static or dynamic stretching, standing frame	Partner stretching, PNF stretching (contract-relax, etc.), standing frame
Joint motions	Scapular adduction, shoulder horizontal abduction and extension, elbow extension, hip extension, knee extension, ankle dorsiflexion	
Frequency	Daily	Twice daily
Intensity	Moderate	Moderate
Duration	30 s/stretch, 10 min/session	30 s/stretch, 30 min/session
Muscular Strength		
Modes	Active assistive, dumbbells, wrist weight, body weight resistance, elastic bands/tubing	Resistance machines, barbells, Smith machine, medicine ball, high-speed isokinetics, plyometrics
Muscle groups	Scapular depressors, elbow extensors, latissimus dorsi, etc. (all innervated muscle groups in balance, if possible)	
Frequency	2 x/wk	Daily
Intensity	15-RM	1–10-RM
Duration	1 set × 15 reps/exercise × 5 exercises	2–3 sets × 1–10 reps/exercise × 15 exercises
Muscular Endurance		
Modes	Same as above for muscular strength, aquatics	Same as above for muscular strength, circuit training, medicine ball
Muscle groups	Same as for muscular strength	Same as above for muscular strength
Frequency	2 ×/wk	Daily
Intensity	Moderate (RPE = 4/11)	Maximal (RPE = 10/11)
Duration	1 set × 1 min/exercise	2–3 sets × 2–5 min/exercise
Aerobic/Cardiopulmonary Fitness		
Modes	Walking, wheeling, seated/standing aerobics, arm/leg cycling, swimming, rowing	Fast walking/jogging/wheeling, arm/leg cycling, swimming, racing, rowing, sports, interval training, fartlek, long distance
Frequency	2 w/wk	1–2 daily
Intensity	Moderate (RPE = 3/11)	Moderate-extremely strong (RPE = 3–10)
Duration	5 min/session	60+ min/session
Coordination/Skill		
Modes	Skill-specific	Skill-specific
Frequency	Daily	Twice daily
Intensity	Low (avoid fatigue)	Low (avoid fatigue)
Duration	20 min/session	60+ min/session

critical to the pursuit of independent productivity (89). However, Figoni et al. (90) identified multiple barriers and inaccessibility of fitness facilities and services. These findings underscore the need for rehabilitation and exercise providers to promote lifelong fitness, to provide instruction and guidelines, and to refer to accessible fitness centers to assist in meeting the identified needs of this population.

With the decline in the duration and reimbursement of (re)habilitation services (91) and the scarcity of frequent adapted physical education in schools, more and more people with SCD are seeking community-based exercise/fitness opportunities (92). Since many people with SCD are marginally independent, deconditioning and activity-related secondary conditions will make independence more difficult or impossible. Along with physical education and fitness education that all students should receive, people with SCD need physical activity/exercise counseling to inform about benefits of activity, identify and remove barriers to exercise, and solve problems related to accessibility/availability of adapted fitness services (93). In particular, the many barriers to physical activity/exercise for people with SCD may not be readily apparent to professionals.

Adherence to physical activity/exercise programs is as important as the programs themselves. People without SCD report that their main barriers (94) are lack of social support, unavailability of facilities, time constraints, and cost. Persons with SCD may face additional barriers such as muscle paralysis, secondary medical conditions and symptoms, need for physical assistance, inaccessibility of facilities, and inappropriateness of equipment and services (90, 95). Table 5.7 summarizes many of these barriers and some potential solutions. One recent publication makes many suggestions for accessibility/universal design of fitness facilities and adaptation of exercise programs/equipment for people with SCD (95).

Less motivated people with or without SCD need structured exercise plans that include behavioral supports to promote adherence. Frequently used supports include self-monitoring (daily activity/exercise log to which they are held accountable), frequent reassessment and tracking of progress with reinforcement, social support (from staff, exercise partner, or fellow members of an exercise group or wheelchair sports team), and provisions for relapse prevention.

All exercise professionals need to be psychologically supportive of efforts made by people with SCD to exercise and remain physically active. They can help them assess their need for specific exercises and activities, set realistic goals, and use effective training methods. Improvements in health, fitness, and function may have profound effects on the lives of people with SCD that professionals may not see in the clinical or fitness setting. If the person with SCD does not seem to be coping with his/her disability, the exercise professional should refer him/her to a clinical psychologist for evaluation. Anxiety and depression is common in the SCD population (96).

Several excellent practical guidelines are recommended concerning fitness/exercise education and training of people with SCD (92–105). Additionally, exercise professionals should be aware that competitive wheelchair sports opportunities are available for potential athletes with SCD. They would fit best in events organized by Wheelchair Sports USA with a classification system based on neurological level of spinal nerve function (106).

CASE STUDY

John sustained a complete spinal cord injury at C8 from a gun shot wound 5 yr ago at age 17. His trunk and leg musculature are paralyzed, with marked spasticity in the hip and knee flexors and ankle plantar flexors. The muscle strength of his upper extremities is normal, but his finger extensors and intrinsics, wrist flexors, pectorals, and latissimus dorsi muscles are weak. John is 180 cm tall and weighs 110 kg (BMI = 34 kg/m^2), with a triceps skinfold of 25 mm. He has gained 50 pounds over the past 5 yr since his discharge from rehabilitation. He uses a manual wheelchair and lives independently in the community and drives an adapted van.

S: John complains of arm muscle fatigue, shoulder pain, dizziness, and shortness of breath when propelling his manual lightweight everyday wheelchair and especially up inclines. He considers himself overweight and out of shape. His posture appears kyphotic with rounded shoulders, forward head, and protruding abdomen.

O: John's resting HR and BP were 65 bpm and 90/60 mm Hg, respectively. During a graded arm-crank exercise test, his peak power output was 45 W. He became progressively more light-headed during the test as his SBP decreased to 70 mm Hg and his DBP was inaudible. His heart rate peaked at 125 bpm just before extreme arm muscle fatigue/exhaustion (RPE = 8 on the Borg CR-11 scale). John takes 20 s to push his chair up a standard (12:1) 4-m ramp. During a 6-min wheeling test, he traveled a distance of 600 m on a flat, smooth indoor surface. In addition to his daily activities, the only formal exercise that John performs on his own is daily stretching.

A: John is physically deconditioned. He needs improved physical fitness to accomplish his daily activities without exhaustion or pain. Specifically, he needs decreased fat body weight, increased triceps and shoulder depressor strength/endurance, and balanced shoulder muscle strength and flexibility. John needs nutritional education and behavior change to manage his body weight over time. John needs medical evaluation to remediate his symptomatic hypotension. He has substantial upper body muscle mass and strength, but profoundly impaired autonomic vasomotor and autonomic control over his cardiovascular system.

P: John will consult a registered dietician to implement an appropriate diet to lose 20 kg of unnecessary fat weight. John will consult his physician to rule out heart disease and a physical therapist concerning his shoulder pain. He will try

Table 5.7. Facilitating Factors and Intrinsic/Extrinsic Alterable/Unalterable Inhibiting Factors Affecting Adherence of Persons with Spinal Cord Dysfunction to Exercise Programs

FACILITATORS	
Dedication to specific goals, intention to exercise	Not currently ill
Belief that benefits will outweigh costs/risks (improved function, health, etc.)	Access to lots of exercise equipment at home or facility
Reliable transportation to facility	Free accessible parking available
Good weather/driving conditions	Accessible facility entrances and halls
Bowels/bladder managed OK today	Accessible scale
Clean exercise clothes	Appropriate accessible equipment
Enjoy fun physical activity/exercise	Appropriate adaptations to equipment
Comfortable with (accepted by) other people at facility	Assistance available
Attendance has priority over other competing activities	Expert staff
Expectation of staff and peers to attend	Social activity (meet friends at facility)
Clean, safe, air-conditioned facility	Service charges covered by project (affordable)
Can participate year-round indoors	Culturally sensitive environment
Competition, adherence	Child care available

INHIBITORS OR BARRIERS	**STRATEGY TO REMOVE BARRIER**
INTRINSIC (DISABILITY, PERSONALITY, BELIEFS, ATTITUDES, PREFERENCES, INTERESTS)	
Alterable	
Exercise is boring	Listen to music, keep mind occupied, wheel/bike outdoors
Muscle or joint soreness	Initial soreness will go away in a few days, build up gradually, stretch after activity, analgesics
Fear of injury	See staff/healthcare provider, education
Frequent temporary illness (cold, flu, allergy, UTI, sores)	See healthcare provider, education
Lack of goal orientation	See staff/healthcare provider, education
Belief that costs/risks will outweigh benefits	See staff/healthcare provider, education
Can't stick with it (low self-efficacy/will-power)	Try it, improve confidence/success/discipline, social support, rewards, benefits, record-keeping, adherence
Prefer outdoors to indoors	Do outdoor activities
Cultural insensitivity of staff/participants	Staff training
Bowel/bladder accident before attendance	See healthcare provider
No previous experience or sport history	Start hobby or enjoyable activity that gets you moving
Don't enjoy exercise	Don't "exercise," try different activities, don't focus on discomfort
Uncomfortable with (not accepted by) other people	See healthcare provider (psychology)
Dislike staff or participants	Be tolerant of diversity (race, gender, level of SCI, athletes), change location of exercise
Persistent hypotensive symptoms (dizzy, sick, weak), poor orthostatic tolerance	Supine posture, aquatics, support hose, binder, orthostatic training (tilt table, standing), see healthcare provider, meds
Too tired, not enough energy, too much effort	Regular activity improves your energy level
Poor balance	Use straps or partner/staff to stabilize
Poor hand grip	Use holding gloves, wraps, or wrist cuffs
Can't use equipment (transfer, change weight, grasp)	Use adapted exercise equipment
Severe arthritis or joint pain	See healthcare provider
Embarrassment (poor body image)	See healthcare provider, psychology
Substance abuse	See healthcare provider
Don't like to ask for help	Assertiveness and social skills training
Like to be alone	Social skills training, use social support
Family does not encourage me to exercise	Convince family of benefits of exercise
Exercise has low priority	See staff/healthcare provider, prioritize and plan
Never see anyone else exercising	Attend a fitness facility or our program
No friends or family who exercise	Find a partner who will exercise, meet other participants
Don't know how to exercise or what to do	See healthcare provider, education
Too old to exercise	See healthcare provider, education
Healthcare provider said not to exercise	See healthcare provider, education
Never had P.E., sport, or activities when I was younger	Never too late to learn and benefit
Unalterable	
Paralysis	Exercise innervated muscles, FES for paralyzed muscles
Incoordination, spasticity	Use simpler/slower exercises, practice skills
Low pain threshold	Build up gradually, analgesics
Occasional illness	Be patient
Cognitive impairment, ADD, mental illness	See healthcare provider

Table 5.7. *(Continued)*

INHIBITORS OR BARRIERS	STRATEGY TO REMOVE BARRIER
"EXTRINSIC" (ENVIRONMENT, SITUATION, ROLES, RESPONSIBILITIES)	
Alterable	
Medications make me drowsy	See healthcare provider
No clean exercise clothes	Do laundry more often; plan ahead
Neighborhood safety	Bring friend, move
Child care unavailable	Plan ahead, have alternatives, bring child
Family demands	Plan ahead, bring family
No role models present	Find one, BBBS
Unreliable transportation to facility, can't drive	Plan ahead, learn to drive, hand controls, repair car, public transport, alternative means of transport
Bad weather/driving conditions	Exercise at home, have alternate plans
Lack of time, takes time from family/job responsibilities	Time management, shorter exercise sessions, watch less TV, make exercise a high priority, exercise improves function and job performance
Inconvenient facility times	Expand facility hours, change facilities
Exercise is hard work and takes too much energy	Build up gradually
Chronic pain	See healthcare provider (education)
Exacerbates an existing medical condition	See healthcare provider (education)
Hours conflict with work/school	Plan accordingly
Music is too loud	Lower the volume, change facilities
Facility is too far away	Make time for commute, find closer facility
Exercise costs too much	Benefits outweigh costs, find less expensive facility, exercise at home
Heavy work schedule	Plan accordingly
Unalterable	
Emergency, death in family, disaster (tornado, flood, fire)	None
Facility closes down, research project ends	Change facilities, have alternate facility and long-term plan

using an elastic abdominal binder, support stockings, leg elevation, or supine posture to maintain his BP during exercise. John will continue all normal daily activities with his manual wheelchair. When tolerable, John will increase his general physical activities to help with weight management. John will exercise at an accessible fitness facility 3 sessions/wk. Assistance will be necessary for postural stability.

John's beginning exercise prescription is as follows.

1. Warm-up (general upper body calisthenics and seated aerobics, dynamic flexibility exercises for upper extremities)
2. Shoulder Balance:
   a. Therapeutic exercises to strengthen the external shoulder rotators and scapular retractors, and stretch the anterior chest and shoulder muscles
3. General Arm Strength, Endurance, and Anaerobic Power Training:
   a. Rickshaw exercise (similar to dips, but on a wheelchair-accessible machine). Two exercises:
      1) with bent elbows (for triceps)
      2) with straight elbows (for shoulder depressors)
   b. Lat Pull-downs (pulleys)
   c. Rowing (pulleys)
   d. Incline Press (against light machine weights)
   e. Bench Press (weight machine)

   Day 1: Assessments: Determine 10-RM for each exercise, and perform Wingate anaerobic power test (maximal work performed during maximal-effort high-intensity arm-cranking for 30 s).

   Day 2: Training: 2 sets × 10 reps at 90% 10-RM

   Progress according to principles of progressive resistive exercise and principles of overload, progression, specificity, regularity, etc.
4. Aerobic Exercise: Choose 2–3 acceptable accessible available modes, e.g., arm-crank ergometry:
   a. Find workload (≈20–30 W) that elicits RPE = 4/11 for at least 5 min or until arm muscle fatigue or dizziness.
   b. Perform at least two assessments to establish training baselines. Example:
      1) Maximal work performed during 6-min period
   c. Progress over time to 30–60 min/workout.
   d. Vary direction of cranking (forward vs. backward).
   e. Vary intensities and durations of workouts, i.e., shorter durations with higher intensity (intervals) vs. long, slow distance.
   f. Watch videos or find partner to combat boredom of arm ergometry.
   g. Repeat assessments every 2 wk.

References

1. Nelson MR, Rott EJ. Chapter 78. Spina bifida. In: Grabois M, Garrison SJ, Hart KA, et al, eds. Physical medicine and rehabilitation: the complete approach. Malden, MA: Blackwell Science, 2000:1414–1432.
2. Cardenas DD, Burns SP, Chan L. Chapter 73. Rehabilitation of spinal cord injury. In: Grabois M, Garrison SJ, Hart KA, et

al, eds. Physical medicine and rehabilitation: the complete approach. Malden, MA: Blackwell Science, 2000:1305–1324.

3. Yarkony GM, Chen D. Chapter 55. Rehabilitation of patients with spinal cord injuries. In: Braddom RJ, ed. Physical medicine and rehabilitation. Philadelphia: W.B. Saunders Co., 1996: 1149–1179.
4. Carpenter MB, Sutin J. Chapter 8. The autonomic nervous system. In: Human neuroanatomy. 8th ed. Baltimore: Wilkins & Wilkins, 1983:209–231.
5. Koizumi K, Brooks CM. Chapter 30. The autonomic system and its role in controlling body functions. In: Mountcastle VB, ed. Medical physiology. Volume 1. 14th ed. St. Louis: C.V. Mosby Co., 1980:893–922.
6. Ditunno JF, Young W, Donovan WH, et al. The international standards booklet for neurological and functional classification of spinal cord injury. Paraplegia 1994;32:70–80.
7. ASIA. International standards for neurological and functional classification of spinal cord injury. Chicago: American Spinal Injury Association, 1996. (accessed online, 5-27-01: http://www.asia-spinalinjury.org/publications/2001_Classif_worksheet.pdf)
8. Consortium for Spinal Cord Medicine. Outcomes following traumatic spinal cord injury: clinical practice guidelines for health-care professions. Washington, DC: Paralyzed Veterans of America, 1999.
9. Furhrer MJ. Rehabilitation and research training center in community-oriented services for persons with spinal cord injury: a progress report. Houston, TX: The Baylor College of Medicine and The Institute for Rehabilitation Research, 1991.
10. Whiteneck GG. Learning from recent empirical investigations. In: Whiteneck GG, Charlifue SW, Gerhart KS, et al., eds. Aging with spinal cord injury. New York: Demos Publications, 1993.
11. Anson CA, Shepherd C. Incidence of secondary complications in spinal cord injury. Int J Rehabil Res 1996;19:55–66.
12. Johnson RL, Gerhart KA, McCray J, et al. Secondary conditions following spinal cord injury in a population-based sample. Spinal Cord 1998;36:45–50.
13. Bauman WA, Spungen AM. Metabolic changes in persons after spinal cord injury. Phys Med Rehabil Clin N Am 2000; 11:109–140.
14. Washburn RA, Figoni SF. Physical activity and chronic cardiovascular disease prevention: a comprehensive literature review. Top Spinal Cord Injury Rehabil 1998;3:16–32.
15. Davis GM. Exercise capacity of individuals with paraplegia. Med Sci Sports Exerc 1993;25:423–432.
16. Figoni SF. Exercise responses and quadriplegia. Med Sci Sports Exerc 1993;25:433–441.
17. Hopman MTE, Nommensen E, van Asten WNJC, et al. Properties of the venous vascular system in the lower extremities on individuals with parapelgia. Paraplegia 1994;32:810–816.
18. Claus-Walker J, Halstead LS. Metabolic and endocrine changes since spinal cord injury. I. The nervous system before and after transection of the spinal cord. Arch Phys Med Rehabil 1981;62:595–601.
19. Kelly LE. Chapter 12. Spinal cord disabilities. In: Winnick JP, ed. Adapted physical education and sport. 2nd ed. Champaign, IL: Human Kinetics, 1997:193–212.
20. Hart AL, Malone TR, English T. Shoulder function and rehabilitation implications for the wheelchair athlete. Top Spinal Cord Injury Rehabil 1998;3:50–65.
21. Winnick JP, Short FX. The physical fitness of youngsters with spinal neuromuscular conditions. Adapted Phys Activity Quart 1984;1:37–51.
22. Shephard RJ. Fitness in special populations. Champaign, IL: Human Kinetics, 1990.
23. Winnick JP, Short FX. The Brockport physical fitness test manual. Champaign, IL: Human Kinetics, 1999.
24. Andrade CK, Kramer J, Garber M, et al. Changes in self-concept, cardiovascular endurance and muscular strength of children with spina bifida aged 8 to 13 years in response to a 10-week physical-activity programme: a pilot study. Child Care Health Dev 1991;17:183–196.
25. Morrison SA, Melton-Rogers SL, Hooker SP. Changes in physical capacity and physical strain in persons with acute spinal cord injury. Top Spinal Cord Injury Rehabil 1997;3:1–15.
26. Hjeltnes N, Jansen T. Physical endurance capacity, functional status and medical complications in spinal cord injured subjects with long-standing lesions. Paraplegia 1990; 428–432.
27. Stewart MW, Melton-Rogers SL, Morrison S, et al. The measurement properties of fitness measures and health status for persons with spinal cord injuries. Arch Phys Med Rehabil 2000;81:394–400.
28. Raymond J, Davis GM, Fahey A, et al. Oxygen uptake and heart rate responses during arm *vs* combined arm/electrically stimulated leg exercise in people with paraplegia. Spinal Cord 1997;35:680–685.
29. Glaser RM. Exercise and locomotion for the spinal cord injured. Exerc Sports Sci Rev 1985;13:263–303.
30. Dreisinger TE, Londeree BR. Wheelchair exercise: a review. Paraplegia 1982;20:20–34.
31. Fuhr L, Langbein F, Edwards LC, et al. Diagnostic wheelchair exercise testing. Top Spinal Cord Injury Rehabil 1997;3: 34–48.
32. Pitetti KH, Barrett PJ, Campbell KD, et al. The effect of lower body positive pressure on the exercise capacity of individuals with spinal cord injury. Med Sci Sports Exerc 1994; 26:463–468.
33. Sawka MN, Latzka WA, Pandolf KB. Temperature regulation during upper body exercise: able-bodied and spinal cord injured. Med Sci Sports Exerc 1989;21:S132–S140.
34. Houtman S, Oeseburg B, Hopman MTE. Blood volume and hemoglobin after spinal cord injury. Am J Phys Med Rehabil 2000;79:260–265.
35. Veeger HEJ, Hajd Yahmed M, van der Woude LHV, et al. Peak oxygen uptake and maximal power output of Olympic wheelchair-dependent athletes. Med Sci Sports Exerc 1991; 1201–1209.
36. Coutts KD, Rhodes EC, McKenzie DC. Maximal exercise responses of tetraplegics and paraplegics. J Appl Physiol 1971; 55:479–482.
37. Gass GC, Camp EM. Physiological characteristics of training Australian paraplegic and tetraplegic subjects. Med Sci Sports Exerc 1979;11:256–265.
38. Van Loan MD, McCluer S, Loftin JM, et al. Comparison of physiological responses to maximal arm exercise among able-bodied, paraplegics, and quadriplegics. Paraplegia 1987;25:397–405.

39. Figoni SF, Boileau RA, Massey BH, et al. Physiological responses of quadriplegic and able-bodied men during exercise at the same $\dot{V}O_2$. Adapted Phys Activity Quart 1988;5: 130–139.
40. Hjeltnes N. Capacity for physical work and training after spinal injuries and strokes. Scand J Rehabil Med 1982;29: 245–251.
41. Hjeltnes N. Control of medical rehabilitation of para- and tetraplegics by repeated evaluation of endurance capacity. Int J Sports Med 1984;5:171–174.
42. Figoni SF, Glaser RM. Arm and leg exercise stress testing in a person with quadriparesis. Clin Kinesiol 1993;47:25–36.
43. Figoni SF, Gupta SC, Glaser RM. Effects of posture on arm exercise performance of adults with tetrapelgia. Clin Exerc Physiol 1999;1:74–85.
44. Hopman MTE, Dueck C, Monroe M, et al. Limits of maximal performance in individuals with spinal cord injury. Int J Sports Med 1998;19:98–103.
45. Ready AE. Responses of quadriplegic athletes to maximal and submaximal exercise. Physiother Can 1984;36:124–128.
46. Hooker SP, Figoni SF, Rodgers MM, et al. Metabolic and hemodynamic responses to concurrent voluntary arm crank and electrical stimulation leg cycle exercise in quadriplegics. J Rehabil Res Dev 1992;29:1–11.
47. Krebs P, Eickelberg W, Krobath H, et al. Effects of physical exercise on peripheral vision and learning in children with spina bifida manifestation. Percep Motor Skills 1989;68: 167–174.
48. Agre JC, Findley TW, McNally MC, et al. Physical activity capacity in children with myelomeningocele. Arch Phys Med Rehabil 1987;68:372–377.
49. Janssen TWJ, van Oers CAJM, van der Woude LHV, et al. Physical strain in daily life of wheelchair users with spinal cord injuries. Med Sci Sports Exerc 1994;26:661–670.
50. Dallmeijer AJ, Hopman MTE, van As HHJ, et al. Physical capacity and physical strain in persons with tetraplegia: the role of sport activity. Spinal Cord 1996; 34:729–735.
51. Davis GM, Shephard RJ, Leenen FH. Cardiac effects of short term arm crank training in paraplegics: echocardiographic evidence. Eur J Appl Physiol Occup Physiol 1987;56:90–96.
52. Davis G, Plyley MJ, Shephard RJ. Gains of cardiorespiratory fitness with arm-crank training in spinally disabled men. Can J Sport Sci 1991;16:64–72.
53. Nilsson S, Staff PH, Pruett ED. Physical work capacity and the effect of training on subjects with long-standing paraplegia. Scand J Rehabil Med 1975;7:51–56.
54. Gass GC, Watson J, Camp EM, et al. The effects of physical training on high level spinal lesion patients. Scand J Rehabil Med 1980;12:61–65.
55. Miles DS, Sawka MN, Wilde SW, et al. Pulmonary function changes in wheelchair athletes subsequent to exercise training. Ergonomics 1982;25:239–246.
56. Knutsson E, Lewenhaupt-Olsson E, Thorsen M. Physical work capacity and physical conditioning in paraplegic patients. Paraplegia 1973;11:205–216.
57. Davis GM, Shephard RJ. Strength training for wheelchair users. Br J Sports Med 1990;24:25–30.
58. McLean KP, Skinner JS. Effect of body training position on outcomes of an aerobic training study on individuals with quadriplegia. Arch Phys Med Rehabil 1995;76:139–150.
59. Lassau-Wray ER, Ward GR. Varying physiological response to arm-crank exercise in specific spinal injuries. J Physiol Anthropol Appl Human Sci 2000;19:5–12.
60. Hooker SP, Figoni SF, Rodgers MM, et al. Physiologic effects of electrical stimulation leg cycle exercise training in spinal cord injured persons. Arch Phys Med Rehabil 1992;73: 470–476.
61. Nash MS, Bilsker S, Marcillo AE, et al. Reversal of adaptive left ventricular atrophy following electrically stimulated exercise training in human tetraplegia. Paraplegia 1992;29: 590–599.
62. Nash MS. Exercise reconditioning of the heart and peripheral circulation after spinal cord injury. Top Spinal Cord Injury Rehabil 1998;4:1–15.
63. Faghri PD, Glaser RM, Figoni SF. Functional electrical stimulation leg cycle ergometer exercise: training effect on cardiorespiratory responses of spinal cord injured subjects at rest and during submaximal exercise. Arch Phys Med Rehabil 1992;73:1085–1093.
64. Janssen TWJ, Glaser RM, Shuster DB. Clinical efficacy of electrical stimulation exercise training: effects on health, fitness, and function. Top Spinal Cord Injury Rehabil 1998;3: 33–49.
65. Figoni SF, Glaser RM, Collins SR. Training effects of hybrid exercise on peak physiologic responses in quadriplegics. Proceedings of the 12th International Congress of World Confederation for Physical Therapy. Alexandria, VA: American Physical Therapy Association, 1995, Paper # PO-SI-0028T on CD-ROM.
66. Cooney MM, Walker JB. Hydraulic resistance exercise benefits cardiovascular fitness of spinal cord injured. Med Sci Sports Exerc 1986;18:522–525.
67. Jacobs PL, Nash MS, Rusinkowski JW Jr. Circuit training provides cardiorespiratory and strength benefits in persons with paraplegia. Med Sci Sports Exerc, 2001;33:711–717.
68. Ekblom B, Lundberg A. Effect of physical training on adolescents with severe motor handicaps. Acta Paediatr Scand 1968;57:17–23.
69. O'Connell DG, Barnhart R. Improvement in wheelchair propulsion in pediatric wheelchair users through resistance training: a pilot study. Arch Phys Med Rehabil 1995;76: 368–372.
70. Yarkony GM, ed. Spinal cord injury: medical management and rehabilitation. Gaithersberg, MD: Aspen Publishers, 1994.
71. Nesathurai S. The rehabilitation of people with spinal cord injury. 2nd ed. Williston, VT: Blackwell Science, 2000.
72. PDR: Physicians' Desk Reference, 2001. Montvale, NJ: Medical Economics Staff, 2001.
73. Stass W, et al. Chapter 42. Rehabilitation of the spinal cord injured patient. In: Delisa JA, Gans BM, Bockenek WL, eds. Rehabilitation medicine: principles and practice. Baltimore: Lippincott William & Wilkins, 1993:891.
74. Figoni SF. Chapter 30. Spinal cord injury. In: Durstine JL, ed. ACSM's exercise management for persons with chronic diseases and disabilities. Champaign, IL: Human Kinetics, 1997:175–179.
75. Kofsky PR, Davis GM, Jackson RW, et al. Field testing—assessment of physical fitness of disabled adults. Eur J Appl Physiol 1983;51:109–120.
76. Franklin BA, Swantek KI, Grais SL, et al. Field test estimation

of maximal oxygen consumption in wheelchair users. Arch Phys Med Rehabil 1990;71:574–578.
77. Pare G, Noreau L, Simard C. Prediction of maximal aerobic power from a submaximal exercise test performed by paraplegics on a wheelchair ergometer. Paraplegia 1993;31:584–592.
78. Glaser RM, Sawka MN, Brune MF, et al. Physiological responses to maximal effort wheelchair and arm crank ergometry. J Appl Physiol 1980;48:1060–1064.
79. Glaser RM. Arm exercise training for wheelchair users. Med Sci Sports Exerc 1989;21(5 suppl):S149–S157.
80. Rimmer JH, Connor-Kuntz F, Winnick JP, et al. Feasibility of the target aerobic movement test in children and adolescents with spina bifida. Adapted Phys Activity Quart 1997; 14:147–155.
81. UDS: Uniform Data System for Medical Rehabilitation. Accessed 6-8-01 at http://www.fimsystem.com
82. Cole B, Finch, Gowland C, et al. Physical rehabilitation outcome measures. Baltimore: Williams & Wilkins, 1995.
83. Hooker SP, Greenwood JD, Hatae DT, et al. Relationship between heart rate and oxygen uptake during submaximal arm cranking in paraplegics and quardriplegics (sic). Ann Physiol Anthrop 1993;13:275–280.
84. Irizawa M, Yamasaki M, Muraki S, et al. Relationship between heart rate and oxygen uptake during submaximal arm cranking in paraplegics and quadriplegics. Ann Physiol Anthrop 1994 Sep;13(5):275–80.
85. Borg G. Borg's perceived exertion and pain scales. Champaign, IL: Human Kinetics, 1998.
86. ACSM. American College of Sports Medicine Position Stand. The recommended quantity and quality of exercise for developing and maintaining cardiorespiratory and muscular fitness, and flexibility in healthy adults. Med Sci Sports Exerc 1998;30:975–1991.
87. Coyle CP, Santiago MC. Aerobic exercise training and depressive symptomatology in adults with physical disabilities. Arch Phys Med 1995;76:647–652.
88. Edwards PA. Health promotion through fitness for adolescents and young adults following spinal cord injury. SCI Nursing 1996;13:69–73.
89. Nichols S, Brasile FM. The role of recreational therapy in physical medicine. Top Spinal Cord Injury Rehabil 1998;3: 89–98.
90. Figoni SF, McClain L, Bell AA, et al. Accessibility of physical fitness facilities in the Kansas City metropolitan area. Top Spinal Cord Injury Rehabil 1998;3:66–78.
91. Morrison SA, Stanwyck DJ. The effect of shorter lengths of stay on functional outcomes of spinal cord injury rehabilitation. Top Spinal Cord Injury Rehabil 1999;4:44–55.
92. Johnson KA, Klaas SJ. Recreation issue and trends in pediatric spinal cord injury. Top Spinal Cord Injury Rehabil 1997;3:79–84.
93. Steadward R. Musculoskeletal and neurological disabilities: implications for fitness appraisal, programming, and counseling. Can J Appl Physiol 1998;23:131–165.
94. Sallis JF, Hovell MF, Hofstetter CR. Predictors of adoption and maintenance of vigorous physical activity in men and women. Prev Med 1992;21:237–251.
95. Howard L, Figoni S, Young LC, et al. Removing barriers to health clubs and fitness facilities. A guide for accommodating all members including people with disabilities and older adults. Chapel Hill: North Carolina Office on Disability and Health, in press.
96. Elliott TR, Rank RG. Depression following spinal cord injury. Arch Phys Med Rehabil 1996;77:816–823.
97. Lowe C. Basic training (fitness, exercise, and sports). In: Lutkenhoff M, Oppenheimer SG, eds. Spinabilities: a young person's guide to spina bifida. Bethesda, MD: Woodbine House, 1997:123–131.
98. Lockette KF, Keyes AM. Conditioning with physical disabilities. Champaign, IL: Human Kinetics, 1994.
99. Miller P, ed. Fitness programming and physical disability. Champaign, IL: Human Kinetics, 1994.
100. Apple DF, ed. Physical fitness: a guide for individuals with spinal cord injury. Washington, DC: VA Rehabilitation Research and Development Service, 1996.
101. Youngbauer J, ed. Deconditioning and weight gain. Secondary conditions prevention & treatment. B Series, No. 3. Lawrence, KS: Research and Training Center on Independent Living, University of Kansas, 1996.
102. Chase TM. Chapter 10. Physical fitness strategies. In: Lanig IS, ed. A practical guide to health promotion after spinal cord injury. Gaithersberg, MD: Aspen Publishers, 1996.
103. Laskin JJ, James SA, Cantwell BM. A fitness and wellness program for people with spinal cord injury. Top Spinal Cord Injury Rehabil 1997;3:16–33.
104. Virgilio SJ. Chapter 6. Fitness education for children with disabilities. In: Virgilio SJ. Fitness education for children. Champaign, IL: Human Kinetics, 1997:47–58.
105. Rimmer JH. Fitness and rehabilitation programs for special populations. Madison, WI: Wm. C. Brown, 1994.
106. Wheelchair Sports USA, 5-27-01. (Website: http://www.wsusa.org)

CHAPTER 6

Postpolio and Guillain-Barré Syndrome

Thomas J. Birk and Kenneth H. Pitetti

EPIDEMIOLOGY AND PATHOPHYSIOLOGY

Postpolio Syndrome

Poliomyelitis is an acute viral disease that attacks the anterior horn cells of the lower motor neurons. This disease reached a peak epidemic period in the United States during the 1950s. Poliomyelitis results in flaccid paresis, paralysis, and atrophy in affected muscle groups with accompanying symptoms of fatigue, weakness, and pain. The acute 2-month phase of the disease is followed by a functional recovery period. A greater degree of functional recovery is expected when the percentage of motor neurons damaged either partially or completely does not exceed 50% (1). The functional period phase is usually stable for 15 years or more after initial diagnosis. During the stable recovery period, skeletal muscle fibers are reinnervated from the lower motor neurons spared by the polio virus. However, at some point, the remaining motor neurons are unable to generate new sprouts, and denervation exceeds reinnervation (see Fig. 6.1). Unable to keep up with reinnervation, symptoms such as fatigue, weakness, pain, muscle atrophy, cold intolerance, muscle spasms, and cramps and the difficulty of completing activities of daily living (ADLs) can appear. These symptoms are similar to the original ones and, therefore, these late or postsymptoms are termed postpolio syndrome (PPS) (2).

Postpolio syndrome (PPS) affects a varyingly large percentage of the almost 1.8 million polio survivors (3, 4, 5). Approximately 40% of these survivors have indicated that fatigue, associated with PPS, significantly interferes with occupational performance, and at least 25% of these survivors reported that PPS-related symptoms also interfered with performance of ADLs (4). PPS conservatively affects up to one-half million polio survivors, 15–40 years after the original diagnosis, with a peak incidence at 30–34 years.

Two subtypes of PPS are recognized: postpolio progressive muscular atrophy (PPMA) and musculoskeletal postpoliomyelitis symptoms (MPPS). PPMA is equated to neurological symptoms (i.e., loss of residual motor units) and, therefore, is regarded as PPS. MPPS, on the other hand, is secondary to "wear and tear" on joints and not due to adverse neurological changes, and its inclusion may be why PPS has a varyingly large incidence.

PPS is more prevalent and more intense in the legs, back, and arms, respectively (5). The increased stress on progressively weakening and wasting muscles heightens joint instability. PPS is hastened when original paralysis affected all four limbs, a ventilator was required, hospitalization was necessary during acute stages, and/or the polio virus was contracted after the age of 10 (6).

In addition to physical fatigue and weakness, difficulty in concentration, memory, and attention span have been reported (4). The brain fatigue generator (BFG) model has been used to explain the cognitive and motor activity problems. The BFG model suggests that viral damage to the reticular formation, hypothalamus, thalamic nuclei, and dopaminergic neurons diminishes cortical activity, thereby reducing information processing as well as inhibiting motor processing. Lower levels of dopamine have been found in individuals with PPS, suggesting that depleted dopamine can contribute to cognitive and motor activity problems in PPS. Credibility to these findings was gained when fatigue, attention span, and memory were improved in PPS patients when they took a dopamine receptor agonist medication.

Guillain-Barré Syndrome

Guillain-Barré syndrome (GBS) is the worldwide leading cause of acute inflammatory demyelinating polyneuropathy (AIDP) and, more significantly, the most fatal. The incidence is estimated between 0.6 and 2.4 per 100,000 population per year (see refs 7 and 8 for review articles). GBS is described as a demyelinating type of neuropathy resulting from an immune attack against a component of myelin on the peripheral nerves. Common events that can precede onset of GBS are a brief antecedent gastrointestinal (e.g., *Campylobacter jejuni*) or respiratory tract illness (e.g., Mycoplasma pneumonia). Neoplasia (e.g., lymphomas), vaccinations (e.g., rabies, flu, and tetanus vaccines) and drugs (e.g., Penicillamine, Streptokinase, Zimelidine) can also be preceding events.

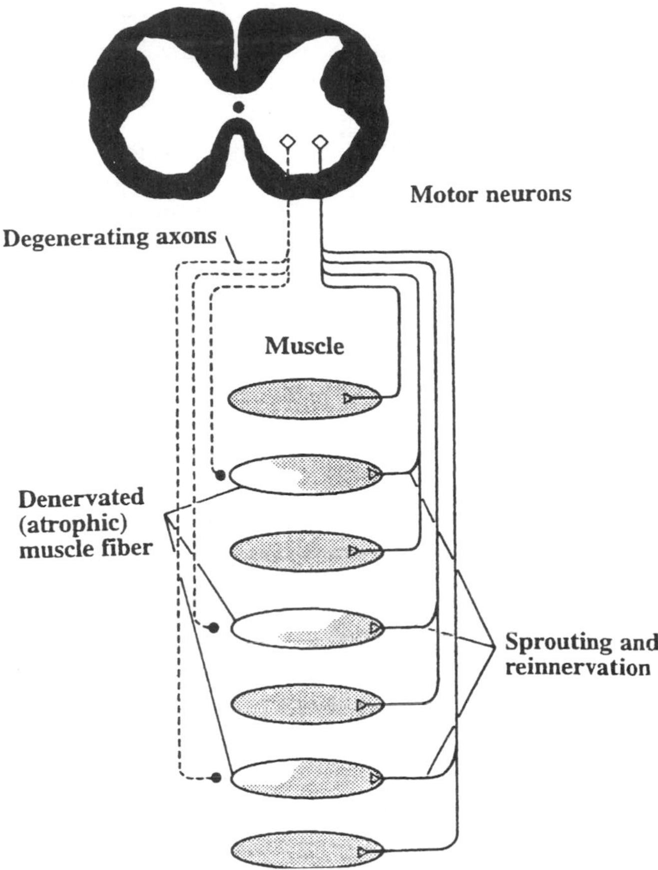

Figure 6.1. Denervation and reinnervation of muscle fibers.

GBS is a self-limiting disorder with a monophasic course. Clinically, GBS is characterized by an "ascending" weakness starting in the lower extremities to the upper extremities and evolving over 1–3 weeks. GBS can move with rapid progression requiring respiratory assistance within 2–3 days. The severity of motor impairment ranges from mild ataxia to complete paralysis of all motor and cranial nerves. Patients are expected to have a favorable outcome (generally, this is equated to mean the ability to ambulate without assistive devices). GBS often begins in both the distal and proximal muscles of the lower extremities and can also start in the upper limbs, but rarely begins as a facial diplegia. Motor recovery is centrifugally oriented (i.e., recovery starts from upper extremities and proceeds to the lower extremities). People of any age can be affected by GBS, although the distribution is bimodal, with peaks in young adults and the elderly. Significant autonomic dysfunction is present in patients along with severe motor weakness and respiratory failure. Autonomic dysfunctions that can be anticipated in patients with GBS are: (1) cardiac arrhythmia (tachyarrhythmia, bradycardia, asystole); (2) changeable blood pressure (orthostatism, hypertension, hypotension); (3) pupillary and sweating abnormalities; and (4) gastrointestinal dysfunction. Pain is common, as either a bilateral sciatica or aching in large muscles of the upper legs, flanks, or back.

AIDP is thought to be synonymous with GBS and together have become the common reference (i.e., AIDP associated with GBS) in the United States, Europe, and Australia. AIDP is thought to be the result of an immune attack on the peripheral nerve that is characterized by macrophage-mediated demyelination. Macrophages have been shown to attack the outer myelin lamellae, often preserving the axon, but it is widely held that intense inflammation and demyelination can result in secondary axonal degeneration. On the other had, GBS in China and Mexico affects predominantly children and young adults, and degeneration of axons without evidence of demyelination has outnumbered cases of AIDP associated with GBS by at least 2:1.

CLINICAL EXERCISE PHYSIOLOGY

Postpolio Syndrome

Studies using a stationary bicycle protocol have reported that aerobic capacity ($\dot{V}O_{2peak}$) was significantly related to muscle strength in the lower extremities (LEs) for persons with "late effects" of polio (9) or "late sequelae" of PPS (10). This strongly suggests that poor exercise performance on the stationary bicycle was limited by weak muscle function and, therefore, low $\dot{V}O_{2peak}$ was secondary to leg strength. In additional, a similar but weaker relationship of leg muscle strength and maximal walking speed was also reported (9). Consequently, the American College of Sports Medicine (11) advocates the use of an ergometer that involves both upper and lower extremities (e.g., Schwinn Air-Dyne ergometer) when evaluating the aerobic capacity of persons with PPS rather than a stationary bicycle or treadmill protocol. For persons with PPS whose condition prevents the use of their legs, arm-crank ergometry is recommended to evaluate exercise capacity (11).

Aerobic capacity for persons with PPS was found to be lower than their able-bodied peers or their peers with polio but without PPS (12). Significant increases in $\dot{V}O_{2peak}$ have been observed following exercise programs of stationary bicycling, walking, and arm cranking (6). These increases occurred in aerobic exercise training programs that ranged from 8–22 weeks and reported no adverse effects from participation.

There is a concern that resistive training of the LEs for persons with PPS could result in loss of strength due to overtaxed motor neurons. However, studies that involved persons with PPS in resistance training regimens of the LEs for a period of 6–12 weeks not only showed significant increases in LE strength, but some participants became more asymptomatic (13, 14, 15). Neither muscle nor joint pain was increased, and evidence of weakness was not seen even though exercise intensity was classified as "moderate to hard." Considering the results of these studies (13, 14, 15), it is recommended that when initiating LE resistance training programs for persons with unstable PPS, a conservative approach should be taken. That is, the person with PPS should begin at a low intensity and gradually (i.e., over 4–6 weeks) increase to a moderate intensity. It is not recommended that high-intensity LE resistance training be performed by persons with PPS (11).

Guillain-Barrè Syndrome

GBS is a significant cause of long-term disability for at least 1,000 persons per year in the United States, and more in other countries. Given the young age at which GBS can occur and the relatively long life expectancies following GBS, it is likely that from 25,000 to 50,000 persons in the U.S. are experiencing some residual effects of GBS. Approximately 40% of patients who are hospitalized with GBS will require inpatient rehabilitation. Issues that affect rehabilitation are dysautonomia (i.e., orthostatic hypotension, unstable blood pressure, abnormal heart rate, bowel and bladder dysfunction), deafferent pain syndrome (pain originating peripherally, not centrally) and multiple medical complications related to length of immobilization, which include deep venous thrombosis, joint contracture, hypercalcemia due to bone demineralization, anemia, and decubitus ulcers.

Rehabilitation therapy strategies are similar to those for other neuromuscular illnesses and diseases (see ref 15 for summary of clinical treatment and inpatient rehabilitation therapy for GBS). GBS patients can display such diverse findings as significant involvement with tetraparesis, or isolated weakness of the arm, leg, facial muscles, or oropharynx. Extreme care should be taken to not over-fatigue the affected motor units during therapy. In fact, overworked muscle groups in patients with GBS have been clinically associated with paradoxical weakening.

Motor weakness in GBS has been associated with muscle shortening and resultant joint contractures and can be prevented with daily range-of-motion exercises. Depending on the amount of weakness, exercise can be passive, active-assistive, or active. Initial exercise should include a program of low-intensity strengthening that involves isometric, isotonic, isokinetic, manual-resistive, and progressive-resistive exercises carefully tailored to the severity of the condition. Orthotics should be incorporated in order to properly position the limbs during exercise and optimize residual function.

Proprioceptive losses (i.e., vibratory sensation and joint position) expressed by GBS patients can cause ataxia (i.e, loss of ability to coordinate muscular movements) and incoordination. Repetitive exercises that involve whole body movements (i.e., picking up an object on a table and placing it onto a shelf) will help improve coordination.

GBS patients who enter inpatient rehabilitation are not usually threatened by cardiac arrhythmias; however, 19–50% will have evidence of postural hypotension. Prevention of hypotensive episodes involves physical modalities such as compression hose, abdominal binders, and proper hydration. Patients who experience long periods of immobilization will find progressive mobilization on a tilt table to be a useful therapeutic tool for treating orthostatic hypotension.

A patient with GBS is still in the recovery phase during inpatient rehabilitation. Changes in the patient's condition should be monitored by nerve conduction velocity and muscle strength testing.

PHARMACOLOGY

Postpolio Syndrome

Medications, such as nonsteroidal anti-inflammatory drugs (NSAIDs) and muscle relaxants, are prescribed for persons with PPS to reduce symptoms and do not usually restrict acute or chronic exercise performance. Medications prescribed for reduction of pain and fatigue include tricyclic antidepressants and serotonin blockers. These medications are not only used to reduce pain but to facilitate anxiety reduction, thus enhancing overall relaxation and restful sleep. Current serotonin blockers have little overall effect on exercise performance, but tricyclic antidepressants have been shown to increase heart rate and decrease blood pressure during rest and exercise. Tricyclic antidepressants can cause ECG abnormalities, resulting in either false-positive or false-negative exercise test results, T-wave changes, and dysrhythmias, particularly in persons with a cardiac history.

Medications such as prednisone, amantadine, pyridostigmine, and bromocriptine mesylate have also been used to diminish fatigue and weakness and enhance physical performance. Prednisone, a corticosteroid, has not significantly increased muscle strength in PPS, and amantadine has not significantly decreased muscle fatigue (17). Pyridostigmine, an anticholinesterase drug, has been investigated and showed muscle fatigue was not significantly diminished (18). Bromocriptine mesylate, a post-synaptic dopamine receptor agonist, did not show effects on diminishing fatigue, but was found to enhance attention, cognition, and memory (5).

These four drugs (prednisone, amantadine, pyridostigmine, and bromocriptine mesylate) should not negatively affect exercise performance. However, chronic use of prednisone can weaken muscle tissue and cause deposition of fat in the muscle cells, and lead to edema.

Guillain-Barré Syndrome

Clinical first-line agents include tricyclic antidepressants or the use of topical capsaicin to the specific well-localized anatomical areas of deafferent pain. These medications should not affect rehabilitation or exercise activities. Second-line agents include anticonvulsants (e.g., carbamazepine), and for patients who have unremitting pain, narcotics may be indicated early in rehabilitation to give relief until the first-line agents can become effective. Rehabilitation should proceed with additional caution when GBS patients are on narcotics.

PHYSICAL EXAMINATION

Postpolio Syndrome

An initial physical exam should include medical history of the person with PPS and a description of both central and peripheral complaints and symptoms, particularly new and/or increased overall fatigue and specific muscle(s) weakness or pain. It is important to understand initial polio problems and to determine whether the new and/or increased fatigue, weakness, and pain are associated with areas of the body affected by the initial polio. Symptoms should be analyzed with reference to type, intensity, duration, and frequency of all physical activities (leisure or recreational), including occupational tasks. Daily body postures and positions should also be analyzed, with specific attention to spinal, pelvic, knee, and ankle areas, to determine any abnormal joint mechanics.

The amount of rehabilitation after the initial polio onset and whether assistive devices were used or are still being used for balance and ambulation is important information to more accurately determine the extent of muscle fatigue and weakness. Also, the length of the functional stability period (see Epidemiology and Pathophysiology section), the highest level of physical function achieved during the stability period, and any psychosocial exacerbating factors are important to note.

An extensive neuromuscular exam should begin with a structural/postural evaluation to determine any adverse structural relationships caused by increased fatigue and weakness. The exam should also evaluate muscle size to indicate atrophy in symptomatic areas and test for light touch, sharp/dull touch, vibration, and temperature. Sensory testing of the symptomatic regions will facilitate determination of possible peripheral nerve dysfunction. Reflex testing should also be included in order to differentiate the extent of lower motor neuron involvement, since decreased responses are indicative of increased flaccidity. However, a hyperactive reflex suggests muscle spasm associated with early poliomyelitis.

The motor portion of the exam should include observation of gait and balance testing, including both static and dynamic challenges. Rapid or alternate movement of symptomatic and asymptomatic limbs should be tested for coordination and timing with the evaluator looking for tremors and/or unsteady movements and visual signs. A goniometer is suggested to assess range of motion (ROM) for all symptomatic limbs and joints, including both active range of motion (AROM) and passive range of motion (PROM). Strength can be measured subjectively by manual muscle testing (MMT) to detect gross motor weakness (19). MMT has five grades corresponding from 0, with no contraction, to 5, which is normal strength. MMT should not be used to differentiate nonfunctional contractions, since this musculature has most likely lost a critical number of motor neurons and will not be involved in exercise programs. The MMT should include either several repetitions and/or single repetitions held for a longer period of time because single-effort maximal contraction will not typically show any strength loss, but repetitive contractions will show additional weakness. Consequently, MMT should involve at least 3, and up to 10, repetitions of near-maximal effort at midrange for the symptomatic musculature. Residual fatigue of the tested muscles should be checked within 30 minutes of the initial test and up to 48 hours posttest. This subjective question assessment provides clinical data relevant to the assessment of PPS for the symptomatic musculature. These physical portions of the exam for symptomatic areas should be performed after the less fatiguing portions of the overall exam to avoid possible confounding effects of exertion.

Guillain-Barré Syndrome

During inpatient rehabilitation, GBS patients can have a relapse of the disease, so close supervision during inpatient rehabilitation is warranted. Detailed daily physical exams should occur involving motor (i.e., strength), sensory, and autonomic tests to identify relapses and/or complications.

MEDICAL AND SURGICAL TREATMENTS

Postpolio Syndrome

Medications, as described under Pharmacology, have not been shown to significantly reduce fatigue or weakness associated with PPS; therefore, management of PPS is based largely on treating symptoms. Soft tissue, joint pain, and fatigue have been treated with various local medications and systemic medications such as serotonin inhibitors and tricyclic antidepressants. Success of these medications to modify pain and fatigue has varied.

Orthotic devices have been successfully used to decrease abnormal, excessive force and motion on LE joints. Certain neuromuscular and orthopedic deficiencies, such as dorsiflexor muscle weakness (i.e., drop-foot), genu valgum (i.e., knock-knee) and genu recurvatum (i.e., hyperextended knee) impose movements that overstress both noncontractile and contractile tissue. For example, ankle-foot orthoses (AFOs) have been fitted to reduce drop-foot and avoid loss of balance and inefficient walking. Gait can be improved with simple heel lifts or shoe inserts, which decrease the amount of dorsiflexion. Knee orthoses, knee-ankle-foot orthoses (KAFOs), and bracing can facilitate balanced compressive forces on the tibia while walking with genu valgum and recurvatum conditions. Abnormal chronic forces on the knee secondary to chronic drop-foot can result in overstretched connective tissue and cartilage shearing. These abnormal changes result in decreased mobility and increased joint-related pain. A KAFO can also spare the other leg from becoming prematurely fatigued and overworked. Lightweight nylon knee braces can be a benefit and less conspicuous. Orthotic devices for persons with PPS need a strong rationale due to early unpleasant memories of braces during the acute polio stage.

Guillain-Barré Syndrome

Plasmapheresis treatment (plasma withdrawn from a donor for the purpose of transfusing a patient in need of fraction plasma replacement) has been shown to shorten not only the time required to walk independently, but also the time the patient stays on respiratory support. Another alternative treatment is the infusion of immunoglobulins (IVIg), which has been associated with similar beneficial outcomes as seen with plasmapheresis. Although controversial, steroids might also be used as a treatment.

DIAGNOSTIC TECHNIQUES

Postpolio Syndrome

PPS is diagnosed by exclusion of multiple sclerosis, amyotrophic lateral sclerosis, myasthenia gravis, chronic infection, hypothyroidism, collagen disorders, neuropathies, and depression. Exclusion or differential diagnosis of painful conditions such as bursitis, tendinitis, myalgias, osteoarthritis, and poliomyositis must also be made because many of these conditions can occur at the same age as late symptoms of polio. Therefore, aging and its effects on the body must also be ruled out when diagnosing PPS. Significant muscle atrophy is a discerning factor since it is not common in aging and is most suggestive of PPS (1).

There are no laboratory procedures that significantly identify PPS, but procedures can rule out other medical conditions. Viral assays can identify the continuance of the polio virus and have been positive in more than 50% of individuals with PPS, but whether the long-term existence of the virus is linked to a progressive onset of PPS is not clear (20). Further evidence has suggested that if the virus remains active, it may not affect the cerebral cortex, and this suggests that fatigue is not of central origin (21).

Electromyography (EMG) and nerve conduction velocity (NVC) assessments have been used to rule out neuropathies and myasthenia gravis and to identify different phases of PPS. EMGs can identify late changes, such as fasciculations, fibrillations, and increased motor unit amplitude and duration (Fig. 6.2)(1). Although nonspecific, these motor unit alterations indicate overall damage to the motor unit. EMG has differentiated new and more severe pathology in PPS and subsequent compensation of the motor unit (22). Even surface EMG has shown good correlation with invasive EMG in identifying enlarged, overburdened motor units (23). While EMG may differentiate new motor unit pathology, it appears to be a poor predictor of muscle strength loss (24).

Subjective complaints of pain, particularly in the hip, are the best correlation to new muscle fatigue and dysfunction (25). Since the hip and pelvis are major weight-supporting structures, it follows that pain in this region could present greater estimation of dysfunction than any other area. Diagnostic techniques such as an EMG can be helpful in diagnosis of PPS, but diagnosis is dependent, at least partially, on a good patient interview.

Guillain-Barré Syndrome

Functional motor recovery should be followed by the admit motor and discharge FIM Rasch motor converted score (16). There seems to be no association between the FIM Rasch motor converted score and proprioception function at admission; therefore, proprioception function should also be evaluated daily. Assessment of GBS during inpatient rehabilitation is usually performed according to the following ordinal scale: 0: healthy; 1: minor symptoms and signs; 2: able to walk 5 m without assistance; 3: able to walk 5 m with assistance; 4: chair-bound or bed-bound; 5: requires assisted ventilation for at least part of the day or night (16).

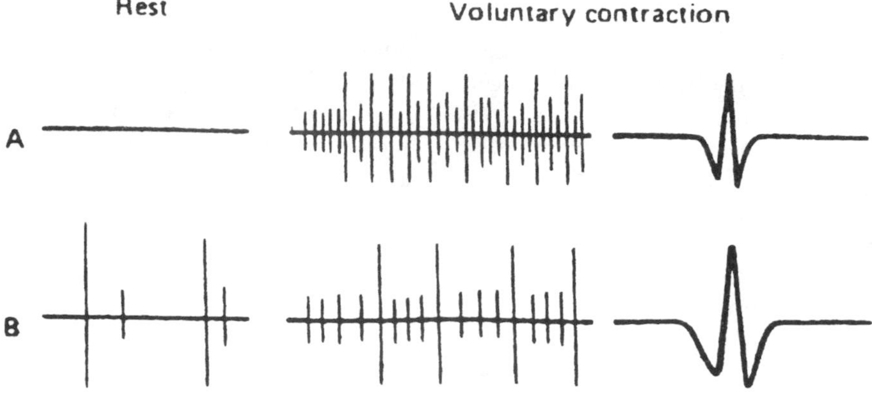

Figure 6.2. EMG responses of: A, normal muscle fiber; B, motor neuron disease (PPS) muscle fiber with chronic denervation.

EXERCISE/FITNESS/FUNCTIONAL TESTING

The basic principles for exercise testing stated in *ACSM's Guidelines for Exercise Testing and Prescription* (26) provide the foundation for this section and the next section, "Exercise Prescription and Programming." When not otherwise stated, these basic principles will apply. In addition, the basic principles for exercise testing and exercise management outlined for polio and postpolio syndrome in *ACSM's Exercise Management for Persons with Chronic Diseases and Disabilities* (11) also provide a foundation for this section and the next section. Special situations created by PPS and GBS will be addressed in these sections.

Postpolio Syndrome

Evaluation of aerobic capacity for persons with PPS should be performed with an ergometer that involves both upper and lower extremities (e.g., Schwinn Air-Dyne ergometer) (11). A discontinuous protocol should be performed, with initial workloads of 10–25 W and incremental increases of 10–25 W every 2 minutes. Rest periods of 2–4 minutes are recommended between each stage. Persons with PPS whose condition prevents the use of their legs should use an arm-crank ergometer, with an initial workload of 5–10 W, incremental increases of 5–10 W every 2 minutes, and rest periods of 2–4 minutes between each stage.

The guidelines established for GBS (see below) are applicable to persons with PPS for muscle strength, endurance, and range-of-motion evaluations.

Muscle strength measurements are used to assess muscle dysfunction, but muscle strength has not been shown to have a good correlation with functional performance (i.e., ADL tasks) (19, 27–29). Consequently, recommendations for evaluating functional performance of such ADL activities as walking, rising from a chair, and rising from supine to standing include: (1) walking capacity—timing a distance of 300 feet with at least three changes in direction and two different grades; (2) stepping capacity—timing the ascent and descent on a flight of 10 steps, twice, using conventional 7-8 inch household steps; and (3) orthostatic capacity—timing 10 repetitions of sit-to-stand from a conventional chair (i.e., 52 cm in height).

These functional tests can be difficult for persons with PPS who have MMT scores of less than 3/5 for knee extension and/or hip abduction for one leg, and extremely difficult for individuals with MMT scores of less than 3/5 for both legs. When persons with PPS are using orthosis or assistive devices, these devices should be worn during functional evaluation.

Guillain-Barré Syndrome

It is important to recognize two distinct phases of rehabilitation for persons with GBS. Testing procedures for inpatient rehabilitation are covered in the sections on clinical exercise physiology and diagnostic techniques. This section and the next section, "Exercise Prescription and Programming," address the "outpatient" phase of rehabilitation and recovery. The outpatient phase is when the patient has been released from a rehabilitation center and is no longer under direct medical care.

The study by Pitetti and colleagues (30) is the only study that has reported methodologies for cardiovascular and strength testing of a GBS patient. Pitetti et al. (30) evaluated the cardiovascular fitness and muscle strength of a 58-year-old male GBS patient, 3.5 years after being released from the hospital. At the time of his discharge from the hospital, this patient had severe muscle atrophy and was unable to ambulate without crutches and ankle orthoses. He also had significant weakness, bilateral foot drop, and some sensory loss in the hands. Three and one-half years later, at the time of exercise evaluation, this patient was able to ambulate with the assistance of one crutch and experienced minimal weakness in the hands and feet.

This patient's peak exercise capacity was evaluated using three different modes of exercise: a Schwinn Air-Dyne ergometer (SAE), an electrically braked bicycle ergometer (BE), and an arm-crank ergometer (ACE). The testing protocol for the SAE and BE was similar, with each exercise starting at an initial workload of 25 W for 2 minutes and increasing workload 25 W every 2 minutes until volitional exhaustion. The protocol for the ACE started the participant with arm cranking at 10 W (50 rpm) for 2 minutes, increasing workload by 10 W every 2 minutes until volitional exhaustion. The peak physiological parameters measured were peak oxygen consumption ($\dot{V}O_{2peak}$, $mL \cdot min^{-1}$ and $mL \cdot kg^{-1} \cdot min^{-1}$), heart rate (HR, bpm), ventilation ($\dot{V}_E$, $l \cdot min^{-1}$), and respiratory exchange ratio (RER, $\dot{V}CO_2$, $\dot{V}O_2$). Peak work capacity (in watts) and length of test time were also measured on the BE. The highest peak physiological parameters were seen using the SAE followed by the BE. The highest work level reached (175 W) was also achieved on the SAE followed by the BE (100 W). Arm-crank ergometry produced the lowest work level of all parameters measured. Blood pressure responses (taken 2 min before, 2 min after exercise, and the last minute of each work level) throughout all three tests were normal.

Knee extension and flexion were evaluated using the Cybex 340 dynamometer. It was the opinion of these authors (30) that, given the physical capacities of this GBS participant, he was capable of performing most any test of flexibility, muscle strength and endurance, or cardiovascular fitness that could be performed by able-bodied individuals, with the exception of a treadmill protocol.

Upper body measurement techniques used to assess range of motion, as well as upper body strength and endurance test protocols used to evaluate able-bodied individuals, should be applicable to most GBS patients. Variations for lower-extremity testing protocols depend on the residual weakness of the lower limbs. Knee flexion and extension and hip measurements (e.g., flexion, extension, adduction, abduction) used to evaluate able-bodied individuals are applicable to GBS patients. As with upper body measurements, GBS patients should be sitting (as with knee or hip flexion and extension measurements) or prone (as in leg press) in order to maintain balance. Standing test measurements, like a squat, should be performed with caution and in the presence of an assistant.

EXERCISE PRESCRIPTION AND PROGRAMING

Postpolio Syndrome

Five classifications of PPS have been developed to facilitate safer and more effective exercise programs (31). If a person is not correctly classified, the exercise program could injure unstable motor units.

Classification I (no clinical polio) is the highest functional and least symptomatic. Individuals with this classification have no history of recent muscle weakness. Their physical exam shows good to normal strength, sensation, and reflexes and no muscle atrophy. EMG and NCV results are normal. Persons in Classification I should be able to exercise aerobically at intensities of 50–70% heart rate reserve (HRR), rating of perceived exertion (RPE) of 12–14 (on the 6–20 scale), or MET levels in the 6–9 range; durations of up to 30 minutes; with frequencies of 3–5 days/week. It is recommended that the mode of exercise involve both upper and lower body musculature (i.e., Schwinn Air-Dyne, swimming).

Classification II (subclinical polio) shows no new weakness but a history of weakness with full recovery. EMG and NCV testing should exhibit chronic denervation or large polyphasic motor unit action potentials but no acute denervation. Exercise for this classification includes similar MHRR and RPE intensities as Classification I, but MET levels should be in the 5–8 range. However, duration periods should include intervals of 5 minutes, with a "rest" period of 1 minute between intervals. Exercise days should alternate with 1 day of rest, and the suggested exercise mode is the same as Classification I.

Classification III (clinically stable polio) shows a history of weakness with variable recovery and no new weakness. Physical exam results include poor to good strength, normal sensation, normal to decreased reflexes, and possible muscle atrophy. EMG and NCV results indicate chronic denervation. Exercise intensity should include an MHRR of 40–60%, RPE of 11–13, with MET levels in the 4–5 range. Duration should be up to 20 minutes total, with intervals of no more than 3 minutes and recovery time of 1 minute. Frequency and modalities are similar to Classification II.

Classification IV (clinically unstable polio) shows a history of weakness with variable recovery and a recent history of new weakness. The physical exam and EMG/NCV results are similar to Classification III. Exercise activities should include durations of 2–3 minutes followed by a 1–2 minute recovery for a total exercise time of 15 minutes, 3 times per week. Intensity level should be HRR of 40–50%, RPE of 11–12, and MET levels at 3. Nonfatiguing resistive exercise can be supplemented.

Classification V (severely atrophic polio) is the lowest functional and most symptomatic, with new weakness and little recovery from the acute stage. The physical exam results show poor muscle strength, normal sensation, areflexic and severe limb atrophy. EMG and NCV tests show decreased insertional activity with few to no motor unit action potentials and acute denervation. Exercise is generally contraindicated. ADL should be the extent of exercise programming. Orthotic and bracing devices are indicated, and often a wheelchair is required for mobility.

Significant increases have been shown in muscle strength of elbow and knee extensors in persons with PPS using concentric contraction training, 3 nonconsecutive times/week, with 3 sets of 20, 15, and 10 repetitions (14). Resistance intensity was 75% of 3-RM with 90 seconds' recovery between sets and 3 minutes' rest between exercises. Another study (13) reported strength gains using isotonic training that consisted of 3 sets, 12 repetitions each, twice a week on nonconsecutive days. Initial weight or resistance was at a differentiated RPE of 13–14.

Guillain-Barré Syndrome

The course of illness can be more prolonged in adults, particularly older adults, than in children. Improvement can continue for up to 2 years after onset, with rate and variability of neurological recovery related to age, requirement for respiratory support, and rate of progression. The course of illness can also result in chronic-relapsing GBS.

Questions regarding the usefulness of exercise to help maintain health for patients with GBS remains unanswered because of the dearth of research regarding the effects of exercise on GBS. The "Medical News" section of the *Journal of the American Medical Association* (32) reported a paper written by Dr. Bensman, who at that time was an assistant professor at the University of Minnesota Medical School. The paper discussed the clinical course of eight GBS patients who were adversely affected by "excessive physical activity" that was part of their inpatient rehabilitation. The phrase "excessive physical activity" was never defined. Three of the eight patients were placed on a nonfatiguing program including passive range-of-motion exercises, which quickly resulted in an increase in muscle strength and no more periods of functional loss. Another three of the eight patients had already been discharged, but loss of function due to weakness and/or paresis reappeared after "exercising too strenuously." These three GBS patients improved after bedrest and limitation of activity, but relapses continued "to be associated with fatigue." The two remaining patients returned to the hospital because of a recurrence of GBS 1 year after the onset of symptoms.

Steinberg (33) noted that excessive exercise, especially fatiguing activity, often causes abnormal sensations for various periods of time. Steinberg (33) suggested that GBS patients be allowed to engage in physical activity up to the point where muscle ache/fatigue begins. Fatigue declined after their activity was "carefully controlled."

The GBS participant in the study by Pitetti et al. (30) performed 40 exercise sessions during a 16-week period on an SAE following initial cardiovascular and strength testing. The GBS participant exercised for 20–30 minutes per session at 70% of peak heart rate as determined by a pre-training exercise test on the SAE. The GBS participant increased cardiopulmonary capacities, peak work level, total work capacity, and isokinetic leg strength following this supervised exercise regimen without any GBS-related complications.

Karper (34) reported the effects of a low-intensity aerobic exercise regimen on a female (18 yr) with chronic-relapsing GBS. The exercise regimen consisted of a 10-week walking phase followed by a 15-week cycling phase. The GBS patient exercised 3 days a week for 20 to 37 minutes as a walking phase and 15 to 32 minutes as a cycling phase. The GBS patient was not allowed to exercise over 45 percent of her HRR (220 − age) reserve. During cycling, the participant stopped every 5 minutes and rested for 2 minutes. No rest periods were reported for the walking phase. Following both exercise phases, the GBS patient improved in walking distance, speed of walking, and riding time (cycle ergometer) without any GBS relapse or side effects.

Given the above reports, a very conservative approach should be taken for both inpatient and outpatient rehabilitation. Once the disease begins to stabilize, inpatient rehabilitation should begin using short periods of non-fatiguing activities (i.e., PROM and AROM). As the patient improves (noted by increase in muscle strength and nerve conduction), light muscle strengthening exercises should be initiated. As the patient continues to improve, more exercises and activities for physical therapy and occupational therapy, as well as training for ADL can be added to the overall rehabilitation plan. During the first 3 to 6 months after onset of the disease, the medical staff should be vigilant to signs of fatigue in their patients, and it is important for the patient to know his/her own limitations and be able to exercise without causing fatigue.

No exercise regimens involving flexibility and muscle strength and endurance exercises, have been reported for GBS patients. However, the GBS patient in the study by Pitetti et al. (30) showed increases in leg strength and the patients in the study by Karper (34) showed improved grip strength following their aerobic exercise regimen. This suggests that an exercise program involving not only aerobic exercise but also resistance training would be beneficial for GBS patients.

In addition to cardiopulmonary improvement, work and strength improvements were seen in the GBS patient in the study by Pitetti et al. (30). The patient also reported subjective improvements in activities of daily living. Housework and yardwork activities had been expanded following the exercise regimen. For instance, the GBS patient was able to mow his yard (self-propelled mower) without rest periods and returned to gardening because weeding, digging up roots, and rototilling were feasible again. He also reported being able to walk up stairs without the use of railings plus an overall reduction in daily fatigue. That is, following the exercise regimen, he seldom took naps, whereas before training, they were daily necessities.

Undoubtedly, a significant number of patients discharged from inpatient rehabilitation who return to their homes could benefit from outpatient rehabilitative services or individualized exercise programs at community health clubs who have someone who is, at the least, certified as a Health Fitness Instructor by the American College of Sports Medicine.

EDUCATION AND COUNSELING

Postpolio Syndrome

Persons with PPS experiencing new and/or increased weakness could employ several strategies to slow further debilitating decline. First, education about ADL and physical activities is important to minimize effects of fatigue, including the pace used in task completion. Second, the use of orthoses can reduce stress and possibly decrease pain and fatigue. Accepting the need for orthoses or accepting the need for assistive devices such as wheelchairs or scooters may require counseling. Assistive devices are particularly helpful when long periods of standing or walking are necessary and when recovery from fatigue has been slow.

A person with PPS can have many adverse problems that surface after many years of status quo. Abrupt changes affecting ADL mobility and independence usually result in increased stress. Consequently, individuals with PPS can be candidates for anxiety and depression. Counseling may be needed along with adequate family support to overcome the changes brought on by PPS.

Guillain-Barré Syndrome

Psychological variables such as symptoms of mild depression occurring after initial disease onset are common. Research is needed to determine the severity of psychological and social issues with severely involved GBS patients (i.e., months to years of ventilatory dependence with chronic-relapsing GBS).

Additionally, the extent and duration of the physically disabling sequelae in GBS has not been adequately described. That is, with regard to motor function and the loss of the active number of motor units with aging, poliomyelitis and GBS have similar clinical issues.

Of note to this issue, a study by Burrows (35) reported on the residual subclinical impact of GBS in four military personnel (3 males and 1 female; ages 19, 21, 58, and 27 yrs, respectively) who were medically pronounced "totally recovered" from the syndrome. Prior to the onset of GBS, all four individuals exceeded requirements to pass the Army Physical Fitness Test (APFT). The APFT includes performing 15 push-ups and 40 sit-ups in 2 minutes and completing a 2-mile run in 21 minutes. All four soldiers were unable to pass the APFT 1 to 3 years following onset of GBS.

Other studies have reported residual long-term disabilities. Melillo and colleagues (36) studied the course of 37 patients following discharge and reported that 13 developed long-term disability. Bernsen et al. (37) reported that 3 to 6 years after onset of Guillain-Barré syndrome, 63% of 122 patients showed one or more changes in their lifestyle, work, or leisure activities due to loss of muscle strength and poor coordination. And Soryal and colleagues (38) reported that residual skeletal problems and complications (i.e., marked joint stiffness and contractures) in GBS patients became major components of disability despite having physiotherapy from the onset and improving neurological status.

Similar residual disabilities were also noted in children and adolescents, which indicates special consideration is needed for children and adolescents recovering from GBS. A report by Berman and Tom (39) indicated that significant and permanent motor loss in extremities was still present 1.5 years following discharge. The authors (39) noted that the late permanent motor paralysis and residual joint deformities secondary to GBS occur in children and adolescents at a higher incidence and severity than in adults. This would suggest that an intensive inpatient and outpatient rehabilitation program is imperative for children and adolescents, including frequent and extended follow-up strength and motor evaluations.

References

1. Thornsteinsson G. Management of postpolio syndrome. Mayo Clin Pros 1997;72:627–628.
2. Dalakas MC, Hallett M. The Post-Polio Syndrome: In: Plum F, ed. Advances in contemporary neurology. Philadelphia: F.A. Davis, 1988;15–95.
3. Widar M, Ahlstrom G. Pain in persons with post-polio. Scand J Caring Sci 1999;13:33–40.
4. Bruno RL, Crenge SJ, Frick NM. Parallels between post-polio fatigue and chronic fatigue syndrome: a common pathophysiology? Am J Med 1998;105:665–738.
5. Aurlien D, Strandjord RE, Hegland O. Postpolio syndrome—a critical comment to the diagnosis. Acta Neurol Scand 1999;100:76–80.
6. Birk TJ. Poliomyelitis and the post-polio syndrome: exercise capacities and adaptation-current research, future directions, and widespread applicability. Med Sci Sports Exerc 1993;25: 466–472.
7. Franco DA, Bashir RM. Current concepts in Guillian-Barré syndrome. Nebr Med J 1996;406–411.
8. Fulgham JR, Wijdicks EFM. Guillain-Barré syndrome. Crit Care Clin 1997;13(1):1–15.
9. Willen C, Cider A, Summerhagen KS. Physical performance in individuals with late effects of polio. Scand J Rehabil Med 1999;31:244–249.
10. Stanghelle JK, Festvag L, Aksnes A. Pulmonary function and symptom-limited exercise stress testing in subjects with late sequelae of postpoliomyelitis. Scand J Rehab Med 1993;25: 125– 129.
11. Birk TJ. Polio and post-polio syndrome. In: ACSM's exercise management for persons with chronic diseases and disabilities. Champaign, IL: Human Kinetics, 1997.
12. Stanghellod JK, Festvag LV. Postpolio syndrome: a 5 year follow-up. Spinal Cord 1997;35:503–508.
13. Agre JC, Rodriquez AA, Franke TM. Strength, endurance, and work capacity after muscle strengthening exercise in postpolio subjects. Arch Phys Med Rehabil 1997;78:681–687.
14. Spector SA, Gordon PL, Feuerstein IM, et al. Strength gains without muscle injury after strength training in patients with postpolio muscular atrophy. Muscle Nerve 1996;19: 1282–1290.
15. Einarsson G, Grindy G. Strengthening exercise program in postpolio subjects. In: Halstead LS, Wiechers DO, eds. Research and clinical aspects of late effects of poliomyelitis. White Plains, NY: March of Dimes Birth Defects Foundation, 1987.
16. Meythaler JM. Rehabilitation of Guillain-Barre syndrome. Arch Phys Med Rehabil 1997;78(8):872–879.
17. Dalakas MC, Bartfeld H, Kurland LT. The pospolio syndrome: advances in the pathogenesis and treatment. Ann N Y Acad Sci 1995;753:1–411.
18. Trojan DA, Collet JP, Shapiro S, et al. A multicenter, randomized, double-blinded trial of pyridostigmine in postpolio syndrome. Neurology 1999;53:1225–1233.
19. Nollet F, Beelen A, Prins MH. Disability and functional assessment in former polio patients with and without postpolio syndrome. Arch Phys Med Rehabil 1999;80:136–143.
20. Julien J, Leparc-Goffart I, Lina B, et al. Postpolio syndrome: poliovirus persistence is involved in the pathogenesis. J Neurol 1999;246: 472–476.
21. Samii A, Lopez-Devine J, Wasserman EM, et al. Normal postexercise facilitation and depression of motor evoked potentials in postpolio patients. Muscle Nerve 1998;21: 948–950.
22. Cywinska-Wasilewaska G, Ober JJ, Koczocik-Przedpelska J. Power spectrum of the surface EMG in post-polio syndrome. Electromyogr Clin Neurophysiol 1998;38:463–466.
23. Roeleveld K, Sandberg A, Stalberg EV, et al. Motor unit size estimation of enlarged motor units with surface electromygraphy. Muscle Nerve 1998;21:878–886.
24. Rodriquez AA, Agre JC, Franke TM. Electromyographic and neuromuscular variables in unstable postpolio subjects, stable postpolio subjects, and control subjects. Arch Phys Med Rehabil 1997;78:986–991.
25. Nordgren B, Falck B, Stalberg E, et al. Postpolio muscular dysfunction: relationships between muscle energy metabolism, subjective symptoms, magnetic resonance imaging, electromyography, and muscle strength. Muscle Nerve 1997;20:1341–1351.
26. American College of Sports Medicine. ACSM's guidelines for exercise testing and prescription, 6th ed. Philadelphia: Lea & Febiger, 2000.
27. Parker TL, Sauriol A, Brouwer B. Fatigue secondary to chronic

illness: postpolio syndrome, chronic fatigue syndrome, and multiple sclerosis. Arch Phys Med Rehabil 1994;75:1122–1126.

28. Einersson G, Grimby G. Disability and handicap in late poliomyolitis. Scand J Rehabil Med 1990;22:113–121.
29. Brimby G, Jonsson G. Disability in poliomyelitis sequelae. Phys Ther 1994;74:415–424.
30. Pitetti KH, Barrett PJ, Abbas D. Endurance exercise training in Guillain-Barrè syndrome. Arch Phys Med Rehabil 1993; 74:761–765.
31. Halstead L, Gawne AC. NRH proposal for limb classification and exercise prescription. Disabil Rehabil 1996;18:311–316.
32. Staff. Strenuous exercise may impair muscle function in Guillain-Barrè patients. JAMA 1970;214, 468–469.
33. Steinberg JS. Guillian-Barrè syndrome (acute idiopathic polyneuritis): an overview for the lay person. Wynnwood, PA: The Guillian-Barrè Syndrome Support Group International, 1987.
34. Karper WB. Effects of low-intensity aerobic exercise on one subject with Chronic Relapsing Guillian-Barrè syndrome. Rehabil Nurs 1991;16(2):96–98.
35. Burrows DS. Residual subclinical impairment in patients who totally recovered from Guillain-Barrè syndrome: impact on military performance. Mil Med 1990;155:438–440.
36. Melillo EM, Sethi JM, Mohsenin V. Guillain-Barré syndrome: rehabilitation outcome and recent developments. Yale J Biol Med 1998;71(5):383–389.
37. Bernsen RA, de Jager AE, Schmitz PI, et al. Residual physical outcome and daily living 3 to 6 years after Guillain-Barré syndrome. Neurology 1999;53(2):409–410.
38. Soryal I, Sinclair E, Hornby J, et al. Impaired joint mobility in Guillain-Barré syndrome: a primary or a secondary phenomenon? J Neurol Neurosurg Psychiatry 1992;22(11): 1014–1017.
39. Berman AT, Tom L. The Guillain-Barrè syndrome in children. Clin Ortho Related Resp 1976;116:61–65.

CHAPTER **7**

Muscular Dystrophy and Other Myopathies

Mark A. Tarnopolsky and Timothy J. Doherty

EPIDEMIOLOGY AND PATHOPHYSIOLOGY

Myopathies encompass a wide range of disorders that can be broadly considered as either congenital or acquired. The congenital forms include the muscular dystrophies, congenital myopathies, channelopathies, and metabolic myopathies (Table 7.1). The acquired myopathies include endocrine myopathies, inflammatory myopathies, toxic myopathies, and primary infectious myopathies (Table 7.2). The incidence and prevalence of muscle disorders varies widely, with myotonic dystrophy and Duchenne dystrophy being about 1/3500 live births (Duchenne only in males) and other disorders such as MELAS 3271 (mitochondrial myopathy) being reported in about 15 people in the world (1, 2).

As expected, most of the congenital myopathies are due to genetic inborn errors of metabolism. These can be categorized as autosomal dominant (AD), autosomal recessive (AR), X-linked recessive (XR), maternally inherited (MI) (mitochondrial disorders), and sporadic spontaneous mutations. In general, the dystrophies are often due to abnormalities in the cytoskeleton (e.g., dystrophin in Duchenne dystrophy), whereas the metabolic myopathies are due to mutations in the energy transduction enzymes (e.g., carnitine palmitoyl transferase deficiency). There are some exceptions to this general rule, such as calpain-3 deficiency (a proteolytic enzyme) seen in a form of autosomal recessive limb girdle dystrophy. The inheritance pattern and gene product of the inherited myopathies are presented in Table 7.3.

The acquired myopathies encountered in North America are usually inflammatory or endocrine. Acute viral myopathies are frequently encountered with a wide spectrum of severity. Fungal and bacterial myopathies are rarely encountered in first-world countries (Table 7.2).

FUNCTIONAL CONSEQUENCES

Progressive muscle weakness is the most common symptom of structural myopathies, and fatigability is the most common symptom of the metabolic myopathies. Most of the congenital myopathies/dystrophies start with weakness in the proximal muscles and eventually spread more distally. Notable exceptions are fascioscapulohumeral dystrophy, where facial weakness is a prominent and early sign, and myopathies with distal weakness including distal myopathies and myotonic muscular dystrophy. In general, the disorders of fat metabolism and mitochondrial cytopathies present with impairment in endurance-type activities, whereas glycogen storage diseases present with symptoms during higher-intensity muscle contractions.

A common outcome from prolonged weakness is joint contracture and secondary bony abnormalities, including osteoarthritis, osteoporosis, and scoliosis. Contractures are most commonly seen at the elbow, ankle, knee, and hip. Many of the myopathies can also affect cardiac muscle with conduction blocks and cardiomyopathy (Table 7.4).

PHYSICAL EXAMINATION

As mentioned above, most patients with myopathy will have significant proximal weakness without any sensory signs or symptoms as primary manifestations of their disorder. Mental status is usually unaffected, with the exception of some children with Duchenne dystrophy, myotonic muscular dystrophy (somnolence is very common and cognitive impairment is seen in more severe forms), and congenital myopathy with central nervous system involvement. Cranial nerve examination is usually normal. However, facial weakness is manifested in fascioscapulohumeral muscular dystrophy and some cases of central nuclear myopathy and myotonic dystrophy. Muscle bulk is reduced in later stages of myopathies and is usually proximal, with the exceptions noted previously. Muscle weakness follows a proximal pattern with the notable exceptions above. Muscle stretch reflexes are normal in the early stages and suppressed later as weakness progresses. Sensory examination is normal and significant sensory abnormalities prompt investigation into acquired causes of neuropathy (compression/entrapment, monoclonal gammopathy of uncertain significance, diabetes, autoimmune disease, B12 deficiency, thyroid abnormali-

Table 7.1. Overview of the Common Congenital Myopathies

MUSCULAR DYSTROPHIES

- Congenital Muscular Dystrophy
- Dystrophinopathies (Becker's and Duchenne)
- Fascioscapulohumeral
- Limb Girdle
- Distal Dystrophies
- Hereditary Inclusion Body Myositis
- Myotonic
- Emery-Dreifuss
- Oculopharyngeal

CHANNELOPATHIES

- Myotonia Congenita (Thomsen's and Becker's)
- Malignant Hyperthermia
- Hyperkalemic Periodic Paralysis
- Hypokalemic Periodic Paralysis
- Potassium Sensitive Myotonia Congenita
- Paramyotonia Congenita

CONGENITAL MYOPATHIES

- Nemaline Rod
- Central Core
- Centronuclear
- Minicore/Multicore

METABOLIC MYOPATHIES

- Glycogen Storage Disease (GSD)
- Fatty Acid Oxidation Defects (FAOD)
- Fatty Acid Transport Defects
- Mitochondrial Myopathies
- Myoadenylate Deaminase Deficiency

ties, toxin exposure, drugs, etc.), as opposed to a myopathic etiology. Orthopedic deformities at birth such as arthrogryposis and talipes equinovarus can be seen in the congenital myopathies due to intrauterine weakness. Secondary orthopedic manifestations include knee, ankle, and hip contractures as weakness progresses. Dermatomyositis and Emery-Dreifuss muscular dystrophy are prone to elbow joint contractures, and the former may also result in subcutaneous calcifications.

MEDICAL AND SURGICAL TREATMENTS

Physical treatment for most myopathies consists of exercise, stretching, and range of motion, as outlined below. Stretching and range-of-motion exercises may be of benefit in the prevention of contractures. When contractures are emerging, serial casting, intensive stretching, and physiotherapy are warranted. If this fails, a surgical procedure such as tendon lengthening may become necessary. Patients with myopathies are very sensitive to the immobility associated with surgery, which may cause a rapid step-wise decline in motor function. Corticosteroids are an accepted mainstay of treatment in patients with dystrophinopathies (3). In spite of their negative side effects, studies show an overall improvement in muscle strength and function (3). Nevertheless, each child must be treated on an individual basis, and we recommend objective and subjective evaluation and follow-up in a tertiary care center familiar with the use of corticosteroids in dystrophinopathy.

Table 7.2. Acquired Myopathies

ENDOCRINE

- Hypothyroidism
- Hyperthyroidism
- Vitamin D deficiency
- Cushing's syndrome-hyper-cortisolemia
- Hypocortisolemia (Addison's disease)
- Acromegaly (growth hormone excess)

INFLAMMATORY MYOPATHIES

- Polymyositis
- Dermatomyositis
- Inclusion body myositis
- Myositis with connective disease
- Transient viral myositis
- Bacterial/fungal myositis

DRUGS

- AZT
- Adriamycin
- Chloriquine
- Corticosteroids

PHARMACOLOGY

Most children with Duchenne and Becker's muscular dystrophy will be treated with corticosteroids (prednisone or deflazacort). Corticosteroids are associated with increased risk of osteoporosis. Therefore, it is important for these individuals to take supplemental calcium, vitamin D, and in many instances, bisphosphates. Corticosteroids can negatively affect therapeutic exercise potential by contributing to proximal weakness and atrophy (steroid myopathy), causing significant weight gain, contributing to hyperglycemia, hypertension, cataracts, and electrolyte abnormalities (hypokalemia/hypernatremia). Some patients with fascioscapulohumeral dystrophy are prescribed β-2 agonists, which can contribute to tachycardia and possibly cardiac dysrhythmia. Many patients are also taking creatine monohydrate, which probably has a positive, as opposed to negative, effect on exercise capacity (4).

DIAGNOSTIC TECHNIQUES

The approach to a patient with suspected myopathy involves a very careful history, physical examination, and family history. Acute and subacute conditions coming on

Table 7.3. Muscular Dystrophies/Congenital Myopathies/Channelopathies

	Inheritance Pattern	Gene Product	Symbol
Duchenne Muscular Dystrophy	XR	dystrophin	DYS-DMD
Becker's Muscular Dystrophy	XR	dystrophin	DYS-BMD
Limb Girdle Muscular Dystrophy (Recessive)	AR	dysferlin	LG-MD2B
	AR	alpha-sarcoglycan	LG-MD2D
	AR	beta-sarcoglycan	LG-MD2E
	AR	gamma-sarcoglycan	LG-MD2C
	AR	calpain-3	LG-MD2A
Limb Girdle Muscular Dystrophy (Dominant)	AD	caveolin-3	LG-MD1C
	AD	laminin A/C	LG-MD1B
Distal Muscular Dystrophy			
- Miyoshi	AR	dysferlin	MM
- Miscellaneous (Nonaka, Udd, and Bethlem)			
Hereditary Inclusion Body Myopathy	AR	?	IBM2
Oculopharyngeal Muscular Dystrophy	AD	poly(A) binding protein	OPMD
Congenital Myopathy/Dystrophy			
- Myotubular Myopathy	XR	myotubularin	MTMX
- Central Core	AD	ryanodine receptor	CCD
- Nemaline Myopathy	AD	α-tropomyosin	NEM1
	AR	nebulin	NEM2
Emery-Dreifuss	XR	emerin	EMD
	AD	laminin A/C	LMNA
Fascioscapulohumeral	AD	?	FSHD
Myotonic Muscular Dystrophy −1	AD	myotonin	DM
Myotonic Muscular Dystrophy −2	AD	?	DM2
Proximal Myotonic Myopathy	AD	?	PROMM
Congenital Muscular Dystrophy	AR	alpha-2 laminin	LAMA2
	AR	integrin α 7	ITG7
Congenital Muscular Dystrophy +CNS abnormality − Fukuyama	AR	fukutin	FCMD
Channelopathies:			
Malignant Hyperthermia	AD	ryanodine receptor	MHS1
Myotonia Congenita	AD	chloride channel	CLC-1 (Thomsen's)
	AR	chloride channel	CLC-1 (Becker's)
Hyperkalemic Periodic Paralysis	AD	sodium channel α subunit	SCN4A
Hypokalemic Periodic Paralysis	AD	dihydropyridine receptor	CACNL1A3

later in life are often acquired. However, some of the metabolic myopathies may present for the first time in later life as well as rather acutely. The pattern of weakness, associated sensory symptoms (pointing more toward a neuropathic disorder), presence or absence of muscle cramping, pigmenturia, and onset of symptoms with endurance or high-intensity exercise are all helpful in the evaluation. More often than not, the tentative diagnosis can be made from the history and physical examination. For example, a classic history of distal weakness, frontal balding, cataracts, hypersomnolence, and grip myotonia would prompt an investigation of lymphoblast culture with DNA extraction for CTG-repeat analysis by southern blot or polymerase chain reaction. In such a case, the finding of expanded CTG-repeat would confirm the diagnosis of myotonic dystrophy, and further testing would not be required to establish the diagnosis. In less classic cases, further testing is required, including serum chemistries for creatine kinase, electrolytes, and thyroid function as an initial screen. The finding of rash, joint involvement, or other autoimmune features would prompt ANA, ESR, C-reactive protein, and extractable nuclear antigens as part of the initial investigations. In suspected metabolic myopathy, forearm ischemic testing may be helpful in showing absence of lactate rise with normal ammonia rise (a classic GSD pattern), or normal lactate rise with absent am-

Table 7.4. Myopathies Associated with Cardiac Abnormalities

Myopathy	Cardiac Defect
Dystrophinopathies (Becker's and Duchenne)	Cardiomyopathy
Myotonic Dystrophy, type 1, 2, and PROMM	Cardiac conduction block
Emery-Dreifuss Muscular Dystrophy	Cardiac conduction block
Nemaline Rod Myopathy	Cardiomyopathy
Centronuclear Myopathy	Cardiomyopathy

neral, resistance exercise in children with DMD n shown to either maintain strength or result in nprovement. There is little consensus among ex- owever, as to the clinical utility of strength training s population. The few studies in the literature are d by: (1) frequent use of nonquantitative, insensi- utcome measures; (2) often poorly defined exercise rams; (3) lack of a control group in many cases or use e opposite limb as a control; (4) heterogeneity in the tment groups regarding age, disease progression, func- nal level, and degree of contracture present; and (5) all sample sizes in the treatment and, when present, ntrol groups. Additionally, any intervention trial di- ected toward DMD must take into account the rapidly progressive nature of this disease.

Two pioneering studies that examined resistance exercise in children with primarily DMD were carried out by Abramson and Rogoff (19) and Hoberman (20). Strength was assessed by manual muscle testing in both studies. Abramson and Rogoff reported slight improvement by about one-half to one grade on the MRC scale in half of their subjects, with the other half remaining unchanged in response to a 7-month program consisting of active, active-assisted, and resistance exercise performed three times per week. Although poorly quantified, mention was also made of improved mobility in 8 of 27 subjects.

Hoberman examined 10 patients over a 4-month daily program of resistance exercise, gait training, and stretching. There were no reported improvements in strength defined as a gain of one full MRC grade. The author noted, however, in some patients for whom there were records, that there was less decline in strength during the program than in the previous year.

The lack of positive results in this study and the failure of one-half of the patients to respond in the former study may have been influenced by the high proportion of subjects in each with severe disease progression. Two-thirds of the patients in both studies were confined to wheelchairs. It has been suggested that, by the time patients with DMD are wheelchair dependent, they have lost half of their muscle mass (9). Additionally, contractures were present in the majority of patients, which further reduces the ability of the muscle to respond optimally to resistance exercise.

Wratney (21) provided a home, unsupervised exercise program to 75 muscular dystrophy patients (majority with DMD) between the ages of 2 and 16 years. The program consisted of arm and leg exercises against gravity for an unspecified length of time within a 3-year period. There were no reported gains in strength; however, it was suggested that a program of this nature may prevent disuse atrophy and maintain range of motion.

Vignos and Watkins (22) attempted to improve upon these earlier studies and examined the effects of a 1-year, home, higher-intensity resistance-training program in a group of still ambulatory patients with muscular dystrophy (14 DMD, 6 LGMD, 4 FSHD). The DMD patients were compared with a nonexercised control group of DMD patients of similar age, strength, and functional ability. As determined by manual muscle testing, measurable increases in strength were reported for all three patient groups. In all three forms of dystrophy, the strength gains occurred in the first 4 months; however, the gains were maintained during the subsequent 8 months. In general, patients with less severe disease improved more so and greater gains were noted in muscles that were initially stronger. The muscle strength had declined in both the exercised and nonexercised DMD patients in the year prior to the study. The control subjects continued to decline during the second year. The exercised group showed no loss in strength and exhibited a minimal increase, thus suggesting some longer-term benefit.

Finally, Delateur and Giaconi (18) isokinetically (Cybex) trained the quadriceps of one leg in four patients with DMD 4 to 5 times per week for 6 months. The non-exercised leg served as a control. All 5 subjects were ambulatory at the onset of the study and had at least grade 3/5 strength in the knee extensors. One subject, however, with rapidly progressive disease became nonambulatory during the study. Strength was tested on the same device at monthly intervals during the 6-month training period and for the first 6 months posttraining, and at 18 and 24 months. Increases in maximal strength in response to this program were modest, and strength was statistically greater in the exercised leg at only the 5- and 9-month test periods. However, it should be noted that the maximal strength of the exercised leg was equal to or stronger than the control leg for all months of follow-up except at 2 years. Additionally, one of the subjects appeared to have deteriorated rapidly during the course of the study, which likely biased this small data set. An important additional conclusion of this study was the lack of any evidence for overuse weakness in the trained legs as compared to the control legs.

In summary, it can be concluded that there is little evidence to support overuse weakness in response to controlled resistance training programs, at least in DMD. For the most part, studies have shown either maintenance of strength and in some cases modest improvements. In general, more significant gains have been noted in patients with less disease progression and in the less-affected muscle groups. These latter points may indicate the need to intervene as early as possible to obtain maximal benefits. Further investigation into the potential benefit of resistance exercise in DMD is required. These studies will require adequate sample sizes, matched controls, carefully designed and monitored programs, and sensitive strength and functional outcome measures. In addition, as noted earlier, most boys with DMD are now treated with either oral prednisone or deflazacort. The additive effect of well-controlled resistance training programs with corticosteroids has not yet been assessed.

Resistance Exercise in Slowly Progressive Myopathy

In more slowly progressive myopathies such as myotonic dystrophy (DM), LGMD, FSHD, and most of the

monia rise (myoadenylate deaminase deficiency). Evaluation of suspected fatty acid (FFA) oxidation defects, FFA transport abnormalities, and mitochondrial cytopathy requires tertiary and quaternary centers that are skilled in the assessment of these disorders. At an initial screen, serum carnitine, urine organic acids, creatine kinese (CK) activity, urine amino acid screen, plasma lactate, pyruvate, ammonia, and urine myoglobin are necessary.

Electrodiagnostic investigation is often helpful in the workup of a potential myopathic disorder. The classic findings on needle electromyographic studies of early recruitment and brief-/low-amplitude polyphasic motor unit action potentials would all point toward a potential myopathy. Alternatively, abnormalities on nerve conduction testing suggestive of sensory involvement, presence of demyelinating features on nerve conduction testing, and neuropathic motor unit action potentials on needle electromyographic testing would all point toward a neuropathic disorder.

The muscle biopsy is an essential part of the workup in most myopathies. We routinely use a 5-mm Bergstrom needle with a custom-made apparatus, such that a 60-mL syringe can provide airtight suction via a plastic hose inserted into the end using a pipette tip. We routinely obtain enough muscle for histochemistry (~40 mg), electron microscopy (~10 mg), and another piece (~60–100 mg) for enzyme and genetic testing. Light microscopy allows for the assessment of morphometry, accumulation of substrates (i.e., glycogen), fiber type, and immunohistochemistry can be used to assess proteins (Table 7.5). Electron microscopy can be useful in the assessment of ultrastructural details such as mitochondrial morphology, Z-disc streaming, and inclusions.

We have found cranial MRI to be particularly helpful in assessment of mitochondrial cytopathies and also in the evaluation of the hypotonic (floppy), particularly if there are developmental delays in more than one sphere. ^{31}-phosphorous MR spectroscopy is also helpful, particularly when combined with exercise and may show delayed phosphocreatine resynthesis rates with fatty acid oxidation defects and mitochondrial cytopathy (5). Near-infrared spectroscopy can contribute significantly to a diagnosis by showing characteristic patterns in metabolic cytopathies (6).

Aerobic exercise testing can be helpful to determine physical fitness of individuals for exercise prescription, but is also very helpful in the evaluation of patients with suspected metabolic disorders. A low $\dot{V}O_{2peak}$ is seen in patients with mitochondrial cytopathies. For example, in our recent study with predominantly MELAS patients, the mean $\dot{V}O_{2peak}$ was approximately 10 mL/kg/min (7). The respiratory exchange ratio also increases rapidly and to a very high level in patients with mitochondrial cytopathies (7).

Table 7.5. Common Microscopy Techniques

Histochemical Analyses	Utility
ATPase	Fiber typing
Hematoxylin and Eosin	Central nuclei, inflammatory cells
Modified Gomori Trichrome	Mitochondria, nemaline rods
Periodic Acid Schiff	Glycogen
Oil red-O	Lipid content
Myoadenylate Deaminase	AMPD1 deficiency
Cytochrome Oxidase	COX deficiency, ragged red fibers
NADH Tetrazolium Reductase	NADH deficiency, ragged red fibers
Succinate Dehydrogenase	CMPLX II deficiency, ragged red fibers
Elastic Van Giesson	Connective tissue

EXERCISE/FITNESS/FUNCTIONAL TESTING

Most physicians and physiotherapists use the MRC Manual Muscle Scale to semiquantitatively categorize muscle strength (Table 7.6). This scale gives a gross picture of the individual's muscle function, and changes from one grade to another require rather substantial objective changes in power. While this is useful clinically, this testing is often not helpful in evaluating an experimental therapeutic substance in a clinical trial (i.e., deflazacort or creatine monohydrate).

More objective strength outcome measures include isokinetic and isometric dynamometry with devices (i.e., Cybex, Biodex, etc.). In our experience, we have found these to be quite helpful in making treatment decisions such as tapering corticosteroids in inflammatory myopathies, and in following patients on a prescribed exercise regimen to ensure that they are not overtraining and losing strength (see later).

Forearm ischemic testing is helpful in the evaluation of suspected myoadenylate deaminase deficiency or GSD. This test requires basal lactate and ammonia determination (both immediately placed on ice and transported to the laboratory). Following this, a sphygmomanometer cuff is inflated to 20 mm Hg beyond the arterial pressure, and the individual performs rhythmic isometric exercise with a 9:1 exercise-to-rest duty cycle. Following 60 sec of contractions, the manometer cuff is released and recovery samples are taken at 1, 3, and 5 min postexercise. Most texts suggest a 10- or even 20-min recovery. However, we have found that this does not add to the sensitivity and

Table 7.6. MRC SCALE

0	=	no contraction
1	=	flicker contraction
2	=	movement through a full range without gravity
3	=	movement through a full range with gravity
4–	=	movement against minimal resistance
4	=	movement against some resistance
4+	=	movement against moderate resistance
5	=	full muscle power

specificity of the test (Tarnopolsky et al., unpublished observations, 2000). The recovery samples must be taken and placed immediately on ice and analyzed rapidly to avoid false elevations in lactate and ammonia from red blood cell metabolism. It is critically important when performing this test to immediately terminate the test if the individual develops a painful muscle contracture and not to proceed with this type of testing if the patient has had definite myoglobinuria with high-intensity exercise in the past. Under these circumstances, semi-ischemic protocols have been developed, although their sensitivity and specificity has not been established.

Submaximal aerobic activity on the cycle ergometer can be helpful to determine the efficacy of a given intervention, i.e., frequent glucose meals for carnitine palmitoyl transferase deficiency, type 2.

EXERCISE PRESCRIPTION AND PROGRAMMING

Introduction

The goal of any therapeutic intervention for patients with progressive diseases involving the neuromuscular system is to maintain independence and the ability to perform normal activities of daily living, including vocational and avocational pursuits, to as full an extent as possible (8, 9). The means of achieving these goals include: (a) the maintenance of maximal muscle mass and strength within the limitations imposed by the disease process, and (b) the prevention or slowing of secondary complications, including disuse weakness and atrophy as well as the development of contractures that lead to the premature loss of ambulation and functional independence. The extent to which exercise therapy is able to improve skeletal muscle strength and function will be reviewed in the following sections.

The hallmark of any progressive myopathy is muscle atrophy and associated weakness. However, in addition to strength losses associated with the underlying disease, most individuals with neuromuscular disorders lead sedentary lifestyles that likely contribute significantly to their degree of impairment and disability (9). The reasons for this are multifactorial and include: (1) concern among parents, educators, physicians, and therapists that exercise may be detrimental to children with progressive myopathic disorders; (2) limited opportunities for children and adults with progressive myopathies to take part in activity due to lack of available, accessible programming in many communities; (3) lack of early development of adequate motor skills in typical sports and games during childhood that limits participation later in life; and (4) minimal positive reinforcement associated with sport and physical activity in these populations. As a result, lack of physical activity likely contributes significantly to the overall disability in patients with progressive neuromuscular disorders and specifically myopathies. Thus, there has been interest in examining the extent to which exercise therapy can reverse or delay some of the maladaptive changes associated with inactivity.

General Issues in Exercise Prescription in Myopathic Disorders

Muscular Dystrophy/Congenital Myopathy

These patients should first be screened for evidence of cardiac conduction defects (i.e., myotonic dystrophy) and cardiomyopathy (i.e., Duchenne dystrophy). We recommend stress testing and echocardiography in all patients in whom cardiac pathology is known to exist (see Table 7.5). It is very important that individuals stretch and warm up prior to exercise. With weight training, we encourage a higher number of repetitions and low percentage of 1-repetition maximum (1-RM) for the first few weeks, with individuals gradually increasing their percentage (1-RM) as they adapt to the activity. It is very important that each patient "listen to his/her body" and report any abnormal muscle or joint pains. We recommend that a muscle group be exercised with weight training no more frequently than every 48 hours. With endurance exercise, most structural myopathies and well-treated inflammatory and recovering endocrine myopathies can follow a standard exercise prescription for otherwise healthy individuals starting an endurance exercise program. A special concern for both endurance and strength training is the individual with a recently diagnosed inflammatory myopathy who is not yet well controlled with corticosteroids and/or other therapies, or has just undergone an exacerbation of his/her condition with increased weakness and elevated creatine kinase. We usually have these individuals reduce their training or delay the initiation of onset, and perform gentle static stretching until the creatine kinase values are returning toward normal, and the individual feels subjective improvements in his/her strength (Table 7.7). All patients who are taking corticosteroids should be taking vitamin D and calcium and, under some circumstances, bisphosphates.

Channelopathies

The main trigger for malignant hyperthermia (MH) is exposure to anesthesia with succinyl choline and/or

Table 7.7. General Resistance Exercise Prescription Guidelines for Patients with Myopathies

WEAKNESS	MRC GRADE	EXERCISE PRESCRIPTION
None to mild	4, 4+, 5	May perform moderate to high intensity resistance exercise with appropriate monitoring (8–12 repetition maximum sets)
Moderate	3, 4−	May perform moderate intensity exercise with appropriate monitoring (15–20 RM sets)
Severe	1, 2	Passive and active assisted range-of-motion exercise to maintain range and prevent contractures

volatile halogenated anesthetic agents. Individuals harboring malignant hyperthermia may also have episodes of potentially fatal hypermetabolic crisis precipitated by prolonged and/or severe exercise in very hot and humid conditions (10). Patients with malignant hyperthermia should follow the ACSM Guidelines for exercise in the heat, and we would recommend avoidance of prolonged or very-high-intensity repeated activities in hot/humid environments. The medication dantrolene sodium has dramatically decreased the mortality from anesthesia-related MH deaths (10) and would certainly be indicated in an MH crisis precipitated by exercise. All patients with malignant hyperthermia should wear a Medic-Alert® bracelet, and if exercise must be performed in hot/humid environments, prophylactic oral dantrolene sodium may be of benefit. Patients with myotonia congenita develop extreme muscle hypertrophy. Most of these patients avoid weightlifting due to precipitation of extreme hypertrophy that can be so extensive that it is disfiguring. Patients tolerate endurance exercise quite well, which does not result in muscle hypertrophy. In patients with paramyotonia congenita, the main issue with exercise is severe symptomatic exacerbation when exposed to the cold. For this reason, these patients should not perform winter activities, where the potential for hypothermia or a severe cold exposure exists. Under no circumstances should these individuals participate in swimming sports in open water, where cold-induced myotonia could be fatal. In paramyotonia and hyperkalemic periodic paralysis, profound muscle weakness occurs in the minutes to hours following exercise. This is exacerbated with complete inactivity (i.e., driving home in a car after a race). For this reason, we recommend that these individuals try to perform a gentle warm-down and keep their legs moving at low intensities following exercise to avoid the paralysis.

Metabolic Myopathies

It is of primary importance for those with fatty acid oxidation defects to avoid fasting and never exercise during a period of concurrent illness. Most patients should start the consumption of carbohydrates at approximately 1 gm/kg/hr in the hour prior to exercise and consume at least 0.25 g/kg at 15-min intervals during endurance exercise. If muscle cramping, shortness of breath, or tachycardia occurs in patients with fatty acid oxidation defects, they should stop their activity, continue to consume fluids with high carbohydrate content, and if symptoms persist, proceed to an emergency department (11). In our experience, we have found that these exercise and dietary strategies have allowed the majority of our CPT2 patients to perform endurance-type activities, some even at rather surprising intensity/duration. For the patient with GSD, it is imperative to perform a long warm-up period in order to mobilize FFAs and proteins to "bypass the defect." Most patients report a very idiosyncratic feeling of "getting their second wind" when the body can aerobically utilize lipids. Studies have shown t
disease (GSD, type 5) may also
of carbohydrate during exercise
the metabolic defect (12). Carb
hour before and during exercise in
7 (Tarui's disease) inhibits fatty acid
lization, and significantly impairs e
(13). Avoidance of carbohydrates befo
cise is also prudent for those with othe
fecting glycolysis (i.e., phospho-glycerate
glycerate kinase).

Specific Concerns during Exercise Traini

Overuse Weakness

Overuse or overwork weakness, a concern firs
in patients recovering from the effects of poliom
major concern among patients, their parents, c
and therapists. There have been anecdotal case re
increased weakness following strengthening exerc
amyotrophic lateral sclerosis, peripheral nerve lesions
Duchenne muscular dystrophy (DMD) (14–16). A
tionally, overuse was suggested in several family memb
with fascioscapulohumeral dystrophy (FSHD) based o
asymmetric weakness in the upper extremities (17). The affected family members showed greater weakness on the dominant side, with the exception of one individual, a heavy equipment operator, who used his nondominant left arm to operate the equipment and exhibited greater weakness on that side. This description is obviously anecdotal and uncontrolled. Additionally, it fails to take into account the common finding of significant asymmetry in the pattern of weakness typically found in patients with FSHD. In one controlled study, patients with DMD performed submaximal knee extension exercise for 6 months and showed no evidence of overuse weakness in comparison to the nonexercised control leg (18). There is no definitive evidence at this time to support overuse weakness in patients with myopathic disorders (see later). It is most prudent, however, that exercise programs be appropriately adapted to the individual needs of the patient and that adequate supervision and monitoring is in place.

Resistance Exercise in Rapidly Progressive Myopathies

In DMD, there is rapid and progressive loss of strength and functional capacity. Boys are typically dependent on wheelchairs for mobility between the ages of 8 and 12 years (9). Because of this rapid progression, these children are limited in the extent to which they can participate with their peers in normal age-appropriate physical activity and play. There is, therefore, considerable risk of isolation and lack of social interaction, as well as the aforementioned additive problem of disuse weakness and atrophy (8). Thus, there has been considerable interest in the potential benefits of strengthening exercise to slow the progression of weakness, improve functional capacity, and allow for more natural development.

congenital myopathies, the goal of resistance exercise programs has been to improve strength and function rather than simply slow the pace of disease progression. The majority of studies in this regard have grouped patients with different disorders to achieve adequate sample sizes.

McCartney and coworkers (23) dynamically trained the elbow flexors of one arm and the knee and hip extensors bilaterally in five patients with slowly progressive neuromuscular disorders (three subjects with spinal muscular atrophy, one with LGMD, and one with FSHD) three times per week for 9 weeks. Strength was objectively determined pre- and posttraining while the extent of motor unit activation was determined with the twitch interpolation technique (24). Force in the trained elbow flexors increased from 19 to 34% and from −14 to +25% in the control arm. Leg strength improved on average by 11%. Three subjects who were unable to completely activate their muscles pretraining, as determined by twitch interpolation, were able to do so posttraining, suggesting a significant neural component to the strength increases.

Milner-Brown and Miller (25) similarly trained a group of patients with slowly progressive neuromuscular disorders (six with FSHD, four with DM, one with LGMD, three with spinal muscular atrophy, and one with polyneuropathy). The elbow flexors and knee extensors were trained with a standard progressive-resistance exercise program, and quantitative measures of strength and fatigue were performed. Significant increases in strength and endurance were noted for markedly to moderately weak muscles. Severely weak muscles (<10% normal), however, generally did not improve.

The impact of a moderate-resistance, home-based exercise program for patients with slowly progressive neuromuscular disease was reported by Aitkens et al. (26). Subjects trained their knee extensors and elbow flexors unilaterally with weights 3 days per week for 12 weeks. A healthy control group was studied for comparison. Training loads were designed to be moderate in intensity and ranged from 10–40% of maximum (except handgrip at 100%). Both the patient and control group demonstrated similar modest increases in strength, and there were similar gains for both the exercised and nonexercised limbs.

This same group of researchers examined the effects of a higher-resistance, home-based, resistance training program (27). The training load for the knee extensors and elbow flexors was based on a 10-RM load (approximately 80% of maximum). The authors expressed concern that a program of this nature may be harmful to patients with neuromuscular diseases as a number of the isokinetic indices for the elbow flexors failed to show any statistical improvement. It should be noted, however, that the healthy control subjects as well failed to show improvement in the majority of isokinetic elbow flexion parameters, perhaps related to the lack of similarity between the training regime and testing condition (isotonic vs. isokinetic). Therefore, the expressed concern over higher-intensity training by the authors in this study may not be valid.

More recently, Tollbäck et al. (28) reported the effects of a supervised high-resistance training program in a small group of patients with DM. Subjects performed supervised unilateral knee extension exercises (3 sets of 10 repetitions at 80% of 1-RM) three times per week for 12 weeks. In the trained leg, the one-repetition maximum load increased significantly by 25%. There were no significant improvements in isokinetic concentric or eccentric values. Muscle biopsy revealed no change in the degree of histopathology, and there was a trend toward increased Type I fiber cross-sectional area. These authors stressed the importance of supervision during programs of this nature to ensure compliance.

Finally, Lindeman and coworkers (29) recently reported the results of a high-quality study that examined the effects of a 24-week strength training program in patients with DM and hereditary motor sensory neuropathy. Matched subjects were randomly assigned to either a training or control group. The training group performed knee extension exercise three times per week with loads increasing gradually from 60 to 80%. Maximal isometric and isokinetic strength, functional tasks, activity of daily living questionnaires, and serum myoglobin were measured pre- and posttraining. Subjects with DM showed no deleterious effects of training, and all subjects progressed with regard to their training loads. None of the less-specific strength or timed functional tasks, however, exhibited any significant improvement. Myoglobin levels were not significantly changed from pretraining levels.

In summary (see Table 7.7), although not all studies have shown consistent positive effects, moderate- to high-intensity resistance training generally has been found to improve strength in patients with a variety of myopathic disorders. As with DMD, strength gains tend to be greatest for muscles with mild-to-moderate weakness and are minimal in muscle groups with severe weakness. Strength training programs for these populations should be designed by experienced, trained personnel, and the program must be specifically tailored to the needs and limitations of the participants. Programs should be supervised, at least during their initial stages, and objective monitoring should be in place. Future high-quality studies are required to better define minimal and optimal training intensities and volumes. These studies should ideally include randomized control groups, completely supervised training programs, blinded assessors, and homogeneous training groups. The latter may require a multicentered approach. Functional, patient-centered outcomes are crucial to examine the potential impact of these interventions on disability and handicap.

Resistance Exercise in Inflammatory Myopathy

Exercise therapy in inflammatory myopathies has traditionally been confined to range-of-motion exercises and stretching in an attempt to prevent contractures and joint limitation. Traditional teaching has promoted rest and energy conservation in these disorders, as it was felt that exercise would potentially harm inflamed muscles. While this may still hold true for the initial stages of treatment in inflammatory myopathies, there is now evidence that a more active approach is safe and of potential benefit in the overall management of these disorders (30).

A single case report was the first indication that resistance exercise could be of potential benefit in the rehabilitation of polymyositis (31). In this case, a 42-year-old male with a stable course of at least 4 months' duration performed isometric resistance exercise (6 × 6-second maximal isometric contractions) for the biceps and quadriceps for 1 month. There was a gradual and significant increase in peak isometric force over the course of the study and if anything a slight decrease in the postexercise CK activity. Thus, there was evidence to suggest potential strength increase and no indication of increased muscle damage.

Escalante et al. (32) similarly reported a small case series of five patients with stable polymyositis or dermatomyositis who underwent successive 2-week periods of generalized rehabilitation and resistance exercise. Four of the five patients had significant increases in strength associated with the periods of resistance exercise. There was a small and likely clinically insignificant 7.7% mean rise in CK postexercise.

Wiesinger et al. (33) reported the results of a randomized controlled trial of progressive bicycle ergometer and step aerobic exercise in a group of patients with stable inflammatory myopathy. As with the resistance training programs described above, there were significant gains in peak isometric strength, and additionally improvements in an activity of daily living questionnaire and maximal oxygen consumption in the trained group in comparison to controls. There was no evidence of any deleterious effects with this type of program.

Finally, Spector and coworkers (34) examined the potential efficacy and safety of resistance training in five patients with inclusion body myositis. Four men and one woman trained 3 days per week for 12 weeks with a program consisting of concentric exercises for the knee flexors and extensors and the elbow flexors. Following the 12-week program, there was no significant increase in MRC scores or the Barthel Index. Three patients, however, reported improved function as a result of the program. Mean 3-RM values were significantly improved for all muscle except the right knee extensors. Strength gains were greatest for the initially stronger muscle groups. Serum CK, B cells, T cells, and natural killer cells (markers of inflammation) remained unchanged. These results were interpreted as suggesting that resistance exercise was safe and may be functionally beneficial in IBM. This is an important finding since, as opposed to PM and DM, there is no proven benefit of immunosuppression or other medical therapy at this point for IBM.

In summary, there is reasonable evidence that resistance training and general conditioning are safe and potentially beneficial in patients with inflammatory myopathy. As with the dystrophies, there is need for appropriate monitoring and follow-up. Patients should be exposed to active exercise programs only when they have been stable for 3 or more months, and programs should initially be supervised.

Respiratory Muscle Training in Myopathies

While limb and trunk muscle weakness is responsible for much of the functional limitation in progressive myopathies, deterioration of respiratory muscle function is primarily responsible for the high mortality among these patients (35). Respiratory insufficiency and associated hypercapnia, loss of lung volume, impaired cough, and pneumonia are leading causes of morbidity and mortality among patients with DMD (35). Thus, along with appropriate respiratory therapy and support, there has been interest in the potential for inspiratory muscle training (IMT) to improve respiratory muscle force and endurance in this patient population. As with other muscle groups, there has been concern over the possibility of overuse weakness with IMT and the extent to which improvement on pulmonary function indices may relate to decreased morbidity.

The results of studies that have assessed the effectiveness of IMT are varied. DiMarco et al. (36) examined the effects of inspiratory muscle resistance training on IM function in 11 patients with dystrophy (DMD, LGMD, FSHD). Following 6 weeks of IM training with inspiratory resistive load, there were improvements in the maximum inspiratory resistance that could be tolerated for 5 minutes and maximal sustainable ventilation. The degree of improvement with training, as noted previously for limb muscles, was directly related to the patient's baseline vital capacity. Smith et al. alternatively found no improvement in inspiratory muscle endurance in 8 patients with DMD following a 5-week crossover single-blinded training study.

Wanke et al. (37) studied the effects of a 6-month IMT program on 15 DMD patients in comparison to a control group of DMD patients. The authors found that the 10 patients who completed the training protocol had improvements in force as measured by maximal transdiaphragmatic pressure and maximal esophageal pressures. There were no changes reported, however, for vital capacity, forced expiratory volume in 1 second, or maximum voluntary ventilation. Again, patients with the most severely reduced function responded less or not at all.

Recently, Gozal and Thiriet (38) examined the effects of a 6-month respiratory muscle training program on respiratory muscle strength and respiratory load perception (RLP) in 21 children with DMD and spinal muscular atrophy type III. They were compared to 20 matched controls. Subjects were randomized to undergo incremental respiratory muscle training against inspiratory and expiratory loads, or against no load. In controls, no change in maximal static pressures or load perception was found. Respiratory training in the neuromuscular patients, alternatively, was associated with improvements in maximal inspiratory and expiratory pressures. Additionally, RLP improved in the group that trained against higher inspiratory and expiratory loads. Static pressures returned to baseline values within 3 months, whereas RLP was still improved after 3 months.

In general, as with the limb muscles, there is some evidence that respiratory muscle training can improve some measures of maximal respiratory muscle function and may decrease the perceived respiratory effort. Those with high pretraining values tend to improve more so, which as with limb muscle training may support the role for early intervention. There is no definite evidence at this time to suggest that respiratory muscle training is able to decrease incidence of chest infection and associated morbidity.

Education and Counseling

With careful monitoring and appropriate treatment, many patients with myopathies live a normal, or only minimally reduced, life span. For these reasons, a healthy lifestyle with respect to nutrition and physical education is important, and general guidelines are not much different than for the otherwise healthy individual with the caveats described above. Barriers to participation are much higher for those who require assistive devices, ranging from orthoses to canes to scooters to wheelchairs. Fortunately, most universities and gyms are now wheelchair accessible, which has removed many of the barriers to participation. Unfortunately, however, many of these patients still feel embarrassed or different when going to a public gymnasium, although these barriers are also falling. A major factor we have encountered, particularly in children with Duchenne dystrophy and most patients with myotonic dystrophy, is disinterest and poor compliance with exercise programs. It is important to make the activities enjoyable and age-specific, and providing time and facilities for those with neuromuscular disability is particularly helpful.

References

1. Dubowitz V. Muscle Disorders in Childhood. 2, 1–133. 95.
2. Tarnopolsky MA, Maguire J, Myint T, et al. Clinical, physiological, and histological features in a kindred with the T3271C melas mutation. Muscle Nerve 1998;21:25–33.
3. Mendell JR, Moxley RT, Griggs RC, et al. Randomized, double-blind six-month trial of prednisone in Duchenne's muscular dystrophy. N Engl J Med 1989;320:1592–7.
4. Tarnopolsky M, Martin J. Creatine monohydrate increases strength in patients with neuromuscular disease. Neurology 1999;52:854–7.
5. Argov Z, Arnold DL. MR Spectroscopy and Imaging in Metabolic Myopathies. Neurol Clin 2000;18:35–52.
6. van Beekvelt MC, van Engelen BG, Wevers RA, et al. Quantitative near-infrared spectroscopy discriminates between mitochondrial myopathies and normal muscle. Ann Neurol 1999;46:667–70.
7. Tarnopolsky MA, Roy BD, MacDonald JR. A randomized, controlled trial of creatine monohydrate in patients with mitochondrial cytopathies. Muscle Nerve 1997;20:1502–9.
8. Kilmer DD. The role of exercise in neuromuscular disease. Phys Med Rehabil Clin N Am 1998;9:115–25, vi.
9. Vignos PJ Jr. Physical models of rehabilitation in neuromuscular disease. Muscle Nerve 1983;6:323–38.
10. Buchthal F, Rosenfalck P. Action potential parameters in different human muscles. Acta Physiol Scand 1955;30:125–131.
11. Tein I. Metabolic myopathies. Semin Pediatr Neurol 1996;3: 59–98.
12. Lewis SF, Haller RG, Cook JD, et al. Muscle fatigue in McArdle's disease studied by 31P-NMR: effect of glucose infusion. J Appl Physiol 1985;59:1991–4.
13. Haller RG, Lewis SF. Glucose-induced exertional fatigue in muscle phosphofructokinase deficiency. N Engl J Med 1991; 324:364–9.
14. Bonsett CA. Pseudohypertrophic muscular dystrophy: Distribution of degenerative features as revealed by anatomical study. Neurology 1963;13:728–738.
15. Hickok RJ. Physical therapy as related to peripheral nerve lesions. Phys Ther Rev 1961;41:113–117.
16. Lenman JA. A clinical and experimental study of the effects of exercise on motor weakness in neurological disease. J Neurol Neurosurg Psychiatry 1959;22:182–194.
17. Johnson EW, Braddom R. Over-work weakness in facioscapulohumeral muscular dystrophy. Arch Phys Med Rehabil 1971;52:333–6.
18. DeLateur BJ, Giaconi RM. Effect on maximal strength of submaximal exercise in Duchenne muscular dystrophy. Am J Phys Med 1979;58:26–36.
19. Abramson AS, Rogoff J. An approach to rehabilitation of children with muscular dystrophy. Proceedings of the First and Second Medical Conferences of the MDAA, Inc. New York, MDAA. 1953, 123–124.
20. Hoberman M. Physical medicine and rehabilitation: its value and limitations in progressive muscular dystrophy. Am J Phys Med 1955;34:109–115.
21. Wratney M J. Physical therapy for muscular dystrophy children. Phys Ther Rev 1958;38:26–32.
22. Vignos PJ, Watkins MP. The effect of exercise in muscular dystophy. JAMA 1966;197:89–96.
23. McCartney N, Moroz D, Garner SH, et al. The effects of strength training in patients with selected neuromuscular disorders. Med Sci Sports Exerc 1988;20:362–8.
24. Belanger AY, McComas AJ. Extent of motor unit activation during effort. J Appl Physiol 1981;51:1131–5.
25. Milner-Brown HS, Miller RG. Muscle strengthening through high-resistance weight training in patients with neuromuscular disorders. Arch Phys Med Rehabil 1988;69:14–9.
26. Aitkens SG, McCrory MA, Kilmer DD, et al. Moderate resistance exercise program: its effect in slowly progressive neuromuscular disease. Arch Phys Med Rehabil 1993;74:711–5.
27. Kilmer DD, McCrory MA, Wright NC, et al. The effect of a high resistance exercise program in slowly progressive neuromuscular disease. Arch Phys Med Rehabil 1994;75:560–3.
28. Tollback A, Eriksson S, Wredenberg A, et al. Effects of high resistance training in patients with myotonic dystrophy. Scand J Rehabil Med 1999;31:9–16.
29. Lindeman E, Leffers P, Spaans F, et al. Strength training in patients with myotonic dystrophy and hereditary motor and sensory neuropathy: a randomized clinical trial. Arch Phys Med Rehabil 1995;76:612–20.

30. Hicks JE. Role of rehabilitation in the management of myopathies. Curr Opin Rheumatol 1998;10:548–55.
31. Hicks JE, Miller F, Plotz P, et al. Isometric exercise increases strength and does not produce sustained creatinine phosphokinase increases in a patient with polymyositis. J Rheumatol 1993;20:1399–401.
32. Escalante A, Miller L, Beardmore TD. Resistive exercise in the rehabilitation of polymyositis/dermatomyositis. J Rheumatol 1993;20:1340–4.
33. Wiesinger GF, Quittan M, Aringer M, et al. Improvement of physical fitness and muscle strength in polymyositis/dermatomyositis patients by a training programme. Br J Rheumatol 1998;37:196–200.
34. Spector SA, Lemmer JT, Koffman BM, et al. Safety and efficacy of strength training in patients with sporadic inclusion body myositis. Muscle Nerve 1997;20:1242–8.
35. McCool FD, Tzelepis GE. Inspiratory muscle training in the patient with neuromuscular disease. Phys Ther 1995;75:1006–14.
36. DiMarco AF, Kelling J, Sajovic M, et al. Respiratory muscle training in muscular dystrophy. Clin Res 1982;30:427A.
37. Wanke T, Toifl K, Merkle M, et al. Inspiratory muscle training in patients with Duchenne muscular dystrophy. Chest 1994;105:475–82.
38. Gozal D, Thiriet P. Respiratory muscle training in neuromuscular disease: long-term effects on strength and load perception. Med Sci Sports Exerc 1999;31:1522–7.

CHAPTER **8**

Peripheral Neuropathy and Neuropathic Pain

Mark T. Pfefer and Kenton C. Freeman

PATHOPHYSIOLOGY

Pain is a common experience, and the capacity to sense pain plays a protective role in warning of current or potential tissue damage. Response to tissue injury (as well as painful stimuli) includes adaptive changes that promote healing and avoid further irritation to the injured tissue.

Peripheral neuropathy is defined as deranged function and structure of peripheral motor, sensory, and autonomic neurons (outside the central nervous system), involving either the entire neuron or selected levels (1). Pain and other sensory changes can be produced in a variety of ways, and in peripheral nerves, motor or sensory fibers may be preferentially affected, but in most neuropathies both are involved, leading to various patterns of sensorimotor deficit (2). Pain is not always associated with peripheral neuropathy. Painful neuropathies are usually a result of damage to the axon, in contrast to demyelinating neuropathies that tend, with some exceptions, to cause pronounced motor or sensory loss without pain (3).

There are two basic mechanisms by which the experience of pain can be evoked: somatic tissue injury (nociceptive) or nerve injury (4). In the typical process of nociceptive pain, stimulation of tissue nociceptors (found throughout the musculoskeletal system) causes action potentials to be propagated along nociceptive axons that ultimately enter the limbic sectors of the cerebral cortex where the pain is perceived. Nociceptive pain is typically described by patients as deep, tender, dull, aching, and diffuse (4). Pain induced by nociceptive pain mechanisms is the most common variety seen in clinical practice (5).

In contrast to nociceptive pain syndromes that are typically related to musculoskeletal damage or injury, damage to the peripheral or central nervous system produces a different type of pain. This type of pain is known as neuropathic pain. Often neuropathic pain is chronic and persistent, and patients are more likely to use adjectives such as shooting, stabbing, lancinating, burning, and searing to describe it and often complain of pain worsening at night (6). Patients with neuropathic pain may appear to have continuous or paroxysmal pain without any detectable relationship to stimulus (7). The symptoms may be divided into those that are unprovoked and those that are provoked by maneuvers such as skin stimulation, pressure over affected nerves, changes in temperature, or emotional factors (2).

One key diagnostic feature of neuropathic pain is the presence of pain within an area of sensory deficit (8). Allodynia is also a commonly seen hyperpathic state in neuropathic pain, in which a normally innocuous stimulus produces a sensation of pain whose quality is inappropriate for the stimulus. An example of this is the patient who cannot tolerate a blanket resting on an affected extremity. Another feature suggestive of neuropathic pain is summation, which is the progressive worsening of pain evoked by slow, repetitive stimulation with mildly noxious stimuli, for example, pinprick (8).

Neuropathic pain can be classified on the basis of the cause of the insult to the nervous system, the disease or event that precipitated the pain syndrome, or the distribution of pain. Certain medical conditions are associated with neuropathic pain, and these commonly include diabetes, HIV infection or AIDS, multiple sclerosis, cancer chemotherapy, malignancy, spinal surgery, alcoholism, herpes zoster, and amputation (6). Cancer patients can develop neuropathy from tumor invasion and also are at higher risk for neuropathic pain following chemotherapy or radiation therapy.

Diabetes is associated with peripheral neuropathy and radiculopathy. HIV is associated with a variety of neuropathies and myelopathies. Multiple sclerosis is associated with neuralgia and neuropathy. Failed spine surgery is associated with radiculopathy. Amputation is associated with neuroma and phantom limb pain (6).

Trauma can lead to the development of entrapment neuropathies, as well as partial or complete nerve transection, plexopathies, and painful scars. Entrapment neuropathies such as carpal tunnel syndrome are usually characterized in the early stages by paresthesia and pain (2).

CLASSIFICATION

A variety of disease processes may cause or contribute to peripheral neuropathy and the possible pain associated with it (9). A working knowledge of these is needed in order to help identify or establish a specific cause or underlying process and develop a prognosis and treatment plan accordingly. Despite a thorough investigation into the cause of peripheral polyneuropathy, the cause often remains unknown in 25–50% of cases (10). It is then the goal of treatment to lesson the patient's symptoms or dysfunction.

Based on anatomical distribution, there are four main types of peripheral nervous system disease. It is useful to know their clinical patterns for diagnosis and treatment (11):

1. Symmetrical polyneuropathy—affects mainly the distal extremities, usually affects the feet with altered sensation. It is the most common chronic type of peripheral polyneuropathy. Diabetes, metabolic causes, or toxin exposures often cause this type of neuropathy.
2. Mononeuropathy—affects a single nerve and is also a common cause of acute or chronic peripheral neuropathy. This type is often from a focal compression of the nerve, but is often found with chronic disease states such as diabetes, which makes the nerve more susceptible.
3. Plexopathy—(dysfunction in the nerve plexus) and is often the result of injury, but can result from an underlying endogenous process, such as might develop after radiation treatment for a tumor. It may affect several peripheral nerves in a nondermatomal pattern with weakness or sensory changes.
4. Radiculopathies—are from involvement or injury to a nerve more proximally (toward the spinal cord) causing nerve root dysfunction, often with weakness, pain, and peripheral sensory deficit in a specific dermatomal pattern (12). Nerve encroachment from spondylitic degenerative changes or disk herniation can commonly cause this.
5. Facial neuralgias—while not classically considered in a discussion of peripheral neuropathies, must also be considered when one is discussing pain in the peripheral nervous system.

CLINICAL EXERCISE PHYSIOLOGY

Basic information about nociception and pain has not received systematic coverage in either exercise science textbooks or the sports medicine literature (13). The patient with a chronic pain problem typically has a complicated medical and psychological history. An adequate comprehensive treatment of the problem requires a careful and multidisciplinary assessment. The goal of the assessment is to identify nociceptive factors that may be correctable, psychological factors that can be addressed (pharmacologically or behaviorally), the contribution of disuse to the pain problem, and the socioenvironmental context in which the pain problem is maintained (14).

Physical exercise is widely used in the treatment of chronic pain patients. Patients with chronic pain have demonstrated highly significant improvements in aerobic fitness measures following a short (4-week) course of exercise intervention (15). Outcomes assessed included $\dot{V}O_{2max}$ and METs, and lower body power output. Possible mechanisms underlying such dramatic improvement include improved physical fitness, learning, or desensitization to symptoms associated with exertion, and improved effort. Patients with chronic pain related to peripheral neuropathy have displayed lower health-related quality of life, and patients placed on a 6-week home exercise program demonstrated slight improvements in this measure as well as increases in muscle strength (16).

Patients with peripheral neuropathy involving the median nerve at the wrist (carpal tunnel syndrome) have been treated with nerve and tendon-gliding exercises. A significant number of patients reported excellent results and were spared the morbidity of a carpal tunnel release procedure (17). Other studies have shown that various exercise interventions may prevent or decrease the incidence of carpal tunnel syndrome and other painful cumulative trauma disorders (18, 19).

Physical activity, including appropriate endurance and resistance training, is a major therapeutic modality for type 2 diabetes. Unfortunately, too often physical activity is an underutilized therapy. Favorable changes in glucose tolerance and insulin sensitivity usually deteriorate within 72 hours of the last exercise session; consequently, regular physical activity is imperative to sustain glucose-lowering effects and improved insulin sensitivity (20). Modifications to exercise type and/or intensity may be necessary for those who have complications of diabetes. Autonomic neuropathy affects the heart rate response to exercise. As a result, ratings of perceived exertion, may need to be used instead of heart rate for moderating intensity of physical activity. Patients with diabetic neuropathy causing sensory loss in the lower extremity may have to alter exercises to focus on the use of non-weight-bearing forms of activity (20).

A recent study demonstrated improvement on several measures of balance in diabetic patients with peripheral neuropathy (21). This study involved a short (3-week) intervention designed to increase lower-extremity strength and balance. Significant improvement was found in unipedal stance time, tandem stance time, and functional reach. Additional studies are needed to determine if this decreases fall frequency in this population.

Pain can be modulated at peripheral sites by opioids, and peripheral blood concentrations of beta-endorphins are increased during exercise (13). Therefore, exercise may play a beneficial role in reducing pain in certain cases, but further research is warranted to understand specific mechanisms. Also, additional research is needed to understand the conditions (e.g., mode, duration, and intensity of exercise, whether or not the exercise itself is painful, and the nature of the noxious stimulus) under which exercise-related analgesia is produced (13).

PHARMACOLOGY

A variety of pharmacological approaches to the management of neuropathic pain are in use, although there is no current consensus on optimal strategy. Pharmacological management is based upon the response of the patient and careful titration of dosage to achieve positive results while minimizing side effects. Pharmacological treatments have generally been selected on the basis of evidence for efficacy in randomized, placebo-controlled trials conducted in disease-based groups of patients, notably in postherpetic neuralgia and diabetic polyneuropathy (22). These studies demonstrate efficacy of tricyclic antidepressants, standard and newer anticonvulsants, and opioids. Evidence for efficacy is less for selective serotonin reuptake inhibitors (SSRIs), antiarrhythmics (mexiletine), and capsaicin. Non-opioid analgesics (aspirin, acetaminophen, and other nonsteroidal anti-inflammatory drugs [NSAIDs]) are often used by patients with neuropathic pain, but they are typically more effective for mild to moderate nociceptive pain.

Many patients with mild to moderate pain are helped by the use of aspirin, acetaminophen, and NSAIDs. Acetaminophen is often used initially due to its lower incidence of gastrointestinal toxicity when taken chronically. It has no anti-inflammatory effect and is not appropriate as a primary therapy for an inflammatory process.

A wide variety of NSAIDs are in use, and many patients respond better to one over another, although this is unpredictable in advance of starting on the drug. NSAID use is associated with an increased incidence of gastrointestinal toxicity and should be avoided in patients who suffer from peptic ulcer disease or bleeding abnormalities (23). NSAIDs should also be avoided in patients over 70 years of age and as unsupervised long-term treatment (24). Patients with neuropathic pain will typically be engaged in low-level exercise programs, but it is important to acknowledge a recent study that demonstrated that use of NSAIDs was found to be a risk factor in exercise-associated hyponatremia in high-level physical activity (25).

Many patients with neuropathic pain experience relief with the use of antidepressants. Pain relief is often achieved at doses that are subtherapeutic for the treatment of depression. The analgesic effects of these agents may result from their ability to block reuptake at presynaptic nerve endings of neurotransmitters, such as serotonin and norepinephrine, which are involved in pain and depression (26). Tricyclic antidepressants remain the class most commonly used, and their use has been documented in a variety of pain-related conditions, including postherpetic neuralgia, diabetic neuropathy, arthritis, low back pain, myofascial pain, cancer pain, migraine and tension-type headaches, central pain, and psychogenic pain (26). Common side effects include sedation and dry mouth. In light of recent reports of sudden death in children being treated with desipramine (tricyclic antidepressant), three of which were associated with physical exercise, the effects of this drug on exercise were evaluated (27). Desipramine was found to have only minor effects on the cardiovascular response to exercise, and the effects did not appear to be age related (27). The authors state that desipramine may increase the risk of exercise-associated arrhythmias in some individuals.

When the previously described drugs are not sufficient, the addition of an anticonvulsant drug to the antidepressant may be useful (28). Anticonvulsants are generally considered to be first-line agents for the treatment of neuropathic pain with a predominantly paroxysmal or lancinating quality, such as trigeminal neuralgia (26). The mechanisms by which anticonvulsants relieve pain may be related to stabilizing neuronal membranes (phenytoin), altering sodium channel activity (carbamazepine), and modulating gamma-a,ompbituroc acod actovotu (clonazepam and valproate) (26). Carbamazepine (anticonvulsant) produced a significant delay in pain increase in patients with peripheral neuropathy that was previously mediated by spinal cord stimulation (29). In this study, the pain-relieving spinal cord stimulation was inactivated prior to introduction of medication. Anticonvulsant medication demonstrated better delay in return of pain compared to an opioid analgesic.

The role of opioid analgesics is controversial in the management of neuropathic pain. Most patients do not respond to these drugs and should not receive them (28). Many patients need detoxification from opioids, sedative-hypnotics, and muscle relaxants (28). There is some evidence that some patients with neuropathic pain do function well while taking low-dose, regularly scheduled opioids (28).

Neuropathic pain with a major cutaneous component may respond well to topical therapy with the substance P depletor, capsaicin, to reduce elevated prostaglandin levels (28). Animal studies are demonstrating a rationale for the selected use of topical capsaicin in the treatment of pain (30).

Chronic pain and depression are often found to coexist. The use of tricyclic antidepressants in higher therapeutic doses is indicated in these cases. SSRIs such as fluoxetine (Prozac), paroxetine (Paxil), and sertraline (Zoloft) have generally replaced tricyclic antidepressants for the treatment of depression (26). Although they are typically well tolerated with fewer side effects, SSRIs have not shown significant efficacy for treatment of pain. Sometimes, patients with chronic pain and depression are placed on bedtime dosing of tricyclics and concomitant daytime dosing of SSRIs. Caution is required since some SSRIs can significantly increase tricyclic antidepressant serum levels (26).

HISTORY AND PHYSICAL EXAMINATION

The history the patient gives can be a very important guide toward diagnosis. Specific attempts should be made to determine the following:

1. The time course of the patient's symptoms: When did they start (acute, subacute, chronic, or relapsing)? Was there a specific event associated with onset? What age did symptoms first occur? How fast have the symptoms progressed?
2. What type of distribution or pattern are the symptoms: symmetrical or asymmetrical, proximal or distal, single nerve, multiple nerves, or diffuse?
3. What type of nerve fibers are affected more: motor (weakness), sensory (pain or anesthesia), or autonomic symptoms (blood pressure, pulse rate, and rhythm changes)?
4. The quality and quantity of pain or sensory change associated (dull ache, sharp, burning, numb) and its effects on daily functions or activities.
5. Does it seem to start in a given area and then radiate?
6. Is there anything the patient can identify that causes the symptom to be worse, or that helps alleviate it (body positions, use, rest, movement)?
7. Is there a certain time of day or night when it worsens or improves?
8. Family history: Attempt to search for possible genetic patterns or links to other family members.
9. Social history: illicit drug use, alcohol use, job history (repetitive strain, toxic exposure, heavy lifting/labor), travel history (exposures and subsequent illnesses), diet changes or patterns (with exposure to toxins or illnesses), and vitamin ingestion (deficiency or toxicities).
10. Past medical history: illnesses or conditions affecting organ systems (infections, diabetes, thyroid or endocrine disease, tumors, kidney disease, connective tissue diseases, metabolic diseases or defects, prior disease treatments or prior medications).
11. Current medications
12. Allergies

Many other conditions may mimic the pain or dysfunction of neuropathy, such as myopathy, arthritides, musculoskeletal pain, myofascial pain, visceral conditions, infections, neoplasms, psychological causes, and pain or weakness from central nervous systems conditions.

Peripheral neuropathy affects lower motor neurons, and the neurological physical exam may uncover any of the constellation of findings that typically result from this. Neurological findings may include weakness, atrophy, loss of sensation, hypersensation, paresthesia, and decreased deep tendon reflexes in the distribution of the affected nerve or nerves (11). In acute neuropathy, there may be nerve tension signs (such as a positive straight leg raise in lumbar radiculopathy) and splinting of muscles, or antalgic body postures. There may be changes in gait due to weakness, pain, or loss of distal sensation. Position sense may be impaired in the extremities and muscles may be atrophied in more chronic nerve disease. In suspected peripheral neuropathy, each of the areas of the neurological physical exam should be evaluated.

It is important, especially with suspected mononeuropathy or radiculopathy, to compare physical exam findings from the affected side of the body to the unaffected side, looking for objective differences or asymmetry in sensation, reflexes, strength, size, and body position.

In peripheral polyneuropathy, there is usually a more symmetrical neurological involvement in the distal limbs. The physical exam will often show decreased deep tendon reflexes, decreased or increased sensation (in a non-dermatomal stocking-type distribution), and possible weakness in the distal extremities (9). The lower extremities are usually most affected in earlier states of involvement, but eventually all extremities may be affected.

Sensory testing for smaller fiber involvement can be performed by pinprick and ice touching. Larger fibers can be tested better with a tuning fork for vibration, two-point discrimination at the fingertips, or by position sense (by lifting a toe or fingertip slightly superiorly or inferiorly with the patient's eyes closed and then asking them to identify what they felt) (31). Strength can be tested manually with resisted joint range of motion against the examiner's own resistance, and with maneuvers that test strength in the lower extremities that the patient can perform (like heel-toe walking, squatting, step-ups or toe raises). Reflexes should be checked with a reflex hammer with the patient's joint in a neutral, relaxed position. To help facilitate a reflex in an areflexic limb, have the patient clasp his hands together in front of his torso and attempt to pull them apart while you retest the reflex. Nerve tension or compression signs may be checked by applying traction to the nerve, by applying focal pressure, or by mechanically tapping over the nerve. Examples would be: (1) the straight leg raise test to stretch the sciatic nerve and lumbar nerve roots in evaluating for suspected lumbar radiculopathy; (2) Spurling's (maximal foraminal compression) test in the cervical spine to check for nerve encroachment in the intervertebral foramen; or (3) compression or tapping over the median nerve at the wrist to reproduce symptoms of carpal tunnel syndrome (median neuropathy at the wrist).

MEDICAL AND SURGICAL TREATMENTS

Treatment of neuropathy of any etiology should be aimed at treating or correcting any underlying identifiable cause, if possible (9, 11). Since there are many etiologies for peripheral neuropathies, there are also numerous approaches to their treatment, whether acute or chronic. Immediate goals of therapy are generally to achieve acceptable pain levels, minimize any functional deficits, and protect from risk of ongoing damage or hypoesthesia.

Acute painful neuropathies (such as acute radiculopathy or acute peripheral nerve trauma) are often treated, depending on severity and cause, with analgesic medications (narcotic and nonnarcotic), appropriate limitations of activity, physical therapy and pain-modulating modalities, appropriate assistive or supportive devices (e.g., upper-extremity sling support, cervical or lumbar support, or functional or static limb bracing), anesthetic nerve blocks, or surgical correction (32, 33). Conservative treatments should be implemented first when possible before attempting more invasive measures. Examples: 1) lancinating sharp pain of trigeminal neuralgia may be treated conservatively with baclofen or anticonvulsant medications (9, 34, 35) (starting at a low dose to minimize more common side effects of drowsiness, dizziness, or gastrointestinal problems), or by more invasive surgical or regional anesthetic techniques (including trigeminal nerve anesthetic block, glycerol gangliolysis injections, or surgical decompression of the trigeminal ganglion). 2) Acute lumbar radiculopathy may often be treated conservatively with relative rest (up to 2–3 days); oral or intramuscular narcotic and nonnarcotic medications (which may include Tylenol, NSAIDs, antispasmodics or muscle relaxants, tramadol, or antidepressants, which may augment other medications effects); intermittent orthotic splinting with a lumbosacral corset; active and passive physical therapy techniques (often with modalities to minimize pain, dysfunction, disuse, spasm, endocrine, or irritation); transcutaneous electrical stimulation; oral steroids; epidural injections with steroids, opioids, anesthetics, or a combination of these drugs; or surgical decompression of the nerve (in severe cases).

In more chronic causes of neuropathy or neuropathic pain that may not be correctable, some of the same techniques and medications may be used, but there is a shift toward more chronic or long-term treatment approaches to help manage the disorder. If there is a chronic underlying disease state causing or contributing to the neuropathy, the initial goal is to medically manage that condition to the best degree possible, as it may often have a positive effect on the neuropathy process and the patient's symptoms (11). Examples: 1) improvement in peripheral polyneuropathy with tight control of blood glucose levels in diabetes mellitus, or 2) appropriate therapeutic control of hypothyroidism with replacement hormone. If the chronic neuropathy has no known underlying cause or cannot be improved by medical intervention, the management of the symptoms or dysfunction is the focus. Often, medications for chronic neuropathic pain may be implemented to help control symptoms (9, 34, 35). These often include sympatholytics; oral anticonvulsants; tricyclic antidepressants or sometimes selective serotonin re-uptake inhibitors; baclofen; topical medications (36) (anesthetics, nonsteroidal drugs, capsaicin, or other neuro-modulating medications that are often used orally, alone, or in combinations with each other), which are less proven, but may be tried alone or with oral medications to lessen their side effects; corticosteroids; oral or intravenous anesthetics; and less often narcotics (usually only used when other methods to control pain have failed).

Anesthetic approaches may be used transiently or more permanently to block sympathetic or somatic nerve transmission. Techniques include infiltration of involved nerves, perineurally, in the epidural space, or intraspinally, with local anesthetics, corticosteroids, sympatholytics, narcotics, or a combination of these drugs, and sometimes neurolytic substances (37, 38). They may be given by single injections or by continuous type of infusion by catheter in patients who fail to obtain sufficient pain relief with less-invasive measures. Examples: (1) lumbar epidural steroid injection for radiculopathy, (2) continual morphine intraspinal infusion for failed low back syndrome. Radio-frequency nerve ablation, cryolysis, or neurosurgical interruptive procedures may also be used as neurodestructive procedures of last resort (39).

Neurostimulatory techniques for neural afferent sensory pathway modulation are other approaches to painful neuropathy. Counter-irritation (rubbing) of the painful area, transcutaneous electrical stimulation, spinal cord stimulation (requires electrode implantation), and acupuncture are examples. Many patients may achieve analgesia soon after their implementation, but often fewer obtain lasting relief (12).

Physical medicine and rehabilitation are often important in patients with significant dysfunctions from neuropathies for their overall outcome and management. Rehabilitation techniques are employed in both acute and chronic neuropathies. They help the patient to accommodate or compensate for deficits; improve strength, coordination, and self-confidence; appropriately use assistive devices (if needed); reduce pain; and help maximize overall functional ability. A vast array of active and passive therapy modalities and techniques may be implemented based on the state and severity of the patient's disease, his dysfunction or pain, comorbidities, and the goals for rehabilitation. Generally speaking, passive therapies are used early in the course of treatment, moving to greater use of active therapy as treatment continues. Passive therapy may include various cold or heat techniques, electrotherapies and stimulation, traction, massage, mobilization, manipulation or manual therapy, and compression. Active therapy may include implementation and training with specific orthoses, therapeutic exercise, gait training, adaptation or training for activities of daily living, vocational adaptation or conditioning, and ergonomic considerations (32). Multiple disciplines may be needed to fully assess and implement many of these strategies to best serve the patient's needs (depending on the disease process). These may include the physician, physical therapist, chiropractor, occupational therapist, orthotist, clinical exercise physiologist, kinesiotherapist, recreational therapist, social worker, and psychologist.

DIAGNOSTIC TECHNIQUES

Diagnostic imaging studies such as computed tomography or MRI may help detect abnormal etiologies contributing to an entrapment neuropathy such as bony encroachments, soft-tissue masses, tumors, infections, vascular lesions, or cysts (40, 41, 42). MRI is the study of choice for imaging most soft-tissue types of suspected lesions, while scanning visualizes many bony processes better (42). These tests provide an anatomical "picture" of the tissues in question and are best used as an extension to a good history and physical exam to provide further information of an already clinically suspected lesion or process. If not used in this manner, their results are less meaningful toward providing accurate diagnostic information and can sometimes mislead the true diagnosis.

Electrodiagnostic studies are physiological tests performed on the specific nerves and muscle they innervate. They are often very valuable in objectively confirming the diagnosis of neuropathy and documenting the type of nerve pathology involved (43–46). They can help classify whether the neuropathy is focal vs. diffuse, sensory vs. motor, or axonal vs. demyelinating types of processes. This helps guide a more accurate diagnosis and treatment. Electrodiagnostic nerve conduction studies do have some limitations. They test the larger-diameter nerve fiber conduction and may be completely normal in patients with painful diffuse peripheral neuropathy involving only the smaller nerve fibers. Electromyographic findings may also be complicated by the process of reinnervation (47).

Laboratory studies are appropriate with undetermined causes of peripheral neuropathy to help further narrow the diagnosis and appropriate treatment (48). Treatment of neuropathies is usually aimed at correcting deficiencies, removing insultive agents, and treating contributing systemic illnesses. Studies of blood, urine, spinal fluid, antibody assays, and sometimes nerve biopsies are needed to help determine a cause (48). Blood, urine, and cerebrospinal fluid (CSF) tests may need to be done to assess for the following conditions: diabetes, liver or thyroid disease, autoimmune processes, collagen-vascular disease, vitamin deficiency or toxicities, toxin exposures or ingestions, prescription and nonprescription or illicit drug use, infections, neoplasms, or hereditary causes.

Anesthetic approaches such as regional analgesia may be implemented in neuropathy to help with diagnosis, prognosis, prophylaxis, or for therapeutic measures (37). Neural blockade (anesthetic) injection procedures may be used to transiently block somatic or sympathetic nerves for diagnostic analysis, or may be used to more permanently block these nerves to abolish the pain (37, 38). Diagnostic (temporary) blocks are directed to affect the afferent pathways involved with pain. They may also be used to prognosticate the affect of a more permanent neurolytic or ablative procedure. Nerve blockade may be performed peripherally in direct proximity of the affected nerve as used with the trigeminal or intercostal neuralgia or sympathetic blocks of the lumbar plexus or stellate ganglion. Regional blockade may be performed intraspinally in the epidural space for conditions such as radiculopathy, or may be performed intrathecally. Repeated blocks may be used therapeutically for patients who obtain relief from an initial trial (37, 38).

PAIN MEASUREMENT

Pain measurement is important to monitor effects of treatment. Measurement of pain poses some difficulties due to the subjectivity of the experience and variations in cognitive and emotional factors from person to person. One of the most common ways to measure and document pain is the use of the visual analog scale (VAS) (49). The patient marks or points to a mark on a 10-centimeter line that corresponds to his/her level of pain with one end point corresponding to "no pain" and the other end point corresponding to "worst pain." The distance in centimeters from the low end of the VAS to the patient's report is used as a numerical index of the severity of pain. High reliability and validity have been reported with this commonly used scaling device (49–53).

Another commonly used instrument is the McGill Pain Questionnaire (54). This questionnaire is designed to assess the multidimensional nature of pain experience and has been demonstrated to be a reliable, valid, and consistent measurement tool (54). A short-form McGill Pain Questionnaire is also available when time limitations are present and there is a need to obtain more than just pain intensity. This questionnaire is widely used and is available in many different languages.

Ongoing assessment of outcomes is vital when dealing with a patient with chronic pain, and quantification of pain is an important part of this process. Providers should periodically assess patients relative to the beginning of care, not just on a visit-by-visit basis. In this way, the risk of losing sight of the overall progress goals in lieu of palliative management can be avoided (55).

EXERCISE/FITNESS/FUNCTIONAL TESTING

Before starting on an exercise program, all patients with peripheral neuropathy or neurogenic pain syndromes should undergo a medical evaluation and graded exercise test to determine their general state of health, the presence and degree of long-term complications, and any limitations or contraindications to exercise. The patient with a chronic pain problem typically has a complicated medical and psychological history. An adequate comprehensive treatment of the problem requires a careful and multidisciplinary assessment. The goal of the assessment is to identify nociceptive factors that may be correctable, psychological factors that can be addressed (pharmacologically or behaviorally), the contribution of disuse to the pain problem, and the socioenvironmental context in which the pain problem is maintained (56).

Exercise tolerance testing in patients with neuropathic pain should be performed only after medical clearance is obtained. Increased activity and exercise may aggravate and increase pain in these patients, so it is important to pay attention to patients undergoing exercise testing and evaluation. Documentation of specific aggravating activities or movement is important.

Muscle weakness, joint contractures, and muscle shortening can occur in patients with peripheral neuropathy. Active and passive range of motion of the trunk and extremities should be evaluated using goniometer or inclinometer assessment. Strength of the trunk and extremities can be evaluated manually or with the use of isokinetic testing equipment. Documentation of pain provoked by active and passive movement, as well as pain produced with resisted range of motion or strength testing, should be noted, including a description of location and character of pain.

EXERCISE PRESCRIPTION AND PROGRAMMING

Therapeutic exercises represent an important part of the treatment program for most patients with pain, keeping in mind that most patients will have varying degrees of deconditioning that can range from mild to severe. Exercises are utilized to increase flexibility, improve strength and endurance, and stabilize weak or lax joints.

Patients with pain often decrease their level of physical activity due to concern that they may exacerbate pain or produce tissue damage. The consequences may include reduced flexibility, decreased muscle strength, muscle wasting, and overall deconditioning (26). Intervention should include exercises specific for the painful area, in addition to general aerobic exercises. The exercises should encourage flexibility and strength improvement while demonstrating to the patient that no harm is being produced.

As discussed above, muscle weakness, joint contractures, and muscle shortening commonly occur in patients with peripheral neuropathy. This should be addressed with ongoing range-of-motion exercises performed both passively and actively. Graded mild resistance training is added as tolerated, keeping in mind that stress on the affected area may produce a hyperpathic pain response or reports of exaggerated pain intensities following exercise or activity.

The guidelines of exercise for the patient with chronic pain differ from those of the acutely injured. Often, medical practitioners use pain as a guideline, telling the patient, "If it hurts, don't do it." This may be appropriate with an acute injury, but not with a chronic condition. As a general rule, exercises that induce more peripheral pain should be avoided, and exercises that centralize the pain should be continued (57).

Prescribed exercises will depend on patient interest and motivation and should minimize risk of exacerbating pain. Examples of appropriate exercises include walking, rapid walking, running, aerobic dance, bicycling, swimming, rowing, and cross-country skiing. The program should be graduated, starting with exercise to tolerance as determined by pain, weakness, or fatigue. Initially, brief daily periods of exercise should be encouraged, with a goal to exercise 15 to 30 minutes at least three times per week. The following specific walking program has been recommended as appropriate for patients with chronic pain (26):

1. Achieve activity level of walking 2000 ft (e.g., 10 laps of 200 ft each) without interruption. If necessary, this goal may be attained by increasing the distance walked by 200–400 ft each day.
2. Increase the distance walked to 2400 ft at previous pace, or decrease time to walk 2000 ft by 30 seconds.
3. When this quota is reached, increase distance another 400 ft, or decrease time another 30 seconds.
4. Continue reduction in time quotas until upper speed limit is reached, as determined by repeated time quota failures.
5. Increase time quota to level previously achieved, and expand distance walked on successive days.
6. Provide positive reinforcement for achieving these goals by documenting increments in speed and distance on performance graphs.

Patients with chronic neuropathies (either focal or diffuse) or with neurogenic pain syndromes may not respond positively to increased exercise. With this group of patients, it may be beneficial to prescribe physical activities not clearly defined as exercise (58). Increased walking may be a useful goal for these patients. Increase in recreational activities such as gardening may also have some beneficial effects in this group of patients. In addition, these patients will often require formal programs to maintain range of motion, improve aerobic conditioning, prevent deconditioning, and enhance strength.

References

1. Dyck PJ. Causes, classification and treatment of peripheral neuropathy. N Eng J Med 1982;307:283–286.
2. Scadding JW. Peripheral neuropathies. In Wall PD, Melzack R, eds. Textbook of pain. Edinburgh: Churchill Livingstone; 1999:1815.
3. Vaillancourt PD, Langevin HM. Painful peripheral neuropathies. Med Clin N Am 1999;83:627.
4. Perle SM, Schneider MJ, Seaman DR. Chiropractic management of peripheral neuropathy: pathophysiology, assessment, and treatment. Top Clin Chiropr 1999;6:6–19.
5. Seaman DR, Cleveland C. Spinal pain syndromes: nociceptive, neuropathic, and psychologic mechanisms. J Manip Physiol Ther 1998;22:458–472.
6. Belgrade MJ. Following the clues to neuropathic pain. Postgraduate Med 1999;106:127–140.
7. Bennett GF. Neuropathic pain. In: Wall PD, Melzack R, eds. Textbook of pain. Edinburgh: Churchill Livingstone; 1994:201–224.
8. Fields HL, Baron R, Rowbotham MC. Peripheral neuropathic pain: an approach to management. In: Wall PD, Melzack R, eds. Textbook of pain. Edinburgh: Churchill Livingstone; 1999:1523–1533.
9. Loar, C. Peripheral nervous system pain. In: Raj P. Pain medicine: a comprehension review. St. Louis: Mosby Year Book: 1996:453–459.
10. Oh SJ, ed. Clinical Electromyography: Nerve Conduction Studies, Baltimore: Williams & Wilkins, 1993.
11. Fisher MA. Peripheral neuropathy. In: Neurology for the non-neurologist. 3rd edition. Philadelphia: J.B. Lippincott Company, 1994:154–170.
12. Hogan QH. Back pain and radiculopathy. In: Abram S, Haddox J, eds. The pain clinic manual. 2nd edition. Philadelphia: Lippincott Williams & Wilkins, 2000:157–166.
13. O'Connor PJ, Cook DB. Exercise and pain: the neurobiology, measurement, and laboratory study of pain in relation to exercise in humans. Exercise and sports science reviews 1999;27:119–166.
14. Cardenas DD, Egan KJ. Management of chronic pain. In: Kottke FJ, Lehmann JF, eds. Krusen's handbook of physical medicine and rehabilitation. Philadelphia: WB Saunders; 1990:1162–1191.
15. Davis VP, Fillingim RB, Doleys DM, et al. Assessment of aerobic power in chronic pain patients before and after a multidisciplinary treatment program. Arch Phys Med Rehabil 1992;73:726–729.
16. Ruhland JL, Shields RK. The effects of a home exercise program on impairment and health-related quality of life in persons with chronic peripheral neuropathies. Phys Ther 1997;77:1026–1039.
17. Rozmaryn LM, Dovelle S, Rothman ER, et al. Nerve and tendon gliding exercises and the conservative management of carpal tunnel syndrome. J Hand Ther 1998;11:171–179.
18. Seradge H, Bear C, Bithell D. Preventing carpal tunnel syndrome and cumulative trauma disorder: effect of carpal tunnel decompression exercises: an Oklahoma experience. J Okla State Med Assoc 2000;93:150–153.
19. Lincoln AE, Bernick JS, Ogaitis S, et al. Interventions for the primary prevention of work-related carpal tunnel syndrome. Am J Prev Med 2000;18:37–50.
20. Albright A, Franz M, Hornsby G, et al. American College of Sports Medicine Position Stand. Exercise and type 2 diabetes. Med Sci Sports Exerc 2000;32:1324–1360.
21. Richardson JK, Sandman D, Vela S. A focused exercise regimen improves clinical measures of balance in patients with peripheral neuropathy. Arch Phys Med Rehabil 2001;82: 205–209.
22. Attal N. Pharmacologic treatment of neuropathic pain. Acta Neurol Belg 2001;101:53–64.
23. Julien RM. A Primer of drug action. A concise, nontechnical guide to the actions, uses, and side effects of psychoactive Drugs. 8th ed. New York: W. H. Freeman and Company, 1998:181–222.
24. Pariente A, Danan G. Gastrointestinal disorders. In: Benichou C, eds. Adverse drug reactions: A practical guide to diagnosis and management. New York: John Wiley & Sons, 1994:77–86.
25. Davis DP, Videen JS, Marino A, et al. Exercise-associated hyponatremia in marathon runners: a two-year experience. J Emerg Med 2001;21:47–57.
26. Hamilton ME, Gershwin ME. Treatment of pain. In: Gershwin ME, Hamilton ME, eds. The pain management handbook. Totowa, NJ: Humana Press: 283–235.
27. Waslick BD, Walsh BT, Greenhill LL, et al. Cardiovascular effects of desipramine in children and adults during exercise testing. J Am Acad Child Adolesc Psychiatry 1999;38:179–186.
28. Lipman AG. Analgesic drugs for neuropathic and sympathetically maintained pain. Clin Geriatr Med 1996;12:501–515.
29. Harke H, Gretenkort P, Ladleif HU, et al. The response of neuropathic pain and pain in complex regional pain syndrome I to carbamazepine and sustained-release morphine in patients pretreated with spinal cord stimulation: a double-blinded randomized study. Anesth Analg 2001;92: 488–95.
30. Minami T, Bakoshi S, Nakano H, et al. The Effects of capsaicin cream on prostaglandin-induced allodynia. Anesth Analg 2001;93:419–23.
31. Ho J, DeLuca KG. Neurologic assessment of the pain patient. In: Benzon H, Raja S, Borsook D, et al, eds. Essentials of pain medicine and regional anesthesia. New York: Churchill Livingstone, 1999:14–15.
32. Tan JC. Practical manual of physical medicine and rehabilitation. St. Louis: Mosby Yearbook, 1998:133–155, 607–644.
33. Williams V, Pappagallo M. Entrapment neuropathies. In: Benzon H, Raja S, Borsook D, et al, eds. Essentials of pain medicine and regional anesthesia. Philadelphia: Churchill Livingstone, 1999:298.
34. Rathmell J, Katz J. Diabetic and other peripheral neuropathies. In: Benzon H, Raja S, Borsook D, et al, eds. Essentials of pain medicine and regional anesthesia. Philadelphia: Churchill Livingstone, 1999:288–294.
35. Backonia M. Anticonvulsants for neuropathic pain syndromes. Clin J Pain 2000;16:S67–S72.
36. Tan JC. Practical manual of physical medicine and rehabilitation. St. Louis: Mosby Yearbook, 1998:133–155, 607–644.
37. Abram SE. Neural blockade for neuropathic pain. Clin J Pain 2000;16:S56–S61.
38. Raj P. Neural blockade in clinical anesthesia and management of pain. St. Louis: Mosby Year Book, 1996:899–934.

39. Levy R. Neuroablative procedures for treatment of intractable pain. In: Benzon H, Raja S, Borsook D, et al, eds. Essentials of pain medicine and regional anesthesia. Philadelphia: Churchill Livingstone, 1999:104–110
40. Kemp SS, Rogg JM. In: Latchaw, ed. MR and imaging of the head, neck, and spine. St. Louis: MosbyYear Book; 1991: 1109–1157.
41. Deutsch AL, Mink JH. Magnetic resonance imaging of musculoskeletal disorders. Radio Clin N Am, 1989;27:983–1002.
42. Daffner RH, Rothfus WB. In Latchaw, ed. MR and imagining of the head, neck, and spine. St. Louis: Mosby Year Book, 1999:1225–1255.
43. Intracosa JH, Christopherson LA. Radiology of the spine. In: Benzon H, Raja S, Borsook D, et al, eds. Essentials of pain medicine and regional anesthesia. New York: Churchill Livingstone, 1999:20–26.
44. Nishida T, Miniek M. Role of neurophysiologic testing for pain. In: Benzon H, Raja S, Borsook D, et al, eds. Essentials of pain medicine and regional anesthesia. New York: Churchill Livingstone, 1999:27–33.
45. Kimura J. Electrodiagnosis in diseases of nerve and muscle principles and practice. 2nd ed. Philadelphia: F.A. Davis Company, 1989.
46. Wilborn AJ. The electrodiagnostic exam of patients with radiculopathies. Muscle Nerve. Amercian Academy of Electrodiagnostic Medicine. Minimonogram. 1998;32:1612–1631.
47. Dumitru D. Electrodiagnostic medicine. Philadelphia: Hanley and Belfus, 1995.
48. Griffin JW, Hiesch ST, McArthur JC, et al. Laboratory testing in peripheral neuropathy. Neurol Clin 1996;14:119–133.
49. Huskisson EC. Measurement of pain. Lancet 1974;2:1127–1131.
50. Huskisson EC. Measurement of pain. J Rheumatol 1982;9: 768–769.
51. Dixon JS. Reproducibility along a 10 cm vertical visual analogue scale. Ann Rheumatol Dis 1981;40:87–89.
52. Scott J, Huskisson EC. Vertical or horizontal visual analogue scales. Ann Rheumatol Dis 1979;38:560.
53. Maxwell C. Sensitivity and accuracy of the visual analogue scale. Br J Clin Pharmacol 1978;6:15.
54. Melzack R, Katz J. Pain measurement in persons in pain. In: Wall PD, Melzack R, eds. Textbook of pain. Edinburgh: Churchill Livingstone; 1999:409–426.
55. Skogsbergh DR, Chapman SA. Dealing with the chronic patient. In: Mootz RD, Vernon HT, editors. Best practices in clinical chiropractic. Gaithersburg, MD: Aspen; 1999:120–129.
56. Cardenas DD, Egan KJ. Management of chronic pain. In: Kottke FJ, Lehmann JF, eds. Krusen's handbook of physical medicine and rehabilitation. Philadelphia: W.B. Saunders; 1990:1162–1191.
57. Yeh C, Gonyea M, Lemke J, et al. Physical therapy. In: Aronoff GM, ed. Evaluation and treatment of chronic pain. Baltimore: Williams & Wilkins. 1985:251–261.
58. Kilmer DD, Aitkens S. Neuromuscular disease. In: Frontera WR, Dawson DM, Slovic DM, eds. Exercise in rehabilitative medicine. Champaign, IL: Human Kinetics; 1999:253–266.

CHAPTER 9

Brain Injury

Karen Palmer McLean, Kimberly Harbst, and Timothy Harbst

EPIDEMIOLOGY AND PATHOPHYSIOLOGY

The term "traumatic brain injury" refers to the condition when a person is hit by, or runs into, an external force great enough to cause damage to the brain (1). Traumatic brain injury (TBI), also known as head injury, is a major cause of disability and death in the United States. Based on data gathered from 1989–1998, the Centers for Disease Control and Prevention estimate that each year 1.5 million Americans incur TBIs (2, 3). As a result of these injuries, various sources estimate that 50,000–75,000 individuals die per year of head trauma, 230,000–500,000 require hospitalization, and 80,000–90,000 experience residual deficits or disability (1, 2, 4, 5). TBI is the leading cause of death and disability in young children and adults. The prevalence of disability due to TBI within the United States is estimated at approximately 5.3 million people (2). According to emergency room data, approximately 525,000 people annually experience "mild" head injuries, an increasing number of whom are being discharged without hospital admission (2, 3, 6, 7). However, approximately 15% of those people having mild head injury experience lasting residual behavioral, emotional, cognitive, and physical (e.g., fatigue, persistent headaches) deficits of the injury.

The typical age of onset of TBI is bimodal with peaks at the 15–24-year and 75-year-and-older age groups. Injuries sustained in the 75+ age group are most often a consequence of a fall and are associated with a high mortality rate (2). Motor vehicle accidents are the most frequent cause of TBI within the 15–24-year-age group (4).

When a person sustains a TBI, the brain is damaged at the point of impact, which is referred to as the "coup" lesion. After the initial impact, the brain rebounds within the bony skull, potentially sustaining an additional impact with the skull opposite the original coup lesion. This damage is referred to as a "contrecoup" lesion (4). Primary damage that may occur to the brain at either of these sites includes bruising and/or tearing of neural tissue and rupture of arteries/veins. The brain may also exhibit secondary damage resulting from pressure associated with edema and/or accumulations of blood within the closed, bony cranial vault. If allowed to persist, this increased pressure can cause the brain to herniate through the dural reflections and/or through the foramen magnum and into the spinal canal. Finally, as a result of the rapid acceleration/deceleration torques that the brain experiences during many of these traumatic occurrences, neurons may be sheared off within the myelin sheaths. This phenomenon is referred to as "diffuse axonal injury." Due to the microscopic nature of diffuse axonal injury, the damage cannot be visualized initially following TBI—unlike the coup or contrecoup sites. However, once the axons begin to die, the brain appears atrophied and shrunken on a computed tomography (CT) or magnetic resonance imaging (MRI) scan. Damage from hypoxic/anoxic brain injuries is similar to diffuse axonal injury in that the impact is diffuse and exhibits similar visualization characteristics. Hypoxic or anoxic brain injuries occur when the brain is subjected to periods with insufficient or no oxygen such as occurs with near-drownings, crush injuries to the chest, and during respiratory arrest.

DIAGNOSTIC TECHNIQUES

Traumatic brain injuries are classified into three general categories (mild, moderate, or severe) depending on the presence, extent, and persistence of deficits following injury. The Glasgow Coma Scale (GCS) is the tool most often used to characterize the patient's level of consciousness and can be used to categorize the patient's injuries as mild, moderate, or severe (8).

The GCS score (Table 9.1) is a sum of the person's eye-opening, verbal, and motor responses with a range of possible total scores from 3 (lowest) to 15 (highest). The GCS is typically obtained as soon as possible after the injury and is monitored periodically thereafter to document any change in status. A GCS score of 13–15 is generally associated with a mild injury. A score of 8 or less defines coma in the majority of cases.

A great deal of controversy exists over the inclusion cri-

Table 9.1. Glasgow Coma Scale

ACTIVITY	SCORE
Eye Opening	
Spontaneous	4
Response to speech	3
Response to pain	2
No response	1
Best Motor Response	
Follows motor commands	6
Localizes	5
Withdraws	4
Abnormal flexion	3
Extensor response	2
No response	1
Verbal Response	
Oriented	5
Confused conversation	4
Inappropriate words	3
Incomprehensible sounds	2
No response	1

teria for "mild" head injury. (The term "concussion" may be used interchangeably with mild head injury.) The presence of any of the following is indicative of a mild head injury (1):

- Loss of consciousness for 30 minutes or less after the injury
- Posttraumatic amnesia (no longer than 24 hours) or retrograde amnesia
- Altered mental state after the injury
- GCS score taken at 30 minutes postinjury ranges from 13 to 15
- Focal neurological deficits that are expected to resolve within 3 months

Moderate TBI is characterized by a GCS of 9–12 during the first 24 hours after injury and posttraumatic amnesia lasting from 1 to 24 hours. Severe TBI is defined by a score of 8 or less, a score defining coma in most cases, during the initial 24 hours postinjury.

OTHER DIAGNOSTIC TECHNIQUES

Physicians typically use either CT or MRI scanning of the brain to localize and determine the current extent of brain injury. As compared with CT scanning, MRI allows improved resolution, decreased exposure to radiation, and detection of smaller areas of injury (4). Accumulation of blood from torn vessels in and around the brain may be observable immediately after injury, depending on the extent of damage to the vessel and the type of vessel injured. If an artery is severed, the increased vascular pressure will force blood out of the vessel more rapidly than if a vein is damaged. Edema accumulation may take place over hours or days; thus, it may not be immediately observable on a scan. Cortical atrophy requires the longest time period to become noticeable on a brain scan.

FUNCTIONAL CONSEQUENCES OF TBI

Sequelae of TBI vary widely, depending on the site and extent of the lesion. Diffuse injuries, including severe diffuse axonal injury and/or hypoxic/anoxic events, are associated with widespread impairments of many body systems. The impact of more focal injuries (i.e., shooting, stabbing) depends on the structure that is affected. A small lesion of the corpus callosum affects the function of a large portion of the body, whereas the same-sized lesion elsewhere in the brain may likely be associated with significantly less damage.

Although deficits following TBI are difficult to predict, characteristic symptoms of even mild head injuries include cognitive, behavioral, and/or emotional changes or deficits. These changes may be transient or persist over months or years and include memory deficits, agitation, frustration, anxiety, depression, impaired executive functions and concrete thinking, and loss of the capability for abstract thinking. The Rancho Los Amigos Scale of Cognitive Function depicts eight behavioral phases of recovery following traumatic brain injury (4, 5). Although this tool is helpful to aid understanding of some typical behavioral and cognitive outcomes, it is important to note that all people with TBI do not experience all eight phases of recovery. Furthermore, some people do not progress past one of the intermediate phases. Finally, people with TBI tend to fluctuate between adjacent phases depending on multiple factors, including fatigue, stress, bodily needs, etc.

Some common cognitive and behavioral sequelae may influence the ability to participate in an exercise program. Examples of such behavioral issues might include deficits of judgment, memory/learning capacity, tolerance for stimulation and/or need for sensory regulation/reduction, and motor planning. The complexity of the brain does not allow one-to-one correspondence between structures and functions. However, lesions in certain areas of the brain are more frequently associated with specific behavioral manifestations. Involvement of the frontal lobe can result in lack of initiation, apathy, easy frustration, loss of inhibition, and impaired cognitive and executive functions. Lesions in the temporal lobe may cause difficulties with new learning, memory deficits, and possible outbursts of aggression. Involvement of the areas of the brain mediating perception and arousal, including the parieto-occipito-temporal area and the reticular activating system, may lead to difficulty screening out irrelevant sensory input in the environment and focusing on important cues.

Sensorimotor impairments following TBI are similar to those experienced by people with other brain lesions (tumor, stroke, cerebral palsy). However, the pattern of body involvement is variable in people with TBI depending on the locations of the lesion(s). The following typical impairments may be experienced:

- Loss of selective, isolated movement patterns
- Loss of variety of the synergy patterns with which to perform functional movement
- Muscle weakness
- Hypertonia or increased resistance of the muscle(s) to passive muscle lengthening
- Hyperactive deep tendon reflexes
- Sensory/perceptual changes (including special senses)

A common consequence of TBI is alteration in bulbar function. Deficits may be attributed to a primary shearing lesion of the cranial nerves during the initial brain injury (9). Additional cranial nerve damage may occur if increased intracranial pressure causes brain herniation through the tentorium and/or into the foramen magnum. Regardless of the cause, the optic, oculomotor, glossopharyngeal, and vagus nerves are commonly affected. Damage to the optic nerve and/or the occipital cortex may result in varying levels of visual impairment. Damage to the oculomotor nerve results in Horner's syndrome, which consists of ptosis of the eyelid, pupillary dilation, and altered parasympathetic function of the affected side of the face, including anhydrosis. These impairments also contribute to visual deficits due to difficulties with conjugate eye movement and the ability to focus/converge. Damage to the glossopharyngeal and vagus nerves causes difficulty swallowing and talking. A person may require a tracheostomy in order to effectively handle secretions and may not be allowed oral feedings if unable to swallow safely and effectively without aspiration. This person would also have a distinctive, nasal vocal quality that may hinder communication. Finally, the olfactory nerve endings are often damaged during head injury. Although the nerves are peripheral at the point of injury, the formation of scar tissue is common, resulting in limited ability to smell and/or taste flavors other than bitter, sweet, salty, and sour.

MEDICAL SEQUELAE

Seizures (Epilepsy)

The risk of developing posttraumatic epilepsy is greatest in the first 2 years following TBI. The seizures may range from petit mal to grand mal in nature. Results of a survey of more than 300 individuals who were about 10 years post-TBI indicate that approximately 15% have a chronic seizure disorder (10). People experiencing grand mal seizures are at risk for falls and injuries.

Neuroendocrine disorders are often associated with chronic seizure activity (10). These disorders may present as changes in eating and appetite regulation that may result in significant weight gain for the patient post-TBI, particularly for women. These disorders are related to impairment of the hypothalamic–pituitary axis. Possible causes include basal skull fractures, implicating direct damage to the pituitary gland. These disorders may also be one of the long-term sequelae of medical interventions during the acute management of TBI when high doses of steroids are administered. Thus, those with post-TBI seizures should be routinely assessed for presence of neuroendocrine disorders.

Heterotopic Ossification

Heterotopic ossification or calcium deposits in soft-tissue structures are found in 11–76% of all people who sustain a severe TBI (11, 12). The etiology of this disorder is unclear, although the incidence seems associated with individuals who experienced multiple traumas requiring open reduction and internal fixation of fractures (10). In the acute stages, the disorder sometimes presents with common inflammatory signs (heat, pain, swelling, redness) leading to contracture formation, but it can be present without overt signs or symptoms. Presence of ectopic ossification can interfere with adequate positioning, passive range of motion, and the ability to perform functional motor activities. Heterotopic ossification can be visualized with a bone scan in the earliest stages or an x-ray at later phases (9).

Cardiopulmonary Impairments

Although a person experiencing a TBI may initially experience hypertension immediately after injury, prolonged hypertension is atypical. Other cardiac impairments are not typical secondary to TBI.

In the acute stages following TBI, many patients require a tracheostomy for ventilation and management of secretions. This procedure is typically reversed when the patient is able to independently manage the airway. However, years after a severe head injury, people have been noted to have a 25–40% reduction in total lung capacity, vital capacity, and forced expiratory volume (9, 13). These limitations may be due to reduced compliance of the chest wall following the limited mobility that typically occurs during the acute phase of recovery. They may also be due to weak or noncoordinated actions of the respiratory musculature.

MEDICAL AND SURGICAL TREATMENTS

Behavioral Deficits

In the acute stages following TBI, psychotropic medications may be used to counteract detrimental effects of behavioral deficits. These medications are typically used to alleviate agitation that interferes with the person's ability to participate in the rehabilitation process. These medications are typically discontinued after agitation resolves (4, 9).

Hypertonia, Hyperreflexia, Clonus

Pharmacological intervention may be necessary to decrease hypertonia that interferes with passive range of motion and/or daily functional abilities. Oral medications (e.g., baclofen, diazepam, tizanidine) can be used to treat generalized hypertonia that occurs throughout the body. However, some people experience side effects of these oral medications, including diminished arousal and cognitive capabilities that may be considered intolerable. An alternative to oral medications includes implantation of an intrathecal pump, which allows smaller doses of baclofen to be administered directly into the spinal canal. Most people experience improved spasticity control with less cortical function impairment using intrathecal medications as opposed to oral medications.

If hypertonia is localized to one extremity or a few muscle groups, a variety of blocks may be used. Phenol blocks are used to denature the myelin sheath surrounding the nerve of hypertonic muscles. Phenol injections may also be used at the motor point to disrupt conductance of neural impulses across the neuromuscular junction. A newer alternative to phenol injections is the injection of specially prepared botulinum toxin (Botox) into the affected muscle belly. The effects of Botox injections are transient, with an average duration of 2–6 months, as opposed to phenol, which typically lasts 6 months.

Seizures (Epilepsy)

Posttraumatic epilepsy may be addressed prophylactically or with medications such as phenytoin or phenobarbital. However, patients may experience cognitive slowing as a side effect of these drugs. The balance between adequate seizure control and adequate arousal for function is often very sensitive and difficult to achieve. Therefore, carbamazepine is an alternative drug that may be used with fewer cognitive side effects. These medications may be withdrawn after 1 or more seizure-free years.

Heterotopic Ossification

Doctors have attempted to prevent the occurrence of heterotopic ossification using diphosphonates with variable results. Maintenance of passive range of motion is encouraged to prevent joint fusion. The ectopic bone can be surgically removed, but recurrence is possible (9).

SOCIAL CONSEQUENCES

Hibbard et al. (10) surveyed 338 individuals who were on average 10 years post-TBI and found that they were more frequently single, divorced, or separated compared with those without disability. Their findings are supported by Gordon et al., who report that individuals post-TBI are less likely to be married (14). Inability to participate in sports with able-bodied children is one of the major sequelae expressed by children who have sustained a TBI (15).

IMPORTANCE OF EXERCISE

Rehabilitation services identify "return to home and community" as the primary goals of treatment. Therefore, program planning should attempt to maximize patients' abilities to integrate socially into the community (16). Participation in an exercise training program is one way to achieve this goal. It should be noted that successful reintegration into sports and leisure activities is particularly important to children and adolescents with TBI (15). Results of a retrospective study that included 240 individuals with TBI (14) suggest that individuals who exercised were less depressed than nonexercisers who sustained a TBI. In addition, exercisers were more productive and more mobile than their nonexercising peers as measured by the Community Integration Questionnaire and Craig Handicap Assessment Capacity Technique, respectively. Those patients with TBI who exercised reported fewer symptoms than those who did not exercise, particularly cognitive symptoms, even though exercisers' initial injuries were more severe as compared to nonexercisers.

The study's authors hypothesized that sustained exercise requires focus and concentration. Perhaps the repeated use of these skills while engaged in exercise training resulted in improved cognitive function. In addition, they questioned whether exercise might increase the production of BDNF or other growth factors that might improve cognitive function.

Grealy and colleagues conducted a prospective exercise training study involving individuals who had sustained a head injury (17). Subjects trained on a nonimmersive virtual reality recumbent ergometer with the virtual environment presented on a color graphics screen. During each exercise session, the subject had to steer around a virtual course or compete in a race against other virtual riders. The authors hypothesized that an exercise program with a high level of interaction is likely to increase the potential for structural change in the brain. Following 4 weeks of training, subjects demonstrated significant improvements in both visual and auditory learning, as well as an improved ability to associate shapes and figures relative to a nonexercise control group.

The findings of these studies certainly argue for the inclusion of fitness training in the overall rehabilitation program for patients who have sustained a TBI. In addition, many of the patients who survive TBI are young and have many years ahead of them. If these individuals do not engage in regular physical activity, they will be at risk for the same diseases as the general population who do not have physical and cognitive impairments.

Due to sensorimotor impairments, some individuals demonstrate decreased locomotor efficiency following a TBI. The combination of low fitness levels and the high energy cost associated with ambulation results in excessive fatigue. Individuals with TBI fatigue at a rate 2.62 times faster than their unimpaired counterparts (18). Some authors have suggested that many individuals with TBI would only be able to work about 3.05 hours of a standard 8-hour day before they were fatigued. The enhanced ability to sustain endurance exercise following an exercise training program reduces fatigability (18). In addition, aerobic capacity is highly correlated (r = 0.81) with worker productivity. Finally, exercise training may be another way to limit the weight gain many individuals, and in particular women, experience after a TBI.

One might assume that only individuals who sustain mild head injuries have the ability to engage in an exercise training program. Gordon et al. conducted a community-based retrospective study of 240 individuals who were post-TBI. They found that exercisers' initial injuries were more severe than the initial injuries of nonexercisers (14). Sullivan et al. found that 88% of the 49 patients they treated for TBI were able to independently ambulate. These data suggest that a large majority of the post-TBI patients have the motor ability to engage in simple conditioning activities (19).

EXERCISE/FITNESS/FUNCTIONAL TESTING

Screening for Health Risk Factors before Initiating a Program

Prior to initiating an exercise program, the client with TBI should be screened for health risk factors that should be considered when designing the program. In addition to using a standard preparticipation screening tool such as the PAR-Q (20), clients should be screened for behavioral factors such as impulsivity, a tendency to display outward aggression, lack of judgment, and misunderstanding of directions (21). A client who lacks judgment may need closer supervision during exercise, while the individual who displays outward aggression may not succeed in certain group exercise settings. A client who is easily agitated/frustrated or highly distractible might be scheduled to exercise at a facility during a quieter time of the day or work out in an area that has fewer distractions. The client who lacks initiative might be more successful in a group setting. Thus, the 31 rehabilitation experts involved in the study by Vitale et al. (21) suggest that it is equally important to consider physiological and behavioral factors to obtain optimal results from an exercise training program.

Exercise Testing Techniques

Since TBI results in varying levels of injury and the typical age of onset is bimodal, selection of exercise testing techniques depends upon the age of the client and the level of physical and cognitive impairment. It is often very difficult to measure maximal aerobic capacity in this population due to cognitive, behavioral, and physical impairments following TBI. Thus, peak $\dot{V}O_2$ is often measured. Some authors have estimated maximal aerobic capacity by plotting the submaximal heart rate (HR) and $\dot{V}O_2$ values and extrapolating the curve to the age-predicted maximal HR (18).

Many individuals with minimal physical impairment can complete progressive exercise tests using a treadmill protocol, such as the Balke (18). Individuals with sensorimotor impairments that result in weakness, loss of movement, or balance deficits may be unsafe on a treadmill. Treadmill testing could still be conducted using a partial body-weight support harness system. In cases of severe weakness, the harness could be used to partially unweight the body during treadmill testing. For other individuals, the harness system could be used simply as a safety measure to prevent a fall should the individual miss a step or experience a loss of balance.

Individuals with sensorimotor impairment could also complete progressive exercise testing using either a bicycle ergometer or a combined arm/leg ergometer. Ergometers may have to be adapted in order to allow the individual with a brain injury to use them effectively. For example, a strap or a mitt may be used to secure the hand of an individual who has difficulty using the handgrip on an arm ergometer or a combination arm/leg ergometer. Similarly, the individual who cannot maintain the foot on the pedal of a bicycle ergometer may need the foot secured with a strap or wrap. The individual should be closely supervised if a strap is used to secure an extremity on a handle or pedal because the individual will be unable to extend the arm or leg to stop a fall in the case of loss of balance. Finally, a step stool may be required for an individual to get on and off of a bicycle ergometer. The client should step up onto the stool with the unaffected leg and step down with the affected leg.

Hunter and colleagues conducted progressive exercise tests on 12 subjects with TBI using three exercise modes—treadmill, bicycle ergometer, and mechanical stairs (22). They found that maximal exercise performance is most accurately assessed on either the treadmill or mechanical stairs. Significantly lower peak $\dot{V}O_2$ values were recorded on the bicycle ergometer, most likely due to the smaller muscle mass involved in this activity. The authors did note that subjects with severe ataxia or hypertonia of the lower limbs required minimal assistance (help directing or guiding a foot to the next step) to complete the exercise test on the mechanical stairs. They also reported that two subjects who were overweight reached very high HRs at very low stepping speeds on the mechanical stairs.

Since treadmills and $\dot{V}O_2$ measurement systems are not available in most rehabilitation centers, field tests have been developed to estimate maximal aerobic capacity in populations following TBI. Vitale et al. (23) developed a reliable field test to estimate aerobic capacity in individuals who sustained a TBI. The test was a progressive, externally paced 20-m shuttle run/walk where intensity was increased every minute until exhaustion. This test appears to have advantages over more traditional self-paced tests, such as the 12-minute walk test, because many individuals following TBI have difficulty measuring their own HR and may not be able to pace themselves to complete a 12-minute run/walk. The shuttle run is also a good field test when motivation is an issue. Similar protocols have been used in adults with mental retardation and individuals with chronic obstructive pulmonary disease. Disadvantages of the test include the locomotor efficiency required at each turn-around that may predispose the subject with balance or coordination problems to falls.

Patients with central nervous system pathology typically demonstrate subnormal aerobic capacities (18). Aerobic capacities have been reported to range from 67% to 74% of the predicted value based on the subjects' height and age (18, 22). These results support the earlier findings of significantly higher submaximal HRs during cycle ergometry among subjects with TBI relative to age-matched controls without physical impairments (13).

Rossi and Sullivan used the standard motor fitness tests administered to children without orthopedic or neurological impairment (sit and reach, hand grip, pull-up, flex-arm-hang, sit-up, 50-yard dash, adapted 20-m shuttle run, standing broad jump, etc.) to test children who had sustained a severe TBI. They found these field tests to be reliable in this population, with intraclass correlation coefficients comparable to or exceeding those observed in children without impairments (15). Children who were an average of 4 years post-TBI ranked only in the 29th percentile relative to motor fitness.

Muscle strength and endurance should also be assessed since it is not uncommon for the client with TBI to demonstrate muscle weakness, hypertonicity, or the loss of the ability to perform isolated movement. Muscular endurance can be measured using the 1-minute sit-up test. Although there are few studies where this parameter has been measured in this population, it appears that muscular endurance is significantly reduced. The 14 sedentary subjects who had sustained a TBI, studied by Jankowski and Sullivan, scored in the 8th percentile on the 1-minute sit-up test (18).

Muscle strength can be measured using a variety of computerized dynamometers (Cybex, Biodex, etc.). A handheld dynamometer can also be used to measure the amount of resistance that can be applied as the individual attempts to maintain a manual muscle testing position. It should be noted that strength testing can be problematic in a population with brain injury. Strength can only be reliably tested when an individual can isolate joint movement. Some individuals may only be able to move in stereotypical patterns and lack the ability to isolate movement. For example, an individual may be able to actively extend the knee if the hip is also moving into extension, but may not be able to extend the knee from a sitting position where the hip is maintained in a flexed position (a position outside of the stereotypical synergy pattern).

Flexibility is a particularly important component of fitness that should be tested in this population. Arthritic complaints are much more common in individuals following TBI relative to individuals without disability (10). An individual with brain injury is more likely to demonstrate limited joint range of motion for several reasons, including the multiple joint trauma that may have accompanied the TBI, reduced mobility during the acute phase of recovery, and the increased risk of heterotopic ossification in this population. Brain injury that results in muscle weakness or hypertonia also has the potential to limit joint range. Limitations in joint motion can be measured with a hand-held goniometer.

EXERCISE PRESCRIPTION AND PROGRAMMING

Aerobic Modes

The selection of mode depends on several factors. First is the individual's level of impairment. Ideally, the selected mode should allow the individual with TBI to exercise a large muscle mass safely with the greatest possible level of independence. This is particularly important if one or more limbs are paretic. As noted earlier, individuals who have sustained a TBI may present in a variety of ways depending on the severity of the injury and the part of the brain that sustained damage. An individual's impairment may be barely noticeable, or the individual may present with hypertonia and severe contractures.

Another factor to consider when selecting a mode of exercise is the specificity of the mode and its consistency with the individual's long-term therapeutic goals. Issues such as the location of the center of mass relative to the base of support, the size of the base of support, the individual's position during exercise with respect to gravity, and the muscle actions required to complete the exercise should be assessed when trying to select a mode of exercise. For example, an individual may be equally independent in completing an exercise session on a bicycle ergometer or a stair-climbing machine. However, a stair-climber, where one exercises in an upright position and is constantly shifting weight from side to side, might be a more specific mode of exercise for the individual who demonstrates inadequate weightshifting during gait and has a long-term goal of improving the ability to ambulate.

Finally, the selected mode should be accessible and should be an activity that the individual enjoys. Accessibility to facilities with exercise equipment is an issue for many individuals who have sustained a TBI. Often, these individuals cannot drive independently and must rely on others or public transportation to get to a fitness facility. There is also the expense of a health club membership to consider, as many of these folks have been involved in accidents in which they received no financial compensation for their injury.

Walking/jogging is an inexpensive mode of exercise for the individual who can ambulate independently and requires no additional equipment. Individuals should be carefully screened prior to prescribing jogging as an exercise mode. Some degree of foot drop is not uncommon in this population; thus, tripping (due to lack of foot clearance) may be a potential problem. Ankle instability, due to sensorimotor impairment, can increase the risk of ankle sprains when the individual increases the pace of walking/jogging. A treadmill offers the option of walking up a grade. This allows an increase in workload for the individual who ambulates independently but does not have the motor ability to run or jog.

If balance or strength impairments preclude walking as a mode of exercise, one might consider a bicycle ergometer, an arm ergometer, or a combination arm/leg ergometer. These modes represent simple, repetitive activities that might be of benefit to the individual who has motor planning and sequencing problems. These are also activities that might provide a physical outlet to alleviate frustration or anxiety in people who become easily agitated. Individuals who have difficulty maintaining their sitting balance independently on the more traditional bicycle ergometer might be able to safely exercise on a recumbent cycle ergometer or a recumbent stepping machine, the seats of which provide greater trunk support for the individual. Seat belts could be added to either of these devices to further increase an individual's stability during the exercise session.

Individuals may be more compliant with an exercise program if the activity is conducted in a group session that promotes social integration. Aerobic exercise classes where individuals exercise with music might further improve compliance. A variety of aerobics classes, including traditional aerobics, water aerobics, or step aerobics, might be appropriate depending on the individual's preferences and abilities. The choreography of the aerobics program can be modified to include specific strengthening, balance, and/or stretching exercise that will address the individual's specific physical impairments. An individual with more severe physical impairments would be able to participate in a chair aerobics program performed from either a wheelchair or a standard straight-back chair. If the individual can stand independently from a sitting position, parts of the exercise program can be performed standing next to the chair, holding on to the chair back if needed.

Resistance Exercise

Previously, it was thought that resistance exercise resulted in further increases in muscle tone in those individuals demonstrating hypertonia. Therefore, resistance exercise training programs were often not included in the rehabilitation programs of many individuals following TBI. These fears appear to be unfounded. Resistance exercises should be prescribed to address any muscle weakness identified during the fitness assessment.

Following TBI, many individuals have difficulty with preparatory postural adjustments and recruiting strength quickly enough to combat the loss of balance. Thus, some of the positions typically used for weight training may need to be modified. For example, many individuals perform dumbbell exercises while standing to increase upper body strength. A person who has difficulty maintaining standing balance should perform these exercises unilaterally while holding onto a bar or other stationary object. They could also perform these exercises from a seated position.

Adaptations to exercise equipment

Exercise equipment may need to be adapted to allow individuals with physical impairments to exercise safely and independently. The use of seat belts, mitts, or straps to stabilize an individual on stationary exercise equipment was discussed in an earlier section. Additionally, during weight training, one might consider adding Velcro™ straps to dumbbells for clients with a weak grasp. Use of straps would minimize the chance of dropping the weight, making it safer for the client and other individuals in the exercise area.

Intensity and Duration of Exercise Training

Exercise intensity should be based on the initial fitness level of the subject. The very deconditioned individual may have to begin at exercise intensities equivalent to 50–60% $\dot{V}O_{2peak}$. Hunter et al. used this lower exercise intensity (60–80% maximal HR—equivalent to 50–65% $\dot{V}O_{2peak}$) in their training study involving 12 subjects who were post-TBI (22). Jankowski and Sullivan in their study involving 14 subjects with TBI utilized a slightly greater intensity, an HR equivalent to 70% of estimated $\dot{V}O_{2peak}$ (18).

Although previous authors have utilized HR as an indicator of exercise intensity, the results of a more recent study suggest that many individuals with TBI cannot accurately measure their radial pulse during exercise. Vitale et al. taught 20 subjects who were 22 months post-TBI to measure their radial pulse at rest (24). All subjects demonstrated the cognitive capacity to complete this task. However, the subjects' self-measured HR after 5 minutes of walking correlated poorly with actual HRs simultaneously obtained from an electronic monitor. Subjects tended to underestimate their HR by 15 bpm, resulting in the subjects exercising at an intensity much higher than desired. The authors of this study suggest that HRs be monitored by either an exercise training buddy or an electronic HR monitor if HR will be used to determine intensity of exercise. As an alternative, rating of perceived exertion (RPE) might be used to monitor exercise intensity. It should be noted that some subjects who have sustained a TBI are also unable to accurately use the RPE scale.

Exercise duration should be set at a minimum of 20 minutes. Once an individual can comfortably complete a 20-minute bout of aerobic exercise, the duration should be gradually increased until the individual can complete an exercise bout equivalent to a caloric expenditure of 300 kcal. As one can see, an individual could complete a shorter exercise bout at a higher intensity or a longer exercise bout at a lower intensity in order to reach the 300-kcal threshold.

Supervision and Monitoring of Exercise Training Sessions

The amount of supervision required during exercise training sessions varies with the person. Some individuals have the ability to exercise safely with little supervision.

Others have slowed reaction times, limited attention spans, visual deficits, perceptual problems, sensory changes, and difficulty recruiting muscles quickly enough to catch their balance. Any of these deficits, particularly when combined with questionable cognition, can result in injury or accident. Thus, the individual who has sustained a TBI should be well supervised during the initial exercise training sessions. Supervision can be relaxed once the client's cognition and physical abilities have been more thoroughly assessed.

One should consider placing exercise equipment in places within the fitness facility to minimize accident or injury. For example, if an individual with TBI tends to frequently use a combination arm/leg ergometer, this piece of equipment should be placed in a location that is easily accessible. Walkways should be clear of clutter and easily negotiated by individuals who may walk with a wide-base gait.

Finally, one should use common sense when working with clients who demonstrate unpredictable behavior or have unexplained emotional outbursts. One might want to avoid having these clients exercise with heavy objects such as hand-held weights. Exercise in an isolated location such as a pool when other staff members are not in the area, should also be avoided.

Results of Exercise Training Studies

Hunter et al. conducted a 12-week training study on individuals who were at least 1 year post-TBI (22). Subjects exercised 50 minutes, 5 times per week. Half of the 50-minute training session was spent engaged in aerobic activities (walking, bicycle ergometer, treadmill, and mechanical stairs), while the remaining 25 minutes was spent on muscle strengthening and flexibility activities. The subjects demonstrated a 14% increase in aerobic capacity (2.1 2.4 L/min). Jankowski and Sullivan reported similar improvements in their 16-week circuit-training program conducted 3 times per week for 14 patients with TBI (18). The circuit included aerobic activities (stationary cycling, rope skipping, jogging, stair climbing) and neuromuscular rehabilitation activities (shooting baskets, ring toss, three-pin bowling, dribbling drills, weight training, and calisthenics). Subjects completed 45 minutes each of aerobic activity and neuromuscular activity during the last 6 weeks of the study. Peak $\dot{V}O_2$ increased 15% (31–36 mL/kg/min), while the number of sit-ups completed in 1 minute increased 92% (15–30).

CASE STUDY

Jane is a 26-year-old woman who sustained a brain injury in a single-car motor vehicle accident 10 years ago when she lost control of her car on an icy road. At the time of injury, Jane was in the middle of her senior year of high school with plans to attend college after graduation. She played volleyball and softball recreationally. She lived at home with her parents and a twin sister. Following her injury, Jane was in a coma for 2 weeks and was hospitalized for approximately 10 weeks. Over the course of the last 10 years, Jane has received periodic outpatient physical and occupational therapy to work on her gait and arm function. Currently, Jane lives alone in a small house next door to her parents. Her sister has moved out of the home and lives in an apartment. Jane has finished an associate's degree in graphic design and photography at the local technical college. She has been unable to secure a full-time job and currently holds three part-time positions—working 2 days per week in her parents' liquor store, 1 day per week retouching photographs, and variable hours per week as a counselor for people seeking financial compensation for disability. Recently, Jane was diagnosed at an annual checkup as having stage I hypertension (155/86), for which she is being monitored. The only medication Jane currently takes is an oral contraceptive. She has taken baclofen in the past to decrease the spasticity in her right arm, but she stopped taking the medication due to the sedative side effects.

SUBJECTIVE

Jane is not involved in any exercise activities and likes to watch television. She thinks she is overweight. She does enjoy a wide variety of music. Jane says that she spends many more than the 8 hours per week for which she is compensated retouching photographs, as certain skills take her longer due to her impairments and because she is a perfectionist. She complains that she has little to no social interaction with peers and does not date. Jane also complains of frequent headaches that began during her recovery from her injury. Her first goal is to improve her functional mobility and coordination to the level required for her to operate a camera and ambulate safely over a variety of surfaces, as she has chosen photography as a vocation. Her second goal is to lose weight.

OBJECTIVE

She is 5 ft 6 in (167.6 cm) tall, weighs 178 lb (80.7 kg), and has a BMI of 28.8 kg/m^2. Her ECG is normal, but her total lung capacity, vital capacity, and expiratory reserve volume are 30% lower than expected. Her $\dot{V}O_{2peak}$ is 21.7 mL/kg/min, and she is able to complete 5 sit-ups in 1 minute.

Flexibility

Her right shoulder and elbow can be passively stretched to 85% of full range of motion.

Motor Function

Jane holds her right arm in a flexed position with her fist clenched. It is difficult for Jane to actively relax her hand and straighten her fingers. She is able to use her right arm to grossly assist function performed with her left arm. She was previously right-handed. The strength of her right arm was not assessed due to her inability to isolate movement.

Functional Mobility

Jane walks slowly with a wide-base gait. Due to weakness, she has difficulty swinging her right leg forward or supporting her body weight during right-leg stance. She fatigues after walking distances of 150–200 feet.

Social /Vocational Integration

Socially, Jane is very outspoken, which her mother describes as a change in her personality.

ASSESSMENT

Jane's current level of functional mobility limits her ability to engage in her chosen vocation. Her aerobic capacity and muscular endurance are greatly reduced, scoring in only the 1st percentile in each of these categories. Her reduced aerobic capacity is most likely due to inactivity, excessive body weight, and her reduced pulmonary function. Jane would benefit from a structured exercise program that would increase her aerobic capacity, improve her muscular endurance, increase caloric expenditure, and allow her an opportunity to socialize with her peers. Increasing Jane's level of physical activity and decreasing her body weight might also reduce her hypertension.

In addition, Jane should engage in some activities that encourage stretching of her right arm, swinging her right leg forward (into hip flexion) while maintaining the knee in an extended position, and partial weight bearing on her right leg. Improvements in the range of motion of her right arm and her ability to ambulate independently would allow her to more fully engage in her photography career.

PLAN

Aerobic Activity Options

Jane's exercise plan is summarized in Table 9.2. Joining a chair aerobics class a few days per week would allow Jane to exercise in a group setting. This would provide Jane with an increased level of social interaction (which is lacking on her photo-retouching job) and may increase her compliance with the activity. Jane might also tend to comply with an aerobics program since she enjoys a variety of music. The choreography of the sitting activities should encourage reaching with the right arm to increase her range of motion. She would also benefit from choreography that allowed her to hold onto the back of the chair while performing standing lower-extremity exercises. These types of movements would encourage weight shift and pelvic stability during one-leg stance. On alternate days, Jane could exercise at home using stationary exercise equipment while she watched a television program. Modes might include a combination upper-/lower-extremity ergometer or a stair-stepper. An ergometer is a relatively safe mode of exercise even for clients with fairly severe motor impairments. The pedaling action might increase the strength of her right leg, thereby improving her gait. A combination upper-/lower-extremity ergometer provides the following advantages over a lower-extremity ergometer:

- If there is significant weakness of the right leg, Jane may exercise primarily with the left leg. During single-extremity exercise, it is difficult to create the oxygen demand required to induce a cardiovascular training effect.
- The upper-extremity action on the ergometer could increase both the range and strength of the right arm.
- The reciprocal action of the upper extremities may increase trunk rotation, thereby increasing gait cosmesis and decreasing her energy expenditure during gait.

A stair-stepper provides Jane the opportunity to exercise in an upright, weight-bearing position. This position more closely simulates the actions required during gait, relative to the position assumed on a recumbent exercise device. Exercise on the stepper also encourages weight shift and hip flexion—two actions that Jane needs to address to improve the quality of her gait.

Table 9.2. Case Study Exercise Program

Type of Activity	Options	Intensity/Frequency/Duration	Comments
Aerobic	Chair aerobics class	• 70% max HR • 3 days/week • 20–60 minutes/session	• Promotes social reintegration • Choreography should include stretching of right arm, standing hip flexion activities of right leg
Aerobic	• Combination arm/leg ergometer • Stair-stepper	• 70% max HR • 2 days/week • 20–60 minutes/session	• Could perform at home while watching television • Stair-stepper more specific to goal of improving gait
Muscle Endurance	• Sit-ups • Heel raises	• 3 days/week	• Begin the heel raise exercise in a standing position, leaning against the wall.
Strength	Multihip machine	• 3 days/week	• Exercise both affected and unaffected leg. • Exercise of the unaffected leg requires use of the affected leg for balance and stability.
Flexibility	• Prone press-ups • Low back flexion exercises	• 5 days/week	

Duration

The duration of the initial exercise sessions should be targeted at 20 minutes. Eventually, the duration should be increased to a level that allows her to expend a minimum of 300 kcal per session.

Intensity

Since Jane is currently inactive, she should begin at an intensity equivalent to 60% of her maximal HR (50% $\dot{V}O_{2peak}$). This lower intensity will allow Jane to successfully complete the 20-minute duration of the initial exercise session. Once she is able to complete about 30 minutes at this intensity, the intensity can be gradually increased.

Muscle Endurance

Jane should include sit-ups as part of her daily exercise program. Even though she does not have the ability to successfully complete more than 1 sit-up, she should be encouraged to complete as much of the sit-up as possible. As her abdominal muscles become stronger and her muscle endurance improves, she will be able to pull herself upright to a position where the scapula clears the floor.

Due to the importance of the push-off phase of gait, Jane should also attempt to increase the muscle endurance of the gastroc/soleus complex in a standing position. An exercise progression for this muscle group might include standing in a foot-flat position while leaning back against a wall. Jane should then attempt to raise her heels while standing in this position and complete as many repetitions as possible until the muscles are fatigued. Symmetry of movement should be stressed. As the strength and endurance of these muscles increases, Jane can progress to performing this exercise from a simple standing position. She may still need to hold onto a chair back or some other stable object in order to maintain her balance

Strength Exercises

Due to the limitations of her right arm, Jane is unable to perform a standard push-up. However, she can increase her upper body strength by working on standing wall push-ups. If she is unable to perform this exercise independently, she can begin an exercise progression by working on isometric exercises in the standing wall push-up position. As her strength improves, she will be able to complete the eccentric component of this exercise, although she may still not have the strength in her left (affected) arm to complete the concentric portion. Again, symmetry of movement should be stressed during the eccentric phase. She can use her unaffected (left) arm with only minimal assistance from her right arm to complete the concentric phase of the exercise. The overflow from her unaffected arm may facilitate action in her affected arm. Jane should not exert herself excessively when trying to perform this exercise, or the effort will produce an exaggerated associated reaction into a stereotypical pattern in the affected arm that should be avoided.

On the days Jane attends a fitness center for her chair aerobics class, she should also spend some time in the weight room working on the multihip machine that allows the user to perform resisted hip flexion, extension, abduction, and adduction in a standing position. She could benefit from performing this exercise bilaterally. When she is exercising her left (unaffected) leg, the right leg will have to work to support her body weight. This exercise should be fairly safe because machines of this type include handrails that could be used to partially support her weight and to maintain her standing balance. Jane should attempt to gradually reduce the weight she places on the handrails and the amount she uses them.

Flexibility

Jane should perform a general stretching program. She might be more compliant with this program if she performed it while watching TV. Her stretching program should include prone press-ups to promote spinal extension and stretch her hip flexor muscles. She should also include low back flexion exercises.

References

1. National Institutes of Health. NIH consensus statement—rehabilitation of persons with traumatic brain injury. U.S. Department of Health and Human Services, 1998.
2. Centers for Disease Control and Prevention (1999 December). Traumatic brain injury in the United States: a report to Congress. Prepared by the Division of Acute Care, Rehabilitation Research, and Disability Prevention; National Center for Injury Prevention and Control; Centers for Disease Control and Prevention; U.S. Department of Health and Human Services. Retrieved July 9, 2000, from the World Wide Web: http://www.cdc.gov/ncipc/pub-res/tbicongress.htm.
3. Thurman D, Alverson C, Dunn KA, et al. Traumatic brain injury in the United States: A public health perspective. J Head Trauma Rehabil 1999;14:602–615.
4. Fulk GD, Geller A. Traumatic brain injury. In: O'Sullivan SB, Schmitz TJ, eds. Physical rehabilitation assessment and treatment. 4th ed. Philadelphia: F.A. Davis Company, 2001.
5. Winkler PA. Head injury. In: Umphred DA, ed. Neurological rehabilitation. 3rd ed. Baltimore: Mosby, 1995.
6. Guerrero JL, Thurman DJ, Sniezek JE. Emergency department visits associated with traumatic brain injury: United States, 1995–1996. Brain Inj 2000;14:181–186.
7. Thurman D, Guerrero J. Trends in hospitalization associated with traumatic brain injury. JAMA 1999;282:954–957.
8. Jennett B, Teasdale G. Management of head injuries. Philadelphia: F.A. Davis, 1981.
9. Rosenthal M. Rehabilitation of the patient with head injury. In: Delisa JA, Gans BM, Bockenek WL, eds. Rehablitation medicine: principles and practice. 3rd ed. Baltimore: Williams & Wilkins, 1998.
10. Hibbard MR, Uysal S, Sliwinski M, et al. Undiagnosed health issues in individuals with traumatic brain injury living in the community. J Head Trauma Rehabil 1998;13:47–57.
11. Anderson D. Management of decreased ROM from overactive musculature or heterotopic ossification. In: Montgomery J, ed.

Physical therapy for traumatic brain injury. New York: Churchill Livingstone, 1995.

12. Hurvitz EA, Mandac BR, Davidoff G, et al. Risk factors for heterotopic ossification in children and adolescents with severe traumatic brain injury. Arch Phys Med Rehabil 1992; 73:459–462.
13. Becker E, Bar-Or O, Mendelson L, et al. Pulmonary functions and responses to exercise of patients following cranio-cerebral injuries. Scand J Rehabil Med 1978;10:47–50.
14. Gordon WA, Sliwinski M, Echo J, et al. The benefits of exercise in individuals with traumatic brain injury: a retrospective study. J Head Trauma Rehabil 1998;134:58–67.
15. Rossi C, Sullivan SJ. Motor fitness in children and adolescents with traumatic brain injury. Arch Phys Med Rehabil 1996;77:1062–1065.
16. Burleigh SA, Farber RS, Gillard M. Community integration and life satisfaction after traumatic brain injury: long-term findings. Am J Occup Ther 1998;52:45–52.
17. Grealy MA, Johnson DA, Rushton SK. Improving cognitive function after brain injury: the use of exercise and virtual reality. Arch Phys Med Rehabil 1999;80:661–667.
18. Jankowski LW, Sullivan SJ. Aerobic and neuromuscular training: effect on the capacity, efficiency, and fatigability of patients with traumatic brain injury. Arch Phys Med Rehabil 1990;71:500–504.
19. Sullivan SJ, Richer E, Laurent F. The role of and possibilities for physical conditioning programmes in the rehabilitation of traumatically brain-injured persons. Brain Inj 1990;4: 407–414.
20. Franklin BA, ed. ACSM's guidelines for exercise testing and prescription. 6th ed. Baltimore: Lippincott Williams & Wilkins, 2000:22–32.
21. Vitale AE, Sullivan SJ, Jankowski LW, et al. Screening of health risk factors prior to exercise or a fitness evaluation of adults with traumatic brain injury: a consensus by rehabilitation professionals. Brain Inj 1995;10:367–375.
22. Hunter M, Tomberlin J, Kirkikis C, et al. Progressive exercise testing in closed head-injured subjects: comparison of exercise apparatus in assessment of a physical conditioning program. Phys Ther 1990;70:363–371.
23. Vitale AE, Jankowski LW, Sullivan SJ. Reliability of a walk-run test to estimate aerobic capacity in a brain-injured population. Brain Inj 1997;11:67–76.
24. Vitale AE, Sullivan SJ, Jankowski LW. Underestimation of subjects' monitored radial pulse rates following traumatic brain injury. Percept Mot Skills 1995;80:57–58.

SECTION TWO

Musculoskeletal Conditions

SECTION EDITOR: *Kenneth H. Pitetti*

CHAPTER **10**

Osteoarthritis, Rheumatoid Arthritis, and Fibromyalgia

Nadine M. Fisher

There are more than 100 rheumatologic conditions that are considered forms of arthritis. Osteoarthritis (OA), rheumatoid arthritis (RA), and fibromyalgia syndrome (FMS) are three of the most common forms. Each is a very distinct arthritic condition. Although there is no cure for OA, RA, or FMS, each condition can be medically and pharmacologically managed with some success. Surgical procedures have been successful, especially for patients with OA and RA. Patient education programs, including exercise, nutritional counseling, and behavior modification techniques, have also had therapeutic benefits for certain patients. These types of arthritis typically result in long-term disability to the patient. Therefore, many patients are interested in therapeutic treatments, especially exercise, to help them manage their disease and decrease their levels of disabilities. In general, rehabilitative exercise has been shown to have a significant impact on decreasing the impairment and disability of arthritis.

EPIDEMIOLOGY AND PATHOPHYSIOLOGY

Osteoarthritis (OA)

Osteoarthritis (OA), also known as degenerative joint disease or osteoarthrosis, is the most common type of arthritis and one of the most common chronic diseases in the United States (1), affecting approximately 40 million people (2). It is the second most common cause of long-term disability in the adult population (1, 3). Contrary to popular myth, it is not a normal characteristic of aging. OA is characterized by localized degeneration of the articular cartilage (the major pathology) and synthesis of new bone at the joint surfaces and/or margins. It typically affects the hips, knees, feet, spine, and hands. Risk factors for OA are age, gender, race, occupation (i.e., repetitive trauma, overuse), obesity, history of joint trauma, bone or joint disorders, genetic mutations of collagen, and a history of inflammatory arthritis (1).

The prevalence of OA differs depending on which joints are considered and how the disease is assessed. The prevalence of OA also differs among different populations. Many individuals may show OA on x-ray, but have no symptoms. Therefore, the prevalence of OA when assessed by x-ray is much higher than when determined by the symptomatology. Ninety percent of the population shows evidence of degenerative changes in weight-bearing joints (hips, knees, feet) by age 40; however, symptoms are generally not present (4). These x-ray changes and the incidence of symptomatic OA continue to progress with increasing age. OA occurs more frequently in women than men after age 50, with evidence of an increase in disease severity and the number of joints affected (5, 6). This disparity becomes larger with age. However, under the age of 45, the prevalence of OA is about the same for men and women. The incidence of OA is not well defined. However, it is known that for hip, knee, and hand OA, the incidence rises with age and is greater in women than men (7). In general, older men are more susceptible to hip OA, while older women are more often diagnosed with OA of the hand and finger joints and the knees. Knee OA is more prevalent in African-American women than Caucasian women (8, 9), as well as in obese persons, nonsmokers, and those who are physically active (10). Women are more susceptible than men to the inflammatory type of OA.

OA is classified into two major types, primary OA and secondary OA (4). Primary or idiopathic OA is the most common type and is diagnosed when there is no known cause for the symptoms. Secondary OA is diagnosed when there is an identifiable cause (e.g., trauma or underlying joint disorders). Each type is further classified into subtypes. For more information on the types and subtypes of OA, see Chapter 105 by Moskowitz in *Arthritis and Allied Conditions: A Textbook of Rheumatology* (4). Specific classification criteria have also been developed by the American College of Rheumatology for OA of the hand (11), knee (12), and hip (13). The common major criterion for each is the presence of pain. Since there is no nerve supply to the articular cartilage, pain may be due to inflammation of the synovium, medullary hypertension or microfractures in the subchondral bone, stretching of periosteal nerve endings by the osteophytes (spurs), or stretching of ligaments and spasming of muscles around the inflamed joint capsule (14).

Common symptoms and features of OA are localized pain and stiffness in and around the joint, osteophytes (bony hypertrophy), cartilage destruction, joint malalignment, movement/gait problems, muscle weakness, activity limitations, morning stiffness lasting less than 30 minutes, gelling (stiffness after inactivity that only lasts a few minutes), and pain that is worse with activity and better with rest. Inflammation is not a typical sign of OA. Specific joint symptoms are instability and buckling of the knees with knee OA, groin pain and radiating leg pain with hip OA, decreased manual dexterity with hand OA, and radiating pain, weakness, and numbness (nerve root compression) in neck and low back OA (1). As pain increases upon joint loading or weight bearing, physical activity and joint mobility decrease. It is not unusual for joint contractures, especially of the weight bearing joints, to occur secondary to the decrease in joint mobility. This leads to an increase in the energy expenditure needed to participate in functional and physical activities. Inactivity due to OA may consequently lead to an increased risk of other comorbid conditions such as heart disease, hypertension, diabetes, depression, obesity, and some cancers.

Rheumatoid Arthritis (RA)

Rheumatoid arthritis (RA) is a chronic, systemic inflammatory disease affecting the synovium of diarthrodial joints. Synovitis or inflammation of the synovial membrane is the dominant pathology. The prevalence of RA is approximately 1–2% in the population, affecting women 2–2.5 times more often than men (1, 15). RA affects all ethnic groups with similar prevalence. RA is most often diagnosed between the ages of 30 and 60 years old, although prevalence increases with age (1). In addition, RA tends to shorten life expectancy (16). The etiology of RA is unknown; however, the progression and pattern of inflammation are related to genetic and environmental factors (1).

RA is typically classified in terms of the functional status of the patient. Functional status is divided into four classes (17). Functional Class I indicates that the individual can completely perform all usual activities of daily living, including self-care activities (e.g., feeding, bathing, grooming, dressing, toileting), recreational/leisure activities, and work/school/home activities. Functional Class II indicates that the individual with RA can completely perform all self-care and work activities, but is limited in performing their recreational/leisure activities. Functional Class III indicates that the individual with RA can completely perform all self-care activities, but is limited in performing their work/school/home and recreational/leisure activities. Lastly, Functional Class IV indicates that the individual with RA is limited in their ability to perform all three types of activities (17). When prescribing exercise for an individual with RA, functional status must be considered.

With RA, it is typical to observe symmetrical and bilateral joint involvement, marked over time by structural damage and deformities (1, 18). Inflammatory synovitis may result in reversible (morning stiffness, synovial inflammation) and irreversible (structural joint damage) signs and symptoms of RA. With synovial inflammation, patients commonly experience prolonged morning stiffness (>2 hours). This is unlike the morning stiffness that is experienced in OA, which typically lasts up to 30 minutes. With a remission of inflammation, the RA patient has a decrease in morning stiffness. During active inflammatory synovitis, the affected joints are usually warm and swollen. There is a linear relationship between the time of active, uncontrolled synovitis and the progression of joint structural damage (1). Joint destruction usually begins within the first 1–2 years of the disease.

Common signs and symptoms of RA are joint pain, swelling, stiffness and contractures, with concomitant muscle weakness and fatigue. The muscles and tendons that surround the inflamed joints tend to spasm and shorten, while the ligaments are weakened by the enzymatic breakdown of collagen. The most common joints affected are the hands, wrists, elbows, shoulders, cervical spine, hips, knees, ankles, and feet. In approximately 20% of RA patients, inflammation of other organ systems occurs. Some of these extra-articular manifestations are skin (e.g., rheumatoid nodules), ocular (e.g., keratoconjunctivitis sicca), respiratory (e.g., pleuritis), cardiac (e.g., pericardial effusion), gastrointestinal (e.g., gastritis, peptic ulcer), renal (e.g., interstitial renal disease), neurological (e.g., cervical spine instability, peripheral nerve entrapment), and hematological (e.g., hypochromic-microcytic anemia with low serum ferritin and low iron-binding capacity) (1).

Fibromyalgia Syndrome (FMS)

Fibromyalgia syndrome (FMS) is a rheumatic syndrome that presents as chronic, diffuse, nonarticular musculoskeletal pain, yet does not appear to be an inflammatory process (1). FMS is not associated with the development of joint deformities (19, 20). It is the most common rheumatic cause of chronic widespread pain (1). FMS is predominantly diagnosed in Caucasian women between 20–60 years of age (approximately 75% of cases) who have middle to upper socioeconomic status (1, 21). The approximate prevalence of FMS in population-based studies indicates rates from 0.7%–13% in women and 0.2%–3.9% in men (21, 22). The prevalence of FMS appears to increase with age. It presents in approximately 15% of rheumatology patients and 5% of the general medical patients (1). The incidence of FMS is unknown. FMS has previously been known as fibrositis, psychogenic rheumatism, nonarticular rheumatism, primary fibromyalgia (no underlying or concomitant condition), and secondary fibromyalgia (other concomitant conditions). However, in 1990, criteria for classifying patients with FMS were published by the Multicenter Committee of the American College of Rheumatology (ACR) (23), and the classifications were abandoned.

The etiology of FMS is unknown. Studies suggest possible factors for the development of FMS; however, none are conclusive. The pain of FMS may be due to (a) genetic factors, including a genetic susceptibility to microtrauma of the musculature or neurohormonal dysfunction; (b) peripheral mechanisms such as muscle tissue abnormalities and microtrauma; and (c) central mechanisms including EEG abnormalities during sleep, neuroendocrine abnormalities (i.e., hypothalamic-pituitary-adrenal axis, low blood serum levels of serotonin, high CSF levels of substance P and low levels of somatomedin C), immunologic factors (i.e., viral infection, Lyme disease), physical trauma, psychological distress/psychiatric disorders, and abnormalities in CNS structures (i.e., thalamus and caudate nucleus) (21).

Common symptoms and features of FMS are diffuse nonarticular (soft-tissue) pain, multiple tender points, fatigue and morning stiffness, and sleep disturbance (1). Fatigue is often due to poor sleep. These patients may also have irritable bowel syndrome (50% of cases), tension headaches, and paresthesias (numbness or tingling sensations) (1). In addition, patients with FMS may have concomitant osteoarthritis, rheumatoid arthritis, Lyme disease, or sleep apnea. FMS symptoms may be exacerbated by inactivity, emotional stress, poor sleep, high humidity, and moderate physical activity (1). It is not unusual for patients with FMS to have an increased incidence of depression.

In general, risk factors associated with all types of arthritis can be considered nonmodifiable and modifiable. The nonmodifiable risk factors are female gender (60% of all cases), genetic predisposition, and age. While arthritis is not considered a normal part of the aging process, the risk does increase with age. Modifiable risk factors are obesity, joint injuries, infections, and certain physically demanding occupations (especially those that require repetitive knee bending) (24).

CLINICAL EXERCISE PHYSIOLOGY

Many studies have shown that patients with OA, RA, and/or FMS have lower neuromuscular and cardiorespiratory function, as well as physical functioning (flexibility, functional performance), than nondiseased individuals. In a very general sense, this is due to the effect that pain has on the ability of the patients to exercise and even perform their activities of daily living. These patients are less active due to the pain on movement. This leads to a neuromuscular deconditioning, followed by a generalized cardiorespiratory deconditioning and, ultimately, difficulty in performing their everyday activities. This downward spiral (loss of physiological reserve) will continue unless appropriate treatments are given.

Significant declines occur in joint range of motion or flexibility (25, 26); neuromuscular function, including EMG activity, muscle strength, muscle endurance, and muscle contraction speed (25, 27–35); cardiorespiratory function, including VO_2, heart rate, blood pressure, and exercise capacity (26, 28, 31, 33, 36–38); functional performance, including walking, climbing stairs (25, 26, 35, 38–45), and physical fitness (46). In addition, increases in arthritis symptoms, including pain, have been documented (25, 26, 35, 36, 38–45). In general, they also show that pain and inflammation limit physical activity and performance on all physiological and functional tests. This is most likely due to motor unit or muscle inhibition (47, 48). For patients with OA, RA, or FMS, incorrectly prescribed or performed exercises may exacerbate arthritis symptoms, especially the pain associated with the microtrauma to the joints and/or musculature.

Many different exercise programs have been studied in the OA, RA, and FMS patient groups. Most have focused on aerobic exercise, resistance exercise, or general conditioning protocols. In general, they have been successful in eliciting some level of improvement in flexibility (49–51), neuromuscular function (27, 32, 38–45, 50–66), cardiovascular function (32, 38, 50, 52, 57, 58, 64, 65, 67–76), functional performance (27, 38–45, 53–55, 58, 62, 64, 66, 69–72, 75, 77–85), pain (38–45, 51–55, 63, 64, 66–70, 72, 73, 76, 77, 79–83, 85, 86), disease symptomatology (27, 49, 57, 63, 64, 67–69, 73, 81, 83, 84), exercise self-efficacy (78, 82, 87), and psychological function (i.e., depression, anxiety) (49, 71, 76, 85).

It is important for the exercise technician to accurately assess physiological function and functional performance in the arthritis patient in order to prescribe an exercise progression that would focus on improving the patient's physiological and functional limitations. When prescribing exercise for patients with arthritis, it is critical to carefully assess baseline exercise capacity (cardiorespiratory, neuromuscular, flexibility, etc.) and functional performance/status in order to individually prescribe the most beneficial program for each patient. Individually prescribed progressive programs, based on physiological and functional deficits, are necessary to ensure that the patients do not fail in the early stages of an exercise program. For the arthritis patient, it is useful to begin the exercise progression slowly, so as to allow the patient to adapt physiologically, prevent early exacerbation, and reduce the potential for noncompliance.

PHARMACOLOGY

Pain reduction or relief is the primary reason for pharmacological treatments in OA, RA, and FMS. Usually, the first line of treatment for OA is simple analgesics such as acetaminophen. At times, topical analgesics such as capsaicin cream may provide pain relief as well. The second line of medications for OA and the first line for RA is nonsteroidal anti-inflammatory drugs (NSAIDs). NSAIDs inhibit the synthesis of proinflammatory prostaglandins (1). Examples of these are aspirin, celecoxib, rofecoxib, ibuprofen, naproxen, and indomethacin. While they generally provide good pain relief, this class of drugs also is known for their increased risk of upper gastrointestinal, renal, hepatic, and central nervous system toxicity (88).

Low-dose oral corticosteroids such as prednisone may be used, especially in active RA. When there is local severe inflammation or a joint effusion, intra-articular corticosteroid injections may be indicated for relief of the painful joint in OA and RA. Adverse reactions to corticosteroids include osteoporosis, myopathy, cataracts, hypertension, and diabetes mellitus (88).

Another class of medications, disease-modifying antirheumatic drugs (DMARDs), is more often used after the other pharmacological treatments have been tried. A relatively new DMARD treatment for OA is intra-articular injections of hyaluronate. DMARDs are more often indicated for patients with RA and are used aggressively early in the disease process in order to prevent disability. Effectiveness of the DMARDs for RA is determined by their ability to change the course of RA for 1 year by increasing physical function, decreasing inflammatory synovitis, and slowing structural damage. Examples of DMARDs are oral gold, etanercept, leflunomide, sulfasalazine, hydroxychloroquine, penicillamine, and methotrexate. As with the other arthritis medications, each DMARD has its related toxic effects. For example, long-term methotrexate use typically results in liver function complications, while sulfasalazine may result in gastrointestinal and central nervous system toxicity.

Recently, certain biological agents (e.g., infliximab) have been used in RA as immunosuppressive agents. Relatively new popular treatments for arthritis, especially OA, are glucosamine sulfate, chondroitin sulfate, or the combination of both. These are nutritional supplements (so-called nutriceuticals) that are currently under study for their effectiveness in providing pain relief.

Specific to FMS, medications are used to improve restorative sleep in order to improve fatigue and decrease the symptomatology of FMS. These pharmacological agents include amitriptyline, cyclobenzaprine, alprazolam, tricyclic antidepressants (nortriptyline), hypnotic agents, S-adenosylmethionine (SAMe), selective serotonin reuptake inhibitors (SSRIs), and NSAIDs. In some cases, tender points are injected with local anesthesia or corticosteroids (1). As is typical with any medication, their effectiveness is not the same for all patients. A meta-analysis of the efficacy of treatment outcomes for FMS indicates that nonpharmacological treatments, especially exercise in combination with cognitive/behavioral therapy, give the best outcomes (89). However, these can be supplemented by pharmacological treatments to reduce pain and sleep disturbances.

Each pharmacological agent for arthritis has side effects and toxicity levels that can impact the different physiological systems. In general, there does not appear to be any more risk of these medications impacting on exercise testing and training than any other class of medications. To find out the specific impact of each drug and its interactions, the reader is referred to the *PDR* (*Physicians' Desk Reference*) (90). For OA, RA, and FMS, it is always recommended that the pharmacological management is used in combination with nonpharmacological treatments.

PHYSICAL EXAMINATION

OA is typically diagnosed by a history and physical exam (1). Several characteristics that may be present upon physical exam (i.e., joint palpation) in a patient with OA are localized symptomatic joints, pain on motion (joint capsule irritation), tenderness at the joint margins and capsules (bony enlargements), decreased range of joint motion (osteophyte formation, contractures), joint instability, joint locking (loose bodies/cartilage fragments in joint), crepitus (irregular joint surfaces), joint malalignment (varus or valgus deformity), and local signs of inflammation (warmth, soft-tissue swelling). A diagnosis of OA is confirmed by radiographs of the affected joints. Osteophyte formation (bony proliferation) at the joint margins is a typical finding on x-ray of a patient with OA. Other findings that indicate OA on the x-ray are asymmetrical joint space narrowing, subchondral bone sclerosis, and possibly subchondral cyst formation. If bone demineralization (periarticular osteoporosis) and erosion of bone at the joint margins is visible on x-ray, the diagnosis is more likely RA than OA (1).

RA is difficult to diagnose early on in the disease process due to the lack of definitive characteristics that are typically present. It generally takes several weeks to several months for RA to be present before it can be diagnosed. The onset is insidious and does not begin with symmetrical joint involvement. The American College of Rheumatology has described the seven criteria for classifying an individual with RA. In order to have a diagnosis of RA, the patient needs to have at least four of the seven criteria, and criteria 1–4 need to be present for a minimum of 6 weeks. The criteria are: (1) morning stiffness lasting a minimum of 1 hour in and around the joints; (2) soft-tissue swelling or fluid in at least three joint areas (especially hands, wrists, elbows, knees, ankles, and feet) simultaneously; (3) at least one swollen hand or wrist joint; (4) concurrent involvement of the same joint area bilaterally; (5) rheumatoid nodules (subcutaneous nodules that typically are located over bony prominences or extensor surfaces); (6) abnormal amount of serum rheumatoid factor; and (7) radiographic evidence of structural changes typical for RA, such as bone erosion or decalcification in or adjacent to the involved joints (especially the hand and wrist) (91). Upon palpation of surface joints (fingers, elbows, knees), joint deformities may be evident. Deformities of the deeper joints (shoulders, hips) may only be evident by range-of-motion limitations. Usually, joint deformities occur in the upper extremity first, as the patient can still function adequately even with a reduced range of motion and less mobility.

In order for a diagnosis of FMS to be made, two specific criteria must be met. First, the patient must have a history of widespread pain for at least 3 months. This means that the patient must have pain on both sides of the body and above and below the waist. There also must be pain in the axial skeletal region, i.e., cervical spine, anterior chest, thoracic spine, or low back. Second, the patient must have pain in 11 of 18 tender point sites (9 bilateral sites) upon digital palpation of approximately 4 kg or by using a calibrated dolorimeter. The tender point sites are: (1) occiput, at the suboccipital muscle insertions; (2) low cervical, at the anterior aspects of the intertransverse spaces of C5–C7; (3) trapezius, at the midpoint of the upper border; (4) supraspinatus, above the medial border of the scapular spine; (5) second rib, at the second costochondral junctions; (6) lateral epicondyle, 2 cm distal to the epicondyles; (7) gluteal, at the upper outer quadrants of the buttocks; (8) greater trochanter, posterior to the trochanteric prominence; and (9) knee, at the medial fat pad proximal to the joint line (23).

MEDICAL AND SURGICAL TREATMENTS

The major goals for treating patients with OA, RA, and FMS are fourfold. They are to relieve the arthritis symptoms (e.g., pain), maintain or increase physical functioning, limit physical disability, and avoid drug toxicity (1). Besides the prescription of medications, medical treatments may include referring the arthritis patient to the appropriate health-care professionals for different nonpharmacological treatments such as joint protection and energy-conservation techniques (including assistive devices), weight loss and maintenance, use of heat and cold modalities, patellar taping techniques (for knee OA), transcutaneous electrical nerve stimulation (TENS) for pain relief, exercise, meditation, acupuncture, biofeedback, and massage (1, 14). In addition, for RA patients, short-term splinting of inflamed joints (hands) may be indicated to decrease inflammation and joint trauma, as well as increase joint alignment. Electrical stimulation of the tender areas, coupled with heat (ultrasound or whirlpool), may be therapeutic for patients with FMS. For patients with FMS and RA, it is important to treat their underlying depression. This can typically be treated by tricyclic antidepressants and/or patient education. It has been shown that patients who are younger and have less severe disease have better outcomes (1).

Cognitive/behavioral therapies have been shown to reduce pain and disability in patients with OA, RA, and to a certain degree in FMS (92–96). Some of these therapies include relaxation training, coping skills training, reinforcement of healthy behaviors, and pain management techniques. The relaxation therapies that have been shown to be more successful for FMS are EMG biofeedback training (97) and hypnotherapy (98).

Surgery for OA and RA is usually not considered a treatment alternative until the patient cannot get pain relief from other methods and there are significant functional impairments. Several surgical options are available for different joints. For the knee, arthroscopic debridement and/or lavage with meniscectomy may be performed to increase joint function and decrease pain by removing loose fragments of cartilage, bone, and menisci (1). Osteotomies for the knee (high tibial) and hip (femoral) may be performed to realign the joints and redistribute the loading on the joints (1). For very advanced disease, arthrodesis or joint fusion may be performed in order to decrease pain and increase stability and joint alignment. This procedure is more frequently performed for the spine (cervical and lumbar), wrists, ankles, and hand and foot joints (1). Joint fusion is not typically recommended since it completely eliminates joint motion and may increase loading on the unfused joints. A surgical treatment that is successful in reducing or eliminating arthritis pain is total joint arthroplasty. This procedure is performed routinely for knees and hips. Total joint replacements, while usually successful, cannot exactly replicate natural articular cartilage and over time may need revision (1). No surgical techniques have been recommended for FMS.

DIAGNOSTIC TECHNIQUES

As mentioned under Physical Examination, section IV, a diagnosis of OA is made by a history and physical exam and confirmed by radiographs of the affected joints. As a routine matter, standard lab tests are conducted; results are typically normal. In addition, tests for rheumatoid factor (RF) and erythrocyte sedimentation rate (ESR) are conducted in order to exclude other joint diseases (1).

There is no one particular test to confirm RA, although inflammatory synovitis must be present. This can be determined by leukocytes in the synovial fluid and/or evidence of joint erosion on x-ray. As mentioned previously, the history and physical exam are important procedures to help in the diagnosis. Lab tests typically ordered to assist with the diagnosis are for RF, ESR, and C-reactive protein. ESR and C-reactive protein are good indicators of synovial inflammation. Contrary to popular myth, RF is not a diagnostic test for RA (99). Some patients with RA are not RF positive, although approximately 85% of RA patients have RF (1). For those patients who are RF positive, their disease is usually severe and they exhibit extra-articular manifestations of RA. Imaging techniques such as x-ray, magnetic resonance imaging (MRI), and scintigraphy are common in RA to assess the degree of joint destruction (including articular cartilage, ligaments, tendons, and bones) (99). Some clinical assessments include tender and swollen joint counts, range-of-motion measurements, walking time, duration of morning stiffness, assessment of fatigue severity, and grip strength.

In general, there are no standard diagnostic tests available for FMS. There are no detectable histologic, laboratory, or radiographic abnormalities. There is also no evidence of deficits in muscle energy metabolism, as measured by phosphorus (^{31}P) magnetic resonance spectroscopy (PCr/P_i) (100). However, in some patients, it is helpful to conduct sleep studies, screening tests for diffuse pain, and/or radiographs and EMGs in symptomatic areas (1). When diagnosing FMS, it is important to exclude other possible conditions such as myofascial pain (more localized pain) and chronic fatigue syndrome (fatigue is primary symptom) that have similar and, at times, overlapping symptoms (1).

EXERCISE/FITNESS/FUNCTIONAL TESTING

In general, it is important for the patient to perform the exercise or functional test protocols in the most pain-free manner possible. Therefore, the exercise technician must consider the positioning of the patient during the testing, as well as the order of the tests to ensure appropriate recovery of the different systems (e.g., cardiorespiratory, neuromuscular) and/or muscle groups. It is not unusual for patients with OA and RA to have joint contractures and, therefore, reduced flexibility or range of motion. Care must be taken with these patients to allow for recovery from fatigue between test protocols and to adjust testing equipment and/or protocols in case of pain or symptom exacerbation. If it is the judgment of the exercise technician that the risks of the testing outweigh the benefits derived from the exercise program, then the patient should not be tested.

Thoughtful planning of testing procedures is important for the different types of arthritis. Usually, there is some assessment of pain, physical limitations, physical function, flexibility, muscle function, and cardiovascular function. As mentioned earlier, taking into consideration the patient's symptoms and exercise goals will allow the exercise scientist to measure the appropriate variables.

Pain and functional limitations are often measured by self-report questionnaires such as visual analog scales for pain, marking painful areas on a diagram of the body. Several specific assessments are valid and reliable for patients with arthritis. The two major assessment tools are the Arthritis Impact Measurement Scales 2 (101) for all types of arthritis and the Western Ontario and McMaster Universities (WOMAC) Osteoarthritis Index for OA (102).

Physical function or performance can be measured in many ways, including a 6-minute walk (distance) plus pulse and rating of perceived exertion, low back flexibility (sit and reach), rising from a chair for 1 minute, climbing stairs, and/or a measured walk for speed. Besides the sit-and-reach test, flexibility can be measured with a goniometer as the subject moves the desired joints through their ranges of motion. For shoulder flexibility, a forward reach test has been shown to be valid.

Muscle function (strength, endurance, contraction speed, power) can be measured isometrically, isotonically, or isokinetically. When conducting these tests, it is important to consider the effect that a painful joint will have on the ability to produce a maximal muscle contraction. Pain will result in neural inhibition, thereby leading to a much lower measure of muscle function. In some cases, EMG activity (surface or invasive) may also be measured.

Work capacity or aerobic function is measured in multiple ways as well. In some cases, depending on the severity of the disease, it may be more practical to estimate aerobic power from a submaximal test (103). Generally, most patients with OA, RA, or FMS will be able to accomplish a symptom-limited graded exercise test, where the major symptoms are pain and peripheral muscle fatigue. It is important to consider the testing equipment that will be used to conduct the test. Using a weight-bearing activity such as walking on a treadmill may result in an abbreviated test due to joint pain in any of the weight-bearing joints. Performing a non-weight-bearing activity such as on a cycle ergometer may allow a more accurate measurement of cardiovascular function if patients can perform to a higher level before they experience pain and stop the test. Due to the possibility of comorbid conditions, especially cardiovascular diseases, it is recommended that all patients be continuously monitored (ECG, heart rate, and blood pressure) throughout the cardiovascular testing (resting, work, and recovery). For patients with FMS, it is usually standard to assess their pain threshold over their tender points using a dolorimeter.

EXERCISE PRESCRIPTION AND PROGRAMMING

As has been shown throughout this chapter, OA, RA, and FMS are very different forms of arthritis. Therefore, it is important to understand the type of arthritis, the characteristic symptoms and limitations, prognosis of the disease, and other comorbid conditions that the patients have when prescribing exercises. Due to the pain, inflammation, fatigue, and limitations in joint movement, these patients are usually more deconditioned peripherally than centrally. This means that the limitations to exercise are usually in the peripheral musculature. Many arthritis patients will stop an exercise test protocol due to muscle fatigue or joint pain, not usually because of dyspnea, angina, or other acute cardiorespiratory events. Therefore, the type of exercise program should focus initially on the primary limitation of each type of arthritis and then progress to more general exercises. For example, if a patient has OA of the knee joint, has pain upon weight-bearing, and quadriceps muscle atrophy, non-weight-bearing resistance exercises would be more appropriate than aerobic exercises.

In general, patients with arthritis can participate in many different types of exercises. With a properly designed program, they will reap the same benefits as anyone who exercises. When designing an exercise program for individuals with arthritis, it is important to distinguish between exercising to improve functional capabilities and exercising to achieve a level of physical fitness. It is essential for the exercise specialist to provide exercises to increase the patient's functional capabilities first and then increase physical fitness. The goal of many patients with arthritis is to engage in their normal everyday activities without undue fatigue or pain. In many cases, they may be more focused on this outcome than achieving a level of physical fitness.

Previous research has shown that patients with OA, RA, and FMS can benefit from aerobic exercises, including walking, stationary cycling, and water exercise (50, 57, 58, 60, 65, 67, 69, 70–78, 80–83, 104), but the benefits over time may be relatively short-lived (50, 69, 105) or sustained above baseline measures for several months (49, 58, 72, 79, 87). While there may be aerobic benefits (e.g. increase in peak oxygen consumption) and improvement in pain (67–70, 77, 81, 82), there is generally not as much improvement in muscle strength and muscle endurance or flexibility from aerobic programs. Water exercises are recommended for patients with arthritis; however, there is no scientific evidence that they improve the patients' aerobic capacity, muscle strength, or endurance. There is slight evidence to support the warm water effects on joint flexibility and overall physical function (49, 78).

In OA and RA patients, research focusing on resistance exercises has shown that these patients have dramatic improvements in muscle strength, muscle endurance, and contraction speed of the muscles that support the arthritic joint (27, 32, 38–41, 43–45, 50, 52–59, 61–64, 66, 71, 72, 80). This type of exercise has also been shown to provide pain relief (38–41, 43–45, 53–55, 63, 64, 66, 68, 71, 72, 80, 82, 83, 85, 86) and increases in muscular efficiency, exercise capacity, and cardiovascular performance (32, 38, 50, 57, 64, 68, 71–74, 80), thereby allowing patients to perform aerobic exercises at a level where they can achieve a cardiovascular/aerobic benefit. In most cases, there is evidence that arthritis patients who participate in resistance exercises can sustain their improvements above baseline measures for several months or more after the completion of the exercise programs (27, 40, 58, 72).

The best exercise prescription for individuals with arthritis appears to be a progression from flexibility exercises, especially of affected joints (to prevent contractures), to muscle function exercises (focusing on muscle strength, endurance, and contraction speed), to aerobic exercises (including non-weight-bearing and weight-bearing alternatives). Built into this prescription may be functional activities (e.g., climbing stairs, rising from a low chair, walking) and relaxation activities (e.g., Tai Chi, yoga). This same type of progression would be useful for prescribing exercise for arthritis patients to improve their everyday function, as well as for improving fitness. Using this rehabilitative strategy, the approach may be more conservative initially in order to monitor any exacerbation of symptoms, to determine the rate of physiological adaptability to the exercise, and to encourage exercise compliance and program adherence.

Table 10.1 provides a general outline of progressive exercise prescriptions for individuals with OA, RA, and FMS. The prescription is basically the same for OA and RA. However, for RA, it is critical to build an appropriate

Table 10.1. General and Progressive Exercise Prescriptions for OA, RA, and FMS*

TYPE OF ARTHRITIS	EXERCISE PROGRESSION		FREQUENCY	INTENSITY	DURATION
OA	Flexibility	• ROM	Daily	Active/gentle	10–15 min.
	Resistance	• strength	2-3×/wk	10–80% max	5–10 reps
		• endurance	2-3×/wk	10–80% max	90–120 sec.
		• speed	2-3×/wk	10–80% max	5–10 reps
	Aerobic	• endurance	3-4×/wk	60–80% peak HR	30–60 min. (cumulative)
	Functional Activities		Daily	Moderate	1-5 reps
RA	Flexibility	• ROM	Daily	Active/gentle	10–15 min.
	Resistance	• strength	2-3×/wk	10–80% max	5–10 reps
		• endurance	2-3×/wk	10–80% max	90–120 sec.
		• speed	2-3×/wk	10–80% max	5–10 reps
	Aerobic	• endurance	3-4×/wk	60–80% peak HR	30–60 min. (cumulative)
	Functional Activities		Daily	Moderate	1-5 reps
FMS	Flexibility	• ROM	Daily	Active/gentle	10–15 min.
	Resistance	• isotonic/isometric	2-3×/wk	5–80% of max	5–30 reps
		• endurance	2-3×/wk	5–80% of max	30–120 sec.
		• speed	2-3×/wk	5–80% of max	5–30 reps
		• strength	2-3×/wk	5–80% of max	3–5 reps
	Aerobic	• endurance	3-4×/wk	40–80% of peak HR	10–60 min. (cumulative 30 min)
	Functional Activities		Daily	Low-moderate	1-5 reps

Note: OA = osteoarthritis; RA = rheumatoid arthritis, FMS = fibromyalgia syndrome; ROM = range of motion; min. = minutes; reps = repetitions; sec. = seconds.

*See text for explanation of progression.

rest/recovery time into the protocol so as not to cause a flare-up, exacerbation, or undo inflammation due to an intense acute bout of exercise. Appropriate rest is also critically important for FMS patients.

Flexibility Exercises

A general program of flexibility and stretching exercises is important for individuals with OA, RA, and FMS. It is important to gently and actively move all joints through the range of motion so as to prevent joint contractures and to stretch the surrounding musculature. This may be performed 3–5 times a day. In order to prevent injury, the joints should never be forced through their range of motion.

Resistance Activities

Resistance exercise programs have become very popular, especially for OA (27, 38–40, 43–45, 53–55, 80, 82) and RA (32, 50, 56–58, 61–64, 66). However, there is very little research to date studying the use of resistance exercises in patients with FMS (52, 68). When prescribing resistance exercises for patients with arthritis, it is important to initially assess each patient's limitations. Whether using a strain gauge, isokinetic device, or the 1-repetition maximum technique, it is important to have a measurement of the patient's maximal capability for any given muscle or muscle group prior to prescribing resistance exercise. Based on the symptomatology, the progression of resistance exercises may be different for patients with FMS than for patients with OA and RA. There are several types of resistance exercises that can be prescribed for arthritis patients, i.e., isometric, isotonic, and/or isokinetic, that can be used in different ways in order to address deficits in muscle strength, muscle endurance, or muscle contraction speed.

Strength

For OA and RA patients who have direct joint involvement, it is important to begin the resistance training with maximal voluntary isometric contractions of the muscles that support the affected joints. An isometric contraction will maximally contract the muscle without joint movement. Ideally, there is no pain. To improve strength, three to five maximal contractions of each muscle group should be performed once a day. Each contraction should be held for 5 to 10 seconds (progression). Patients can perform isometric contractions using a variety of methods (e.g., resistance bands, overloaded weight bench, bicycle tire or surgical tubing, another person). Strength can also be improved by progressing to higher-resistance, low-repetition isotonic muscle contractions. It is recommended that the progression for resistances begins very low (approximately 10% of the patient's maximum) and progresses at a maximal rate of 10% per week. While this may appear conservative, it allows the exercise technician to monitor the patient's progress and ability to adapt to the exercise without an exacerbation of symptoms. Patients should perform the isotonic contractions three times per week. They do not need to do more than 5–10 repetitions with any muscle group per day. If the patients have access to a clinic with isokinetic equipment, they can perform the isometric and isokinetic contractions with supervision. In all cases, regardless of where the patients go to exercise, they need to be taught the proper mechanics of performing each exercise so as not to become injured or progress at too rapid a rate.

Endurance

There are several ways to improve muscle endurance. Traditionally, muscle endurance has been addressed using a low-resistance, high-repetition model. While this may improve the endurance of the slow twitch or Type I muscle fibers, it does not train all fibers within the muscle. In order to address multiple muscle fiber types, it is important to sustain a muscle contraction over time. One way to do this is by having the patient lift the prescribed resistance (beginning at 10% of maximal and increasing by 10% each week) and holding it for a period of time. Depending on the type of arthritis, the patient may progressively increase the amount of time the resistance is held or always hold it for a predetermined amount of time. For example, patients with OA and RA can sustain the contraction for 90 seconds at each training session, while the FMS patients may initially hold the contraction for 30 seconds and eventually work up to 90 seconds using the same resistance before increasing to a higher resistance.

Contraction Speed

Another aspect of muscle physiology that is frequently overlooked when exercising individuals with arthritis is their ability to contract their muscles quickly. It is important to improve their muscle contraction speed in order to improve their ability to do certain functional activities (e.g., cross the street before the traffic light changes) and to help prevent falls. In many people with arthritis, their gait becomes affected over time due to joint deformities, pain, fatigue, and/or possible contralateral limb compensation strategies. Contraction speed can be improved by having the patient lift the prescribed resistances as rapidly as possible in a controlled manner through the range of joint motion. If this exercise is performed isotonically with no supervision, it is extremely important to teach the patient how to lift the resistances in a controlled manner in order to protect the arthritic joint and/or to prevent muscle injury and undue pain. These exercises can also be performed safely using isokinetic equipment. Patients with FMS will be able to add contraction speed exercises into their exercise progression earlier in their programs than patients with OA and RA due to the fact that, with FMS, there is not as much concern for joint effusions. It is recommended that for patients with OA and RA, contraction speed exercises should be added to the progression last, after the muscles around the affected joints have begun to adapt and help support the joint. It is recommended that this higher impact activity be performed 3 days per week and using lower resistances initially. Within 6–12 weeks, the musculature should be trained to a level where the patient starts to notice significant improvements in function and, in many cases, a reduction in pain and/or fatigue levels.

Cardiovascular Activities

Once the musculature has been trained sufficiently and the muscles can be used more efficiently, it is recommended that aerobic exercises and functional activities be added to the exercise progression. Again, if the potential exists to measure the patients' maximal or peak aerobic power, this will provide the tools to prescribe the best aerobic program. An important consideration when prescribing an aerobic training program for persons with arthritis is to consider the types of aerobic activity they are comfortable doing. For instance, many individuals with OA and RA are overweight and will not do water exercises because they are uncomfortable in public wearing a bathing suit. It is also important to consider if a non-weight-bearing or weight-bearing aerobic exercise would be more appropriate. Generally, whatever exercise the patient is willing to perform regularly will suffice. It is recommended that the exercise progression begin conservatively by allowing the patient to adapt to aerobic activity by using lower target heart rate ranges and then progress up to the cardiovascular training ranges.

Functional Activities

Functional activities can be defined as basic physical activities that an individual does to participate in his/her daily leisure, recreational, family, and work activities. Examples of these activities are walking, climbing stairs, rising from a chair, and bending. As part of an overall exercise program, it is important to include functional activities. It has been shown that although there is physiological adaptation with the traditional types of exercise, it does not translate into better functioning unless the person can use his/her improved physiology to increase the efficiency of their actual functional activities.

EDUCATION AND COUNSELING

Other than the medical, pharmacological, and surgical management of the different types of arthritis, patient self-management is critical. It has been shown that arthritis patients with higher self-efficacy report less pain and impairment during physical activities (78, 82, 106). Group programs, combining strategies to improve fitness and flexibility with stress-reduction techniques and support groups, seem to hold promise as community or outpatient programs for individuals with arthritis (107). Generally, any programs to promote physical activity and weight reduction that the patient will comply with are recommended. The Arthritis Foundation offers several community-based programs for individuals with arthritis. These include the land-based PACE (People with Arthritis Can Exercise) program and the warm-water–based Arthritis Foundation YMCA Aquatics program. Both programs focus on low-level flexibility and endurance activities. Another educational intervention sponsored by the Arthritis Foundation is the Arthritis Self-Help Course (ASHC). ASHC gives the patients information on their disease, medications and side effects, dealing with their physicians, pain management, energy-conservation techniques, nutrition and weight management, relaxation techniques, and exercise and physical activity (24). This program has been shown to reduce the costs associated with arthritis care as well as reduce the patients' perceptions of pain by 20% (108, 109). Infrequently, patients are referred to physical and/or occupational therapy.

CASE STUDY

CASE HISTORY

The patient is a 76-year-old retired ironworker who is married, has four children, and lives in a ground floor apartment. He has an eighth grade education. He complains of occasional pain and some stiffness in his knees, with his left knee worse than the right. He has had difficulty going up and down stairs for the last year. He also has some problems/pain in his left shoulder and back for more than 15 years that have never been diagnosed. Currently, he is not on any medications. He weighs 77 kg and is 167 cm tall.

Medical History

Physician Report—The patient has high blood pressure (168/78 mm Hg resting), but is not on any antihypertensive treatment. He takes some kind of "nerve" medication to keep from smoking. He denies any other medical problems. He had prostate cancer and is checked annually. He cannot remember any other illnesses. He has some mild memory deficits and is allergic to aspirin.

Medical Exam

The patient has an abnormal gait. He can follow commands well and has good coordination. He has slight thoracolumbar scoliosis but has good back mobility. His range of motion is good throughout, except for his left shoulder, where he has pain on abduction and extension. His muscle strength, determined by manual muscle testing, is 5/5 throughout. He has no abnormal reflexes, and his deep tendon reflexes are uniformly active. He has crepitus and bony hypertrophy around the left knee.

Radiographic Review

Radiologist Report—Upon bilateral weight-bearing AP (anterior-posterior) view x-rays of the knees, the patient has evidence of osteoarthritic changes involving the medial compartments of both knees, but more pronounced on the left. There are also early degenerative changes in the lateral compartments of both knees. There is no evidence of acute osseous (bony tissue) abnormalities.

RESTING AND BASELINE EXERCISE RESPONSES

Prior to a quantitative progressive resistance exercise training program (QPER) for his knee OA, his resting and baseline exercise data were as follows:

Functional Assessment

When walking, he has a constant aching pain on every step in his left knee. When rising from a standard height chair, he has mild aching in both knees and severe pain in his back. When climbing up and down a flight of stairs, he leans heavily on the handrail and climbs one step at a time. He has aching in both knees, especially when going down the stairs.

Muscle Function Assessment

His average maximal voluntary isometric strength contractions for the quadriceps and hamstrings for the right and left legs were 18.5 kg and 15.8 kg (quads) and 3 kg and 5.8 kg (hams), respectively. He complained of pain in the left knee during the quadriceps activity. His maximal voluntary isometric endurance over 90 seconds for the quadriceps and hamstrings for the right and left legs were 643 kg· sec and 622 kg· sec (quads) and 120 kg· sec and 190 kg· sec (hams), respectively.

Metabolic/Cardiovascular Function Assessment

Results of a baseline graded exercise test on a cycle ergometer were as follows:

At rest, VO_2 = 4.7 mL/min/kg; BP = 168/78 mm Hg; HR = 96 bpm
At 25 W, VO_2 = 13 mL/min/kg; BP = 189/73 mm Hg; HR = 108 bpm
At 50 W, VO_2 = 16 mL/min/kg; BP = 215/80 mm Hg; HR = 120 bpm

Test was stopped due to fatigue in the peripheral musculature and knee pain.

POSTTRAINING EXERCISE RESPONSES

The patient's results after the 2-month QPER resistance training program were as follows:

Functional Assessment

The patient stated that he required less assistance and had less pain during activity. His walking time over 50 feet was 11% faster, and he had no knee pain when walking. He was able to climb up and down the stairs normally with no knee pain. When rising from a chair, he had no knee pain and only slight back pain. He claimed that he had less cramping in his legs during the night, was able to now cross his legs and bend them easier, had less pain when walking long distances, and had better balance.

Muscle Function Assessment

He had average improvements of 33% and 117% in quadriceps and hamstring strength, respectively, and of 72% and 104% in quadriceps and hamstring endurance, respectively.

Metabolic/Cardiovascular Assessment

The GXT results on the cycle ergometer were as follows:

At rest, VO_2 = 4.8 mL/min/kg, BP = 145/73 mm Hg, HR = 90 bpm
At 25 W, VO_2 = 11.3 mL/min/kg, BP = 168/74 mm Hg, HR = 107 bpm
At 50 W, VO_2 = 13.6 mL/min/kg, BP = 186/70 mm Hg, HR = 114 bpm
At 75 W, VO_2 = 17.2 mL/min/kg, BP = 210/64 mm Hg, HR = 126 bpm

Test was stopped when the patient could not maintain the pedaling frequency with a workload of 100 W.

He had, on average, a 14% decline in submaximal VO_2 and an 8% increase in VO_2"peak." His maximal workload increased by 25 W.

INTERPRETATION

His resting and baseline responses prior to the exercise program are typical for an elderly individual with OA. Due to the joint pain, he is less active and experiences muscular fatigue easily. This is evidenced by the low leg muscle strength and endurance, as well as the low exercise VO_2s and exercise workloads. The joint pain and physical inactivity work in combination to decrease his functional performance on such activities as walking, climbing stairs, and rising from a chair. Although the resting BP and HR are elevated, increases with increasing exercise are still evident. The quantitative progressive resistance exercise program improved all measures (functional performance, muscle, and metabolic/cardiovascular), including those that would traditionally be trained using aerobic training programs. In particular, it appears that the increase in maximal workload and VO_{2peak} are due to an overall improvement in lower-extremity muscular efficiency. More importantly for the patient, there was a significant decrease in knee pain at rest and during physical activity.

CLINICAL IMPLICATIONS

The primary patient complaint with knee OA is pain. Therefore, when conducting exercise testing and training programs, it is important to consider how the knee pain will impact the patient's ability to perform the testing and training protocols. For example, for this patient, it was decided to conduct the GXT on a cycle ergometer to provide a non-weight-bearing activity so that the patient would be able to reach a higher workload before having to stop the test due to knee pain. Also, since his gait was reported as abnormal, the stationary cycling was a safer form of exercise than walking on a treadmill (weight-bearing activity). Although the patient had overall decreased physiological function, it was decided to prescribe a resistance training program initially, instead of an aerobic training program, not only because of his decreased muscle strength and endurance and increased joint pain, but also because of his response to the GXT. Since he stopped the GXT because of peripheral muscle fatigue and not because of any type of cardiorespiratory distress, it seems apparent that the condition of his musculature was the limiting factor in his ability to continue the test. In general, for patients with OA, isometric muscle contractions can be performed maximally without joint pain since the joint is stationary. The order of progression from isometric to low-resistance isotonic to higher-resistance isotonic, endurance, and speed contractions allows the musculature to adapt, as well as lower the risk of increased pain and joint swelling.

References

1. Klippel JH, ed. Primer on the rheumatic diseases. 11th ed. Atlanta, GA: Arthritis Foundation, 1997.
2. Iversen MD, Liang MH, Bae SC. Selected arthritides. In: Frontera WR, Dawson DM, Slovik DM, eds. Exercise in rehabilitation medicine. 1st ed. Champaign, IL: Human Kinetics, 1999:227–252.
3. Peyron JG, Altman RD. The epidemiology of osteoarthritis. In: Moskowitz RW, Howell DS, Goldberg VM, et al., eds. Osteoarthritis: diagnosis and medical/surgical management. 2nd ed. Philadelphia, PA: WB Saunders Inc., 1992:15–37.
4. Moskowitz RW. Clinical and laboratory findings in osteoarthritis. In: Koopman WJ, ed. Arthritis and allied conditions: a textbook of rheumatology. 13th ed. Baltimore, MD: Williams & Wilkins, 1997:1985–2011.
5. Kellgren JH, Lawrence JS, Bier F. Genetic factors in generalized osteo-arthrosis. Ann Rheum Dis 1963;22:237–255.
6. Felson DT, Naimark A, Anderson JJ, et al. The prevalence of knee osteoarthritis in the elderly: the Framingham Osteoarthritis Study. Arthritis Rheum 1987;30:914–918.
7. Felson DT. Epidemiology of the rheumatic diseases. In: Koopman WJ, ed. Arthritis and allied conditions: a textbook of rheumatology. 13th ed. Baltimore, MD: Williams & Wilkins, 1997:3–34.
8. Peyron JG. Epidemiologic and etiologic approach to osteoarthritis. Semin Arthritis Rheum 1979;8:288–306.
9. Anderson J, Felson DT. Factors associated with knee osteoarthritis (OA) in the HANES I survey: evidence of an association with overweight, race and physical demands of work. Am J Epidemiol 1988;128:179–189.
10. Felson DT, Zhang Y, Hannan MT, et al. Risk factors for incident radiographic knee osteoarthritis in the elderly: the Framingham study. Arthritis Rheum 1997;40:728–733.
11. Altman R, Alarcón G, Applerouth D, et al. The American College of Rheumatology criteria for classification and reporting of osteoarthritis of the hand. Arthritis Rheum 1990; 33:1601–1610.
12. Altman R, Asch E, Bloch D, et al. Development of criteria for classification and reporting of osteoarthritis. Classification of osteoarthritis of the knee. Arthritis Rheum 1986;29:1039–1049.
13. Altman R, Alarcón G, Applerouth D, et al. Criteria for classification and reporting of osteoarthritis of the hip. Arthritis Rheum 1991;34:505–515.
14. Brandt KD. Nonsurgical management of osteoarthritis, with an emphasis on nonpharmacologic measures. Arch Fam Med 1995;4:1057–1064.
15. Albani S, Carson DA. Etiology and pathogenesis of rheumatoid arthritis. In: Koopman WJ, ed. Arthritis and allied conditions: a textbook of rheumatology. 13th ed. Baltimore, MD: Williams & Wilkins, 1997:979–992.
16. Wolfe F, Mitchell DM, Sibley JT, et al. The mortality of rheumatoid arthritis. Arthritis Rheum 1994;37:481–494.
17. Hochberg MC, Chang RW, Dwosh I, et al. The American College of Rheumatology 1991 revised criteria for the classification of global functional status in rheumatoid arthritis. Arthritis Rheum 1992;35:498–502.
18. Hale LP, Haynes BF. Pathology of rheumatoid arthritis and associated disorders. In: Koopman WJ, ed. Arthritis and allied conditions: a textbook of rheumatology. 13th ed. Baltimore, MD: Williams & Wilkins, 1997:993–1016.
19. Goldenberg DL. Treatment of fibromyalgia syndrome. Rheum Dis Clin N Am 1989;15:61–71.
20. Buckelew SP. Fibromyalgia: a rehabilitation approach. Am J Phys Med Rehabil 1989;68:37–42.
21. Bradley LA, Alarcón GS. Fibromyalgia. In: Koopman WJ, ed. Arthritis and allied conditions: a textbook of rheumatology. 13th ed. Baltimore, MD: Williams & Wilkins, 1997:1619–1640.
22. Wolfe F, Ross K, Anderson J, et al. The prevalence and characteristics of fibromyalgia in the general population. Arthritis Rheum 1995;38:19–28.
23. Wolfe F, Smythe HA, Yunus MB, et al. The American College of Rheumatology 1990 Criteria for the Classification of Fibromyalgia: Report of the Multicenter Criteria Committee. Arthritis Rheum 1990;33:160–172.
24. Arthritis Foundation, Association of State and Territorial Health Officials, and Centers for Disease Control and Prevention. National Arthritis Action Plan: a public health strategy. Arthritis Foundation National Office, 1999.
25. Mannerkorpi K, Burckhardt CS, Bjelle A. Physical performance characteristics of women with fibromyalgia. Arthritis Care Res 1994;7:123–129.
26. Minor MA, Hewett JE, Webel RR, et al. Exercise tolerance and disease related measures in patients with rheumatoid arthritis and osteoarthritis. J Rheumatol 1988;15:905–911.
27. Hurley MV, Scott DL. Improvements in quadriceps sensorimotor function and disability of patients with knee osteoarthritis following a clinically practicable exercise regime. Br J Rheumatol 1998;37:1181–1187.
28. Ettinger WH Jr, Afable RF. Physical disability from knee osteoarthritis: the role of exercise as an intervention. Med Sci Sports Exerc 1994;26:1435–1440.
29. Slemenda C, Brandt KD, Heilman DK, et al. Quadriceps weak-

ness and osteoarthritis of the knee. Ann Intern Med 1997;127: 97–104.
30. Tan J, Balci N, Sepici V, et al. Isokinetic and isometric strength in osteoarthrosis of the knee. Am J Phys Med Rehabil 1995;74:364–369.
31. Beals CA, Lampman RM, Banwell B, et al. Measurement of exercise tolerance in patients with rheumatoid arthritis and osteoarthritis. J Rheumatol 1985;12:458–461.
32. Danneskiold-Samsøe B, Lyngberg K, Risum T, et al. The effect of water exercise given to patients with rheumatoid arthritis. Scand J Rehab Med 1987;19:31–35.
33. Ekdahl C, Broman G. Muscle strength, endurance, and aerobic capacity in rheumatoid arthritis: a comparative study with healthy subjects. Ann Rheum Dis 1992;51:35–40.
34. Hsieh LF, Didenko B, Schumacher HR Jr, et al. Isokinetic and isometric testing of knee musculature in patients with rheumatoid arthritis with mild knee involvement. Arch Phys Med Rehabil 1987;68:294–297.
35. Fisher NM, Pendergast DR. Reduced muscle function in patients with osteoarthritis. Scand J Rehab Med 1997;29: 213–221.
36. Mengshoel AM, Vollestad NK, Forre O. Pain and fatigue induced by exercise in fibromyalgia patients and sedentary healthy subjects. Clin Exp Rheumatol 1995;13:477–482.
37. Philbin EF, Groff GD, Ries MD, et al. Cardiovascular fitness and health in patients with end-stage osteoarthritis. Arthritis Rheum 1995;38:799–805.
38. Fisher NM, Pendergast DR. Effects of a muscle exercise program on exercise capacity in subjects with osteoarthritis. Arch Phys Med Rehabil 1994;75:792–797.
39. Fisher NM, Gresham GE, Pendergast DR. Quantitative progressive exercise rehabilitation for osteoarthritis of the knee. Phys Med Rehabil Clinics NA 1994;5:785–802.
40. Fisher NM, Pendergast DR, Gresham GE, et al. Muscle rehabilitation: its effects on muscular and functional performance of patients with knee osteoarthritis. Arch Phys Med Rehabil 1991;72:367–374.
41. Fisher DR, Pendergast DR. Application of quantitative and progressive exercise rehabilitation to patients with osteoarthritis of the knee. J Back Musculoskeletal Rehabil 1995; 5:33–53.
42. Fisher NM, Gresham GE, Abrams M, et al. Quantitative effects of physical therapy on muscular and functional performance in subjects with osteoarthritis of the knees. Arch Phys Med Rehabil 1993;74:840–847.
43. Fisher NM, Gresham G, Pendergast DR. Effects of a quantitative progressive rehabilitation program applied unilaterally to the osteoarthritic knee. Arch Phys Med Rehabil 1993; 74:1319–1326.
44. Fisher NM, Kame VD, Rouse L, et al. Quantitative evaluation of a home exercise program on muscle and functional capacity of patients with osteoarthritis. Am J Phys Med Rehabil 1994;73:413–420.
45. Fisher NM, White SC, Yack HJ, et al. Muscle function and gait in patients with knee osteoarthritis before and after muscle rehabilitation. Disabil Rehabil 1997;19:47–55.
46. Bennett RM, Clark SR, Goldberg L, et al. Aerobic fitness in patients with fibrositis: a controlled study of respiratory gas exchange and ^{133}xenon clearance from exercising muscle. Arthritis Rheum 1989;32:454–460.
47. McNair PJ, Marshall RN, Maguire K. Swelling of the knee joint: effects of exercise on quadriceps muscle strength. Arch Phys Med Rehabil 1996;77:896–899.
48. Hurley MV. The role of muscle weakness in the pathogenesis of osteoarthritis. Rheum Dis Clinics NA 1999;25:283–298.
49. Hall J, Skevington SM, Maddison PJ, et al. A randomized and controlled trial of hydrotherapy in rheumatoid arthritis. Arthritis Care Res 1996;9:206–215.
50. van den Ende CH, Hazes JM, le Cessie S, et al. Comparison of high and low intensity training in well controlled rheumatoid arthritis. Results of a randomized clinical trial. Ann Rheum Dis 1996;55:798–805.
51. Dellhag B, Wollersjo I, Bjelle A. Effect of active hand exercise and wax bath treatment in rheumatoid arthritis patients. Arthritis Care Res 1992;5:87–92.
52. Mengshoel AM, Komnaes HB, Forre O. The effects of 20 weeks of physical fitness training in female patients with fibromyalgia. Clin Exp Rheumatol 1992;10:345–349.
53. O'Reilly SC, Muir KR, Doherty M. Effectiveness of home exercise on pain and disability from osteoarthritis of the knee: a randomized controlled trial. Ann Rheum Dis 1999;58: 15–19.
54. Røgind H, Bibow-Nielsen B, Jensen B, et al. The effects of a physical training program on patients with osteoarthritis of the knees. Arch Phys Med Rehabil 1998;79:1421–1427.
55. Maurer BT, Stern AG, Kinossian B, et al. Osteoarthritis of the knee: isokinetic quadriceps exercise versus an educational intervention. Arch Phys Med Rehabil 1999;80:1293–1299.
56. Machover S, Sapecky AJ. Effect of isometric exercise on the quadriceps muscle in patients with rheumatoid arthritis. Arch Phys Med Rehabil 1966;47:737–741.
57. Lyngberg KB, Danneskiold-Samsøe B, Halskov O. The effect of physical training on patients with rheumatoid arthritis: changes in disease activity, muscle strength and aerobic capacity. A clinically controlled minimized cross-over study. Clin Exp Rheumatol 1988;6:253–260.
58. Ekdahl C, Andersson SI, Moritz U, et al. Dynamic versus static training in patients with rheumatoid arthritis. Scand J Rheumatol 1990;19:17–26.
59. Brighton SW, Lubbe JE, van der Merwe CA. The effect of a long-term exercise programme on the rheumatoid hand. Br J Rheumatol 1993;32:392–395.
60. Hansen TM, Hansen G, Langgaard AM, et al. Long-term physical training in rheumatoid arthritis. A randomized trial with different training programs and blinded observers. Scand J Rheumatol 1993;22:107–112.
61. Lyngberg KB, Ramsing BU, Nawrocki A, et al. Safe and effective isokinetic knee extension training in rheumatoid arthritis. Arthritis Rheum 1994;37:623–628.
62. Hakkinen A, Hakkinen K, Hannonen P. Effects of strength training on neuromuscular function and disease activity in patients with recent-onset inflammatory arthritis. Scand J Rheumatol 1994;23:237–242.
63. Rall LC, Meydani SN, Kehayias JJ, et al. The effect of progressive resistance training in rheumatoid arthritis. Increased strength without changes in energy balance or body composition. Arthritis Rheum 1996;39:415–426.
64. Komatireddy GR, Leitch RW, Cella K, et al. Efficacy of low load resistive muscle training in patients with rheumatoid arthritis functional class II and III. J Rheumatol 1997;24: 1531–1539.

65. Lyngberg KK, Harreby M, Bentzen H, et al. Elderly rheumatoid arthritis patients on steroid treatment tolerate physical training without an increase in disease activity. Arch Phys Med Rehabil 1994;75:1189–1195.
66. McMeeken J, Stillman B, Story I, et al. The effects of knee extensor and flexor muscle training on the timed-up-and-go test in individuals with rheumatoid arthritis. Physiother Res Int 1999;4:55–67.
67. McCain GA, Bell DA, Mai FM, et al. A controlled study of the effects of a supervised cardiovascular fitness training program on the manifestations of primary fibromyalgia. Arthritis Rheum 1988;31:1135–1141.
68. Martin L, Nutting A, MacIntosh BR, et al. An exercise program in the treatment of fibromyalgia. J Rheumatol 1996; 23:1050–1053.
69. Wigers SH, Stiles TC, Vogel PA. Effects of aerobic exercise versus stress management treatment in fibromyalgia. A 4.5 year prospective study. Scand J Rheumatol 1996;25:77–86.
70. Mangione KK, McCully K, Gloviak A, et al. The effects of high-intensity and low-intensity cycle ergometry in older adults with knee osteoarthritis. J Gerontol:Med Sci 1999; 54A:M184–190.
71. Minor MA, Hewett JE, Webel RR, et al. Efficacy of physical conditioning exercise in patients with rheumatoid arthritis and osteoarthritis. Arthritis Rheum 1989;32:1396–1405.
72. Ekblom B, Lovgren O, Alderin M, et al. Effect of short-term physical training on patients with rheumatoid arthritis I. Scand J Rheumatol 1975;4:80–86.
73. Harkcom TM, Lampman RM, Banwell BF, et al. Therapeutic value of graded aerobic exercise training in rheumatoid arthritis. Arthritis Rheum 1985;28:32–39.
74. Baslund BK, Lyngberg K, Andersen V, et al. Effect of 8 weeks of bicycle training on the immune system of patients with rheumatoid arthritis. J Appl Physiol 1993;75:1691–1695.
75. Minor MA, Hewett JE. Physical fitness and work capacity in women with rheumatoid arthritis. Arthritis Care Res 1995; 8:146–154.
76. Noreau L, Martineau H, Roy L, et al. Effects of a modified dance-based exercise on cardiorespiratory fitness, psychological state and health status of persons with rheumatoid arthritis. Am J Phys Med Rehabil 1995;74:19–27.
77. Burckhardt CS, Mannerkorpi K, Hedenberg L, et al. A randomized, controlled clinical trial of education and physical training for women with fibromyalgia. J Rheumatol 1994; 21:714–720.
78. Gowans SE, deHueck A, Voss S, et al. A randomized, controlled trial of exercise and education for individuals with fibromyalgia. Arthritis Care Res 1999;12:120–128.
79. Deyle GD, Henderson NE, Matekel RL, et al. Effectiveness of manual physical therapy and exercise in osteoarthritis of the knee. A randomized, controlled trial. Ann Intern Med 2000;132:173–181.
80. Ettinger WH Jr, Burns R, Messier SP, et al. A randomized trial comparing aerobic exercise and resistance exercise with a health education program in older adults with knee osteoarthritis. The Fitness Arthritis and Seniors Trial (FAST). JAMA 1997;277:25–31.
81. Kovar PA, Allegrante JP, MacKenzie CR, et al. Supervised fitness walking in patients with osteoarthritis of the knee. A randomized, controlled trial. Ann Intern Med 1992;116:529–534.
82. Rejeski WJ, Ettinger WH, Martin K, et al. Treating disability in knee osteoarthritis with exercise therapy: a central role for self-efficacy and pain. Arthritis Care Res 1998;11:94–101.
83. Perlman SG, Connell KJ, Clark A, et al. Dance-based aerobic exercise for rheumatoid arthritis. Arthritis Care Res 1990;3: 29–35.
84. Stenstrom CH, Arge B, Sundbom A. Dynamic training versus relaxation training as home exercise for patients with inflammatory rheumatic diseases. A randomized controlled study. Scan J Rheumatol 1996;25:28–33.
85. Stenstrom CH, Arge B, Sundbom A. Home exercise and compliance in inflammatory rheumatic diseases—prospective clinical trial. J Rheumatol 1997;24:470–476.
86. van Baar ME, Dekker J, Oostendorp RA, et al. The effectiveness of exercise therapy in patients with osteoarthritis of the hip or knee: a randomized clinical trial. J Rheumatol 1998;25:2432–2439.
87. Buckelew SP, Conway R, Parker J, et al. Biofeedback/relaxation training and exercise interventions for fibromyalgia: a prospective trial. Arthritis Care Res 1998;11:196–209.
88. Semble EL. Rheumatoid arthritis: new approaches for its evaluation and management. Arch Phys Med Rehabil 1995;76:190–201.
89. Rossy LA, Buckelew SP, Dorr N, et al. A meta-analysis of fibromyalgia treatment interventions. Ann Behav Med 1999;21:180–191.
90. *Physicians' Desk Reference (PDR)*. 55th ed. Montvale, NJ: Medical Economics Company, 2001.
91. Arnett FC, Edworthy SM, Bloch DA, et al. The American Rheumatism Association 1987 revised criteria for the classification of rheumatoid arthritis. Arthritis Rheum 1988;31:315–324.
92. Bradley LA, Young LD, Anderson KO, et al. Effects of psychological therapy on pain behavior of rheumatoid arthritis patients. Treatment outcome and six-month followup. Arthritis Rheum 1990;30:1105–1114.
93. Keefe FJ, Caldwell DS, Williams DA, et al. Pain coping skills training in the management of osteoarthritis knee pain: a comparative study. Behav Ther 1990;21:49–62.
94. Nielson WR, Walker C, McCain GA. Cognitive behavioral treatment of fibromyalgia syndrome: preliminary findings. J Rheumatol 1992;19:98–103.
95. Goldenberg DL, Kaplan KH, Nadeau MG, et al. A controlled study of a stress-reduction, cognitive-behavioral treatment program in fibromyalgia. J Musculoskeletal Pain 1994;2:53–66.
96. White KP, Nielson WR. Cognitive-behavioral treatment of fibromyalgia syndrome: a follow-up assessment. J Rheumatol 1995;22:717–721.
97. Ferraccioli G, Ghirelli L, Scita F, et al. EMG-biofeedback training in fibromyalgia syndrome. J Rheumatol 1987;14: 820–825.
98. Haanen HC, Hoenderdos HT, van Romunde LK, et al. Controlled trial of hypnotherapy in the treatment of refractory fibromyalgia. J Rheumatol 1991;18:72–75.
99. Fuchs HA, Sergent JS. Rheumatoid arthritis: the clinical picture. In: Koopman WJ, ed. Arthritis and allied conditions: a textbook of rheumatology. 13th ed. Baltimore, MD: Williams & Wilkins, 1997:1041–1070.
100. Simms RW, Roy SH, Hrovat M, et al. Lack of association between fibromyalgia syndrome and abnormalities in muscle energy metabolism. Arthritis Rheum 1994;37:794–800.

101. Meenan RF, Mason JH, Anderson JJ, et al. AIMS2. The content and properties of a revised and expanded Arthritis Impact Measurement Scales health status questionnaire. Arthritis Rheum 1992;35:1–10.
102. Bellamy N, Campbell J, Stevens J, et al. Validation study of a computerized version of the Western Ontario and McMaster Universities v3.0 Osteoarthritis Index. J Rheumatol 1997;24:2413–2415.
103. King S, Wessel J, Bhambhani Y, et al. Validity and reliability of the 6 minute walk in persons with fibromyalgia. J Rheumatol 1999;26:2233–2237.
104. Chamberlain MA, Care G, Harfield B. Physiotherapy in osteoarthritis of the knees. A controlled trial of hospital versus home exercises. Int Rehab Med 1982;4:101–106.
105. Sullivan T, Allegrante JP, Peterson MGE, et al. One-year followup of patients with osteoarthritis of the knee who participated in a program of supervised fitness walking and supportive patient education. Arthritis Care Res 1998;11: 228–233.
106. Buckelew SP, Murray SE, Hewett JE, et al. Self-efficacy, pain, and physical activity among fibromyalgia patients. Arthritis Care Res 1995;8:43–50.
107. Bennett RM, Burckhardt CS, Clark SR, et al. Group treatment of fibromyalgia: a 6 month outpatient program. J Rheumatol 1996;23:521–528.
108. Lorig K, Mazonson PD, Holman HR. Evidence suggesting that health education for self-management in patients with chronic arthritis has sustained health benefits while reducing health care costs. Arthritis Rheum 1993;36:439–446.
109. Kruger JMS, Helmick CG, Callahan LF, et al. Cost-effectiveness of the Arthritis Self-Help Course. Arch Intern Med 1998;158:1245–1249.

CHAPTER 11
Exercise and Activity for Individuals with Nonspecific Back Pain

Maureen J. Simmonds

Low back pain (LBP) is an enigma. It remains a common, complex, and controversial problem. It is one of the most widely experienced health-related problems in the world. It is incredibly costly in both human and economic terms, and its presentation and consequences are characterized by variability. LBP may be sudden or insidious in onset; result from major trauma or multiple episodes of microtrauma; have muscular, articular, nociceptive, and/or neuropathic components; involve single or multiple sites of pain; and persist for weeks, months, or a lifetime.

Some individuals experience an acute episode of LBP as a temporary inconvenience that has little effect on their regular activity. Others with a similar level of impairment enter a downward spiral of distress, disability, and dependence on the health-care system (1). Most individuals with LBP adapt to, and cope with, persistent and recurrent symptoms of pain and temporary activity limitation (2). Clearly, LBP is a simple label for a complex, multidimensional (biopsychosocial) problem that is *managed rather than cured.* Clinical guidelines now recommend that this management should be based on exercise/activity and education (3, 4). The purpose of this chapter is to review the problem of LBP and its management using an expanded conceptual framework and best available evidence.

EPIDEMIOLOGY AND PATHOPHYSIOLOGY

Impairment and disability are key terms in any discussion of LBP. The World Health Organization defined the terms as follows (5). *Impairment* is any loss or abnormality of psychological, physiological, or anatomical structure or function (e.g., decreased range of motion or strength). *Disability* is any restriction or lack (resulting from an impairment) of ability to perform an activity in the manner or within the range considered normal (e.g., the inability to work). Nagi (6) recognized the need for a concept that bridged impairment and disability, and proposed the term *functional limitation. Functional limitation* is defined as compromised ability to perform activities of daily living (ADLs). Nagi proposed a model that illustrated the linkage from pathology, through impairment and functional limitation, to disability.

Pathology ⟶ Impairment ⟶ Functional Limitation ⟶ Disability

A shortcoming of this model is the implied unidirectional and linear progression from pathology to disability that is not entirely accurate. Rather, each of the constructs is complex and is influenced by a myriad of factors. Depending on when and how the different constructs are measured, and on the influence of mediating factors (e.g., psychosocial factors), the relationships among the constructs (pathology, impairment, functional limitation, and disability) may be trivial. Nevertheless, the disablement model provides an expanded conceptual framework for understanding, assessing, and managing LBP.

The lifetime prevalence of LBP is between 58 to 70 percent (7–10), and the yearly prevalence rate is between 15 and 37 percent in industrial countries (7, 8, 11). Although interesting, these data do not provide much information about the nature or the effect of the problem. The data frequently don't distinguish between a single episode of mild backache that lasts less than a day and severe back pain that is permanently incapacitating. Croft (12) noted that, although an episode of LBP may resolve quickly, recurrence rates are approximately 50% in the following 12 months. Andersson (7) reported that approximately 2 percent of the population with LBP are temporarily disabled or become chronically disabled.

Von Korff et al. (13) reported that 41% of adults between 26 and 44 years of age reported having back pain in the previous 6 months. The majority had occasional episodes of pain that lasted a few days, was mild or moderate in intensity, and did not limit activities. However, 25% of these individuals in Von Korff's study (13) had back pain more often than not, and that limited their activity. Wahlgren et al (2) showed that in a cohort of 76 individuals, who had a first episode of LBP, 78% still experienced pain at 6 months and 26% were disabled by LBP. It was also reported that, at 12 months, 72% still experienced pain and 14% were disabled by LBP. These results suggest that although a high percentage of individuals have persistent LBP, the majority (75 percent) self-manage their problem, and a minority become significantly disabled.

The cost of care for those who enter the health-care system due to LBP is tremendous. Frymoyer and Durret (14) estimated the cost of LBP in the United States to range between $38 and $50 billion a year. This includes the cost for approximately 50 million chiropractic visits and more than 5 million physical therapist visits each year (14). In addition, there are also about 300,000 operations annually (15), including back and neck operations, which are the third most common form of surgery in the United States (16).

Pain

Pain is a multidimensional (biopsychosocial) experience that is one of the most misunderstood and mismanaged health problems (1, 15, 17, 18). A comprehensive review of the complex physiological mechanisms (e.g., transduction, central processing, modulation, and neural plasticity), psychological factors (e.g., personality characteristics, emotional states, and cognitive processes), and social circumstances (e.g., family and work interactions) involved in the pain experience is beyond the scope of this chapter. This chapter will focus on some of the key elements and common misconceptions about LBP and the relationships between tissue injury, pain, and physical dysfunction, and the ameliorating role of activity and exercise.

An extensive plexus of nerve fibers supplies the spine (osseous and non-osseous tissues), the surrounding facet joints, soft tissues (muscle and ligaments), and the neurovascular tissues. The extensive plexus is one reason why the source of pain is frequently enigmatic. Any innervated structure can trigger a nociceptive signal, and most structures in the back are well innervated, relatively small, and in close proximity to each other.

The sensory system that transmits nociceptive signals includes sensory receptors in the periphery, processing circuits in the dorsal horn, and ascending pathways in the spine that lead to the brain, where the signal is interpreted. In the brain, however, a nociceptive signal may or may not be interpreted as painful because a myriad of factors such as past experience, current mood, and social context influence interpretation. Thus, an important distinction exists between nociception and pain.

Clearly, the nociceptive signal that arrives at the cortex is distinctly different from that generated in the periphery. Whether the signal is enhanced or inhibited as it travels from the periphery to the brain depends upon the relative strength of the opposing neuromodulatory processes. Again, the interpretation of the signal is influenced by the individual's mood, attention, sense of control, current activity, past experience, and the social and environmental context in which the signal is received. Indeed, the meaning that the individual attaches to the pain will influence his/her emotional response and subsequent behavior, and that behavior can outlast the sensory signal and may contribute to disability. Interested readers are referred to the excellent review by Vlayen and Linton on this topic (19).

The beliefs that an individual has about his/her pain will influence what he/she does about it. Some individuals will consider the pain a minor inconvenience and attempt to ignore it, whereas others will worry about the pain and its meaning and immediately seek professional help. If their pain is aggravated by activity, they may avoid activity, even simple activity if they anticipate it will be painful. Although this action may be appropriate in the short term for acute pain, it is not appropriate for chronic pain when *pain pathology* rather than *spinal impairment* is the problem.

In summary, LBP is a multidimensional experience. It has sensory, emotional, cognitive, and behavioral components. The relative magnitude of each component helps determine how an individual's problem should be managed (i.e., modify sensory input, address misunderstandings about the meaning of the pain and the relationship to injury, and/or address anxieties about pain and activity). The simple adage "let pain be the guide" belies the complexity of the construct.

CLINICAL EXERCISE PHYSIOLOGY

See the discussion below under "Exercise Prescription and Programming."

PHARMACOLOGY

Medications most commonly used for symptom control by individuals with nonspecific LBP for symptom control are nonsteroidal anti-inflammatory medications (NSAIDS), and/or nonnarcotic analgesics. These may be obtained over the counter or by prescription. Common NSAIDS include aspirin, ibuprofen, indomethacin, phenylbutazone, naproxen, and others. Cox-2 inhibitors (e.g., Celebrex or Vioxx) have analgesic and anti-inflammatory properties with fewer gastrointestinal side effects. Acetaminophen, a common nonnarcotic analgesic used by persons with LBP, does not have anti-inflammatory properties. None of these medications should have a significant effect on exercise capacities and physical performance, with the exception that they can allow an individual to exercise more comfortably and, therefore, more effectively.

PHYSICAL EXAMINATION

The physical examination supplements the information obtained in the medical history. The basic elements of a physical examination include observation of posture, measurement of spinal range of motion, tests of muscle strength, and the presence and location of pain at rest or during specific movements. Neurological dysfunction is evaluated in the physical examination through testing straight leg raising, myotome strength, and dermatome sensitivity. In addition, sacroiliac joint tests are often included in the physical examination.

Although this type of assessment has been standard practice for many years, and is well described in any orthopedic text, it is frequently not helpful diagnostically because many components of the exam have questionable validity (sensitivity and specificity), and most provide minimal information regarding the individual's level of function. For example, spinal posture and active and passive joint motions are key components of a physical examination. However, except in extreme cases, they have limited clinical value because of the high level of individual variability and the frequently weak relationship with disability. In addition, Mellin (20) found lumbar spine mobility to have few significant correlations, none higher than r = 0.19, with the modified Oswestry questionnaire for LBP. Also, generally weak correlations between lumbar flexion and physical performance tests have been reported. Noteworthy is the correlation between range of lumbar flexion and the speed of lumbar flexion (r = 0.16). The latter is a more useful indicator of function than the former (21).

Although the physical examination provides limited information about diagnosis and function, it can help eliminate misgivings or concerns the individual has regarding the performance of simple movements. It can also identify gross deficiencies in flexibility and strength so treatment can be implemented.

Pain

Pain is a common presenting symptom, and it should be assessed using standardized methods. Pain is a subjective phenomenon and, therefore, self-report should be the primary form of assessment. Assessment should include a measure of pain intensity, pain affect, and pain distribution.

Pain intensity and pain affect can easily be measured using numeric rating scales (NRS) or visual analogue scales (VAS). Research studies provide support for the reliability, validity, and responsiveness of these measures (22). For a measure of pain intensity using the NRS, the individual is asked to select a number between 0 and 10 that best describes the intensity of his/her pain (i.e., 0 = no pain and 10 = most severe pain imaginable). The VAS consists of a 10-cm line with descriptors at the endpoints (e.g., 0 = no pain and 10 = most severe pain imaginable). The individual places a mark on this line, and a level of pain intensity score is computed by measuring the distance from the 0 point to the mark made by the individual.

A second important dimension of the pain experience is pain affect. Pain affect refers to the unpleasantness of pain. It can be measured at the same time as pain intensity using 0–10 NRS or ***10-cm*** VAS with different endpoint words. Endpoints for pain affect are: 10 cm = not at all unpleasant and 10 cm = most unpleasant pain imaginable. Pain intensity and affect are related, but certain treatments, such as certain medications and physical therapies, can contribute to a reduction in pain affect rather than pain intensity (23).

Pain location is most easily assessed using a body map, which is an outline of a human figure on which the individual is asked to shade the painful area.

Functional Assessment

LBP can have a major impact on a person's functional ability. Standard clinical assessments of LBP, however, are traditionally limited to measures of *impairment.* Although restoration of function is one of the most common aims of treatment, Jette and colleagues (24) reported that function is not always directly assessed but is inferred from the level of impairment. In the last two decades, it has become increasingly obvious that impairment does not have a strong or stable relationship with functional limitation or disability (17). This is partly due to the complexity of the constructs and partly due to the difficulties in measuring them. Functional measurements assess at the level of the whole person, whereas impairment measurements (e.g., range of motion, muscle strength) assess at the level of a "part" of the person.

Traditional assessments based on impairment measures are now often complemented with functionally based measures, which assess the impact of any impairment and, in that respect, are more meaningful to the patient. The assessment methods include patient self-report questionnaires and clinician-measured tasks (25).

An advantage of questionnaires is that they sample a range of different activities, including mobility, the performance of household chores, and other work-related activities. They can be relatively quick, simple, and practical to administer and score. They are widely used, norms are available, and clearly they have superior face validity when compared to health professionals' estimates of function. The most commonly used self-report questionnaires for functional assessment of LBP are the Oswestry Disability Questionnaire (26), Roland and Morris Questionnaire (27) and the SF-36 (28). The SF-36 is a multidimensional measure of general health status, whereas the Oswestry and Roland and Morris Questionnaires are both LBP specific.

Simmonds and colleagues (21) developed a comprehensive but simple battery of performance tests to complement the functional assessment of individuals with LBP. It is known that individuals with LBP have difficulty withstanding spinal loads (compressive and shear), and velocity and acceleration of motion is generally slower compared to pain-free individuals (21, 23, 29). Therefore, performance on the task battery is generally measured on how far a participant can reach forward (i.e., an indirect measure of spinal load) and how quickly a task can be performed (i.e., an indirect measure of velocity and acceleration of motion). The indirect measure of spinal load is how far forward the person can reach while holding a 4.6 kg

Table 11.1. Red Flags for Potentially Serious Conditions

- Features of cauda equina syndrome (especially urinary retention, bilateral neurological symptoms and signs, saddle anesthesia)—this requires very urgent referral
- Significant trauma
- Weight loss
- History of cancer
- Fever
- Intravenous drug use
- Steroid use
- Patient over 50 years old
- Severe, unremitting nighttime pain
- Pain that gets worse when patient is lying down

weight, and the timed tasks include repeated trunk bending, sit to stand, 50-foot speed walk, and a 5-minute walk.

In the study by Simmonds and colleagues (21), all measures had an excellent inter-rater reliability (i.e., Intraclass correlation coefficients were all equal or greater than 0.95). Face validity, convergent, discriminant, and predictive validity have also been established (21). Noteworthy is another report by Simmonds and colleagues (30), that the physical performance measures in 66 patients with LBP outperformed impairment factors as predictors of disabilities (i.e., $R^2 = 0.61$ compared to $R^2 = 0.47$, respectively).

MEDICAL TREATMENT

Despite the cost and extent of health care for individuals with LBP who seek professional care, there has been little consensus and less evidence supporting many specific treatment techniques and regimens for most cases of LBP. Indeed, treatment regimens have been based on historical tradition, practitioners' knowledge, skills and biases, available resources, and payers' regulations, rather than the needs of the individual (15–19).

In recent years, clinical guidelines have been published in the United States, the United Kingdom, and New Zealand (3, 4, 31). The guidelines are based on systematic reviews and consensus statements and focus on the assessment and management of back pain in primary care. Most guidelines promote the use of a screening assessment of "red flags" to identify serious physical pathology. Some (e.g., New Zealand [31]), also promote the use of a psychosocial screening assessment of "yellow flags" to identify those at risk of chronic disability (Figure 11.1 and Table 11.2). All guidelines promote the use of patient education and exercise in the management of LBP. However, the U.K. guidelines emphasize and promote self-management, whereas the U.S. guidelines reflect a balance between traditional health care and self-management. This difference probably reflects cultural variance but may also reflect the evidence available when the guidelines were produced (17). The U.K. guidelines were published 4 years after the U.S. guidelines.

DIAGNOSTIC TECHNIQUES

Diagnostic terms used for LBP are usually descriptive, anatopathological, or physiological, whereas *classification* of LBP is usually based on duration of trouble, signs and symptoms, treatment, or consequences (32). A variety of diagnostic labels are applied to LBP (e.g., facetogenic, myofascial, discogenic, muscle strain, and sprain). The labels are based on hypothesized injuries or pathologies of specific structures. However, most are not verifiable due to problems with the sensitivity and specificity of clinical assessment and imaging measurements. Grazier et al. (33) estimated that of the 11 million outpatient visits made to physicians for LBP each year, 9 million were soft-tissue problems, "diagnosed" as strains and sprains (33). However, Nachemson (23) has estimated that a specific *verifiable* diagnosis is only possible in less than 5% of acute cases. Indeed, Waddell (17) astutely noted that although some doctors and therapists claim to be able to diagnose the site and nature of the lesion, such a label reveals more about the practitioner than the patient's back.

Regardless of such diagnostic issues, it is unlikely that injuries are as tissue-specific as many diagnostic labels imply. Tissue injury leads to an increased sensitivity of both the injured tissues and adjacent tissues, thereby confounding a tissue-specific "diagnosis." If significant or definitive spinal "red flags" (e.g., fracture, spinal stenosis, nerve root compression, or visceral pathologies) have been ruled out, a generic term such as "nonspecific" LBP is probably the most useful and accurate "diagnostic term." The term does not conjure worrisome images of spinal disintegration for patients and does not provide a false sense of diagnostic knowledge to practitioners.

The U.S. clinical practice guidelines recommend the use of three classifications based on medical history and clinical findings (3). These are: (1) potentially serious spinal condition (e.g., spinal tumor, infection, fracture, or cauda equina syndrome); (2) sciatica: back-related lower limb symptoms suggesting nerve root compromise; and (3) nonspecific back symptoms, which are symptoms occurring primarily in the back that suggest neither nerve root compromise, nor a serious underlying condition. Nonspecific back pain thus includes but is not limited to pain of muscular origin.

Grouping individuals with LBP based on pain distribution and pain duration is the simplest and the most reliable classification method. Pain distribution groups are determined according to whether they have: (1) back pain alone, (2) back pain with radiating pain into the thigh, (3) back pain with pain radiating into the leg below the knee (35). Pain distribution has been shown to influence levels of pain, disability, and physical performance (36, 37). Pain duration groups are usually determined as follows: (1) acute—less than 6 weeks, (2) subacute—6–12 weeks, (3) chronic—more than 12 weeks of

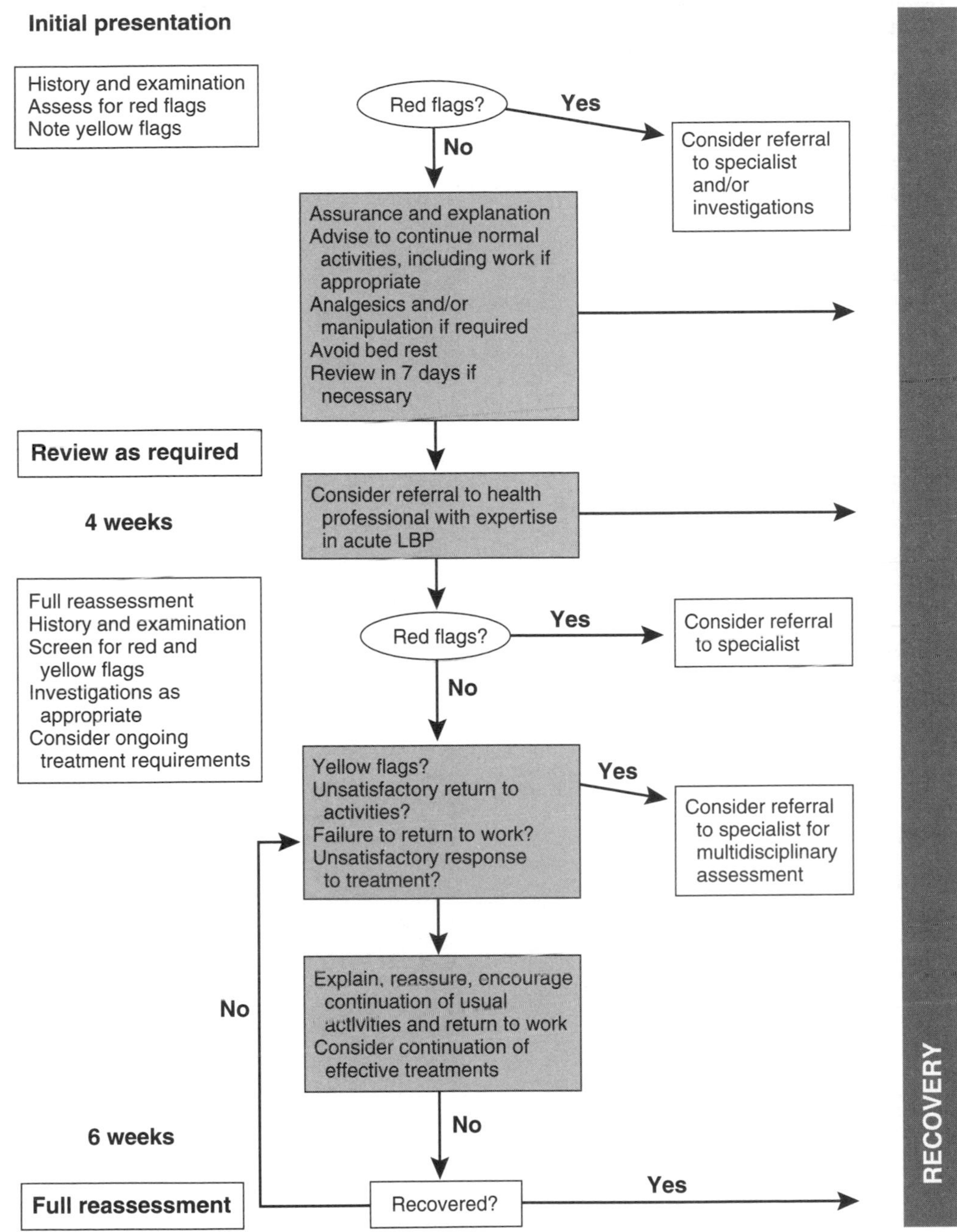

Figure 11.1. Management of acute low back pain. Reproduced with permission from the Accident Rehabilitation and Compensation Insurance Corporation of New Zealand and the National Health Committee, Wellington, New Zealand, 1997.

continuous symptoms (34). Duration of symptoms can be a problematic basis for classification because of the recurrent, episodic nature of LBP. However, the problem can be ameliorated by the inclusion of a "recurrent" category. Thus, the New Zealand LBP guidelines classify LBP as acute, chronic, or recurrent. Recurrent LBP is defined as: episodes of acute low back problems lasting less than 3 months but recurring after a period of time without low back symptoms sufficient to restrict activity or function (31).

EXERCISE/FITNESS/FUNCTIONAL TESTING

Individuals with LBP can perform the same graded exercise/fitness tests as pain free unimpaired individuals. The tests are outlined in the ACSM Guidelines (38). Because individuals may limit their exercise performance due to an actual or anticipated increase in pain, testers should identify and record the limiting factor so that the data from the test is interpreted correctly. It is noteworthy that prediction equations that estimated maximum oxy-

Table 11.2. Yellow Flags for Potential Risk of Chronic Incapacity, Distress, and Work Loss

- Attitudes and beliefs about back pain
  - Belief that pain is harmful or disabling resulting in fear and avoidance of movement
  - Belief that all pain must be abolished before return to normal activity or work
  - Expectation of increased pain with activity or work, lack of ability to predict capability
  - Catastrophising, thinking the worst, misinterpreting bodily symptoms
  - Belief that pain is uncontrollable
  - Passive attitude towards rehabilitation
- Behaviors
  - Use of extended rest
  - Reduced activity level with significant withdrawal from activities of daily living
  - Irregular participation with physical exercise, poor pacing
  - Avoidance of normal activity and progressive substitution of lifestyle away from productive activity
  - Report of extremely high intensity of pain
  - Excessive use on the use of aids or appliances
  - Sleep quality reduced since onset of back pain
  - Smoking
- Compensation/litigation issues
  - Lack of financial incentive to return to work
  - Delay in accessing income support and treatment costs, disputes over eligibility
  - History of claims for other pain problems
  - Previous experience of ineffective claims management
- Diagnostic and treatment
  - Health professional sanctioning disability, not providing interventions that will improve function
  - Experience of conflicting diagnoses or explanations for back pain, leading to confusion
  - Diagnostic language leading to catastrophising and fear
  - Dramatization of back pain by health professional producing dependency on treatments, and continuation of passive treatment
  - Number of visits to health professionals in the previous year
  - Expectation of a quick fix
  - Lack of satisfaction with previous treatment for back pain
  - Advice to withdraw from job
- Emotions
  - Fear of increased pain with activity or work
  - Depression, loss of sense of enjoyment
  - More irritable than usual
  - Anxiety about and heightened awareness of body sensations
  - Feeling under stress and unable to maintain a sense of control
  - Presence of social anxiety or disinterested in social activity
  - Feeling useless and not needed
- Family
  - Over-protective partner/spouse, emphasizing fear of harm (usually well-intentioned)
  - Solicitous behavior from spouse
  - Socially punitive behavior from spouse
  - Extent to which family members support return to work
  - Lack of support person to talk to about problems
- Work
  - History of manual work
  - Work history, frequent job changes, dissatisfaction, poor relationships with peers, lack of vocational direction
  - Belief that work is harmful
  - Unsupportive or unhappy work environment
  - Low educational background, low socioeconomic status
  - Job involves significant biomechanical demands such as lifting and handling heavy items, extended sitting, extended standing, driving, vibration, inflexible work schedule
  - Shift work or unsociable hours
  - Minimal availability and/or unsatisfactory implementation of selected duties and graduated return to work pathways
  - Negative experience of workplace management of back pain
  - Absence of interest from employer

Reproduced with permission from the Accident Rehabilitation and Compensation Insurance Corporation of New Zealand and the National Health Committee, Wellington, New Zealand, 1997.

gen consumption (VO_{2max}) for healthy, nondisabled men and women have been shown to be valid for persons with chronic low back pain (39).

EXERCISE PRESCRIPTION AND PROGRAMMING

Physical inactivity can have a detrimental effect on cardiovascular and musculoskeletal systems. It can also have a detrimental effect on psychosocial well-being (40). *A consequence of LBP, regardless of its genesis, is a temporary or permanent reduction in activity.* Therefore, maintenance of, or early return to, normal activity is a fundamental aim of management. What is less clear is whether a particular exercise or activity regimen will facilitate resumption of normal activity, and, if so, whether the specific mechanisms of the effects are biological, psychological, sociological, or all of the above.

Physical activity is an umbrella term that includes concepts such as fitness, exercise, training, and conditioning (41). Essentially, any bodily movement that increases energy expenditure above the resting level is physical activity (42). Exercise is frequently used interchangeably with physical activity. However, exercise and exercise training is purposeful activity specifically designed to improve or maintain a particular component of physical fitness (e.g., flexibility, strength, or endurance—cardiovascular or musculoskeletal).

The treatment of LBP incorporates a variety of different regimens and specific types and intensity of exercise that have been used in clinical practice with the aim of preventing and/or treating LBP and its consequences. Most regimens have been based on a biomedical impairment model and have thus focused on improving specific trunk strength, endurance, and/or flexibility and aerobic fitness (e.g., 43–45). The implied rationale of this assessment and management approach is that trunk muscles are weak and the spine is stiff. However, trunk strength and mobility neither predict LBP (43, 46–48) nor disability (30, 47). Moreover, these measures frequently don't discriminate between individuals with and without LBP because of the large range of interindividual variability (21, 49, 50).

Other treatment regimens focus on general exercises and aerobic conditioning. Jette et al. (24) reported that endurance exercises were included in 52% of treatment plans of 739 individuals with LBP. Again, the implied and oft stated rationale (51) is that individuals with LBP are deconditioned, or become deconditioned, due to LBP. However, the evidence supporting that notion is weak and contradictory (31, 41, 58). In 1994, the Agency for Health Care Policy and Research (AHCPR) recommended the use of low-stress aerobic exercise, endurance, and conditioning exercise (3). However, the report acknowledged the evidence supporting that recommendation was moderate to weak.

Although the AHCPR guidelines were associated with political and scientific controversy following their release, the guidelines served to shake clinical complacency regarding the evidence, or lack thereof, supporting common clinical practices for LBP. One result has been systematic investigations into the *mechanisms* of action, the *efficacy*, and the *effectiveness* of specific exercise regimens in acute, subacute, and chronic nonspecific LBP.

A serious review and critique of the literature on LBP is a daunting task. The literature is voluminous and highly variable in terms of scientific quality. Moreover, the natural history of the condition and the many methodological differences among research studies make it difficult to compare their outcomes. For example, participants are heterogeneous or are not well described; exercise interventions are often inadequately described in terms of type, intensity, or duration; and outcome measures vary from specific impairment measures (e.g., pain reduction) to social measures such as return to work. Although social measures are a very important outcome, they are influenced more strongly by the individuals' beliefs about their back problem, their education and job skills, and by the unemployment rate rather than by the severity of their LBP. Finally, studies differ in their length of follow-up that can vary between immediate postintervention and up to 2 years postintervention. The length of follow-up is an important consideration in LBP because of its recurrent nature. Also, individuals seek health care when symptoms are at their worst, which favors early resolution, or at least reduction in symptoms, despite any treatment intervention. Therefore, in future studies, long-term follow-up is essential in order to establish the effectiveness of an exercise intervention.

Given the voluminous and variable nature of the literature, the lag between research and the clinical application of research findings is understandable. This is why government agencies, scientific societies, and research groups have formed task forces (clinicians and researchers) to appraise the evidence and publish treatment guidelines. Dissemination of findings to key decision makers and consumers of health-care services is expected to assist health-care professionals and managers ensure that their practice reflects best available evidence. The final section of this chapter will review the evidence and discuss the guidelines regarding exercise for nonspecific LBP. Acute and chronic LBP will be discussed in terms of understanding: (1) how the condition became chronic and (2) whether the acute phase was managed appropriately. Moreover, all patients with chronic LBP will have recurrent episodes of acute LBP, which may be the time at which they seek professional care. Therefore, practitioners must understand the role of exercise in all phases of nonspecific LBP.

For a significant *acute* back injury (where pain and injury are related) it is reasonable to reduce activity, treat the pain (e.g., with analgesic medication and/or a physical modality such as ice) and be guided by pain intensity and duration as normal activity is resumed (1–2 days). However, the period of inactivity should be limited by time, not pain. An early return to normal activities should be encouraged and expected. *Any advice to rest must be accompanied by advice on activity resumption.*

For *chronic* or *recurrent* LBP, this approach is inappropriate and could be harmful. Pain is not indicative of ongoing tissue injury and is likely to persist; therefore, it cannot be used to guide the amount of activity. However, practitioners must be sensitive to the amount of pain and to the effect of that pain on the individual's psychological and physical state. Measurement of pain and disability due to LBP, using reliable and valid assessment tools, is an essential component of LBP management. *You can't manage what you don't measure.* This does not imply that practitioners should focus on pain and pain behavior. It does mean that practitioners should acknowledge the presence of pain; address misconceptions or fears about pain, tissue injury; and activity, and motivate patients to resume appropriate activity.

Exercise for Acute Low Back Pain

Acute nonspecific LBP is defined as symptoms that are less than 6 weeks in duration, with no evidence of serious pathology or nerve root irritation. The history, rather than the physical examination, provides the most useful categorization information to the clinician (3, 53). Some investigative teams have examined the effects of rest, exercise, education, and other interventions in individuals with acute LBP (54–56), while others have conducted systematic or critical reviews of the evidence (57–60).

The AHCPR guidelines were published in 1994. They contain three recommendations against the use of bed rest for acute LBP (two of which were supported by moderate evidence) and six recommendations regarding exercise for acute LBP (all of which were supported by limited or no research evidence). The recommendations and the evidence that supports them are as follows.

1. Low-stress aerobic exercise can help prevent debilitation due to inactivity and may help patients return to their highest level of function that is possible for their circumstances. *Strength of evidence: Limited (at least one adequate scientific study).*
2. Aerobic (endurance) exercise programs (walking, biking, or swimming) minimally stress the back can be started during the first 2 weeks for most patients with acute low back problems. *Strength of evidence: No research basis.*
3. Conditioning exercises for trunk muscles (especially back extensors) that gradually increase in duration are helpful for patients with acute back pain. *Strength of evidence: Limited (at least one adequate scientific study).*
4. Back-specific exercises performed on machines provide no benefit over traditional exercises. *Strength of evidence: No research basis.*
5. Stretching exercises (for back muscles) are not recommended. *Strength of evidence: No research basis.*
6. Exercises using quotas yield better outcomes than exercises using pain as a guide to progression. *Strength of evidence: Limited (at least one adequate scientific study).*

Thus, there is consensus and evidence that rest is detrimental for LBP. Based on that evidence, it seems reasonable to believe that exercise is beneficial for LBP. However, the guideline recommendations regarding exercise are primarily based on consensus rather than evidence. Subsequent systematic reviews (57–59) and a report from the International Paris Task Force (61) do not support the use of specific exercise regimens in acute LBP, based on available evidence. Faas et al. (59) identified four randomized controlled trials on acute LBP that met the criteria for inclusion in their systematic review. They reported that the trials with the highest method score reported no efficacy of flexion or extension exercises. For example, Detorri et al. (45) compared outcomes in 149 individuals with LBP assigned to a trunk flexion exercise group, a trunk extension exercise group, or a no exercise group. They reported no differences in outcomes (impairment, pain, and disability) at 8 weeks between the exercise groups. Moreover, there were no differences in recurrence rates between any of the groups at 6 and 12 months. This is a finding that questions the value of exercise in preventing LBP, albeit evidence suggests that physical activity mediates disability due to LBP (62).

In a later (2000) Cochrane review, Van Tulder (63) reported that when exercise therapy for LBP was compared to inactive treatment and other active treatments, there was strong evidence showing no difference in effectiveness. Effectiveness was judged on the basis of reduction in pain intensity, an increase in functional status, overall improvement, and return to work.

Although specific exercises have not clearly been shown to be useful, it is recommended to continue usual daily activity (54). The U.K. guidelines assert that there are "generally consistent findings in the majority of acceptable studies . . ." that ". . . advise to continue ordinary activity can provide for a *faster* symptomatic recovery from an acute episode. . . ."

The majority of people with nonspecific LBP are expected to recover within days or weeks, regardless of management strategy. Analgesics and anti-inflammatory medications are appropriate to control symptoms and allow people to remain reasonably active. An important component of acute care is to provide reassurance, promote self-care, and identify individuals at risk of disability. The New Zealand guidelines suggest that a preliminary screening for psychosocial yellow flags is appropriate at the time of initial presentation. Others suggest the screening should be used for those individuals with LBP who still have significant pain and disability after 4 weeks. Finally, excess disability can result from the attitude and beliefs of the treatment provider as well as those of the patient. "Reliance on a narrow medical model of pain; discouragement of self care strategies and failure to instruct the patient in self management; sanctioning of disability and not providing interventions that will improve function; and over-investigation and perpetuation of belief in the 'broken part hypothesis'" will contribute to chronic disabling LBP (31). The "broken part hypothesis" is the belief that part of the spine is actually broken and therefore needs a definitive medical or surgical "fix."

Exercise for Chronic Low Back Pain

Chronic nonspecific LBP is characterized by the persistence of symptoms beyond 12 weeks. However, with the exception of sharing persistent symptom duration, individuals with chronic LBP are characterized by heterogeneity. The majority of individuals with chronic and persistent symptoms of LBP do not seek health care but, in fact, continue to work and are generally not distressed about their back. Those who do seek professional care vary widely in terms of their total duration of symptoms, the severity of symptoms, the level of disability, distress, and overall physical condition resulting from those symptoms. Clearly, the approach to management has to be individualized, holistic, and rational, with consideration given to biological, psychological, and sociological factors.

At present, there are no government-sponsored clinical guidelines that address the assessment and management of chronic LBP. However, in the U.K., the Clinical Standards Advisory Group (4) has suggested that as LBP becomes chronic, psychological factors become more important and physical management alone should be avoided in favor of active exercise and multidisciplinary rehabilitation based on a biopsychosocial model. The 2000 report from the International Paris Task Force on Back Pain (61) recommends the prescription of physical, therapeutic, or recreational exercise in cases of chronic nonspecific back pain.

A number of randomized controlled trials and systematic reviews have addressed exercise and activity in individuals with chronic nonspecific LBP. The trials and reviews suggest that exercise and activity are beneficial for individuals with LBP as they can reduce the perception of pain and enhance the sense of well-being. It is less clear whether the type, intensity, frequency, or duration of exercise or activity is important. The Paris Task Force recommends that exercise programs should combine strength training, stretching, and/or fitness. But perhaps the most effective exercise or activity regimen is the one the individual actually performs.

Individuals with LBP contend with barriers to, and motivators of, physical activity similar to individuals in the general population (e.g., lack of time, inclement weather, family commitments) (64). However, it is interesting that back problems are identified as both barriers to, and motivators of, activity. In a qualitative study, Keen and colleagues (64) interviewed 27 individuals who were participants in a randomized control trial of a progressive exercise program. He reported that some individuals believed that being more physical helped ease their back pain and made them feel better. They were worried about stopping exercise for fear that their back pain would return. Others did not exercise on a regular basis but resumed exercise when reminded by their back pain. Still others avoided physical activity for fear of aggravating of their LBP. Although all participants identified the avoidance of some physical activity (e.g., lifting, gardening), not all were fearful or anxious about such activity. It appears that those individuals not fearful or anxious about physical activity reported that their confidence was restored over time through: (1) reassurance and advice from health professionals; (2) modifying the way an activity was done (e.g., less vigorous); and (3) a progressive exercise program (64). It appears that a change in behavior led to a change in belief about the ability to be active.

Participation in exercise/activity is essential if benefits are to accrue, whether those benefits are physical or attitudinal. Friedrich and colleagues (65) conducted a double-blind randomized study and evaluated the effect of a motivation program on exercise compliance (adherence) and disability. Ninety-three patients with LBP were randomly assigned to either a standard exercise program (n = 49) group or a combined exercise and motivation group (n = 44). The exercise program included individual submaximal gradually increased training sessions. Each patient was prescribed 10 sessions that each lasted about 25 minutes. The specific exercises were aimed at "improving spinal mobility, as well as trunk and lower limb muscle length, force, endurance, and coordination, thereby restoring normal function." The flexibility exercises for the trunk and lower limbs preceded the strengthening exercises for the trunk. The motivation program consisted of five sessions that included counseling, providing information about LBP and exercise, reinforcement, forming a treatment contract between patient and therapist, and keeping an exercise diary.

The combined exercise and motivation group increased their rate of attendance and reduced their level of disability and pain in the short term (4 and 12 months). However, there was no difference in exercise adherence in the long term. Long-term adherence to exercise is an acknowledged problem in the general population and is no different for individuals with LBP. Exercise benefits may not be immediate or even apparent for individuals with LBP, and recurrence of LBP is inevitable, so it is hardly surprising that adherence to exercise is problematic. Encouraging and facilitation of a more active lifestyle may be more beneficial for these individuals than prescribing a specific exercise regimen that is not performed. And the fact that there is no evidence that any specific regimen is more beneficial than another supports this position. There is some evidence that supervised activity is more effective than nonsupervised activity (55–56). However, the mechanisms through which supervision is effective are not established and may not be as obvious as they seem. Although supervision ensures that the prescribed exercises and activities are carried out, the nonspecific effects (e.g., reduction of anxiety) cannot be ruled out.

A number of studies have shown that the exercise groups do better than the control groups. However, there was no clear indication that any specific exercise regimen was superior. The Paris Task Force reviewed 10 scientifically rigorous randomized control trials of exercise that studied exercise for chronic LBP. The patient groups did better than control groups in terms of functional improvement in seven of the 10 trials. However, the regimens were characterized by variability of type, intensity, and duration. Moreover, some treatment programs included additional components such as education and/or behavior modification. For example, Frost et al. (55) tested a supervised general fitness program. Eighty-one individuals with chronic LBP were randomly assigned to either a fitness program group or a control group. Both groups were taught exercises and attended an educational program about LBP. The exercise group also attended eight sessions of a supervised fitness program extending over 4 weeks. Cognitive behavioral principles and a normal model of human behavior rather than a disease model was followed. Participants were encouraged to compare themselves to sports participants who had been laid off from training and who needed to get back to previous activity levels. They were also reminded that unaccustomed exercise might lead to muscle aches, and that pain and injury (hurt and harm) were not synonymous. Finally, participants were encouraged to improve their own performance record (not compete with others) and to complete an activity diary. The fitness program is included in Table 11.3. A mean reduction of 7.7% (pain and disability) was obtained in the exercise group compared to a 2.4% reduction in the control group. This difference was statistically significant and was maintained at the 2-year follow-up. However, the authors note that the confidence interval of the differences between groups was large, indicating a wide variation in treatment effect. Moreover, the use of percentage change can bias results in favor of individuals who have an initial low level of pain and disability. Therefore, it is not possible to determine from the article whether those who responded optimally were in fact those with a relatively low level of pain and disability at baseline.

Table 11.3. Fitness Program Circuit of Exercise

1. Static cycling. Gradually increase resistance, not speed.
2. Free arm weights while in lying. Increase and record weight.
3. Alternate knee raise while in standing (right knee toward left hand and v.v. Progress by lifting legs higher toward opposite elbow.
4. Repeated sit-to-stand.
5. Press-ups against wall, progressing through half press-ups to full press-ups on a mat.
6. Bridging.
7. Step-ups.
8. Medicine ball lifts while in lying.
9. Jogging on a bouncer.
10. Rounding and hollowing back in four-point kneeling.
11. Walking—back and forth between two markers on the floor. Gradually increase speed.
12. Arm raising while in standing, gradually increase speed.
13. Straight leg lifting while in lying.
14. Abdominal crunch while in lying.
15. Skipping with a rope.

Participants record the number of repetitions or weights used as appropriate.

The studies suggest that when comparing relatively active and relatively passive intervention, the active intervention is more effective. However, in a recent study, Mannion and colleagues (66) compared three active therapies for chronic low back pain. One hundred and forty eight participants were randomly assigned to (1) an active physiotherapy program, (2) a muscle-reconditioning program using training devices, and (3) a low-impact aerobics program. Participants attended their program twice a week for 3 months. All programs led to a reduction in pain and disability that was maintained at 6 months. There were no differences between groups, suggesting a lack of treatment specificity.

The studies suggest that the specific type of exercise or exercise regimen is much less important than once thought. Although this notion may be an anathema to traditional thinking clinicians who are entrenched in a narrow structurally focused biomedical (impairment) model, it is less surprising to those who recognize the biopsychosocial nature of chronic LBP. Exercises targeted at a specific biological or structural impairment may affect changes in impairment, but the actual impairment may contribute relatively little to the individual's LBP problem. Although speculative at present, it is plausible to suggest that exercise is beneficial for those with chronic LBP because it reduces psychosocial distress (40), leads to improvement in mood, reduces anxieties about the LBP, and changes the perception of self as disabled. Thus, the primary benefits of exercise or activity for individuals with chronic LBP are central rather than peripheral or structural.

Summary

The title of Waddell's recent book, *The Back Pain Revolution*, captures the profound change in the conceptualization and thus assessment and management of LBP (17). Recognition of a broad psychosocial model of health, the positive role of activity, the reliance on clinical evidence, and the application of clinical guidelines has the potential to transform the assessment and management of LBP into one that has a more rational basis (67). Primary management of LBP must include education and advice on staying active. The approach should be individualized, holistic, and rational, with consideration given to biological, psychological, and sociological factors.

Clearly, it is not possible to recommend evidence-based specific exercises or activity regimens for individuals with nonspecific LBP. However, it is possible to recommend exercise and activity guidelines. The Paris Task Force (61) recommends exercise programs that should combine strength training, stretching, and/or fitness. Thus, the exercise and activity principles are essentially no different from those applied to individuals without LBP. Perhaps the enigma of LBP is the fact that there is no enigma after all.

EDUCATION AND COUNSELING

A myriad of personal, physical, and psychosocial factors are associated with the presence and impact of LBP. This is evidence of the multidimensional nature of the problem. Personal factors associated with LBP include age and gender, some anthropometric characteristics (e.g., height and body build), spinal abnormalities, and previous history of low back problems. Previous history is one of the most reliable predictors of subsequent LBP (68). None of the foregoing factors are modifiable, whereas other personal risk factors such as overweight/obesity, physical fitness, and smoking can be modified (68). In a 1-year longitudinal survey of 2715 adults, Croft et al. (69) reported that poor general health was the strongest predictor for a new episode of LBP. However, he also noted that self-reported low levels of physical activity were not consistently linked with subsequent LBP.

A number of social or work-related factors are also associated with LBP. These include physical factors such as heavy physical work, lifting and forceful movements, awkward postures, and whole body vibration. Work-related risk factors account for 28 to 50 percent of the low back problem in the adult population (68).

Although there is no evidence to suggest that psychological factors predict the initial occurrence of LBP, these factors do predict the impact of LBP and the response to treatment. Therefore, practitioners need to understand and address such treatment confounders. Excessive attention to the biological domain at the expense of psychological and sociological domains is destined to lead to treatment failure and frustration for both patient and practitioner. Factors that are predictive of disability or poor outcome include depressed mood, negative or passive coping strategies, and fear of pain and reinjury (18). Social factors predictive of negative outcome include dissatisfaction with current work, low educational level, and solicitous behavior of significant others (18).

CASE STUDY

Mr. A. is a 40-year-old, male university professor with a 10-year history of recurrent back pain. His first episode of back pain occurred when he was helping a friend move furniture. He was unable to work for 2 weeks following that incident. Since then, he has frequent "grumbling" backache. He has also had about six episodes of acute back pain over the last 10 years that have each significantly disrupted his activity for at least 1 week. These episodes usually seem to coincide with relatively busy times at work. Years ago, he was advised by a physician to "take it easy" because of his back. He followed that advice but is concerned that his back is getting worse and he is able to tolerate a decreasing amount of physical activity. Mr. A. has been referred for assessment and an exercise program.

CLINICAL EXAMINATION

The interview showed Mr. A. denied recent weight loss, severe night-time pain, bowel and bladder problems, or any other "red flags" indicative of a potentially serious condition. His physical examination revealed no other medical complications. He describes his back pain as "2" on average, and "5" at worst, on a 0–10 numerical rating scale. His pain never radiates below the buttocks. He scored 4 out of 24 on the Roland and Morris Disability Scale, indicative of a relatively minor level of disability. His performance on the Time and Distance tasks on the Simmonds Performance Battery (21) is indicative of mild to moderate compromise in physical function. He expresses some concern about participating in an exercise program because he doesn't want to hurt his back.

RESTING DATA

ECG showed normal sinus rhythm with a heart rate of 72 bpm and a blood pressure of 134/80 mm Hg.

EXERCISE RESPONSE

Mr A. performed a modified Bruce Protocol (2-minute stages), and the test was terminated after 6 minutes due to fatigue.

INTERPRETATION

The results of the interview, clinical examination, and exercise test suggest that Mr. A. does not have serious spinal or visceral pathology. The presentation is suggestive of simple, nonspecific mechanical back pain that has led to mild physical dysfunction. Noteworthy is the comment made by Mr. A. that he is following the advice given by a physician years ago, that he should "take it easy" because of his back. The implied belief therefore is that activity is potentially harmful to the back. This belief has led Mr. A. to reduce his level of activity. Of concern is the fact that it appears he is gradually becoming intolerant of activity.

CLINICAL IMPLICATIONS

Several clinical implications arise from this scenario. First and foremost is the recognition that Mr. A. does not have any serious pathological "red flags" that are leading to his symptoms. A second important piece of clinical information is the recognition that although Mr. A. has some concern about his back problem, especially in relation to activity, he does not exhibit any serious psychosocial issues, or "yellow flags," that are risk factors for chronic incapacity. He is well educated, employed, and has only mild physical dysfunction and activity intolerance despite a long history of back pain.

Clearly, there are no contraindications to exercise and activity for Mr. A. In fact, there is a potential for improvement in Mr. A.'s activity tolerance if he participates in an exercise and conditioning program. The first step should be to address the inaccurate belief that Mr. A. has about the negative effect of activity on back pain. In regards to exercise participation, general advice about exercise is probably adequate. That is, he should be advised about warm-up exercises, flexibility and strengthening exercises, and aerobic-type activities. Mr. A. should be advised about pacing himself and also to participate in those aerobic-type activities (e.g., walking, cycling, swimming) that he most prefers because this will increase the likelihood that he will participate in that activity.

Finally, Mr. A. should be advised on how to deal with future acute episodes of back pain. Key elements of this advice are as follows. (1) Exacerbation is likely to occur; it is also likely to be temporary, and he can "handle" it. (2) Temporary relief of symptoms can be aided by the application of ice or over-the-counter analgesics. (3) Temporary modification of activity is acceptable but early resumption of activity is important. (4) If a totally "new set of symptoms" occurs (e.g., red flags, or pain that is very different from "usual" either in quality or distribution), then he should seek a medical opinion.

References

1. Pither CE, Nicholas MK. The identification of iatrogenic factors in the development of chronic pain syndromes: abnormal treatment behaviour? In: Bond MR, Charlton JE, Woolf CJ, eds. Proceedings of the VIth World Congress on Pain. Netherlands: Elsevier Science, 1991:429–434.
2. Wahlgren DR, Atkinson JH, Epping-Jordan JE, et al. One-year follow-up of first onset low back pain. Pain 1997;73: 213–221.
3. Bigos S, Bowyer O, Braen G, et al. Acute Low Back Problems in Adults. Clinical Practice Guideline No. 14. AHCPR Publication No. 95-0642. Rockville, MD: Agency for Health Care Policy and Research, Public Health Service, U.S. Department of Health and Human Services, 1994.
4. CSAG (Clinical Standards Advisory Group). Back Pain: Report of a CSAG Committee on Back Pain, HMSO, London, 1994.
5. World Health Organization (1980) International classification of impairments, disabilities and handicaps. WHO, Geneva.
6. Nagi SZ. Disability concepts revisited: implications for prevention. In: AM Pope, AR Tarlov (Eds.) Disability in America: Toward a National Agenda for Prevention. Washington, D.C.: Division of Health Promotion and Disease Prevention, Institute of Medicine, National Academy Press. 1991: 309–327.
7. Andersson GBJ. The epidemiology of spinal disorders In: JW Frymoyer Ed. The Adult Spine: Principles and Practice 2nd ed, Lippencott-Raven Philadelphia, 1997:93–142.
8. Walsh K, Cruddas M, Coggon D. Low back pain in eight areas of Britain. Journal of Epidemiology and Community Health 1992;46:227–230.
9. Papergeorgiou AC, Croft PR, Ferry S, et al. Estimating the prevalence of low back pain in the general population. Evidence from the South Manchester back pain survey. Spine 1995;20:1889–1894.
10. Skovron ML, Szpalski M, Nordin M, et al. Sociocultural factors and back pain. A population based study in Belgian adults. Spine 1994;19:129–137.
11. Mason V. The prevalence of back pain in Great Britain. Office of Population Censuses and Surveys, Social Survey Division. HMSO, London, 1994:1–24.
12. Croft P, editor Low Back Pain. Oxford: Radcliffe Medical Press, 1997.
13. Von Korff M, Dworkin SF, Le Resche LA, et al. An epidemiologic comparison of pain complaints. Pain 1988;32:173–183.
14. Frymoyer JW, Durret CL. The economics of spinal disorders. In: JW Frymoyer Ed. The Adult Spine: Principles and Practice 2nd ed, Lippencott-Raven Philadelphia, 1997:143–150.
15. Waddell G Low back pain: a twentieth century health care enigma. Spine 1996;21:2820–2825.
16. Cherkin DC, Deyo RA, Loeser JD, et al. An international comparison of back surgery rates. Spine 1994;19:1201–1206.
17. Waddell G. The Back Pain Revolution. Edinburgh, Churchill Livingstone, 1998.
18. Wennburg JE. Practice variations and the challenge to leadership. Spine 1996;21:910–916.
19. Vlayen JWS, Linton SJ. Fear-avoidance and its consequences in chronic musculoskeletal pain:a state of the art. Pain 2000; 85: 317–332.
20. Mellin G. Correlations of spinal mobility with degree of chronic low back pain after correction for age and anthropometric factors. Spine 1987;12:464–468.
21. Simmonds MJ, Olson SL, Jones S, et al. Psychometric characteristics and clinical usefulness of physical performance tests in patients with low back pain. Spine 1998;23:2412–2421.
22. Jensen MP, Karoly P. Self-report scales and procedures for assessing pain in adults. In: Turk DC, Melzack R (eds) Handbook of pain assessment, Guilford Press New York. 1992: 135–151.
23. Simmonds MJ, Claveau Y. Measures of pain and physical function in patients with low back pain. Physiother Theory Prac 1997;13:53–65.
24. Jette AM, Smith K, Haley SM, et al. Physical therapy episodes of care for patients with low back pain. Phys Ther 1994; 74:101–115.
25. Lee CE, Simmonds MJ, Novy DM, et al. A comparison of self-report and clinician measured physical function among patients with low back pain. Archives of Physical Medicine and Rehabilitation, 2000. In press
26. Fairbank JCT, Couper J, Davies JB, et al. The Oswestry low back pain disability questionnaire. Physiotherapy 1980; 66:271–273.
27. Roland M, Morris R. A study of the natural history of back pain. Part I: Development of a reliable and sensitive measure of disability in low-back pain. Spine 1983;8:141–144.
28. Ware J, Sherbourne C. The MOS 36-item Short Form Health Survey (SF-36). Med Care1992;30:473.Van Tulder MW.

Evidence-based physical therapy for low back pain: A promising future. Dutch Journal of Physical Therapy 1999; 109: 29–32.
29. Marras WS, Wongsamm PE. Flexibility and velocity of normal and impaired lumbar spine. Arch Phys Med Rehabil 1986;67:213–217.
30. Simmonds MJ, Olson S, Jones SC, et al. Disability prediction in patients with back pain using performance based models. Joint Meeting North American Spine Society and American Pain Society, Charleston South Carolina, April 26–29, 1998.
31. New Zealand acute low back pain guide, and Guide in assessing psychosocial yellow flags in acute low back pain. January 1997. Accident Rehabilitation and Compensation Insurance Corporation of New Zealand and the National Health Committee, Wellington, NZ.
32. Cedraschi C, Nordin M, Nachemson AL, et al. Health care providers should use a common language in relation to low back pain patients. Baillieres Clin Rheumatol 1998;12:1–15.
33. Grazier KL, Holbrokk TL, Kelsey JL, et al., eds. The frequency of occurrence, impact, and cost of musculoskeletal conditions in the United States. Chicago: American Academy of Orthopedic Surgeons, 1984.
34. Nachemson AL. Exercise, fitness and back pain. In: Scientific Proceedings of the International Conference on Exercise, Fitness and Health. Champaign, Ill: Human Kinetics Publishers Inc, 1988.
35. Spitzer W, LeBlanc F, Dupuis M, et al. Scientific approach to the assessment and management of activity-related spinal disorders. Spine 1987;7S:S1–S55.
36. Selim AJ, Ren SR, Fincke G, et al. The importance of radiating leg pain in assessing health outcomes among patients with low back pain: results from the Veterans Health Study. Spine 1998;23: 470–474.
37. Simmonds MJ, Lee CE, Jones S. Pain distribution and physical function in patients with low back pain. 13th International Congress of World Confederation for Physical Therapy, May 23–28, Yokohama Japan, 1999.
38. ACSM Guidelines 6th edition 2000 Lippincott Williams and Wilkins Philadelphia pp 33–114.
39. Wittink H, Hoskins MT, Wagner A, et al. Deconditioning in patients with chronic low back pain: fact or fiction? Spine 2000;25:2221–2228.
40. Simmonds MJ, Kumar, S. and Lechelt, E. Psychosocial factors in low back pain: Causes or consequences? Disabil Rehabil 1996;18:161–168.
41. Protas EJ. Physical activity and low back pain. In: Pain 1999 An updated review M.Max (ed) IASP Press Seattle, 1999:145–152.
42. U.S. Department of Health and Human Services. Physical Activity and Health: A report of the surgeon general. Atlanta, GA: U.S. Department of Health and Human Services, Centers for Disease Control and Prevention, National Center for Chronic Disease Prevention and Health Promotion, 1996.
43. Helewa A, Goldsmith CH, Lee P, et al. Does strengthening the abdominal muscles prevent low back pain—a randomized controlled trial. J. Rheumatol 1999;26:1808–1815.
44. Jette AM, Smith K, Haley SM, et al. Physical therapy episodes of care for patients with low back pain. Phys Ther 1994; 74:101–115.
45. Dettori JR, Bullock SH, Sutlive TG, et al. The effects of spinal flexion and extension exercise and their associated postures in patients with acute low back pain. Spine 1995;20:2303–2312.
46. Battie MC, Bigos SJ, Fisher LD, et al. The role of spinal flexibility in back pain complaints within industry. Spine 1990; 15:768–773.
47. Waddell G. A new clinical model for the treatment of low back pain. Spine 1987;12:632–644.
48. Nelson RM, NIOSH Low back atlas of standardized tests and measures, National Technical Information Service, Springfield, VA, 1988.
49. Pope MH. A critical evaluation of functional muscle testing. In Weinstein JN (Ed): Clinical Efficacy and Outcome in the Diagnosis and Treatment of Low Back Pain. Raven Press, New York 1992:101–113.
50. Newton M, Thow M, Somerville D, et al. Trunk strength testing with Iso-machines. Part 2: Experimental evaluation of the Cybex II Back testing system in normal subjects and patients with chronic low back pain. Spine 1993;18(7):812–824.
51. Mayer TG, Gatchel RJ. Functional restoration for spinal disorders: The Sports Medicine Approach. Philadelphia: Lea and Febiger, 1988.
52. Protas EJ. Aerobic exercise in the rehabilitation of individuals with chronic low back pain: a review. Critical reviews in Physical and Rehabilitation Medicine 1996;8:283–295.
53. Jackson DA, Llewelyn-Philips H, Klaber-Moffett J. Categorization of back pain patients using an evidence based approach. Musculoskeletal Management. 1996;2:39–46.
54. Malmivaara A, Hakkinen U, Aro T, et al. The treatment of acute low back pain—bed rest, exercises, or ordinary activity? New Eng J Med 1995;332:351–355.
55. Frost H, Lamb SE, Klaber-Moffett JA, et al. A fitness programme for patients with chronic low back pain: 2-year follow-up of a randomized controlled trial. Pain 1998;75: 273–279.
56. Tortensen TA, Ljungggren AE, Meen HD, et al. Efficiency and costs of medical exercise therapy, conventional physiotherapy, and self-exercise in patients with chronic low back pain. Spine 1998;23:2616–2624.
57. Maher C, Latimer J, Refshauge K. Prescription of activity for low back pain: what works? Australian Journal of Physiotherapy 1999;45:121–132.
58. Faas A, Battie MC, Malmivaara A. Exercises: which ones are worth trying for which patients and when? Spine 1996;21: 2874–2879.
59. Nordin M, Campello M. Physical therapy. Exercises and the modalities: when, what and why? Neurologic Clinics 1999; 17:76–89.
60. Abenhaim L, Rossignol M, Valat JP, et al. The role of activity in the therapeutic management of back pain. Report of the International Paris Task Force on Back Pain Spine 2000:25(4 Suppl):1S–33S.
61. Videman T, Sarna S, Battie MC, et al. The long-term effects of physical loading and exercise lifestyles on back-related symptoms, disability, and spinal pathology among men. Spine 1995;20:699–709.
62. van Tulder MW, Malmivaara A, Esmail R, et al. Exercise therapy for low back pain (Cochrane Review). The Cochrane Library, Issue 2,2000. Oxford:Update Software.
63. Keen S, Dowell AC, Hurst K, et al. Individuals with low back pain: how do they view physical activity? Family Practice 1999;16:39–45.
64. Friedrich M, Gittler G, Halberstadt Y, et al. Combined exercise and motivation program: effect on the compliance and

level of disability of patients with chronic low back pain: a randomized controlled trial. Arch Phys Med Rehabil 1998; 79(5):475–87.

65. Turk DC. The role of demographic and psychosocial factors in transition from acute to chronic pain. In Jensen TS, Turner JA, Wiesenfield-Hallin Z. (Eds.). Proceedings of the 8th World Congress on Pain, Progress in Pain Research and Management, IASP Press, Seattle, 1997;185–213.
66. Mannion AF, Muntener M, Taimela S, et al. A randomized clinical trial of three active therapies for chronic low back pain. Spine 1999;24:2435–2448.
67. Simmonds MJ, Harding V, Watson PJ, et al. Physical therapy assessment: expanding the model. In: Proceedings of the 9th World Congress on Pain. Progress in Pain Research and Management. Vol 16. Eds Devor M, Rowbotham MC, Wiesenfield-Hallin, IASP Press, Seattle, 2000:1013–1030.
68. Shelerud, R. Epidemiology of Occupational Low Back Pain. In: Occupational Medicine: State of the Art Reviews. Philadelphia, PA: Hanley and Belfus 1998:1–22.
69. Croft PR, Papageorgiou AC, Thomas E, et al. Short-term physical risk indicators for new episodes of low back pain. Spine 1999;24:1556–1561.

CHAPTER **12**

OSTEOPOROSIS

David L. Nichols, Marianna Horea, and Elaine Jackson

EPIDEMIOLOGY AND PATHOPHYSIOLOGY

Osteoporosis is the most common disease that affects the skeleton. It is estimated that between 7 and 10 million women in the United States currently have osteoporosis (1), although the estimate varies based on which skeletal sites are measured to diagnose osteoporosis. In addition, although osteoporosis is thought of primarily as a disease of women, an estimated 2 million men in the United States have osteoporosis, and 3 million more may be at risk (2). Approximately 1.3 million osteoporotic fractures occur in the U.S. each year, and of these, half are spinal fractures and a quarter are hip fractures. Fractures of the hip and spine result in disability, decreased independence and quality of life, and increased risk of death (3). A 50-year-old woman has a lifetime fracture risk of 54%. Her risk of sustaining a spinal fracture is 32–35%, 16–18% for a hip fracture, and 15–17% for a wrist fracture. The majority of hip fractures occur as a consequence of traumatic falls, making falls the number one cause of accidental death in people over the age of 75. There are approximately 50,000 deaths each year as a result of complications from hip fracture. Although men are at a lower risk for sustaining a hip fracture than women, the mortality associated with hip fracture is higher in elderly men compared to women (4). The current cost of osteoporosis to the health-care system is estimated at $10–15 billion per year (5, 6), with approximately 20% of that cost attributable to fractures in men. This cost is expected to rise to $30 billion by the year 2020.

Definition and Classification

Osteoporosis, often called "brittle-bone disease," is defined as a systemic skeletal disease characterized by low bone mass and microarchitectural deterioration of bone tissue with a consequent increase in bone fragility and susceptibility to fracture (7). There are two categories of osteoporosis: primary osteoporosis and secondary osteoporosis (8). Primary osteoporosis is due to a disruption in the normal cycle of bone turnover. Postmenopausal osteoporosis (formerly known as Type I osteoporosis) is categorized as primary osteoporosis. Other types of primary osteoporosis include senile osteoporosis (formerly known as Type II osteoporosis) and idiopathic osteoporosis (8). Secondary osteoporosis occurs when bone loss is a consequence of diseases such as Cushing's disease, hyperthyroidism, and prolonged treatment with corticosteroids (8).

Bone Physiology

Bone tissue has three main functions. First, bones provide structural, mechanical, and protective support for soft tissues, serving as attachment points for skeletal muscle and acting as levers for locomotion. Second, the skeleton is responsible for maintaining calcium homeostasis, as well as serving as a storage site for phosphate, magnesium, potassium, and bicarbonate. Finally, the skeleton is the primary site of hemopoiesis (9).

There are two types of bone tissue, cortical bone and trabecular bone. Cortical bone, also known as compact bone, is found in the shafts of the long bones and comprises approximately 80% of the skeleton. Trabecular, or cancellous, bone constitutes the remaining 20% of the skeleton. Trabecular bone is arranged in a honeycomb pattern of trabeculae and is found in the flat bones, such as the pelvis and vertebral bodies, and in the ends of the long bones, such as the head and neck of the femur. Trabecular bone is more metabolically active than cortical bone and, therefore, is more sensitive to changes in biochemical, hormonal, and nutritional status. Because of this, trabecular bone is more susceptible to being lost and trabecular sites are typically where age-related losses in bone are first detected. It is for this reason that a majority of osteoporotic fractures occur in areas with a large proportion of trabecular bone: the lumbar spine, proximal hip (femoral neck and greater trochanter), and distal radius and ulna (10).

The adult skeleton is a dynamic organ that undergoes a constant process of resorption and deposition, referred to as remodeling. Remodeling serves to maintain the architecture and strength of the bone, maintain mineral homeostasis, and prevent fatigue damage. Remodeling is also important during periods of growth when the majority of adult bone mass is laid down (11). Bone remodeling should be distinguished from bone modeling. Modeling and remodeling often occur simultaneously, and distinctions between them are not always apparent, but in general, bone modeling refers to alterations in the shape of the bone such as changes in length. Bone modeling usually ceases around the age of 18–20 when the skeleton stops growing. Remodeling occurs throughout the life span (11).

Bone resorption is carried out by osteoclasts, large multinucleated cells originating from stem cells in the bone marrow. Resorption involves the dissolving of bone mineral by proteolytic enzymes and organic acids released from the osteoclasts. The result is a cavity of approximately 60 μm within the surface of the bone. The deposition of new bone matrix in the cavity created by the osteoclasts is carried out by osteoblasts. Bone matrix is composed of collagen fibers and calcium salts known as hydroxyapatite.

Osteoporosis results when the rate of bone resorption exceeds that of deposition. During young adulthood, these two processes are balanced, and bone loss is minimal or bone mass is maintained. During perimenopause, women lose bone mass at a rate of approximately 1% per year. At menopause, when ovarian function ceases, estrogen deficiency ensues and results in rapid bone loss for up to 5 years after menopause (12, 13). There also appears to be some age-related bone loss (approximately 0.5–1.0% per year) experienced by both men and women (13, 14), although the exact age of onset of this loss is not known. Osteoblasts seem to be more greatly affected by aging than osteoclasts, and thus, bone formation decreases more than bone resorption, resulting in this age-related bone loss (15).

Risk Factors and Pathophysiology

There are several risk factors associated with osteoporosis, some of which are immutable and others that may be modifiable. Immutable risk factors include family history of osteoporosis, gender, advanced age, and race. Risk factors that might be modifiable, to some extent, include dietary factors, physical activity, body weight, smoking, gonadal hormone status, and use of certain medications (16).

As with many diseases, including cancer and cardiovascular disease, osteoporosis tends to be genetically related. Peak bone density and/or rate of bone loss are dependent on genetic components as well as shared environmental factors. Women are at greater risk than men for developing osteoporosis. This is mostly due to the postmenopausal loss of estrogen, but is partly due to the facts that women tend to be less physically active than men, have a smaller bone size, and most women also have inadequate calcium intakes. It appears Caucasians and Asians may be at greater risk for osteoporosis, but this is debatable (17).

Dietary factors that can influence the risk of osteoporosis include inadequate calcium and vitamin D intake and excessive consumption of caffeine and alcohol. Adequate calcium intake is necessary for the attainment of peak bone mass as well as being effective in reducing postmenopausal bone loss. Vitamin D is required for calcium absorption from the gut and for the maintenance of bone calcium (18). Caffeine causes a short-term increase in urinary calcium loss and is associated with an increased risk of hip fracture in elderly women (19). Similarly, alcohol is associated with increased urinary loss of calcium, and excessive alcohol intake may reduce absorption of calcium from the intestine. Alcohol is also toxic to osteoblasts (20).

Body weight is directly correlated to bone density (21) and is the greatest determinant of bone density in adults (20). Smoking is associated with low bone mineral density (BMD), an increased risk of fracture (22), and is thought to interfere with estrogen metabolism (23). The gonadal hormones, particularly estrogen, are essential for maintaining bone mass. Estrogen directly affects bone turnover by binding to estrogen receptors on the osteoblasts. Estrogen also enhances calcium absorption from the intestines (18). Several medications, in particular the glucocorticoids, have adverse effects on the skeleton that include increased urinary excretion and decreased intestinal absorption of calcium, reduced levels of gonadal hormones, inhibition of osteoblast function, and increased bone resorption (18).

Several of these risk factors are interrelated. For example, peak bone mass is largely determined by genetic factors; however, failure to reach one's genetic potential is often the result of inadequate calcium intake and exercise (20). Also, risk of osteoporosis increases with advancing age, particularly after menopause in women, and an even greater risk is seen with early menopause, either natural or surgical. Postmenopausal bone loss is largely the result of estrogen deficiency, but hormone replacement therapy can dramatically attenuate postmenopausal bone loss.

CLINICAL EXERCISE PHYSIOLOGY

The primary purposes of acute exercise testing are typically to aid in the diagnoses of coronary artery disease (CAD) and/or to determine appropriate levels of exercise training. There are no specific studies regarding acute physiological responses to exercise in an osteoporotic population, but for those patients who can tolerate the exercise, there is no reason to believe their cardiovascular responses would be different from those individuals without osteoporosis. Osteoporosis can sometimes mask the presence of heart disease because it can prevent an individual from achieving the adequate heart rate and blood pressure necessary for accurate diagnoses. In addition, severe thoracic kyphosis can sometimes impair respiration and limit the test. Nonetheless, there are no specific recommendations from the American College of Sports Medicine that would suggest that osteoporosis is an absolute contraindication to exercise testing (24). If an exercise stress test is to be performed with an osteoporotic individual, one utilizing a cycle ergometer protocol would probably be the best choice, since that would involve the least trauma and impact on the bones. However, caution must still be taken when utilizing a cycle ergometer. An upright posture should be maintained by the patient at all times, as any sort of spinal flexion is contraindicated in people with osteoporosis. Treadmill protocols can be utilized, but a walking protocol is recommended, and care must be taken to ensure the patient does not trip or fall.

Chronic responses to exercise in the osteoporotic population and in postmenopausal women have been studied (25–30). The primary purpose of prescribing exercise for these populations is to increase, or at least maintain, BMD and to increase overall fitness and balance to aid in fall prevention. In this regard, the majority of studies have shown positive results. A number of studies with postmenopausal women have shown that exercise can increase bone density or prevent further bone loss when compared to nonexercising controls (27–29, 31, 32). However, these studies have also pointed out that exercise without concomitant estrogen replacement will generally result in further bone loss. There have been some studies that have shown that exercise alone will increase bone mass in postmenopausal women (27, 33), although the increases were greater when estrogen and exercise were used in combination.

Although research has been primarily directed toward the adult population, a recent review of the literature highlights the importance of exercise in establishing optimal levels of bone mineral during the growing years when bone modeling accompanies growth (34). Retrospective studies of children generally report a positive association between BMD and weight-bearing, but not non–weight-bearing, activities (35–37). Further, the timing of exercise intervention during childhood has been demonstrated to affect bone mineral status in adulthood. Female tennis and squash players who started their playing careers before or at menarche were found to have a two- to threefold greater dominant arm BMC than those who had started playing more than 15 years after menarche (38). This point is further illustrated by examining two separate studies on athletes. Courteix et al. (39) and Taaffe et al. (40) each examined BMD in gymnasts and controls. In the first study, gymnasts were prepubertal with an average age of 10.4 years and had been training for only 3 years. In the second study, gymnasts were 19.3 years of age and had been training for 12 years. Despite the 9 years of difference in training time of the gymnasts in the two studies, the percentage difference in BMD between gymnasts and controls was the same for both studies. Results from these studies would suggest that the optimal time to begin exercise training to increase BMD is before puberty.

There are a number of recent intervention studies in children and adolescents that point out the potential for exercise to increase bone mass (41–44). Participation in athletics also has the potential for increasing bone mineral density. A number of studies, both cross-sectional and longitudinal, have found positive effects for bone health from the training associated with sports participation (45–49). However, sufficient evidence does not exist to suggest that one type of exercise or athletic activity is better than another with regard to osteogenic effect. It does appear that those sports or exercises that involve a high degree of impact (gymnastics or volleyball) are more beneficial to bone than those without impact loading (swimming or cycling) (40, 45, 50).

PHARMACOLOGY

The majority of women diagnosed with osteoporosis, and postmenopausal women in general, take some form of calcium and vitamin D supplements. Other common drugs available, that have FDA approval for treatment or prevention of osteoporosis, include estrogen alone or in combination with progesterone, bisphosphates, calcitonin, and selective estrogen receptor modulators (SERMs). Other less common agents include isoflavones (natural and synthetic), sodium fluoride, and parathyroid hormone (see Table 12.1 for a complete list). Isoflavones are plant-derived compounds that have a chemical structure similar to estrogen and thus have physiological affects that may also be similar to estrogen. The effects of any of these drugs or nutrients on acute or chronic exercise responses have not been extensively studied. However, there is no clear reason why any of these agents would affect exercise responses, with the possible exception of estrogen. Estrogen (and its cousins the isoflavones) has acute vasodilator action and thus may alter responses to exercise during a treadmill test. Although this effect has been seen in studies using larger doses of estrogen (51), it has not been demonstrated with doses normally used in estrogen-replacement therapy (52).

PHYSICAL EXAMINATION

The physical assessment of the client with osteoporosis should include a detailed medical history, including information about all medications and supplements used by the client. A pain history also provides useful information along with a careful assessment of height and observation of posture.

Pain Assessment

Although osteoporosis frequently presents with no pain until a fracture has occurred (16), pain history is an important part of the physical examination of the client with osteoporosis. The most common fractures that occur in individuals with osteoporosis are hip, wrist, and vertebral fractures. Fractures of the hip and wrist are easily identified on x-rays and usually occur as a result of a fall. Vertebral fractures, however, often cannot be visualized on x-rays and frequently occur during routine daily activities such as lifting a grocery bag or sneezing. Sharp and persistent back pain may be the only physical finding to suggest vertebral fracture (16). Although a bone scan may be performed to confirm the fracture, the nature of the pain experienced and the circumstances leading up to the pain are often considered sufficient to make the diagnosis of vertebral fracture. History of any previous fractures should also be noted, along with the mechanics and circumstances leading up to these fractures.

Assessment of Stature

Loss of height that may range from 1 inch to as much as 4 or 5 inches is an important physical finding because a loss of height occurs with each spinal compression fracture sustained by the individual with osteoporosis. In a compression fracture of the vertebra, the bone within the vertebral body collapses, resulting in a loss of height of the vertebra. An individual can sustain multiple fractures to the same vertebra or fractures to multiple vertebra that can result in several inches of lost height. These compression fractures may be accompanied by severe pain or minimal pain that may be ignored by the individual. In any case, loss of height is always a significant finding and should be monitored closely. The use of a stature board allows precise measurement of height and is useful in monitoring changes.

Postural Assessment

Spinal compression fractures often occur specifically in the anterior portion of the vertebral body. When the anterior portion of the vertebral body collapses, the loss in anterior vertebral height results in a wedge-shaped vertebra (hence the name, wedge fracture). Wedge fractures cause a change in the overall curvature of the spine that is seen as an increased thoracic kyphosis, sometimes referred to as "dowager's hump." As the thoracic kyphosis progresses, the head is thrust forward and the ribs approach the pelvic bones, resulting in further loss of height. Additionally, as the kyphosis progresses, there is less room for lung expansion. If the kyphosis is severe enough, respiration will be affected. Degree of forward head, thoracic kyphosis, and lumbar lordosis should be noted in the postural assessment. Additionally, there are simple tools that can be used to obtain objective measurements of thoracic kyphosis and lumbar lordosis. A surveyor's flexicurve provides a simple, inexpensive method of assessing thoracic kyphosis and lumbar lordosis (53). The flexicurve is a plastic "ruler" that bends in one plane and holds its shape. It can be molded to a subject's spine, then lifted and laid on a ruled sheet to be traced. Objective measurements can then be obtained from the tracing. Accuracy and precision of the flexicurve, however, are somewhat limited.

MEDICAL AND SURGICAL TREATMENTS

All of the current drugs with an FDA approval for osteoporosis are considered antiresorptive drugs. They halt the loss of bone, or even increase bone mass, by inhibiting bone resorption, while bone formation remains the same. The majority of the drugs available are presented in Table 12.1. It must be pointed out, however, that all drug therapies approved by the FDA for treatment or prevention of osteoporosis are approved for use in postmenopausal women only. Estrogen replacement therapy (ERT) has been used for several years in the treatment and prevention of osteoporosis in postmenopausal women. Studies have shown that estrogen therapy can halt the loss of and often increase bone mass, but its effect on fracture risk is less well established (54–58). Estrogen use is contraindicated in women who are pregnant, have any history or suspected history of breast cancer, or have thrombo-

Table 12.1. Medical Therapies Available in the Treatment or Prevention of Osteoporosis

Drug Class	Name of Drug	Brand Name
Estrogens[1]	Estrone Sulfate	Ogen®
	Conjugated Estrogen	Premarin®
	Transdermal Estrogen	Estraderm®
	Estropipate	Ortho-Est®
	Esterified Estrogen	Estratab®
	Conjugated Estrogen +	Premphase®
	Medroxyprogestrone Acetate[2]	PremPro®
		Activella®
Calcitonin[3]	Synthetic Salmon Calcitonin	MiaCalcin®
		Calcimar®
Bisphosphonates	Alendronate[4]	Fosamax®
	Risedronate[4]	Actonel®
	Etidronate[5]	Didronel®
	Ibandronate[6]	
	Zolendronate	
	Tiludronate[6]	
	Pamidronate	Aredia®
SERMs	Raloxifene[7]	Evista®
	Tamoxifene	Nolvadex®
	Droloxifene[6]	
	Levormeloxifene	
Others	Isoflavones (natural flavonoids)	
	Tibolone or Ipriflavone (synthetic flavonoids)	
	Calcitriol[8]	
	Sodium Fluoride[9]	
	Parathyroid Hormone[7]	

[1]All estrogens have FDA approval for prevention of osteoporosis, but only Premarin® is approved for treatment.

[2]Premphase®, PremPro® and Activella® are estrogen and progesterone taken in combination; Premphase and PremPro are FDA approved for treatment of osteoporosis; Activella is approved for prevention.

[3]Both calcitonins are approved for prevention, but only MiaCalcin® is approved for treatment of osteoporosis.

[4]Alendronate and risedronate have FDA approval for both prevention and treatment of osteoporosis.

[5]Etidronate has FDA approval but not with an osteoporosis indication.

[6]In clinical trials for treatment or prevention of osteoporosis.

[7]FDA approved for prevention and treatment of osteoporosis.

[8]Calcitriol is a vitamin D metabolite with FDA approval, but not for osteoporosis.

[9]Approval pending for an osteoporosis indication.

embolic disorders. Side effects include breakthrough bleeding, breast tenderness, thrombophlebitis, and cramps. As many as 70% of women will discontinue estrogen therapy within a year (59). Dosages vary for estrogen depending on the exact type used but range from 0.3 to 2.5 mg, with 0.625 mg probably the most commonly prescribed for osteoporosis.

Calcitonin is a hormone used for calcium regulation by the body. Salmon calcitonin, either in an injectable or nasal spray preparation, has proved effective in both increasing low bone mass and decreasing fracture risk in postmenopausal women (60–63). Side effects are rare but may include headaches or flushing. The most common dosages are 200 IU for the nasal spray preparation and 100 IU for the injectable form.

Bisphosphonates are one of the newer classes of drugs now being used in the prevention and treatment of osteoporosis. They are probably the most powerful of the antiresorptive drugs available. Several different bisphosphonates have been shown to be effective in reducing bone loss and decreasing fracture risk in postmenopausal women (64–69). Recent studies have also indicated that combining estrogen and bisphosphonates may be better than either treatment alone (70). Gastrointestinal problems may occur with improper administration of the drug (71), and contraindications to bisphosphonate use include esophageal stricture, difficulty swallowing, active esophageal ulcer, esophagitis, or renal insufficiency or failure (71). Bisphosphonates are typically given in either 5 or 10 mg doses.

Selective estrogen receptor modulators (SERMs) are another antiresorptive agent under investigation for use in osteoporosis. Raloxifene has FDA approval for use in prevention of osteoporosis, but there are very little data on other SERMs with regard to their effects on low bone mass. The advantages of SERMs include favorable effects on bone and lipids, much like estrogen, but they do not have the stimulatory effect on breast or endometrial tissue seen with estrogen (72). The increases in BMD that are shown when taking raloxifene or other SERMs are generally less than seen with estrogen (73, 74), and unlike ERT, SERMs appear to have no beneficial effect on HDL cholesterol (73, 74). However, for the woman with a history of breast cancer, SERMs would be a good alternative to ERT. Raloxifene is commonly prescribed in 60 mg tablets, and side effects include hot flashes and leg cramps.

The effectiveness of calcium and/or vitamin D supplementation on increasing bone density in postmenopausal women is unclear. Some studies have shown increases in BMD (75, 76), while others have shown no effect (77, 78). The number of years past menopause may play a role in the effectiveness of calcium and/or vitamin D (79). An important thing to consider with regard to calcium and vitamin D is that the vast majority of studies investigating other therapeutic modalities for osteoporosis (bisphosphonates, estrogen, exercise) have given calcium and/or vitamin D supplementation to the treatment groups. Thus, the effectiveness of these therapies may be reduced without the inclusion of calcium or vitamin D supplementation.

Surgery is often necessary to repair the fractures that occur as a result of osteoporosis. However, surgical interventions aimed at preventing or treating the disease itself are virtually unavailable. The one possible exception is the use of acrylic bone cements. This is a minimally invasive procedure in which some form of polymethylmethacrylate bone cement is injected into the fractured vertebrae (80). Pain relief in patients has been reported to be as high as 75% (81). In addition, *in vitro* studies have demonstrated increased strength in vertebrae augmented with bone cement (82). Although this procedure shows promise, there have not been any good randomized studies on its effectiveness or any possible long-term consequences.

Falls are one of the major causes of fracture, and thus, fall prevention is important in the health management of the patient with osteoporosis. To help offset the chance of fracture if a fall does occur, the use of hip protectors has some possibilities (83).

DIAGNOSTIC TECHNIQUES

Diagnosis of osteoporosis involves the measurement of BMD. Several methods for measuring BMD have been used in the past, including radiogammetry, single-photon absorptiometry, and dual-photon absorptiometry. However, these techniques lacked the precision and accuracy necessary for broad clinical use. Dual-energy x-ray absorptiometry (DXA) is considered the gold standard for assessing bone mineral density. Quantitative computed tomography (QCT) and ultrasound are also used for the measurement of bone.

Dual-energy x-ray absorptiometry is the most commonly used technology for measuring BMD and is the primary technique used to diagnose osteoporosis. DXA uses low-dose x-ray to emit photons at two different energy levels. BMD is calculated based on the amount of energy attenuated by the body. DXA measurements are reported in g/cm^2, so are not a true density, but rather an area density. DXA is capable of differentiating between bone and soft tissue and therefore can also be used to measure regional and total body composition. The advantages of DXA, as compared to other methods, include the capability of measuring small changes in BMD over time, measuring with a low precision error of 0.5–2.0%, requiring short exam times (5–10 minutes), and providing low radiation exposure.

Quantitative computed tomography has two advantages over DXA in that it provides a three-dimensional anatomical localization for direct measurement of true bone density and QCT is also capable of differentiating between trabecular and cortical bone and is used to examine the anatomy of trabecular regions within the spine. This makes QCT quite attractive in certain research applications. However, QCT is less practical than DXA for routine screening for osteoporosis due to expense, higher radiation exposure, and less precision, and thus QCT is rarely used in diagnosing osteoporosis.

Another emerging technology for assessing bone health is quantitative ultrasound (QUS). Ultrasound does not measure bone density, but rather measures two parameters called speed of sound (SOS) and broadband ultrasound attenuation (BUA) that are related to the structural properties of bone. Some manufacturers will then use BUA and/or SOS to derive other indices or even estimate bone mineral density. However, since the use of QUS is relatively new in the field of bone health, not all manufacturers use the same technology. Speed of sound measured on one device may be a different type of measurement on an ultrasound unit from another manufacturer. Nevertheless, studies have shown that QUS measures have the ability to distinguish fracture patients from controls (84), as well as predict future fracture (85, 86). The advantages for ultrasound devices are that they are small, portable, and use no ionizing radiation.

Bone mineral density is reported not only in g/cm^2 (DXA) or g/cm^3 (QCT), but also in terms of standard deviations, or z-scores. The likelihood of sustaining a fracture increases 1.5- to 3-fold for each standard deviation decrease in BMD (87, 88). The World Health Organization Consensus Development Conference has developed diagnostic criteria for osteoporosis based on this relationship (89). Normal BMD is less than 1.0 standard deviation below the mean for young adults. A BMD that is between 1.0 and 2.5 standard deviations below the young adult mean is considered low bone mass, or osteopenia. Osteoporosis is defined as BMD more than 2.5 standard deviations below the young adult mean and is considered "severe" if accompanied by one or more fractures. Although these criteria were originally developed for diagnosis of osteoporosis at the proximal femur in postmenopausal women, they are commonly used for men and women of all ages and are applied to the lumbar spine and distal radius and ulna.

EXERCISE/FITNESS/FUNCTIONAL TESTING

Exercise recommendations for individuals with osteoporosis or those who are at risk for developing osteoporosis generally include an aerobic, weight-bearing exercise program (such as walking) and a resistive exercise program to promote bone health. Non–weight-bearing exercises (such as swimming or water aerobics) do not seem to provide the osteogenic effect seen with weight-bearing exercise, but their use might be recommended for those individuals who cannot tolerate the higher impact associated with weight-bearing exercise. Additionally, if an individual has osteoporosis, that individual is at increased risk of fracturing a bone. Because falls are associated with most hip and wrist fractures, and are a leading cause of injury in older adults, a falls-intervention program should be instituted in all older adults who are diagnosed with osteoporosis. The following exercise testing should be conducted in order to provide each individual with a safe, effective training program.

Aerobic Fitness Testing

Graded exercise testing is recommended for individuals who are considered to be at risk for heart disease according to American College of Sports Medicine guidelines (24). The results of the graded exercise test can be used to determine the appropriate intensity for the walking or jogging exercise included within the training program. When graded exercise testing is not deemed necessary or is contraindicated, age-predicted maximal heart rate is used to determine training intensity based on a target heart rate (24).

Muscle Strength Testing

Muscle strength testing is used to determine training intensity of the resistance exercise program. Determination of the 1-repetition maximum (RM) is generally used for strength assessment in healthy persons, but use of the 1-RM is discouraged in the client with osteoporosis because of the increased possibility of fracture. Assessment of the 10-repetition maximum is recommended for strength assessment in the osteoporotic client.

Because deficits in lower-extremity muscle strength are associated with an increased incidence of falls (90, 91), maximal isometric muscle strength assessment can be used to identify muscle strength deficits as part of the overall evaluation of fall risk. Hand-held dynamometry is sometimes used because it provides an easy, objective measurement of isometric strength and a useful indication of overall muscle strength. It can also be used for monitoring change in muscle strength in response to an exercise program; however, its use is not advised in hypertensive individuals. The use of a normative muscle strength database is recommended to help identify strength impairments.

Balance Testing

A deficit in balance has also been shown to be a predictor of falls (90), and is therefore, a critical component in the evaluation of fall risk. The ability to stand on one leg is a simple clinical test frequently used to assess balance function. Although force platform systems can provide more information about the nature of the balance impairment, single stance time has been shown to distinguish fallers from nonfallers among the elderly (92 ,93).

Gait speed and tandem gait ability have been reported to be independent predictors of hip fracture risk (94). While these factors are a function of both balance and muscular fitness, they are not properly tested for by either balance or muscular strength testing and therefore should be independently assessed. Testing for other fall-related factors such as visual acuity and cognitive ability should also be considered.

Flexibility Testing

General flexibility tests such as the sit-and-reach and shoulder elevation tests are not performed in clients with osteoporosis. Primarily, flexibility of muscles that have the potential to adversely affect posture should be assessed. Decreases in length of muscles that cross more than one joint have the greatest potential to cause problems in posture (for example, hamstrings and hip flexors). Insufficient length in the hamstrings or hip flexors will produce a posterior pelvic tilt or anterior pelvic tilt, respectively. Such postural alterations affect how weight is borne through the bones in the spine and lower extremities. Other muscles that frequently lose flexibility and can lead to postural problems include the pectoral muscles and the gastrocnemius muscles. Flexibility is assessed by measuring joint range of motion (ROM) when the muscle is fully elongated over each joint crossed by that muscle. For example, flexibility of the gastrocnemius muscle is assessed by measuring dorsiflexion of the ankle when the knee is kept fully extended.

Contraindications for Exercise

Impact exercises that impart high loads to the skeleton, such as jumping, running, or jogging, are contraindicated for people with osteoporosis (95). These exercises cause high compressive forces in the spine and lower extremities, and can cause fractures in weakened bones. Impact exercises such as two-footed jumping, however, have been shown to be effective for increasing bone mineral density in nonosteoporotic women and can be used to help prevent osteoporosis in a nonosteoporotic population (96).

People with osteoporosis should not perform exercises that require bending forward at the waist or excessive twisting at the waist. Bending and twisting motions at the waist produce very high compressive forces over an area of the spinal bones that is most susceptible to fracture. For this reason, exercises such as toe touches, sit-ups, or rowing machines, as well as activities such as golf, tennis, or bowling, should be avoided by people with osteoporosis (16). Resistive exercises are not contraindicated for people with osteoporosis, but resistance should be used cautiously when the osteoporosis is severe.

EXERCISE PRESCRIPTION AND PROGRAMMING

Although studies have shown that several forms of exercise training have the potential to increase BMD, the optimal training program for skeletal integrity has yet to be defined. Based on current experimental knowledge, it has been proposed that an osteogenic exercise regimen should have load-bearing activities at high magnitude (force) with few repetitions, create versatile strain distributions throughout the bone structure (load the bone in directions to which it is unaccustomed), and be long term and progressive in nature (50, 97). Resistance training (weight lifting) probably offers the best opportunity to meet these criteria on an individual basis, requires little skill, and has the added advantage of being highly adaptable to changes in both magnitude and strain distribution. In addition, strength and muscle size increases have been demonstrated following resistance training, even in the elderly (98).

There are no known studies that have specifically examined cardiovascular adaptations in osteoporotic patients, but older adults can increase their fitness levels 10–30% with prolonged endurance training (99). A good number of older women with osteoporosis will not be on estrogen replacement therapy (59) and thus will be receiving none of the cardiovascular benefits associated with ERT (100). Since exercise endurance training can decrease cardiovascular disease risk factors such as high blood pressure and cholesterol, it is recommended for the osteoporotic woman.

Thus, resistance training combined with cardiovascular training (bicycling or walking) is the best recommendation for an exercise program for the patient with osteoporosis. Not only will such a program increase overall fitness and perhaps bone mineral density, it will aid greatly in reducing the risk of falling (99, 101, 102), which is one of the primary causes of fracture in osteoporosis.

Although osteoporosis occurs in young amenorrheic women, it is still a disease that primarily occurs in older women. Currently, the American College of Sports Medicine recommends that anyone over the age of 50 who wants to begin a vigorous exercise program should have a medically supervised stress test (24). However, for osteoporotic older women who simply want to begin a walking and/or resistance training program, this recommendation may be both impractical and unnecessary. Careful screening should be undertaken to identify which individuals need further evaluation by a physician (103).

There are recommendations, specific to the patient with osteoporosis, to consider when developing an exercise program. Impact activities such as running, jumping, or high-impact aerobics should be avoided with osteoporotic patients due to their risk of a fracture with little or no trauma. Another activity that absolutely must not be done by people with osteoporosis is spinal flexion, including things such as sit-ups or toe touches (104). Spinal flexion drastically increases the forces on the spine, increasing the likelihood of a fracture (105). Other activities to avoid are those that increase the chance of falling such as trampolines, step aerobics, skating (ice or in-line), or exercising on slippery floors (95).

From the other perspective, there are certain exercises that are quite beneficial for the osteoporotic patient. These include exercises designed to help with balance and agility in order to reduce falls. For instance, exercises that strengthen the quadriceps are helpful. However, squats with free weights should be avoided because of the excess load that might be applied to the spine as well as the potential for spinal flexion during the squat lift. A specific exercise that helps build hip and low back strength as well as improve balance is standing on one foot for 5 to 15 seconds. Initially, the patient should be encouraged to place his/her hands on a counter for support until he/she develops the strength and/or balance needed to perform the exercise without danger of falling. The osteoporotic patient should also be encouraged to do spine extension (but NOT spinal flexion) exercises (104). Spine extension exercises can be performed in a chair and can help strengthen the back muscles, which can help reduce the development of a dowager's hump and possibly reduce the risk of vertebral fracture (106). However, these and all exercises done by patients with osteoporosis should be performed with slow and controlled movements, avoiding jerky, rapid movements. More complete information can be found on these and other exercises for the osteoporotic patient (95, 107).

As stated, the physiological responses to exercise in an osteoporotic population have not been specifically investigated, but they should not be substantially different from an age-matched person without osteoporosis. Similarly, the goals of an exercise program for a person with or without osteoporosis should also be the same. For someone just beginning an exercise program, those goals should include an increase in cardiovascular fitness, increased muscular strength, and an increase (or at least no decrease) in bone mineral density. Heart disease remains the number one killer of both women and men by a wide margin. So, the goal of everyone should be to increase their physical activity to reduce the risk of heart disease, and in that regard, physical activity may be a better recommendation than hormone replacement therapy for women (108). The 1996 Surgeon General's report on health and physical activity recommends approximately 30 minutes of moderate physical activity accumulated on most if not all days of the week (109). This would be a worthwhile goal for anyone, including those with osteoporosis. However, if the person with osteoporosis is just beginning an exercise program, the duration of exercise might need to be shortened initially to allow time for adjustment to the exercise. As the person's fitness level increases, the duration of exercise can be increased. For an osteoporotic person, or for that matter any man or woman just beginning an exercise program, a walking program should provide the needed benefits along with being a safe mode of exercise.

Weight training appears to offer the most benefits for increases in muscular strength and bone density. Current recommendations suggest a single set of 15 repetitions of 8–10 exercises performed at least 2 days per week (110). Again, this is a worthwhile goal for the person with osteoporosis, but a less strenuous program may be needed initially, with care taken to avoid the exercises mentioned above that are dangerous. In addition, some resistance training exercises have a tendency to cause spinal flexion, especially exercises for the upper and lower extremities, so it is important that during resistance training all exercise be done with an upright posture.

A program to increase flexibility can also benefit the osteoporotic patient since decreased flexibility can cause problems with posture. Muscles that cross more than one joint such as the hamstring are particularly important. However, many of the commonly prescribed exercises for increasing flexibility, especially of the hamstring, involve spinal flexion and must be avoided. There is little consensus on the optimal training program for increasing flexibility, but good suggestions are available from many sources (95, 111).

Thus, exercise may be beneficial for both increasing bone density to help prevent osteoporosis and as a therapeutic modality for those patients in whom osteoporosis is already present. However, caution must be observed in the type of exercise program to be used and the specific exercises performed. Patients with severe osteoporosis who are just beginning an exercise program should be supervised until it is determined that they can properly perform the exercises without danger to themselves.

EDUCATION AND COUNSELING

Activity/Exercise

Following instructions in an appropriate exercise program is important, and in order to encourage compliance with the recommended exercise program, these two points should be emphasized:

- Gains made in bone density will only be maintained as long as the exercise is continued (28).
- Approximately 9 months to 1 year are required to detect a significant change in bone mass (11).

Safety Hazards in the Home

Falls are a frequent cause of fracture, and thus, fall prevention is important to the osteoporotic patient. The reasons falls occur are varied, but identified risk factors include environmental hazards, muscle weakness, poor balance, and medication-related side effects (112, 113). Eliminating as many of these risk factors as possible can greatly reduce the danger of falling. A discussion of safety hazards in the home and suggestions to remove these hazards is an integral part of any falls-prevention program. Completing a falls risk assessment form such as the one developed by the World Health Organization (WHO) can help identify hazards in the home. The examiner may then make suggestions on how to remove the hazards or how to modify the home to make it safer. These suggestions may be as simple as moving a telephone and light to within reach of the bed to avoid falls when getting up in the dark, eliminating slippery floors, or installing safety features for the bathtub (114, 115). Educating patients on the side effects of medications, such as those that cause dizziness, is also an important step in fall prevention, as is improving muscle weakness and balance with the use of a properly structured exercise program.

Activity Modification

Although proper body mechanics during lifting should be encouraged in all individuals, it is absolutely critical in patients with osteoporosis. Attempting to lift an object with the back flexed is a common mechanism of vertebral fracture in people with osteoporosis. Instructions on how to bend the knees while keeping the back straight in order to pick up an object from the floor must be provided.

Daily activities such as sweeping, vacuuming, or mopping can also present problems for people with osteoporosis because these activities are typically performed by using a lot of bending and twisting of the spine. These activities, however, can be modified to avoid spinal twisting and bending, and instead can provide beneficial loading to the spine and hips. People with osteoporosis should be encouraged to mop, sweep, or vacuum by placing one foot in front of the other, and shifting weight from one foot to the other in a rocking motion (16). The knees are bent and the back is kept straight during this rocking motion. The rocking motion from one foot to the other takes the place of bending and twisting of the spine in order to reach forward when mopping, sweeping, or vacuuming.

Dietary Modifications and Calcium Supplements

The National Institutes of Health recommends a daily calcium intake of 1500 mg for all women over the age of 64 and for any postmenopausal woman not on ERT. A review of foods that are a good source of calcium should be provided along with instructions stating how to read food labels. Food labels show what percentage of the recommended daily requirement is provided by the food item. Unfortunately, these percentages are based on the inaccurate assumption that the recommended daily requirement is 1000 mg for everybody, regardless of age or gender. Converting from percentages to actual quantity of calcium in milligrams is not difficult. People simply need to be educated on how to do the conversion.

A discussion about the different types of calcium supplements is also valuable because people often take their supplements incorrectly and therefore reduce the effectiveness. Calcium comes in many different forms, but the two most common forms are calcium citrate (Ex. Citracal) and calcium carbonate (Ex. Os-Cal, Caltrate, Viactiv). Studies show that calcium citrate is more readily absorbed (116) but has less calcium per tablet than calcium carbonate. That means that more tablets of calcium citrate must be taken per day in order to attain the recommended requirement of 1200 to 1500 mg/day. In any case, if a person chooses calcium carbonate because they can take fewer tablets per day, they should take part of their requirement after each meal. Taking calcium carbonate after a meal improves the absorption, but it still will not be absorbed as well as calcium citrate. Vitamin D will help increase calcium absorption, and all osteoporotic patients should be encouraged to take in at least 400 IU/day of vitamin D.

Patients should also be made aware of the fact that caffeine causes more of their calcium to be lost in the urine. That doesn't mean that people with osteoporosis must give up all caffeine, however. A good rule of thumb is to restrict the number of servings that contain caffeine to no more than 2 or 3 per day. This recommendation is based on two studies that showed 400–600 mg of caffeine did not cause significant loss in calcium as long as the individual consumed at least 600 mg of calcium per day (117, 118).

CASE STUDY

Jane is a 53-year-old, postmenopausal, Caucasian woman diagnosed in April 1998 with osteoporosis at the femoral neck ($Z = -2.53$) and osteopenia at the lumbar spine (L2–4) ($Z = -1.48$). Jane has no family history of osteoporosis, or history of amenorrhea, has been physically active throughout childhood and adult life, and never abused alcohol nor consumed excessive caffeine. She is 175 cm (69 inches) tall and weighs 50 kg (110 lb). She has never smoked, but as a flight attendant for 32 years was exposed to second-hand smoke from 1967–1997. She has supplemented her diet with 1000 mg of calcium for 20 years. At age 43, Jane initiated hormone replacement therapy. Immediately following diagnosis, Jane increased her calcium supplementation to 1500 mg daily. She also increased her walking program from 30 min, 3–4 days/week to 50 min, 7 days/week and began performing isometric exercises for the abdominals and upper back twice daily. Jane also began a resistance training program consisting of 10 free-weight and machine exercises performed in 2 sets of 8–15 repetitions, 2–3 days/week. Six months after diagnosis, Jane began treatment with 10 mg of alendronate daily. In 18 months of resistance training, Jane has experienced an average increase in strength of 250%. Follow-up bone density scans in October 1999 revealed an increase in BMD of 9.28% at the femoral neck ($Z = -1.99$) and 10.49% at the lumbar spine ($Z = -0.88$). Based on Jane's outcome, it appears that the combination of an aggressive resistive and weight-bearing exercise regimen in the treatment of osteoporosis may be effective in increasing BMD above that expected from calcium supplementation and antiresorptive therapy alone.

References

1. Looker AC, Johnston CCJ, Wahner HW, et al. Prevalence of low femoral bone density in older U.S. women from NHANES III. J Bone Miner Res 1995;10:796–802.
2. Orwoll ES. Osteoporosis in men. Endocrinol Metab Clin North Am 1998;27:349–367.
3. Chrischilles EA, Butler CD, Davis CS, et al. A model of lifetime osteoporosis impact. Arch Intern Med 1991;151:2026–2032.

4. Poor G, Atkinson EJ, O'Fallon WM, et al. Determinants of reduced survival following hip fractures in men. Clin Orthop 1995;319:260–265.
5. Ray NF, Chan JK, Thamer M, et al. Medical expenditures for the treatment of osteoporotic fractures in the United States in 1995: report from the National Osteoporosis Foundation. J Bone Miner Res 1997;12:24–35.
6. Chrischilles EA, Shireman T, Wallace R. Costs and health effects of osteoporotic fractures. Bone 1994;15:377–385.
7. Peck WA. Consensus development conference: diagnosis, prophylaxis, and treatment of osteoporosis. Am J Med 1993; 94:646–650.
8. Riggs BL, Melton LJ. Evidence for two distinct syndromes of involutional osteoporosis. Am J Med 1983;75:899–901.
9. Rodan GA. Introduction to bone biology. Bone 1992;13: S3–S6.
10. Buckwalter JA, Glimcher MJ, Cooper RR, et al. Bone biology. Part I: Structure, blood supply, cells, matrix, and mineralization. J Bone Joint Surg 1995;77-A:1256–1275.
11. Buckwalter JA, Glimcher MJ, Cooper RR, et al. Bone biology. Part II: Formation, form, modeling, remodeling, and regulation of cell function. J Bone Joint Surg 1995;77-A:1276–1289.
12. Ensrud KE, Palermo L, Black DM, et al. Hip and calcaneal bone loss increase with advancing age: longitudinal results from the study of osteoporotic fractures. J Bone Miner Res 1995;10:1778–1787.
13. Jones G, Nguyen T, Sambrook P, et al. Progressive loss of bone in the femoral neck in elderly people: longitudinal findings from the Dubbo osteoporosis epidemiology study. BMJ 1994;309:691–695.
14. Glynn NW, Meilahn EN, Charron M, et al. Determinants of bone mineral density in older men. J Bone Miner Res, 1995; 10:1769–1777.
15. Eriksen EF, Langdahl BL. The pathogenesis of osteoporosis. Horm Res 1997;48:78–82.
16. National Osteoporosis Foundation. Boning up on osteoporosis: A guide to prevention and treatment. 1997. Washington, DC, National Osteoporosis Foundation.
17. Pollitzer WS, Anderson JJB. Ethnic and genetic differences in bone mass: A review with a hereditary vs environmental perspective. Am J Clin Nutr 1989;50:1244–1259.
18. Krall EA, Dawson-Hughes B: Osteoporosis. In: Modern Nutrition in Health and Disease. Shils M, Olson J, Shike M, Ross AC, eds. Baltimore: Williams and Wilkins, 1999.
19. Kiel DP, Felson DT, Hannan MT, et al. Caffeine and the risk of hip fracture: the Framingham Study. Am J Epidemiol 1990;132:675–684.
20. Heaney RP. Pathophysiology of osteoporosis. Am J Med Sci 1996;312:251–256.
21. Cummings SR, Nevitt MC, Browner WS, et al. Risk factors for hip fracture in white women. N Engl J Med 1995;332: 767–773.
22. Slemenda CW, Christian JC, Reed T, et al. Long-term bone loss in men: effects of genetic and environmental factors. Ann Intern Med 1992;117:286–291.
23. Michnovicz JJ, Hershcopf RJ, Naganuma H, et al. Increased 2-hydroxylation of estradiol as a possible mechanism for the anti-estrogenic effect of cigarette smoking. N Engl J Med 1986;315:1305–1309.
24. American College of Sports Medicine: ACSM's Guidelines for Exercise Testing and Prescription. Philadelphia, PA: Lippincot, Williams & Wilkins, 2000:1–373.
25. Bassey EJ, Ramsdale SJ. Weight-bearing exercise and ground reaction forces: a 12-month randomized controlled trial of effects on bone mineral density in healthy postmenopausal women. Bone 1995;16:469–476.
26. Hatori M, Hasegawa A, Adachi H, et al. The effects of walking at the anaerobic threshold on vertebral bone loss in postmenopausal women. Cal Tiss Inter 1993;52:411–414.
27. Kohrt WM, Snead DB, Slatopolsky E, et al. Additive effects of weight-bearing exercise and estrogen on bone mineral density in older women. J Bone Miner Res 1995;10: 1303–1311.
28. Dalsky GP, Stocke KS, Ehsani AA, et al. Weight-bearing exercise training and lumbar bone mineral content in postmenopausal women. Ann Intern Med 1988;108:824–828.
29. Prince RL, Smith M, Dick IM, et al. Prevention of postmenopausal osteoporosis: A comparative study of exercise, calcium supplementation, and hormone-replacement therapy. N Engl J Med 1991;325:1189–1195.
30. Nelson ME, Fiatarone MA, Morganti CM, et al. Effects of high-intensity strength training on multiple risk factors for osteoporotic fractures. A randomized controlled trial. JAMA 1994;272:1909–1914.
31. Notelovitz M, Martin D, Tesar R, et al. Estrogen therapy and variable-resistance weight training increase bone mineral in surgically menopausal women. J Bone Miner Res, 1991;6: 583–590.
32. Pruitt LA, Jackson RD, Bartels RL. Weight-training effects on bone mineral density in early postmenopausal women. J Bone Miner Res 1992;7:179–185.
33. Kohrt WM, Ehsani AA, Birge SJJ. HRT preserves increases in bone mineral density and reductions in body fat after a supervised exercise program. J Appl Physiol 1998;84:1506–1512.
34. Bailey DA, Faulkner RA, McKay HA. Growth, physical activity, and bone mineral acquisition. Exerc Sport Sci Rev 1996; 24:233–266.
35. Cassell C, Benedict M, Specker B. Bone mineral density in elite 7- to 9-yr-old female gymnasts and swimmers. Med Sci Sports Exerc 1996;28:1243–1246.
36. Grimston SK, Morrison K, Harder JA, et al. Bone mineral density during puberty in western Canadian children. Bone Miner 1992;19:85–96.
37. Slemenda CW, Miller JZ, Hui SL, et al. Role of physical activity in the development of skeletal mass in children. J Bone Miner Res 1991;6:1227–1233.
38. Kannus P, Haapasalo H, Sankelo M, et al. Effect of starting age of physical activity on bone mass in the dominant arm of tennis and squash players. Ann Intern Med 1995;123:27–31.
39. Courteix D, Lespessailles E, Peres SL, et al. Effect of physical training on bone mineral density in prepubertal girls: A comparative study between impact-loading and non-impact-loading sports. Osteoporos Inter 1998;8:152–158.
40. Taaffe DR, Snow-Harter C, Connolly DA, et al. Differential effects of swimming versus weight-bearing activity on bone mineral status of eumenorrheic athletes. J Bone Miner Res 1995;10:586–593.
41. McKay HA, Petit MA, Schutz RW, et al. Augmented trochanteric bone mineral density after modified physical education classes: a randomized school-based exercise intervention

study in prepubescent and early pubescent children. J Pediatr 2000;136:156–162.
42. Witzke KA, Snow CM. Effects of plyometric jump training on bone mass in adolescent girls. Med Sci Sports Exerc 2000;32:1051–1057.
43. Bradney M, Pearce G, Naughton G, et al. Moderate exercise during growth in prepubertal boys: changes in bone mass, size, volumetric density, and bone strength: a controlled prospective study. J Bone Miner Res 1998;13:1814–1821.
44. Morris FL, Naughton GA, Gibbs JL, et al. Prospective tenmonth exercise intervention in premenarcheal girls: Positive effects on bone and lean mass. J Bone Miner Res 1997;12: 1453–1462.
45. Fehling PC, Alekel L, Clasey J, et al. A comparison of bone mineral densities among female athletes in impact loading and active loading sports. Bone 1995;17:205–210.
46. Kirchner EM, Lewis RD, O'Connor PJ. Effect of past gymnastics participation on adult bone mass. J Appl Physiol 1996;80:226–232.
47. Lee EJ, Long KA, Risser WL, et al. Variations in bone status of contralateral and regional sites in young athletic women. Med Sci Sports Exerc 1995;27:1354–1361.
48. Nichols DL, Sanborn CF, Bonnick SL, et al. The effects of gymnastics training on bone mineral density. Med Sci Sports Exerc 1994;26:1220–1225.
49. Taaffe DR, Robinson TL, Snow CM, et al. High-impact exercise promotes bone gain in well-trained female athletes. J Bone Miner Res 1997;12:255–260.
50. Snow CM. Exercise and bone mass in young premenopausal women. Bone 1996;18:51S–55S.
51. Rosano GM, Sarrel PM, Poole-Wilson PA, et al. Beneficial effect of oestrogen on exercise-induced myocardial ischaemia in women with coronary artery disease. Lancet 1993;342: 133–136.
52. Holdright DR, Sullivan AK, Wright CA, et al. Acute effect of oestrogen replacement therapy on treadmill performance in postmenopausal women with coronary artery disease. Eur Heart J 1995;16:1566–1570.
53. Cutler WB, Friedmann E, Genovese-Stone E. Prevalence of kyphosis in a healthy sample of pre- and postmenopausal women. Am J Phys Med Rehabil 1993;72:219–225.
54. Ettinger BF, Genant HK, Cann CE. Long-term estrogen replacement therapy prevents bone loss and fractures. Ann Intern Med 1985;102:319–324.
55. Hillard TC, Whitcroft SJ, Marsh MS, et al. Long-term effects of transdermal and oral hormone replacement therapy on postmenopausal bone loss. Osteoporos Int 1994;4:341–348.
56. Kohrt WM, Birge SJJ. Differential effects of estrogen treatment on bone mineral density of the spine, hip, wrist and total body in late postmenopausal women. Osteoporos Int 1995;5:150–155.
57. Lees B, Pugh M, Siddle N, et al. Changes in bone density in women starting hormone replacement therapy compared with those in women already established on hormone replacement therapy. Osteoporos Int 1995;5:344–348.
58. Prestwood KM, Pilbeam CC, Burleson JA, et al. The short term effects of conjugated estrogen on bone turnover in older women. J Clin Endocrinol Metab 1994;79:366–371.
59. Keating NL, Cleary PD, Rossi AS, et al. Use of hormone replacement therapy by postmenopausal women in the United States. Ann Intern Med 1999;130:545–553.
60. Grigoriou O, Papoulias I, Vitoratos N, et al. Effects of nasal administration of calcitonin in oophorectomized women: 2-year controlled double-blind study. Maturitas 1997;28: 147–151.
61. Kapetanos G, Symeonides PP, Dimitriou C, et al. A double blind study of intranasal calcitonin for established postmenopausal osteoporosis. Acta Orthop Scand Suppl 1997; 275:108–111.
62. Overgaard K, Hansen MA, Jensen SB, et al. Effect of salcatonin given intranasally on bone mass and fracture rates in established osteoporosis: a dose-response study. BMJ 1992; 305:556–561.
63. Reginster JY, Deroisy R, Lecart MP, et al. A double-blind, placebo-controlled, dose-finding trial of intermittent nasal salmon calcitonin for prevention of postmenopausal lumbar spine bone loss. Am J Med 1995;98: 452–458.
64. Ensrud KE, Black DM, Palermo L, et al. Treatment with alendronate prevents fractures in women at highest risk: results from the Fracture Intervention Trial. Arch Intern Med 1997;157:2617–2624.
65. McClung M, Clemmesen B, Daifotis A, et al. Alendronate prevents postmenopausal bone loss in women without osteoporosis. A double-blind, randomized, controlled trial. Ann Intern Med 1998;128:253–261.
66. Mortensen L, Charles P, Bekker PJ, et al. Risedronate increases bone mass in an early postmenopausal population: two years of treatment plus one year of follow-up. J Clin Endocrinol Metab 1998;83:396–402.
67. Reid IR, Wattie DJ, Evans MC, et al. Continuous therapy with pamidronate, a potent bisphosphonate, in postmenopausal osteoporosis. J Clin Endocrinol Metab 1994;79:1595–1599.
68. Thiebaud D, Burckhardt P, Kriegbaum H, et al. Three monthly intravenous injections of ibandronate in the treatment of postmenopausal osteoporosis. Am J Med 1997;103: 298–307.
69. Wimalawansa SJ. A four-year randomized controlled trial of hormone replacement and bisphosphonate, alone or in combination, in women with postmenopausal osteoporosis. Am J Med 1998;104:219–226.
70. Bone HG, Greenspan SL, McKeever C, et al. Alendronate and estrogen effects in postmenopausal women with low bone mineral density. J Clin Endocrinol Metab 2000;85:727–733.
71. Francis RM. Bisphosphonates in the treatment of osteoporosis in 1997: A review. Curr Therap Res 1997;58:656–678.
72. Khovidhunkit W, Shoback DM. Clinical effects of raloxifene hydrochloride in women. Ann Intern Med 1999;130:431–439.
73. Delmas PD, Bjarnason NH, Mitlak BH, et al. Effects of raloxifene on bone mineral density, serum cholesterol concentrations, and uterine endometrium in postmenopausal women. N Engl J Med 1997;337:1641–1647.
74. Lufkin EG, Whitaker MD, Nickelsen T, et al. Treatment of established postmenopausal osteoporosis with raloxifene: a randomized trial. J Bone Miner Res 1998;13:1747–1754.
75. Baeksgaard L, Andersen KP, Hyldstrup L. Calcium and vitamin D supplementation increases spinal BMD in healthy, postmenopausal women. Osteoporos Int 1998;8:255–260.
76. Dawson-Hughes B, Harris SS, Krall EA, et al. Effect of calcium and vitamin D supplementation on bone density in men and women 65 years of age or older. N Engl J Med 1997;337:670–676.

77. Dawson-Hughes B, Dallai GE, Krall EA, et al. A controlled trial of the effect of calcium supplementation on bone density in postmenopausal women. N Engl J Med 1990;323: 878–883.
78. Riis B, Thomsen K, Christiansen C. Does calcium supplementation prevent postmenopausal bone loss: A double blind, controlled clinical trial. N Engl J Med 1987;316:173–177.
79. Heaney RP. Effect of calcium on skeletal development, bone loss, and risk of fractures. Am J Med 1991;91:23S–27S.
80. Cotten A, Boutry N, Cortet B, et al. Percutaneous vertebroplasty: state of the art. Radiographics 1998;18:311–320.
81. Cyteval C, Sarrabere MP, Roux JO, et al. Acute osteoporotic vertebral collapse: open study on percutaneous injection of acrylic surgical cement in 20 patients. AJR Am J Roentgenol 1999;173:1685–1690.
82. Tohmeh AG, Mathis JM, Fenton DC, et al. Biomechanical efficacy of unipedicular versus bipedicular vertebroplasty for the management of osteoporotic compression fractures. Spine 1999;24:1772–1776.
83. Lauritzen JB, Petersen MM, Lund B. Effect of external hip protectors on hip fractures. Lancet 1993;341:11–13.
84. Schott AM, Weill-Engerer S, Hans D, et al. Ultrasound discriminates patients with hip fracture equally well as dual energy X-ray absorptiometry and independently of bone mineral density. J Bone Miner Res 1995;10:243–249.
85. Bauer DC, Gluer CC, Cauley JA, et al. Broadband ultrasound attenuation predicts fractures strongly and independently of densitometry in older women. A prospective study. Study of Osteoporotic Fractures Research Group. Arch Intern Med 1997;157:629–634.
86. Hans D, Dargent-Molina P, Schott AM, et al. Ultrasonographic heel measurements to predict hip fracture in elderly women: the EPIDOS prospective study. Lancet 1996;348:511–514.
87. Ross PD, Genant HK, Davis JW, et al. Predicting vertebral fracture incidence from prevalent fractures and bone density among non-black, osteoporotic women. Osteoporos Int 1993;3:120–126.
88. Faulkner KG, Cummings SR, Black D, et al. Simple measurement of femoral geometry predicts hip fracture: the study of osteoporotic fractures. J Bone Miner Res 1993;8: 1211–1217.
89. Kanis JA, Melton LJ, Christiansen C, et al. The diagnosis of osteoporosis. J Bone Miner Res 1994;9:1137–1141.
90. Guralnik JM, Ferrucci L, Simonsick EM, et al. Lower-extremity function in persons over the age of 70 years as a predictor of subsequent disability. N Engl J Med 1995;332:556–561.
91. Whipple RH, Wolfson LI, Amerman PM. The relationship of knee and ankle weakness to falls in nursing home residents: an isokinetic study. J Am Geriatr Soc 1987;35:13–20.
92. Gehlsen GM, Whaley MH. Falls in the elderly: Part II, Balance, strength, and flexibility. Arch Phys Med Rehabil 1990; 71:739–741.
93. Heitmann DK, Gossman MR, Shaddeau SA, et al. Balance performance and step width in noninstitutionalized, elderly, female fallers and nonfallers. Phys Ther 1989;69: 923–931
94. Dargent-Molina P, Favier F, Grandjean H, et al. Fall-related factors and risk of hip fracture: the EPIDOS prospective study. Lancet 1996;348:145–149.
95. Bonnick, S. L. The Osteoporosis Handbook 1997;1: 1–180. Dallas, Texas, Taylor Publishing.
96. Bassey EJ, Ramsdale SJ. Increase in femoral bone density in young women following high-impact exercise. Osteoporos Int 1994;4:72–75.
97. Kannus P, Sievanen H, Vuori I. Physical loading, exercise, and bone. Bone 1996;18:1S–3S.
98. Harridge SD, Kryger A, Stensgaard A. Knee extensor strength, activation, and size in very elderly people following strength training. Muscle Nerve 1999;22:831–839.
99. American College of Sports Medicine. American College of Sports Medicine Position Stand. Exercise and physical activity for older adults. Med Sci Sports Exerc 1998;30: 992–1008.
100. Aygen EM, Karakucuk EI, Basbug M. Comparison of the effects of conjugated estrogen treatment on blood lipid and lipoprotein levels when initiated in the first or fifth postmenopausal year. Gynecol Endocrinol 1999;13:118–122.
101. Campbell AJ, Robertson MC, Gardner MM, et al. Randomised controlled trial of a general practice programme of home based exercise to prevent falls in elderly women. BMJ 1997;315:1065–1069.
102. Gregg EW, Cauley JA, Seeley DG, et al. Physical activity and osteoporotic fracture risk in older women. Study of Osteoporotic Fractures Research Group. Ann Intern Med 1998;129:81–88.
103. Evans WJ. Exercise training guidelines for the elderly. Med Sci Sports Exerc 1999;31:12–17.
104. Sinaki M, Mikkelsen BA. Postmenopausal spinal osteoporosis: flexion versus extension exercises. Arch Phys Med Rehabil 1984;65:593–596.
105. Bouxsein ML, Myers ER, Hayes WC: Biomechanics of age-related fractures. In: Osteoporosis. Marcus R, Feldman D, Kelsey JL, eds. San Diego, CA: Academic Press, Inc, 1996; 373–393.
106. Sinaki M, Wollan PC, Scott RW, et al. Can strong back extensors prevent vertebral fractures in women with osteoporosis? Mayo Clin Proc 1996;71:951–956.
107. Sinaki M. Postmenopausal spinal osteoporosis: physical therapy and rehabilitation principles. Mayo Clin Proc 1982;57:699–703.
108. Wong S, Wong J. Is physical activity as effective in reducing risk of cardiovascular disease as estrogen replacement therapy in postmenopausal women? Int J Nur Studies 1999; 36:405–414.
109. U.S. Department of Health and Human Services, Physical Activity and Health. A report of the Surgeon General. 1996:22–29. Atlanta, GA.
110. Feigenbaum MS, Pollock ML. Prescription of resistance training for health and disease. Med Sci Sports Exerc 1999;31:38–45.
111. Fredette DM: Exercise recommendation for flexibility and range of motion. In: ACSM's Resource Manual for Guidelines for Exercise Testing and Prescription. American College of Sports Medicine, ed. Baltimore, MD: Lippincott, Williams and Wilkins, 1998:456–471.
112. Robbins AS, Rubenstein LZ, Josephson KR, et al. Predictors of falls among elderly people. Results of two population-based studies. Arch Intern Med 1989;149:1628–1633.
113. Wickham C, Cooper C, Margetts BM, Barker DJ. Muscle strength, activity, housing and the risk of falls in elderly people. Age Ageing 1989;18:47–51.

114. Province MA, Hadley EC, Hornbrook MC, et al. The effects of exercise on falls in elderly patients. A preplanned meta-analysis of the FICSIT Trials. Frailty and Injuries: Cooperative Studies of Intervention Techniques. JAMA 1995;273: 1341–1347
115. Hornbrook MC, Stevens VJ, Wingfield DJ. Seniors' Program for Injury Control and Education. J Am Geriatr Soc 1993;41:309–314.
116. Heller HJ, Stewart A, Haynes S, et al. Pharmacokinetics of calcium absorption from two commercial calcium supplements. J Clin Pharmacol 1999;39:1151–1154.
117. Heaney RP, Recker RR. Effects of nitrogen, phosphorus, and caffeine on calcium balance in women. J Lab Clin Med 1982;99:46–55.
118. Massey LK, Bergman EA, Wise KJ, et al. Interactions between dietary caffeine and calcium on calcium and bone metabolism in older women. J Am Coll Nutr 1994;13: 592–596.

CHAPTER 13
VERTEBRAL DISORDERS

Sue Smith

In both form and function, the human spine is an elegant and intriguing structure. Because the spine is critical in posture, movement, and protection, pain and loss of function hinders an individual's ability to perform routine activities. As with any complex structure, the potential for problems is great. Although "vertebral disorders" can occur in any part of the spine (cervical, thoracic, lumbar, sacral, and coccygeal), most vertebral disorders are lumbar. Lumbar disorders result in the highest medical, financial, legal, and psychosocial costs to society. Consequently, lumbar disorders have attracted international medical, scientific, economic, and popular attention. This chapter, therefore, focuses on lumbar disorders, and specifically, on what is termed nonspecific, mechanical low back pain.

EPIDEMIOLOGY AND PATHOPHYSIOLOGY

Low back pain afflicts nearly everyone at some stage in life. A 60–80% overall lifetime prevalence of low back pain has been reported (1, 2). Furthermore, the recurrence rate after an episode of low back pain has been estimated at 60% within the first year (3). Low back pain is one of the most prevalent and costly health problems in industrialized countries. In 1990, direct medical costs for low back pain exceeded $24 billion. When disability costs are included, the total annual costs for low back disorders increase from $35 to $56 billion (4, 5). Low back pain is among the leading reasons people seek health-care intervention.

Pain is considered "an unpleasant sensory and emotional experience associated with actual or potential tissue damage or described in terms of such damage" (6). Nociceptive nerve endings (pain fibers) are activated with mechanical, thermal, or chemical stimuli. Mechanical pain is caused by deformation of tissues and varies with physical activity. That is, certain movements or positions increase mechanical pain, while other movements or positions relieve mechanical pain.

In general, pain can be *somatic* (arising from stimulation of nerve endings in a musculoskeletal site [joint, muscle, ligament, bone]), *visceral* (arising from a body organ), *neurogenic* (arising from irritation of the axons or cell bodies of peripheral nerves, spinal nerves, or nerve roots), or *psychogenic*. Pain resulting from irritation of spinal nerves or roots is more specifically called *radicular pain*. Furthermore, pain can be referred to and perceived in an area remote from the source of the pain. Pain referred elsewhere from the viscera is called *visceral referred pain*, and pain from somatic sources is described as *somatic referred pain*. An example of visceral referred pain is the arm pain sometimes associated with a myocardial infarction. An example of somatic referred pain might be the diffuse pain in the buttock or leg associated with low back pain.

The etiology of spinal pain is frequently elusive. As Bogduk (7) points out, any structure with nociceptors is capable of producing irritation that manifests as the perception of pain. These structures in the spine include, but are not limited to, the intervertebral discs, zygapophysial joints, bones, muscles, ligaments, dura mater, dorsal and ventral ramus, and mixed spinal nerves. Of these anatomical sources of pain, the most common are the intervertebral discs and the zygapophysial joints (8, 9).

Given the various anatomical sites that can be associated with spinal pain, a number of labels, or diagnoses, for vertebral disorders have evolved. Some frequently used diagnoses for vertebral disorders are as follows: low back pain, fractures, ligamentous sprains, spondylolysis, spinal stenosis, strain, zygapophysial joint locking, sacroiliac dysfunction, trigger points, zygapophysial osteoarthritis, disc gradation/degeneration, spondylolisthesis, scoliosis, instability, and herniated discs, or herniated nucleus pulposus. The latter, intervertebral disc lesions, have been further subclassified based on the extent to which the nuclear material has herniated, or externalized. In one classification system, these disc pathologies have been called disc protrusions (bulges with no migration of nuclear material and no neural compromise), prolapses (migration of the nucleus, with no externalization, that can manifest with neural and dural signs), extrusions (externalized nuclear material with neurological deficit), and sequestrations (extruded nuclear material fragmented into the spinal canal; the size and location of the fragment determines the clinical findings). Another classification system merely divides disc lesions into those contained within the outer layer of the disc (the anulus) and those not contained within the anulus. Contained lesions usually have minimal neurological deficits while uncontained disc lesions tend to demonstrate greater neurological deficits (10).

However, spinal pain is rarely the result of a single event, or it emanates from a single tissue type. As Sahrmann (11) points out, the question is not what is the source of the pain, but what caused the tissues to become painful. Frequently, the precipitating event was preceded by accumulated incidents of microtrauma from sustained or repetitive loading. Lumbar disorders are typically nonspecific and theoretically result from a combination of events leading to segmental articular dysfunction.

Kirkaldy-Willis (12) proposed a three-stage degenerative cascading process that begins with injury and cumulative trauma and leads to changes in the intervertebral disc, zygapophysial joints, supporting ligaments, joint capsules, and vertebral end plates that ultimately results in the pain and dysfunction. Stage I of this process (the stage of dysfunction) is characterized by joint synovitis, subluxation, early cartilage degeneration, radial and linear annular tears within the disc, local ischemia, sustained local muscle hypertonicity, and ligamentous strain. Stage II (the stage of instability) manifests in further cartilage degeneration and capsular laxity that permits increased rotational movement and further annular disruption and joint stress. Typical osteoarthritic changes, including joint space narrowing, fibrosis, osteophyte (bone spur) formation, and loss of joint cartilage, characterize Stage III (the stage of stabilization). These changes can contribute to central and spinal stenosis. This degenerative cascade model helps explain the age-related incidences of spinal disorders. Discogenic sources of pain are more common in the fourth and fifth decades (stages of dysfunction and instability), and stenosis is more common in the sixth and seventh decades (stage of stabilization).

Thus, a pathoanatomic diagnosis is often not possible. Indeed, the symptoms are frequently caused by movement disorders rather than structural, morphologic disorders. Because back pain is difficult to diagnose, various classification systems have evolved. Waddell (13) suggested a three-category triage system consisting of "simple backache," "nerve root pain," and "serious spinal pathology." Simple, nonspecific low back pain includes a variety of disorders and is the most common type of back pain. Nerve root pain could be attributed to disorders such as disc prolapse or spinal stenosis and is present less than 5% of the time. Serious spinal pathology includes diseases such as tumors, infections, and inflammatory disorders, such as ankylosing spondylitis, and represents less than 1% of the persons presenting with low back pain.

The Quebec Task Force developed 11 activity-related diagnostic categories consisting of (a) localized spinal pain, (b) pain radiating to an extremity proximally, (c) pain radiating to an extremity distally, (d) pain radiating to an extremity with positive neurologic signs, (e) radicular compression presumed, (f) radicular compression confirmed, (g) spinal stenosis confirmed, (h) post surgery less than 6 months, (i) post surgery greater than 6 months, (j) chronic pain syndrome, and (k) other (14). Note that, once again, this system is not based on identifying the precise anatomic structure involved. The value of selected classification systems will be discussed later in this chapter.

Because low back pain is a multifactorial disorder with a number of potential etiologies, determination of risk factors is difficult. Hence, a multitude of risk factors for low back pain has been identified. None of these factors is considered causal, and the strength of the evidence supporting each factor is variable. Risk factors can be categorized generally into personal, health behavior, and occupational risk factors. Table 13.1 lists commonly identified risk factors associated with low back pain as reviewed by Manchikanti (15).

CLINICAL PICTURE

Typically, individuals with vertebral disorders present with one or more of the following physical complaints: back pain, leg pain, neurologic symptoms, and spinal deformity. Pain is usually the primary complaint.

According to Waddell (13), persons with "simple backache" are usually healthy individuals between 20 and 55 years of age, who present with pain in the lumbosacral region, buttocks, and thighs. Pain varies in intensity and may be produced, aggravated, or relieved with general or specific spinal movements, activities, positions, and time. Morning stiffness or pain is common, and pain may worsen over the course of the day. A lateral spinal shift can be present, where the spine is pulled to one side, and the lordotic lumbar curve can be lost. Individuals presenting with "nerve root pain" complain of unilateral leg pain

Table 13.1. Potential Risk Factors Associated with Spinal Low Back Pain (15)

Personal risk factors	*Estimated strength of the evidence of risk*
Heredity/genetic	Strong
Sex	Moderate
Age	Strong
Height	Weak
Postural "deformities"	Weak
Psychosocial factors	Moderate
Prior back pain history	Moderate
Health behavior risk factors	***Estimated strength of the evidence of risk***
Physical fitness	Weak
Smoking	Strong
Obesity	Moderate
Occupational risk factors	***Estimated strength of the evidence of risk***
Physical work	Moderate
Lifting and twisting	Moderate
Static work postures	Moderate
Vibration	Moderate
Job dissatisfaction	Moderate

that is worse than their back pain, pain that radiates below the knee, numbness or altered sensation in the same distribution, nerve root signs (such as a positive straight leg raise test), and motor, sensory, or reflex changes in one nerve root. Frank "nerve root compression" signs are reflex changes, muscle weakness, muscle atrophy, and sensory loss over a defined area. Red flags for "potential serious pathology" are presented in Table 13.2.

Pain involves more than the transmission of sensory input. In addition to one or more of the physical complaints, people with low back pain can also present with varying amounts of anxiety, fear, anger, frustration, preoccupation with bodily sensations, irritability, decreased concentration, fatigue, and depression secondary to the physical disorder and pain. These emotions are common and normal responses to pain. However, these same emotions can become harmful and perpetuate symptoms if prolonged or excessive. Pain, fear, and anxiety seem particularly interrelated. Response to the stress of back pain often influences the response to intervention. Therefore, these emotions need to be considered and dealt with appropriately in any plan of care. Pain reinforced by secondary gain, inappropriate treatment, job dissatisfaction, pending litigation, and Worker's Compensation can manifest in symptom-magnification behaviors and disability.

Table 13.2. Red Flags Potentially Suggestive of More Serious Pathology and Need for Medical Consultation or Referral

Saddle (anal, genital, or perineum) anesthesia*
Unsteadiness, gait disturbances, fainting spells, or falling*
Difficulty or incontinence with urination or fecal incontinence*
Progressive weakness or incoordination in arms or legs**
Poor general health***
- Unexplained weight loss
- Loss of appetite
- Unusual fatigue or general malaise
- Chest pain or heaviness
- Frequent or severe abdominal pain
- Nausea and vomiting
- Fever
- Severe headaches or dizziness
- Shortness of breath
- Unusual lumps, growths, or unexplained swelling
- Changes in vision, hearing, swallowing, or speech

Onset before 20 or after 55 years of age
Severe trauma (e.g., falls, motor vehicle accidents)
Constant, nonmechanical pain
Unrelenting night pain
Thoracic pain
History of cancer, systemic steroids, osteoporosis, recent infections, rheumatologic disorders, HIV
Major persisting spinal deformity
Severe spasm
Severe lumbar flexion limitation
Psychologic overlay (yellow flags)
Inflammatory disorders
- Gradual onset before age 40
- Marked morning stiffness
- Persisting limitations in spinal movement in all directions
- Peripheral joint involvement
- Iritis, skin rashes, colitis, urethral discharge
- Family history

*Urgent referral: combination of signs suggests cauda equina lesion.
**Urgent referral: suggests serious spinal pathology
***May require urgent referral depending on findings (e.g., cardiac)

Another important consideration is the stage of the disorder. Symptoms vary within the same low back pain episode over the course of time. "Acute" to the patient frequently means "intense." However, to the health-care provider, acute is usually defined in terms of the duration of symptoms in months, weeks, days, and even hours. Most commonly, acute describes pain lasting less than 6 weeks. Presumably, the acute stage reflects the characteristics of the inflammatory process accompanying the disorder. Acute pain may be present at rest, aggravated by most activities, and felt over a diffuse area.

The subacute stage is considered the period of time between 6 and 12 weeks after the event. Pain in the subacute stage is more localized, associated with specific movements, and not present at rest. Notably, some authors do not distinguish between acute and subacute stages and consider the acute stage as less than 3 months' duration.

Chronic pain is defined as continuous pain lasting longer than 3 months or beyond the expected recovery time. Some people have frequent recurrences, such that the condition appears chronic, but might be better classified as recurrent (16). "True" chronic pain is modulated differently within the nervous system and becomes dissociated from the original physical disorder. Chronic pain can be intractable and self-perpetuating. Chronic pain is usually not amenable to the same kinds of treatment interventions used in the acute, subacute, or recurrent stages. Patients with chronic pain can become depressed and manifest with symptom magnification and chronic pain-related disability.

Considering the stage of the disorder is important when developing a treatment regimen. However, as noted, intermittent exacerbations of symptoms and recurrent episodes cloud the distinction among stages.

A distinction should also be made between pain and disability. Disability is the inability or restricted capacity to perform activities. Disability refers to patterns of behavior that have emerged over time, during which functional limitations could not be overcome to maintain usual role performance (17). Persons seeking medical attention often present with some limitation in activity, postures, or both. In their survey, Cassidy et al. (18) used four classifications for persons experiencing low back pain: (a) low pain intensity and disability, (b) high pain and low disability, (c) high pain intensity and moderate disability, and (d) high pain intensity and severe disability. Patients and some health-care providers assume that disability will be eliminated when pain is relieved. However, pain does not always lead to disability, nor does the intensity of pain reported reflect the amount of perceived disability. Pain intensity does not necessarily signal that tissue damage is occurring, i.e., pain can occur in structurally normal tissues. Simply put, hurt does not always mean harm. Stretching one's hamstrings is uncomfortable, but is not typically harmful. Patients and clinicians need to make this distinction in order to help prevent disability by keeping generally active.

DIAGNOSTIC TECHNIQUES

Accurate diagnosis is, of course, the cornerstone of effective intervention. But, as previously pointed out, in the case of low back pain, diagnosis does not always identify the tissue causing the pain. Waddell's (13) triage system gives a clinical picture of low back pain and offers a screening system that can be used to guide in further diagnostic testing. The key points in diagnosing low back pain are determining whether the pain is indeed coming from the back, ruling out more serious disorders, and acquiring information necessary to develop a plan of care. Diagnostic procedures always include a clinical examination and evaluation, and may include movement system, radiologic, electrodiagnostic, and laboratory testing when further information is needed. Each of these diagnostic techniques is discussed briefly in the following paragraphs.

Clinical Examination and Evaluation

The primary diagnostic procedure in the case of low back pain is the clinical examination and evaluation. The clinical examination consists of two parts, the subjective examination, or history, and the objective examination, or physical. Based on the results of the examination, the clinician evaluates (or assesses) the findings of the examination and either makes a diagnosis or determines the need for further testing. Typical components of a clinical examination are outlined in Table 13.3. Magee (19) provides a comprehensive text on this subject.

History

The history, or subjective examination, consists of gathering information from patient reports in five major areas: the present condition, previous incidents, medical history, personal information, and patient goals.

Information about the present condition can be further subdivided into information about the mechanism and date (or time period) of onset, area of symptoms, nature and intensity of pain, behavior of the symptoms, and types of functional limitations. Each of these sources of information is discussed in the following paragraphs.

The onset of pain could be an injury or it could be a gradual onset with no discernible precipitating event. Gradual onset may have been triggered by predisposing activities such as a change in habits, work duties, work environment, chair, etc. The date or time frame suggests the stage of the disorder, and the area (or anatomic distribution) of symptoms directs the extent and type of examination. Particularly important is whether the pain is centrally located, peripherally located, or both.

The nature or quality of the symptoms is helpful in determining the general source of the problem. Different

Table 13.3. Outline of Typical Components of a Clinical Examination of a Patient with Low Back Pain*

CLINICAL EXAMINATION
History
(Subjective Examination)
Present condition
Mechanism and date of onset
Area of symptoms
Nature and intensity of pain
Behavior of symptoms
Types of disabilities
Previous incidents
Prior treatment and outcomes
Medical and surgical history
Medications
Personal information
Demographic
Occupational
Social
Living environment
Patient goals
PHYSICAL EXAMINATION*
(Objective Examination)
Part 1: Systems review
Systems review and observations
General appearance
Communication ability, affect, and behavior
Gross symmetry, structure, and skin integrity
Locomotion, balance, and transitional movements
Heart and respiratory rate and blood pressure
Height and weight
Other
Part 2: Tests and measures to verify lumbar spine involvement and the general nature of involvement
Posture/alignment
Movement examination: Active, passive, and resistive lumbar movements
Quantity (range) of movement
Quality and pattern of movement
Effect of movement on symptoms
Neurological screening of lower quarter
Cutaneous sensation in dermatomes
Myotome (groups of muscles supplied by a single nerve root) testing
Deep tendon reflexes
Upper motor neuron screen (e.g., pathological reflexes)
Neurodynamic tests (e.g., straight leg raising, dural mobility tests)
Vascular screening of lower quadrant (e.g., pulses)
Peripheral and sacroiliac joint screening
Special tests (as indicated based on symptoms)
Palpation
Temperature
Tenderness
Tissue condition: tension, texture, thickness, etc.
Intervertebral joint movement screening (movement and end feel)
Functional assessment screening (task performance ability)

*Content and extent of the physical examination varies with the practitioner's discipline, background, and experience, the results of the subjective examination, and the purpose of the examination.

sources of pain give rise to different types of sensation. For example, as noted previously, somatic referred pain is typically deep, diffuse, achy, hard to localize, and varying in intensity. Pain intensity or severity is typically assessed either verbally or diagrammatically using a pain scale. When using a numeric pain scale, the patient is asked to express the intensity of the pain from 0 to 10, with 0 being no pain and 10 suggesting that the pain is as bad as it could possibly be or requires going to the emergency room. A visual analog scale (VAS) can also be used. A VAS typically consists of a 100-mm line with the extremes of pain denoted at each end of the line, i.e., no pain to the worst possible pain. The patient is then asked to mark the pain intensity on the line. Alternatively, the patient may be asked to circle adjectives describing the nature of the pain.

The behavior of the symptoms is especially important in helping to rule out more serious pathology, gauging the intensity of the physical examination, and ultimately developing an intervention strategy. Specifically, the patient is asked to describe what makes the pain better or worse. The clinician is particularly interested in the postures, movements, and activities that affect the nature, location, and intensity of the pain when evaluating mechanical pain.

Other information needed about the present condition is knowledge of any functional limitation or disability the patient is encountering because of the low back pain. The patient can simply be asked about his/her activity restrictions, or a functional status questionnaire can be used. Typical assessment includes inquiry about bending, lifting, standing, walking, sitting, sleeping, dressing, sexual activity, traveling, and performing household chores, childcare, work, leisure, and social activities. Two of the more widely used measures of low back disability are the Oswestry (20) and Roland-Morris (21) questionnaires.

The patient is also asked about the nature, duration, and frequency of any previous episodes of low back pain. Medical history questions are generally designed to identify red flags suggestive of more serious pathology and to alert the clinician to factors that may confound the problem or that need to be considered in treatment (such as diabetes). Personal questions include questions about age, occupation, leisure activities, and social history. Lastly, the patient is asked about his/her goals and expected outcome of care.

The examiner usually makes a *preliminary* diagnosis based on the history. In addition, the examiner judges the *irritability* of the disorder, that is, how easy or difficult it is to provoke the symptoms. An irritable condition will be easy to reproduce and may require a gentle physical examination. A less irritable condition can be difficult to evoke and may require a more extensive, vigorous physical examination.

Physical Examination

The second part of the clinical examination is the physical or objective examination. The physical examination is used to confirm or refute the *preliminary* diagnosis by reproducing the "comparable sign." The comparable sign is the collection of signs and symptoms that reproduce *the* pain or dysfunction that caused the patient to seek the services of a health-care provider (22). The content and extent of the physical examination vary with the practitioner's discipline, background, and experience; the results of the subjective examination; and the purpose of the examination. A physician may only need to decide whether the patient has nonspecific low back pain, nerve root irritation, pain from a source other than the spine, or red flags signaling potential serious pathology. This may be sufficient information to decide on a course of action. However, a diagnosis of nonspecific low back pain (or one of the many diagnostic labels suggesting essentially the same thing, e.g., sprain/strain, degenerative disc or joint disease, and so on) is insufficient for a physical therapist, for example, to initiate intervention. A physical therapist needs detailed information about the quality and quantity of active and passive movements and the effect of movements and positions on pain and function. Assessment of these movements is used in conjunction with other information to direct treatment.

Potential components of a physical examination are outlined in Table 13.3. The examination consists of two parts. The first part is the *systems review* used primarily to confirm or refute any red flags suggested by the history. The second part of the examination is to determine the presence of signs of nerve irritation, decide whether the pain actually involves the lumbar spine, and obtain further clarifying information in order to make a differential diagnosis and develop a plan of care. The general intent of the physical examination is to reproduce the comparable sign through selected tests, measures, and patient responses, and to determine the nature and extent of impairments, function, and disability.

Evaluation

Based on evaluation (interpretation) of the results of the history and physical examinations, the clinician can usually decide on one of two courses of action:

- Diagnose the disorder (see section entitled, *Medical and Clinical Diagnosis*), make a prognosis, and design and implement the plan of care, or
- Tentatively diagnose the disorder and determine the need for further testing to confirm or refute this working diagnosis. Trial treatment, based on the tentative diagnosis, may not be initiated at this time.

If further diagnostic procedures are indicated, this testing might consist of more in-depth movement system testing, diagnostic imaging, electrodiagnostic testing, or laboratory testing to clarify the diagnosis. The tests depend on the discipline and background of the practitioner and the needs of the patient.

Movement System Testing

Movement is a physiological system with several contributing systems. Movement system impairments are theorized to lead to pain, functional limitations, disability, and pathology (11). Movement system testing is performed when the examination failed to yield an adequate medical diagnosis and/or additional information on movement system impairments is needed in order to make a clinical diagnosis and develop a plan of care. *Impairments* are defined as alterations in anatomical, physiological, or psychological structures or functions (17). For the purposes of this discussion, movement dysfunctions are as follows: reduced motion, excessive motion, aberrant motion, or malalignment. Movement dysfunctions can occur because of impairments in elements of the movement system at the neuromusculoskeletal level (e.g., extensibility, mobility, strength, endurance), neuromuscular control level (e.g., muscle recruitment and feedback), biomechanical level (e.g., static and dynamic forces), support level (e.g., cardiovascular and cardiopulmonary) (11), or a combination. The movement system evaluation is used to determine which, or which combination of these elements, is causing or perpetuating the pain and dysfunction. Examples follow.

The routine clinical examination may have included screening of passive physiological intervertebral mobility as listed in Table 13.3. If indicated by the screen, more in-depth and specialized testing of articular (joint) mobility [termed a *biomechanical examination* by Meadows (23)] may be needed. When restricted physiological intervertebral movements are found, specific passive arthrokinematic (movement at the level of the joint surface) intervertebral movement tests are used to detect articular dysfunctions potentially amenable to manipulation or mobilization. When excessive movement is detected with physiological intervertebral movement testing, segmental stability is examined to test for articular integrity. Hypermobility (clinical instability) is potentially amenable to segmental stabilization, which is discussed later in this chapter.

Movement system impairments occurring primarily at the musculoskeletal and neuromuscular levels (e.g., problems with muscle strength, muscle extensibility, muscle length-tension properties, endurance, mobility, alignment, stability, coordination, or muscle recruitment patterns) may also cause movement-related disorders. More in-depth movement system testing is likely to include examination and evaluation of the impairments hypothesized to relate to the patient's functional limitations and disability. This testing might consist of traditional testing of muscle force or torque capacity, such as with a dynamometer, mobility testing using goniometry, etc. (see section on *Exercise, Fitness, & Functional Testing*). Or, regional, integrated, standardized movement impairment syndrome assessment protocols, such as that developed by Sahrmann (11), can be used. The latter helps identify interrelationships among systems that affect movement quality and detect the offending "directional susceptibility to movement (DSM)." Specific movement system disorders are corrected with individualized exercise and retraining programs.

Diagnostic Imaging

Diagnostic imaging may be indicated in certain circumstances and in recommended time frames. Because anatomic anomalies and aging changes will be present on diagnostic images, the patient's clinical findings must be correlated with radiologic findings. Typical imaging used to assist in diagnosis might include one or more of the following: plain film radiography, myelography, computed tomography, bone scans, discography, fluoroscopy, and magnetic resonance imaging. Each of these procedures is briefly discussed, based mostly on Magee (19).

Plain film radiography (x-ray) is a primary means of diagnostic imaging for musculoskeletal disorders. The primary purpose of plain film radiography is to rule out fractures, infection, serious disease, and structural abnormalities. Radiographs poorly differentiate most soft-tissue structures.

Computed tomography (CT) scans produce cross-sectional images taken at specific levels and axial projections. CT is particularly useful for visualizing bone and has good resolution of soft-tissue structures such as the paravertebral muscles. CT scans can detect disc protrusions, spinal stenosis, joint disease, tumors, epidural scarring after surgery, and fractures.

Bone scans (radionuclide imaging) consist of intravenous injections of radioactive tracers (isotopes) to localize specific areas of high level turnover of bone. These areas of high turnover are then detected, usually with radiographs, as "hot spots." Bone scans are used to detect bone loss, active bone disease, fracture, infection, arthritis, and tumors. Bone scans are sensitive to bone abnormalities, but do not identify the specific abnormality.

Discography is an invasive and relatively uncommon technique that involves injection of radiopaque dye into the nucleus pulposus of an intervertebral disc under radiographic guidance. Discography is used to determine internal disc derangement especially when magnetic resonance imaging and myelography are normal. Discography is also used to determine whether the injection reproduces the patient's symptoms.

Myelography is an invasive imaging procedure used to visualize soft tissues within the spine. A radiopaque dye is injected into the epidural space and allowed to flow to different levels of the spinal cord. A plain film or a computed tomograph (CT is then taken. The procedure is used to detect such disorders as disc herniation, spinal stenosis, osteophytes, tumor, and nerve root entrapment. MRI has largely replaced myelography, but myelography is used as a surgical screen when the MRI or CT is equivocal.

Fluoroscopy is an infrequently performed technique used to show motion in joints using x-ray imaging. Fluoroscopy, however, is frequently used to direct the needle in injection therapy.

Magnetic resonance imaging (MRI) is a noninvasive, multiplanar imaging technique that uses exposure to magnetic fields to image bone and soft tissue. MRI has the advantage of no exposure to x-ray. Delineation of soft tissues is greater with MRI than with CT. MRI is the preferred technique for imaging disc disease. MRI can be used to detect tumors, disc pathology, infection, and soft-tissue lesions. MRI can also be used with contrasts, for example, to enhance imaging of intrathecal nerve roots. Emerging developments in MR imaging, including imaging in weight-bearing positions, such as standing, and use of cinematographic MRI, may yield even more sophisticated diagnostic capabilities for low back disorders, especially for identifying movement disorders.

Electrodiagnostic Testing

Electrodiagnostic testing (e.g., electromyography [EMG] and nerve conduction velocity [NCV] studies) is sometimes indicated to localize dysfunction along lower motor neurons. Specifically, disease processes can be localized to the level of the anterior horn cell, nerve root, plexus, or peripheral nerve, neuromuscular junction, or muscle.

Laboratory Testing

Sometimes laboratory-screening tests, such as erythrocyte sedimentation rate (ESR), blood count, or urinalysis, are requested when there are clinical red flags suggesting disease or infection. Otherwise, use of laboratory tests in the case of low back pain is not common.

MEDICAL AND CLINICAL DIAGNOSIS

A diagnosis, even one made on interpretation of the most reliable and valid tests and measures, is largely provisional and subject to change. A diagnosis is both a process and a product. A *medical diagnosis* is the identification of a patient's pathology or disease from the symptoms, signs, and test results. Physicians diagnose and treat diseases and pathologies. However, frequently, no significant underlying disease or pathology can be identified, or the identified disease or pathology may be insufficient upon which to develop an intervention strategy. As noted, sometimes a diagnosis is simply "low back pain." In these cases, a *clinical diagnosis* is made. A clinical diagnosis is a classification, or a label, encompassing a cluster of signs and symptoms commonly associated with a disorder, syndrome, or category of impairment, functional limitation, or disability (17). Subclassification of patients based on diagnostic classification paradigms is essential in determining appropriate interventions and outcomes.

Clinical Diagnosis or Classification of Low Back Disorders

Because of the recognized need to develop classifications to characterize low back pain, a number of these systems have evolved. The Quebec classification system, mentioned earlier in this chapter, is one such diagnostic classification system. Sahrmann (11) proposed a movement impairment-based classification system for clinically diagnosing clusters of impairments in quality of movement. Other efforts have been directed toward developing treatment-based, clinical diagnoses that direct the precise intervention (e.g., traction, extension movement, and manipulation). Delitto et al. (24) published a treatment-based classification system specifically for conservative management of persons with low back syndrome. Such classification systems are based on the concept that, although the majority of patients with low back pain are without a specific diagnosis, they are not a homogeneous population. Clinically differentiating patients generally categorized with nonspecific low back pain is a prerequisite to determining effective intervention and suc-cessful, cost-controlled outcomes. Otherwise, decisions about conservative intervention for low back pain are largely "hit or miss." Much work remains in developing and validating classification systems for low back disorders. Riddle (25) reviewed a number of these classification systems.

Prognosis and Plan of Care

Once a diagnosis is established, the expected optimal level of improvement in the desired outcomes is predicted, and the amount of time required to reach these outcomes is estimated. Based on the diagnosis, stage, and severity of the disorder, prognosis, and patient goals, an individualized plan of care is developed specifying the goals, outcomes, specific interventions, and the proposed timing for managing the disorder. The *general* anticipated goals and expected outcomes may be one or more of the following: affect pathology/pathophysiology, reduce function-related impairments (including pain), restore function, prevent disability, promote health, reduce risk and prevent recurrences, and satisfy patients, all accomplished in a measurable, timely, and cost-effective manner. Interventions can be generally classified as medical, pharmacologic, physical, educational and counseling, alternative, and surgical. Of course, several intervention strategies can be used concurrently, or specific interventions may follow the successful or unsuccessful outcome of previous interventions.

MEDICAL, PHARMACOLOGIC, PHYSICAL, EDUCATIONAL AND COUNSELING, ALTERNATIVE, AND SURGICAL INTERVENTIONS

Management of spinal pain is dependent on the presumed cause or classification, severity, stage of the disorder, the presence of comorbidities, practitioner experience and judgment, and individual patient factors (e.g., age, values, motivation, activity level, goals). Discussion of the management of nerve root disorders and serious spinal pathology (e.g., inflammatory diseases, cauda equina syndrome, and spinal tumors) is beyond the scope of this chapter. *The focus in this section is on intervention strategies for nonspecific, activity-related or mechanical back pain.*

The strength of evidence for different intervention strategies varies; however, none of the evidence is particularly strong. Therefore, it should be noted that **no intervention has been shown to be unequivocally effective in the treatment of nonspecific acute and chronic low back pain.** Some of the people are helped some of the time. As noted, part of the problem in determining effectiveness is lack of adequate methodology for subclassifying this large heterogeneous population of persons with nonspecific low back pain. In order to research the effectiveness of various interventions, more homogeneous groupings are needed. The Agency for Health Care Policy and Research (AHCPR) *Clinical Practice Guideline for Acute Low Back Pain in Adults* (26) provides the current status of the information on the effectiveness of various management strategies for adults with *acute* low back pain. To expand on Kane (27), the ultimate key to successful intervention and patient outcome at all levels is to do the right things for the right people at the right time and to do them well. We just don't yet know with certainty the right things, the right people, the right time, or perhaps, even the right way.

Medical Intervention

Medical intervention typically consists of dispensing information, advice, reassurance, and psychological support; making referrals; and managing pharmacologic intervention. Dispensing information, advice, reassurance, and psychological support is discussed in the subsection on educational and counseling interventions. Recognizing the need for appropriate referrals is essential for each practitioner dealing with persons with low back pain. Pharmacologic intervention is discussed in the next subsection.

Pharmacologic Intervention

Pharmacologic intervention for low back pain is common. Drugs may be nonprescription or prescription, and oral, topical, or injected. Medication types used in the treatment of low back pain are anti-inflammatories (nonsteroidal anti-inflammatory drugs [NSAIDs] and steroids), muscle relaxants, analgesics (opioids and non-opioids), antidepressants, and anesthetics.

Commonly used nonprescription medications are acetaminophen or paracetamol (Tylenol), aspirin, and ibuprofen (Motrin). Acetaminophen is primarily used as an analgesic in treating low back pain. Aspirin and ibuprofen are NSAIDs and analgesics.

NSAIDs are widely prescribed for low back pain (28) and purportedly reduce swelling and inflammation and promote healing. Examples of prescription NSAIDs are Celebrex, Naprosyn, and Vioxx. NSAIDs have a number of potential side effects, especially gastrointestinal irritation, and must be used with discretion. NSAIDs are sometimes augmented with a muscle relaxant (29) (e.g., Flexeril, Robaxin) and acetaminophen. Drowsiness is a common side effect of muscle relaxants. Oral steroids (e.g., Prednisone, Medrol) have similar general effects to NSAIDs and are occasionally used short term for more severe inflammation. Likewise, a short course of opioid analgesics (e.g., Darvocet, Tylenol with codeine, Vicodin) is occasionally prescribed for more severe pain, but less likely with nonspecific low back pain. Opioid analgesics are addictive and usually avoided.

In addition, injection therapy is sometimes used for symptom control. Typical injections consist of myofascial trigger point, intra-articular (facet), or epidural injections and nerve blocks. Myofascial trigger point injections are injections of anesthetic into muscles for the purpose of relieving pain and spasm. Intra-articular injections, epidural injections, and nerve blocks consist of local injections of a mixture that typically includes steroids and anesthetics into a specific area under x-ray (fluoroscopic) guidance. These injections are used both diagnostically and therapeutically. That is, if the symptoms are relieved, the injection was treatment. If the symptoms were not affected, then presumably the injection sites were not the source of pain. Intra-articular injections are made directly into the offending lumbar joints in order to relieve pain and inflammation. Epidural injections consist of injecting into the epidural space close to the affected area. Epidural injections are used for patients with nerve root irritation or compromise and presumably decrease inflammation of nerve roots and relieve pain. A lumbar sympathetic nerve block involves injecting around the sympathetic nerves in order to "block" neuropathic pain. Blocks can also be selective nerve root blocks for specific spinal roots. In severe cases, injections are used to permanently destroy nerves in order to relieve pain. The efficacy of injection therapy is not well established.

Physical Intervention

Physical intervention consists of a broad range of treatments that might be categorized as physical agents, electrotherapeutic modalities, mechanical modalities, orthotics, protective and supportive devices, manual therapy, and exercise. In general, the evidence supporting use of various physical interventions is inconclusive or found to be useful only during specific stages, i.e., acute or chronic.

Physical agents use heat, cold, sound, or light energy to decrease pain, increase tissue extensibility, reduce soft-tissue inflammation, decrease swelling, remodel scar tissue, etc. Ultrasound, hydrotherapy, hot packs, and cold packs are examples of physical agents used in treatment of low back pain. Typically, physical agents, if used, are used in the acute stages of low back pain and/or as adjunctive interventions to other physical interventions, such as using heat combined with stretching.

Electrotherapeutic modalities consist of physical agents that use electricity to decrease pain, reduce soft-tissue inflammation, decrease muscle spasm and guarding, and assist in muscle reeducation. Examples of electrotherapeutic modalities include alternating direct and pulsed current, transcutaneous electrical nerve stimulation (TENS), low-level laser, neuromuscular electrical stimulation (NMES), and surface electromyography (SEMG).

Mechanical modalities include traction, compression, taping, and continuous passive motion. Mechanical modalities are typically intended to decrease pain, stabilize or mobilize an area, apply distraction or compression, and/or increase range of motion.

Orthotics, and protective and supportive devices used in treating low back pain primarily consist of shoe inserts or lifts and various back supports, corsets, and braces. Corrective foot orthotics are sometimes prescribed for patients who have back pain while standing or walking and who do so for long periods. Shoe lifts might be used to correct a leg length discrepancy. Back supports, corsets, and braces can be used as adjunctive treatment to restrict movement and provide support. The selection of the type of brace depends on the amount of immobilization required and the region of the spine requiring stabilization.

Manual therapy consists of several techniques including, but not limited to, spinal manipulation/mobilization, muscle energy technique, myofascial release, and soft-tissue mobilization. Manual therapy is practiced by a number of different practitioners, primarily osteopathic physicians, physical therapists, and chiropractors. Massage therapists also may perform some deep-tissue techniques. **Manipulation/mobilization** is defined as a continuum of skilled passive movements to joints and/or related soft tissues that are applied at varying speeds and amplitudes. *Manipulation* is typically thought of as a localized thrust of high velocity and small amplitude therapeutic movement (17), whereas *mobilization* is usually considered a nonthrust technique. The general objectives of manipulation/mobilization are to regain pain-free movement and restore function. Manipulation may be helpful for selected patients with low back pain. Use of manipulation with patients with radiculopathy is controversial. **Muscle energy technique** is an active procedure in which the patient helps correct a movement by contracting muscle in a controlled direction against a counterforce supplied by a clinician. Muscle energy technique can be used to mobilize joints and relax, lengthen, or strengthen muscle (30). **Myofascial release and soft-tissue mobilization** may serve as a prelude to other procedures. These techniques are used to mechanically stretch skin, fascia, and muscle to improve extensibility, increase circulation, and decrease muscle guarding and spasm.

Exercise includes physical activities to increase mobility, stability, muscle performance, balance, coordination, posture, neuromuscular control, cardiovascular and muscular endurance, and movement patterns. Exercises are used to relieve pain, improve physical function and health status, and prevent complications and future impairments or functional loss (31). Exercises will be discussed in more detail in the section titled *Exercise Prescription and Programming*.

Educational and Counseling Intervention

Educational and counseling interventions can take many forms: informal or formal, group or individual, verbal or written, solicited or unsolicited, individualized or generic, to name a few. Nonspecific low back pain may seem common and routine for the clinician, but the patient fears pain, damage, harm, and permanent functional limitations and disability. Information is one key in allaying these fears that naturally accompany low back pain. Another key to relieving fear is providing reassurance, comfort, and caring. Pain is, after all, a sensory and emotional experience for people, not their spines.

The AHCPR *Clinical Practice Guideline for Adults with Acute Low Back Pain* indicates that patient education should include an explanation of the diagnosis, natural history of the disorder, prognosis, safe and effective methods of symptom control, use of diagnostic procedures, methods of limiting recurrence, and general course of care (26). Advice might consist of the use, discontinued use, or presumed effectiveness of various treatments or products (e.g., supports, mattresses, herbals), and the *do's and don'ts* of general, occupational, social, and leisure activity modifications, positions, and rest. Bed rest is not recommended for most cases of simple, nonspecific backache (32). If used, rest should not exceed 2 days for persons without neuromotor deficits (33).

To paraphrase a saying attributed to Hippocrates, healing is often a matter of time and opportunity. Modifying various positions and activities is frequently recommended as a means of providing the opportunity for healing. It is difficult to heal that which is constantly being irritated. Patients may need *individualized* guidance on the position and activity modifications appropriate to their disorder, behavior and severity of symptoms, age, general health, and typical physical demands. For example, merely teaching a patient who experiences pain with spinal extension to initiate movement from the hips versus the spine when returning to upright from spinal flexion, may relieve all symptoms associated with that activity. Some positions and activities may be deemed irritating, and therefore, temporary or permanent lifestyle changes may be recommended.

Specific position and activity modifications are based primarily on the patient's report of the behavior of the symptoms and on known mechanical spine stressors, such as lifting. For example, if patients complain of pain *during* sitting, they may be advised to temporarily limit or interrupt periods of sitting. Likewise, if patients complain of pain *during* running, they may be advised to limit running. However, patients complaining of symptoms *after* running may be able to continue running, but may need to modify the activity they do after running, that is, when they feel the pain (frequently sitting). Patients are generally encouraged to continue ordinary activity and working and to gradually increase their physical activities over a period of a few days or weeks (32).

Another area of patient education focuses on ergonomic and work/home site recommendations. Patients may need information on chair types and adjustments, sitting supports (e.g., lumbar rolls), pillows, shoes, standing surfaces, seating and desk arrangements, computer heights, lifting, etc.

In addition to individualized education, various pamphlets, books, magazines, and information from relatives, friends, strangers, and websites is readily available. Frequently, patients need help in interpreting this information relative to their situation and in judging the quality of the information.

Structured patient education through back schools has been somewhat effective in the workplace (26) and may include work-site–specific education. Behavioral interventions, cognitive therapies, and pain management clinics are more often recommended for patients dealing with chronic pain.

Alternative (Complementary) Intervention

An ever-increasing number of alternative, or complementary, interventions for treating low back pain have evolved largely based on anecdotal and extrapolated evidence and on failures of conventional medical care. Some of the more common complementary interventions for low back pain at this time are acupuncture, acupressure, biomagnets, selected mind–body techniques, herbs, and supplements (such as glucosamine–chondroitin sulfates). Increased popular use of these complementary interventions has sparked interest in scientific circles. However, most of these interventions have not yet been studied sufficiently to warrant recommendation.

Surgical Intervention

Surgical intervention is not typically indicated for nonspecific low back pain but is indicated with progressive neurologic deficit and with some serious disorders. Surgery is also used in some cases of severe pain and in cases with significant neurologic deficit. A number of different surgical approaches and techniques are available and are constantly evolving. Common types of surgeries are fusions, decompressions, and other procedures.

Spinal fusion is performed to eliminate motion at one or more vertebral segments. Spinal fusion involves adding a bone graft to an area of the spine that then grows between the segments to eliminate motion. Fusions may also be augmented by implanting fixation implements, such as screws and rods, to further stabilize the area. Examples of types of fusions include posterolateral, interbody, anterior–posterior, and lumbar cage fusion. Fusions may be performed for conditions such as degenerative disc disease, iatrogenic segmental instability, and spondylolisthesis.

The general purpose of **decompressive spinal surgery** is to relieve neural impingement by creating more space. Decompressive laminectomy is a common procedure to treat lumbar spinal stenosis. Two examples of decompressive surgeries for neural impingement caused by disc herniation are microdiscectomy and discectomy via laminectomy. Percutaneous and endoscopic discectomies and intradiscal electrothermal therapy (IDET) are other less-invasive surgical techniques for lumbar disc herniation.

Outcomes of Intervention

Successful outcomes from management of an episode of low back pain are typically measured using minimally clinically important differences (MCID) on standardized pain and disability scales, and with patient-specific functional scales and patient satisfaction questionnaires. Scales used should be validated for individuals as well as groups. Given the high rate of recurrence, patients should also be provided with knowledge of warning signs and self-management strategies, or first aid (e.g., ice, specific movements), for future episodes. In addition, patients should be informed of individualized risk reduction (see Table 13.1) and preventive strategies (see section on *Preventing Low Back Pain*). True success would be a happy, fully functioning client without recurrence or future reliance on the health-care system.

EXERCISE, FITNESS, AND FUNCTIONAL TESTING

A variety of tests exist for measuring exercise, fitness, and function for patients with low back pain. The reliability and validity of these tests and measures is variable and is, in all cases, population specific. Therefore, the selection of tests should be based on the purpose of the test and applicability to the patient. Selected tests and measures associated with low back disorders are presented in Table 13.4.

CLINICAL EXERCISE PHYSIOLOGY

In order to understand the exercise prescription and programming, a brief description of trunk muscle function is included, followed by a brief description of acute and chronic responses to exercise.

Functionally, the lumbopelvic muscles can be divided into local stabilizing (or deep) muscles and global stabilizing muscles. Two of the primary local stabilizing muscles are the transversus abdominis and the multifidus. These muscles have been hypothesized to contribute to lumbar spine stiffness and to control intersegmental motion. A contraction of the transversus abdominis normally precedes movement of an extremity (34, 35). Onset of premovement activity in the transversus abdominis is delayed in patients with low back pain. Evidence suggests that poor endurance of the multifidus and segmental fibers of the erector spinae may be a predictor for recurrent low back pain (36). Further, and importantly, the multifidi do not automatically recover full strength after the first episode of low back pain without specific exercise (37).

Muscles of the global stabilizing system consist of the erector spinae, quadratus lumborum, rectus abdominis, and internal and external obliques. These muscles not only move the spine but also function to transfer external loads applied to the trunk in order to minimize load on the lum-

Table 13.4. Potential Tests and Measures for Determining Exercise, Fitness, and Function of Patients with Nonspecific, Mechanical Low Back Pain*

TESTS	MEASURES	COMMENTS
Aerobic capacity and endurance		
• Treadmill • Cycle (bike or recumbent) • Arm ergometer	• 12-lead ECG, heart rate, RPE, blood pressure	• Testing may be warranted if risk or symptoms of CAD • Usually select low-impact test methods • Choice of test method may be dictated by patient symptoms • Testing is usually not applicable within the first 2–6 weeks of onset when activity may be curtailed
• 6- or 12-minute walk test	• Distance walked	• Fitness indicators
• 1-meter walk test	• Time	
Posture & anthropometry		
• Alignment and position (dynamic and static)	• Symmetry, curvature, flexicurve measures	
• Body composition	• Body mass index	
Extremes/range of motion		
Spinal		
• Dual goniometry	• Lumbar extremes of motion (deg)	
• BROM	• Schober's Lumbar Flexion Method; Attraction Extension Method (cm)	
• Tape measure		
Extremities		
• Goniometry	• Joint angle	
Flexibility/extensibility		
• Goniometry	• Joint angle	• Especially 2-joint muscles in lower extremities
Strength (trunk & extremities)		
• Isometric, isotonic, or isokinetic dynamometry	• Peak torque/force	
• Weight lifted	• 1 repetition maximum (RM)	
Muscular endurance		
• Isometric, isotonic, or isokinetic dynamometry • Weight lifted	• Maximum repetitions at 60% peak torque/force or 10 RM	• Isometric tests need a minimum 5-sec holding contraction.
• Trunk extensor endurance	• Specific timed trunk extensor endurance tests (e.g., Sorenson's, Ito's)	
Neuromuscular		
• Gait analysis	• Observational analysis	
• Locomotion	• Observations, ADL (activities of daily living) scales	
• Stability (balance)	• Balance scales, force platforms, timed tests	
• Transitional movements (e.g., sit-and-stand)	• Observations, ADL scales, and indexes	
• Motor control	• Recruitment patterns, substitutions, movement quality, compensations	
Functional performance		
• Ergonomics	• Work simulations, impairment ratings, task analysis	• Useful for determining work capacity, estimating job or sport restrictions
• Body mechanics	• ADL scales, observations	
• Functional capacity	• Functional capacity evaluations (FCEs)	
• ADL	• ADL scales and indexes	
• Lifting	• Lift capacity (with different types of lifts) and projections	
• Sports performance	• Screening, simulations, observations, task analysis	
• Functional status	• Roland-Morris Questionnaire, Oswestry Low Back Pain Disability Questionnaire, Patient-Specific Functional Scale	

***SPECIAL CONSIDERATIONS**

- Testing may not be reliable in the presence of pain owing to submaximal patient effort.
- Testing may need to be modified owing to age, stage of the disorder, comorbidities, severity of pain, and patient needs.
- Testing may need to be terminated or deferred in the presence of increasing pain.
- Testing should be terminated with progressive sensory or motor deterioration.
- Timing of testing postoperatively is at the surgeon's discretion based on patient status and type of surgery.

bar spine and its segments. The global stabilizing system needs strength and endurance; however, the global muscles cannot control shear forces at the segmental level. Overemphasis on exercising the global system in the presence of an inadequate local stabilizing system creates a potentially harmful imbalance. Evidence suggests that stabilization exercise programs should be based on assessment of need and should target the appropriate stabilizing system or systems (38). Furthermore, the rectus abdominis is primarily a trunk flexor and of less importance in rehabilitating patients with low back pain.

Acute and chronic responses to exercise are usually not altered by nonspecific low back pain without concomitant diseases; however, the stage of the disorder, severity of symptoms, goals, and positions for exercising are important considerations. Certain exercises may aggravate the symptoms, especially in the first 2–3 weeks after onset of low back pain. Nonetheless, patients should be kept as active as possible to prevent debilitation secondary to inactivity. More specific exercise guidelines are discussed in the next section.

EXERCISE PRESCRIPTION AND PROGRAMMING

A consumer publication survey (39) of 46,000 readers recently reported that 66% of the respondents with back pain had tried exercise and ranked exercise "among the treatments receiving the highest marks for back pain." Interestingly, a recent systematic review of the use of exercise in acute, nonspecific low back pain (40) did not find that exercise was successful in relieving low back pain. Certainly, this is not the first time that popular opinion differed from research-based evidence. However, exercise is apparently helping some people. Perhaps the problem is definitions and lack of specificity, i.e., "back pain" is generic, "exercise" is generic, and "relieving" is generic.

What exactly is *back pain?* As discussed in the section on pathophysiology, spinal pain has numerous causes and may even arise from different areas: lumbar, thoracic, or sacral. Not all causes of nonspecific spinal pain can be helped by exercises. To further complicate the problem, the effectiveness of exercise interacts with the stage of the disorder. Abdominal strengthening may not help acute low back pain, but a chronic problem might be helped. And what is *exercise?* Exercise could be walking, weight training, stretching, self-manipulation, a standardized routine (like Williams' flexion exercises), stabilization exercises, a self-directed program, or a specifically prescribed regimen. And, as noted, exercises appropriate for one type of disorder may not be appropriate for another. Further, exercises appropriate for the disorder, but applied at the inappropriate time in the stage of the disorder may not be effective. Compliance also affects the reported success of exercise. And finally, what is *relief?* Is relief the absence of pain, occasional pain not interfering with activities, or even continued pain but the ability to return to work and leisure activities? And is the goal of exercise to relieve pain or also to restore function, prevent disability, and promote health? We have a lot to learn. The question, then, is not only does exercise work or not, but also on whom, to what extent, and under what conditions?

Management of persons with certain red flags (e.g., inflammatory conditions) and some nerve root involvement may at times include exercise. However, the exercise intervention for people with these conditions needs to be relegated to practitioners with specific knowledge and expertise. Exercise for patients with nonspecific low back pain is based on patient needs, severity of symptoms, and functional limitations (see Table 13.5).

Patients with nonspecific low back pain need subclassifying, staging, and individualizing in order to design an appropriate intervention. Therefore, general exercise intervention strategies are difficult to describe. Further, in the absence of better guidelines, the clinician is required to "integrate" information from a number of sources, each diverse, yet similar, and each with varying scientific and empirical support. Figure 13.1 presents this author's algorithm for exercise intervention for patients with nonspecific low back pain. The algorithm was compiled and integrated from several sources (11, 13, 24, 41) in an attempt to reconcile and consider seemingly different approaches, all of which appear to offer credible (albeit limited) evidence for clinical effectiveness. Not all patients need to proceed through each stage of rehabilitation. Patients should "enter" the model at the appropriate stage. Therefore, guidelines to staging, based loosely on Fritz and George (42) will be discussed first.

Staging Nonspecific Low Back Pain

With the current absence of evidence-based criteria for accurate staging, appropriate staging is mostly a matter of patient self-assessment and clinician judgment. Although insurance company representatives and others prefer to consider stages as merely the passage of time, passage of time is not the sole consideration. This is analogous to advancing students in school based on passage of time (i.e., grade levels) without meeting the criteria for passing the grade level.

Table 13.5 General Guidelines for Exercise Prescription for Low Back Pain

GENERAL CATEGORIZATION	GENERAL RECOMMENDATION
Red flagged serious conditions	Follow exercise recommendations by qualified practitioners
Nerve root pain	Follow exercise recommendations by qualified practitioners
Nonspecific low back pain	Consider stage, acuteness, degree of severity, functional limitations, functional capacity, and individual patient needs, but, in general, continue and gradually increase activity*

*See Table 13.6

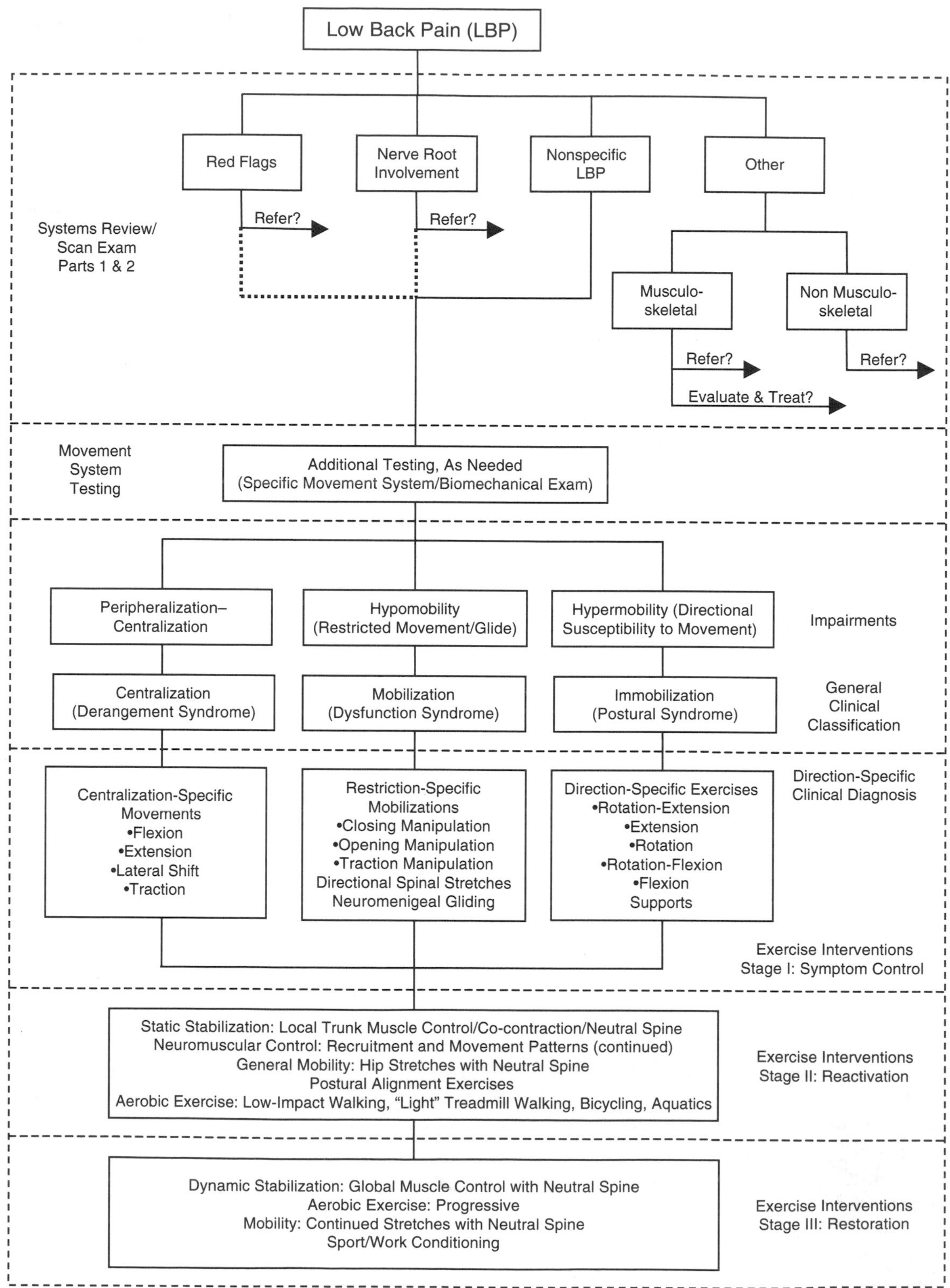

Figure 13.1 Algorithm for clinical diagnosis and exercise intervention for persons with nonspecific, mechanical low back pain.

Patients may need to learn to control somatic symptoms (stage I) regardless of the duration of their symptoms. Perhaps "graduating" from each stage *(if needed)* is necessary to decrease the recurrence rate of low back pain. The length of time a patient spends in each stage varies according to severity and the speed with which the patient accomplishes the goals of each stage. Some people need only spend a few days in each stage. Three stages of rehabilitation are identified–Stage I: Symptom Control, Stage II: Reactivation, and Stage III: Restoration (see Figure 13.1). Persons with chronic pain syndrome with dissociated symptoms and symptom-magnifying behaviors need a different type of intervention program than is presented in this chapter.

Stage I (Symptom Control) **may** correspond to the "acute" stage in the sense of passage of time and with persons presenting with higher symptom severity and more major functional limitations. Persons in stage I **might** have problems performing basic ADL (activities of daily living) such as sitting, standing, bending, and walking. However, stage I can better be considered appropriate for patients who demonstrate consistent direction-specific symptoms with active or passive movements or with prolonged positions of the spine and/or extremities. *Stage II* (Reactivation) **might** include persons with medium symptom severity and more moderate functional limitations. With regard to duration, this stage **might** represent the early part of the "subacute" or "recurrent" stage. However, again, passage of time may not be an important consideration. Persons in stage II **might** have difficulty performing more demanding home, occupational, and recreational activities (e.g., vacuuming, lifting, gardening). However, once again, stage II represents persons with difficulty with local static trunk ("core") stabilization and control. *Stage III* (Restoration) **may** be chronologically in the latter part of the "subacute" or "recurrent" stage. Persons in stage III **may** have low symptom severity (and typically more intermittent symptoms) and more minor functional limitations. Exercises in stage III are started as the goals of stage II are accomplished in order to help patients return to full activity.

Goals and Exercises for Each Stage

Providers or clinicians, for the most part, are ethically responsible for judging their own qualifications for subclassifying and staging persons with low back pain and for determining their ability to prescribe, assess, and progress exercise. Persons presenting with high symptom severity and major functional limitations (stage I) may need referral to clinicians with specific training. Staging, the general goals for each stage, and examples of exercises for selected stages are provided in Table 13.6.

Stage I: Symptom-Control Exercises

The goals of stage I are to relieve symptoms, increase function, prevent disability, and progress to stage II exercises. Stage I interventions include self-performed movements to centralize peripheral symptoms if the centralization phenomenon is present, manipulation for movement restrictions, if present, or stabilization via supports and/or direction-specific exercises for hypermobilities, if present. A common thread among interventions in stage I is that they are direction specific, that is, specific movements aggravate symptoms and others ease symptoms. As the goal

Table 13.6 Examples of Various Exercises by Rehabilitation Stages and General Goals

Stage	General Goals & Examples	Examples of Potential Exercises & Progressions
I. Symptom Control	Centralization	
	• Extension	Prone lying, prone-on-elbows, press-ups, & standing backbends
	• Flexion	Supine single and double knees-to-chest, sitting flexion
	Immobilization	
	• Extension–rotation	Must be individualized to impairments, but might include an abdominal progression starting supine with leg sliding with abdominal stabilization, supine bent knee fall-outs with abdominal stabilization, side-lying hip lateral rotation with stationary pelvis, prone knee flexion with abdominal stabilization, quadruped backward rocking with movement correction, wall slides with abdominal stabilization (11)
II. Reactivation	Static Segmental Stabilization (local muscles)	
	• Recruit transversus abdominis	Abdominal drawing in or hollowing, hollowing with arm and leg movements, hollowing with bridging
	• Recruit lumbar multifidi	Quadruped co-contraction with transversus abdominis, quadruped with single arm/leg lifts, quadruped with opposite arm/leg lifts
	Global Muscle Stabilization	
	• Recruit quadratus lumborum	Horizontal side support lifts with abdominal hollowing knees flexed, progress to knees extended
	• Recruit oblique abdominals	Horizontal side support lifts with abdominal hollowing, bent knee fall-outs, curl-ups with trunk rotation, leg lowering, hanging leg lifts
	Hip flexibility	Static stretching with neutral spine (co-contraction) as needed for hamstrings, hip flexors, etc. Standing flexion from hip with neutral spine
	Aerobic Conditioning	Low impact; walking or cycling
III. Restoration	Dynamic Stabilization	Neutral spine (co-contraction) with progressive gymnastic ball exercises, e.g., arm and/or leg lifts, bridging on ball, upper back lifts over ball, etc. Can be combined with weights, pulleys
	Work/Sport Conditioning	Simulations

at this stage is more symptom relief, repetitions and prolonged holding of stabilizing muscle contractions are typically emphasized versus loading or resistance training.

With patients exhibiting the centralization phenomenon, pain or paresthesia is abolished or moves from the periphery toward the spine with specific movements, usually spinal flexion or extension. The test movements are part of the musculoskeletal scan exam and consist of the effect of standing, supine, prone, and perhaps quadruped movements on symptoms. Movements that centralize symptoms are used as the patient's initial exercise program. For example, if extension movements centralize symptoms from the leg to the lumbar spine, prone lying, or prone press-ups may be prescribed. The patient's response to the movements determines the exercises and the progression. Exercises that centralize the symptoms are continued, and those that cause peripheralization to the leg, in this example flexion, are initially avoided. In other cases, flexion movements may centralize the symptoms, and extension is initially avoided. Flexion movements might consist of double knees to the chest, progressing to sitting flexion. Once symptoms are centralized, the patient can progress through the initially offending movements and on to stage II. For more information on centralization and mechanical treatment, the reader is referred to McKenzie (41) and Donelson, et al. (43).

Some patients in stage I will benefit from manipulation, which is beyond the scope of this chapter. Other patients will benefit from movement system rebalancing exercises to restore alignment and precise movement of specific segments in order to relieve musculoskeletal pain (11). Test movements of the spine and extremities during the movement system examination will identify the primary movement impairment. These movement impairment syndromes are subclassified in the overall category of hypermobilities by this author (see Figure 13.1) (with apologies to Dr. Sahrmann), because although the identified movement impairments can be caused by stiff, short, weak, or imbalanced muscles or by poor patterns of muscle recruitment, the pain is presumably caused by the hypermobile segments or the area of compensatory movement, i.e., the directional susceptible movement (DSM) (11).

Unlike the centralization-specific movement subcategories (flexion, extension, etc.), where the syndrome is named for the curative movement, the low back impairment syndromes are named by the offending movement(s). Therefore, in a person with a lumbar flexion DSM, flexion activities such as bending forward would be avoided and appropriate exercises such as standing forward bending at the hip with a neutral spine would be prescribed. The specific exercises are suggested from the movement examination. When a patient is unable to perform a test movement without compensatory painful movement, correct performance of the test movement without the compensatory movement becomes the exercise. Further information on the diagnosis and treatment of movement impairment syndromes can be found in Sahrmann's text (11).

Stage II: Reactivation Exercises

The goals of stage II are to develop static trunk stabilization and endurance of the local stabilizing muscles, learn the neutral spine position, control of the stabilizing muscles during progressive hip mobility and limb movements, return to low-impact aerobic conditioning activities, increase function, prevent disability, and progress to stage III activities. Static stabilization is retraining the local stabilizing muscles, primarily the transversus abdominis and the multifidi. According to Richardson and Jull (44), functional demands suggest that isometric exercise [a prolonged tonic holding at a low maximum voluntary contraction (MVC)] is most beneficial for reeducating these local stabilizing muscles. Initial positions used to recruit these muscles are quadruped and prone. Further, exercise for the local stabilizing muscles is to be repeated several times a day. The progression is to first increase the holding time of the co-contraction (arbitrarily to 10 seconds) and to increase the number of repetitions to at least 10. Second, the next progression is to perform these exercises with gradually increasing external loads; and then third, to co-contract these deep muscles during dynamic functional movements of the trunk. Asking the patient to "draw in," or hollow, the lower abdomen activates the transversus abdominis. No movement of the spine, ribs, or pelvis should occur, and the patient should be able to breathe normally. The multifidus is thought to co-contract when the patient is able to maintain the normal lumbosacral curve during the exercise. Asking the patient to "swell out," or contract, the muscles in the lumbar spine while the practitioner palpates the multifidi can encourage further, isolated contraction of the multifidi. Substitution of global muscles, such as breath holding and spinal movement, should be corrected.

When the patient can perform these contractions in quadruped and prone, this retraining is practiced in other positions, e.g., standing, during low levels of leg loading, and in light functional tasks. Examples of exercises might be supine bent-knee fall-outs, supine single or double leg sliding in supine, bridging, and opposite arm and leg lifts from a quadruped position while maintaining the neutral spine position. Patients also learn to contract these deep stabilizing muscles while performing trunk movements that usually aggravate their pain.

Again, the noteworthy implication reported previously is that activating the global muscles with poor local muscle control actually inhibits the deep stabilizing muscles and is potentially harmful. This finding suggests that performing exercises using the global muscles without proper local stabilization is actually contraindicated (38).

After patients have developed adequate lumbar stabilization, hip stretching (e.g., of the hip flexors, hamstrings, etc.) may be added while the patient activates the deep stabilizing muscles. In other words, traditional stretching techniques can be used, but the patient is taught to perform the stretches with the spine maintained in the neutral posture.

Additional stage II exercises may include continuation, progression, or initiation of the movement rebalancing exercises from stage I; postural alignment; and additional stabilizing exercises emphasizing the static stabilizing elements. For example, exercises to recruit the quadratus lumborum and the oblique abdominals (also stabilizing muscles), such as the horizontal side support lifts, can be initiated. In this exercise, the patient lies on the side with knees bent and the upper body supported on the elbow and forearm. The patient incorporates the "drawing in" contraction of the transversus abdominis and then lifts the body upward from the surface. Extending the knees increases the difficulty of the exercise. Oblique abdominal exercises can gradually be incorporated and might consist of curl-ups with trunk rotation and unilateral or bilateral leg lowering.

Low-impact aerobic activities such as walking; "light," or de-weighted, treadmill walking (i.e., using a harness system to reduce the amount of compressive forces during walking); bicycling; and aquatic exercises are encouraged. Even at this stage, the choice of activities may have some directionality. For example, if symptoms occurred with sitting, bicycling may not be the best choice for an aerobic activity. Likewise, not all patients can tolerate walking because of the more extended lumbar spine. The guidelines for aerobic exercises in this stage are similar to those of a healthy individual resuming an activity or for individuals new to aerobic exercise.

Stage III: Restoration Exercises

Persons with low back pain have been shown to have deficits in dynamic control of the trunk, such as decreased spinal proprioception, increased reaction time, and increased postural sway (45). The goals of stage III are to develop dynamic trunk stabilization and trunk strength using the local and global stabilizing muscles, using the neutral spine position in dynamic activities, progressing aerobic conditioning activities, preventing disability, and returning to full function, if possible. In stage III, isometric exercises for the deep stabilizing lumbar muscles are combined with dynamic exercise for other parts of the body, that is, local muscle retraining is incorporated into more dynamic activities that require both local and global trunk muscles. Dynamic stabilization programs often use unstable surfaces, such as large gymnastic balls. Here again, the patient should maintain the neutral spine by contraction ("drawing in") of the transversus abdominis during all exercises. The patient can sit on the ball and perform arm and leg movements while maintaining the neutral spine. Additionally, the patient can lie supine on a surface and put his or her legs on the ball and bridge, or the patient can maintain a bridging position lying with his or her back on the ball and feet on the floor. Catching and throwing activities, wobble boards, and trampolines can be used. Activities should also incorporate patient-specific sport, leisure, or work activities, such as lifting and weight training.

Evidence suggests that it may take several months to accomplish the goals of an exercise program and further, that low back exercises may be more effective when performed daily (46).

PREVENTING LOW BACK PAIN

Interestingly, just as much of the evidence for clinical care of persons with low back pain is of unproven effectiveness; interventions to prevent low back pain are also of unproven effectiveness. However, higher levels of fitness have been associated with a decreased incidence of low back pain (47) and with effective interventions for both acute and chronic low back pain (26, 48). Therefore, patients are typically encouraged to continue with an aerobic exercise program. This may reduce the likelihood of recurrence, and it provides general health benefits.

In addition, some patients should be encouraged to continue other specific exercises based on their individual movement impairments, and to use the protective neutral spine position, especially in activities that stress the lumbar spine, such as lifting.

SUMMARY

General recommendations for treatment of adults with acute low back pain currently consist of individualized patient education, acetaminophen, NSAIDs, spinal manipulation for patients without radiculopathy, activity modifications, rest for 2–4 days for patients without leg pain, gradual resumption of activity, trunk exercises, and aerobic activities. Although evidence from large, randomized controlled trials indicating the role of specific exercise in the treatment and prevention of low back pain is limited, research in this area is a high priority because of the high cost of low back pain.

Thus far, the key points with respect to specific exercise programs seem to be to: (a) relieve symptoms with individualized direction-specific movements, mobilizations, and/or exercises; (b) retrain and increase the endurance of the deep stabilizing muscles, if needed; (c) introduce more dynamic stabilization activities only after successfully training the patient to recruit the deep stabilizing muscles; (d) maintain a neutral spine position with co-contraction of the rectus abdominis and lumbar multifidi during activities that stress the spine; (e) develop extremity mobility; and (f) condition aerobically.

Meanwhile, we continue our quest for the right thing for the right person at the right time done the right way.

References

1. Frymoyer JW, Cats-Buril WL. An overview of the incidences and cost of low back pain. *Orthop Clin North Am* 1991;22: 263–271.

2. Walker BF. The prevalence of low back pain: A systematic review of the literature 1966 to1998. *J Spinal Disord* 2000;13: 205–217.
3. Troup JD, Martin JW, Lloyd DC. Back pain in industry: a prospective survey. *Spine* 1981;6:61–69.
4. Frymoyer JW. Can low back pain disability be prevented? *Baillieres Clin Rheumatol* 1992;6:595–606.
5. Pope MH, Andersson GB, Frymoyer JW, eds. Occupational Low Back Pain. St. Louis: Mosby-Year Book, 1991.
6. Pain terms: a list with definitions and notes on usage. Recommended by the IASP Subcommittee on Taxonomy. *Pain* 1979;6:249–252.
7. Bogduk N. Clinical Anatomy of the Lumbar Spine and Sacrum. 3rd ed. New York: Churchill Livingstone, 1997.
8. Kuslich SD, Ulstrom CL, Michael CJ. The tissue origin of low back pain and sciatica: a report of pain response to tissue stimulation during operations on the lumbar spine using local anesthesia. *Orthop Clin North Am* 1991;22:181–187.
9. Schwarzer AC, Aprill CN, Derby R, et al. The relative contributions of the disc and zygapophyseal joint in chronic low back pain. *Spine* 1994;19:801–806.
10. Jönsson B, Strömqvist B. Clinical appearance of contained and noncontained lumbar disc herniation. *J Spinal Disord* 1996;9:32–38.
11. Sahrmann SA. Diagnosis and Treatment of Movement Impairment Syndromes. St. Louis: Mosby, 2001.
12. Kirkaldy-Willis WH. Three phases of the spectrum of degenerative disease. In: Kirkaldy-Willis WH, Burton CV, eds. Managing Low Back Pain. 3rd ed. New York: Churchill-Livingstone, 1992.
13. Waddell, G. The Back Pain Revolution. Edinburgh: Churchill Livingstone, 1998.
14. Scientific approach to the assessment and management of activity-related spinal disorders. A monograph for clinicians. Report of the Quebec Task Force on Spinal Disorders. *Spine* 1987;12:S1-S59.
15. Manchikanti L. Epidemiology of low back pain. *Pain Physician* 2000;3:167–192.
16. DeRosa CP, Porterfield JA. A physical therapy model for the treatment of low back pain. *Phys Ther* 1992;72:261–269.
17. American Physical Therapy Association. Guide to physical therapist practice. 2nd ed. *Phys Ther* 2001;8:9–744.
18. Cassidy JD, Carroll LJ, Cote P. The Saskatchewan health and back pain survey. The prevalence of low back pain and related disability in Saskatchewan adults. *Spine* 1998;23:1860–1866.
19. Magee DJ. Orthopedic Physical Assessment. 3rd ed. Philadelphia: WB Saunders Co., 1997.
20. Fairbank JC, Couper J, Davies JB, et al. The Oswestry low back pain disability questionnaire. *Physiotherapy* 1980;66:271–273.
21. Roland M, Morris R. A study of the natural history of back pain. Part I: development of a reliable and sensitive measure of disability in low back pain. *Spine* 1983;8:141–144.
22. Maitland GD. Vertebral Manipulation. 5th ed. London: Butterworths, 1986.
23. Meadows JTS. Orthopedic Differential Diagnosis in Physical Therapy: A Case Study Approach. New York: McGraw-Hill, 1999.
24. Delitto A, Erhard RE, Bowling RW. A treatment-based classification approach to low back syndrome: identifying and staging patients for conservative treatment. *Phys Ther* 1995; 75:470–485.
25. Riddle DL. Classification and low back pain: a review of the literature and critical analysis of selected systems. *Phys Ther* 1998;78:708–737.
26. Bigos S, Bower O, Braen G, et al. *Clinical Practice Guideline for Acute Low Back Pain in Adults.* US Department of Health and Human Services. Public Health Service. Agency for Health Care Policy and Research (AHCPR) Guideline No. 14. AHCPR Publication No. 97-N012. Rockville, MD, February 1997.
27. Kane RL. Looking for physical therapy outcomes. *Phys Ther* 1994;74:425–429.
28. van Tulder MV, Scholten RJ, Koes BW, et al. Nonsteroidal antiinflammatory drugs for low back pain: a systematic review within the Cochrane Collaboration Back Review Group. *Spine* 2000;25:2501–2513.
29. Cherkin DC, Wheeler KJ, Barlow W, et al. Medication use for low back pain in primary care. *Spine* 1998;23:607–614.
30. Greenman PE. Principles of Manual Medicine. Baltimore: Williams & Wilkins, 1989.
31. Hall CM, Brody LT. Therapeutic Exercise: Moving Toward Function. Philadelphia: Lippincott Williams & Wilkins, 1999.
32. Waddell G, Feder G, Lewis M. Systematic reviews of bed rest and advice to stay active for acute low back pain. *Br J Gen Pract* 1997;47:647–652.
33. Deyo RA, Diehl AK, Rosenthal M. How many days of bed rest for acute low back pain? A randomized clinical trial. *N Engl J Med* 1986;23:1064–1070.
34. Hodges PW, Richardson CA. Contraction of the abdominal muscles associated with movement of the lower limb. *Phys Ther* 1997;77:132–142.
35. Hodges PW, Richardson CA. Feedforward contraction of the transversus abdominis is not influenced by the direction of arm movement. *Exp Brain Res* 1997;114:362–370.
36. Sihvonen T, Lindgren KA, Airaksinen O, et al. Movement disturbances of the lumbar spine and abnormal back muscle electromyographic findings in recurrent low back pain. *Spine* 1997;22:289–295.
37. Hides JA, Richardson CA, Jull GA. Multifidus muscle recovery is not automatic after resolution of acute, first-episode low back pain. *Spine* 1996;21:2763–2769.
38. Richardson C, Jull G, Hodges P, et al. Therapeutic exercise for spinal segmental stabilization in low back pain: scientific basis and clinical approach. Edinburgh: Churchill Livingstone, 1999.
39. The mainstreaming of alternative medicine. *Consumer Reports.* May 2000:17–25.
40. van Tulder MV, Malmivarra A, Esmail R, et al. Exercise therapy for low back pain (Cochrane Review). In: The Cochrane Library, Issue 2, 2001. Oxford: Update Software.
41. McKenzie RA. The Lumbar Spine: Mechanical Diagnosis and Therapy. Waikanae, New Zealand: Spinal Publications, 1981.
42. Fritz JM, George S. The use of a classification approach to identify subgroups of patients with acute low back pain. Interrater reliability and short-term treatment outcomes. *Spine* 2000;25:106–114.
43. Donelson R, Silva G, Murphy K. Centralization phenomenon. Its usefulness in evaluating and treating referred pain. *Spine* 1990;15:211–213.
44. Richardson CA, Jull GA. Muscle control—pain control. What exercises would you prescribe? *Manual Ther* 1995;1:2–10.

45. Gill KP, Callaghan MJ. The measurement of lumbar proprioception in individuals with and without low back pain. *Spine* 1998;23:371–377.
46. McGill SM. Low back exercises: evidence for improving exercise regimens. *Phys Ther* 1998;78:754–765.
47. Cady LD, Bischoff DP, O'Connell ER, et al. Strength and fitness and subsequent back injuries in firefighters. *J Occup Med* 1979;21:269–272.
48. van Tulder MV, Koes BW, Bouter LM. Conservative treatment of acute and chronic nonspecific low back pain. A systematic review of randomized controlled trials of the most common interventions. *Spine* 1997;22:2128–2156.

Suggested Reading

Liemohn W. Exercise prescription and the back. New York: McGraw-Hill, 2001.

CHAPTER 14
AMPUTATION

Kenneth H. Pitetti and Robert C. Manske

EPIDEMIOLOGY AND PATHOPHYSIOLOGY

Amputations have historically been described in two major categories: upper extremity and lower extremity. A large majority (i.e., 80%) of lower-extremity (LE) amputations is the direct result of peripheral vascular disease and diabetes (1), with trauma (e.g., vehicular accidents or job-related accidents) being the second most prevalent cause. Major causes of upper-extremity (UE) amputations are vehicular accidents, severe lacerations from tools or machinery, and frostbite (2). Curative treatment of tumors, such as a malignant osteogenic sarcoma that has not yet metastasized, is an additional cause of both upper- and lower-extremity amputations. Amputations caused by infection have been significantly reduced due to the advent of antibiotics, improved aseptic surgical techniques, and sepsis control.

Lower-Extremity Amputations

Lower-extremity amputations are commonly classified into the following categories: (a) toe and partial foot amputation; (b) unilateral (i.e., involvement of only one leg) below-knee (transtibial); (c) unilateral above-knee (transfemoral); (d) hip disarticulation and hemipelvectomy; (e) bilateral (i.e., involving both legs) below-knee; (f) bilateral above-and-below knee (i.e., one leg amputated above the knee, the other below the knee); and (g) bilateral above-knee (i.e., both legs amputated above the knee).

Toe disarticulation causes little functional disability, unless the big toe (first phalange) is lost, which is vital for balance during the propulsive phase of gait. A *Symes* amputation is an amputation of the forefoot or midfoot usually leaving the heel bones (calcaneus and talus) intact. The Symes amputation creates full weight bearing onto the heel of the foot.

The most frequently performed LE amputation is the below-knee amputation caused by peripheral vascular disease. This amputation retains the knee joint, which is critical to lower-extremity function. The center of axis for knee flexion and extension will remain very similar to an able-bodied person once a proper prosthetic device is fitted.

It is important to note that the energy expenditure of ambulation is higher for LE amputees when compared to either nondisabled peers or UE amputees. In fact, the increased energy cost is directly related to the level of amputation. Huang and colleagues (3) reported that even when LE amputees choose their own comfortable walking speed, the mean energy cost was 9% higher in unilateral below-knee, 49% higher for unilateral above-knee, and 280% higher for bilateral above-knee amputees when compared to their able-bodied peers. Other researchers have reported similar findings (4–6). Although design improvements of prostheses since these studies were conducted have decreased the energy cost of ambulation (7), LE amputees have a higher risk for developing cardiovascular disease and hypertension than the general population due to a sedentary lifestyle (8, 9).

Upper-Extremity Amputations

Amputations of the upper extremity are commonly categorized as either below-elbow or above-elbow amputation. Within these two major categories are several subcategories that are listed in Table 14.1. Upper-extremity amputations have little effect on the individual's ambulatory capacity and, therefore, have much less effect on activity level. Upper-extremity amputees have no greater risk of cardiovascular disease, hypertension, obesity, or adult-onset diabetes than able-bodied individuals (8, 9).

CLINICAL EXERCISE PHYSIOLOGY

Risks and complications from amputations are divided into ***preprosthetic*** (or postoperative) and ***postprosthetic*** types. Preprosthetic complications include delayed healing, which can be caused by inappropriate amputation-level selection, suboptimal operative technique, inadequate postoperative management, and infection. The closure site of the amputation must have an adequate amount of soft-tissue envelope to decrease the risk of the underlying bone adhering to the skin on the residual limb (i.e., stump). The risk of flexion contractions increases when the patient maintains a flexed limb posture for long periods, which is

Table 14.1. SubCategories of Below-Elbow and Above-Elbow Amputations

CATEGORY AND SUBCATEGORY	DESCRIPTION
Below Elbow	
Partial Hand	One or more digits, could include the radial or ulnar borders of the hand
Wrist Disarticulation	Removal of all portions of the hand distal to the radioulnar joint
Long Below-Elbow	Residual limb approximately 8–10 inches from center of the lateral epicondyle
Medium Below-Elbow	Residual limb approximately 6–8 inches in length
Short Below-Elbow	Residual limb approximately 2–4 inches from the center of the lateral epicondyle
Above Elbow	
Elbow Disarticulation	Spares the entire length of the humerus
Long Above-Elbow	Residual limb 50–90% original length of humerus
Short Above-Elbow	Residual limb 30–50% original length of humerus
Shoulder Disarticulation	Amputation of the arm from 30% of length of original humerus through the shoulder

generally the position of comfort. Flexure contracture of the knee and hip is common for both below-knee amputations and above-knee amputations, respectively. Contracture of the shoulder to a position of glenohumeral adduction and forward flexion is common in UE amputees. Flexion contracture of the elbow is common in a below-elbow amputation. Early, aggressive range-of-motion exercises must be instituted as soon as the postoperative pain has decreased to a tolerable level in order to prevent these contractures.

It is important to improve muscular strength of the residual limb to prepare for the prosthesis. This can be done by manual resistive isometric and isotonic training. In most cases, it is best to begin treatment with a static isometric hold, progressing to submaximal isotonic exercise. Isotonic exercise training allows the patient to move the residual limb through the full range of motion as the assistant provides manual hand resistance to the movement. This improves muscular strength at the knee or elbow for extension and flexion movements for below-knee and above-elbow amputations, respectively. Adduction and abduction movements, as well as flexion and extension movements, should also be performed for the hip and shoulder muscles on the involved side for above-knee and above-elbow amputations, respectively.

Postprosthetic complications can be the result of residual limb pain, adherence of skin to bone, insensitive skin leading to overuse and tissue breakdown, poor prosthetic fit, and body/bone overgrowth in children. These complications for LE amputations present a major obstacle for weight-bearing movements and, therefore, limit activities of daily living. Although these complications may only be temporary (i.e., days to weeks), the patient's overall physical capacities (aerobic power, muscle strength, and endurance of uninvolved limbs) could significantly deteriorate. It is recommended that in addition to range-of-motion exercises, limited or partial weight-bearing exercises (e.g., upper/lower-body ergometers such as the Schwinn Air-Dyne, arm crank ergometers, swimming) be performed to prevent overall physical deconditioning during recovery times.

Prosthetic use for UE amputation is encouraged as soon as pain is tolerable to enable the individual to have prehension (grabbing or seizing of an object) from the involved extremity and to ultimately restore body image. Functional use of the upper extremity is paramount to most UE amputees. Normal functioning of the involved upper extremity, including dexterity and coordination of the prosthetic arm and hand, involves daily training and practice. In addition to dexterity and coordination, the ability to learn tactile sensation, proprioception, pressure, and position sense of the involved limb is equally important. As with LE amputations, the greater the length of the UE residual limb, the better the prosthetic fit and, therefore, more functional ability is maintained. Therefore, a patient with a below-elbow amputation will fare better than a patient with an above-elbow amputation.

One biomechanical problem of concern for the amputee is the change in his/her center of gravity. The center of gravity is the one single point in the body where every portion of body mass is equally distributed. This point for an able-bodied adult is positioned slightly anterior to the second sacral vertebra (10). The loss of a limb will shift this position to the contralateral side of the body (i.e., the side opposite the amputated limb). This shift in the center of gravity will require greater muscular strength and endurance as well as better balance on the opposite side of the body to compensate for this shift.

Regardless of the level of amputation, therapeutic exercise is needed to help decrease pain and swelling; increase residual limb muscular strength, endurance, and range-of-motion; and maintain neuromuscular patterns, kinesthesis, proprioception, and balance.

Therapeutic exercise for LE amputations that incorporates the involved extremity should be performed for cardiovascular endurance, muscular strength, and endurance and for range of motion, proprioception, and balance. An LE amputation will hinder, to varying extents, the amputee's ability to run or jog, and in some cases, walk. Therefore, cardiovascular fitness is generally more affected by an LE amputation than by a UE amputation because the UE amputee still has full function of his/her lower extremities. LE amputees who find it difficult to perform LE cardiovascular exercise with a prosthesis can perform such modes of exercise as swimming, combined upper/lower-body cycle ergometers, or arm ergometry.

One of the most important, yet most overlooked, regions of the body, which also needs strength and range-of-motion exercises for LE amputees, is the abdomen, hip girdle, and upper thigh musculature. The strength of this body region is crucial for LE amputations because it provides a base that maintains both static and dynamic stability. Without proximal stability of the abdomen, hips, and upper thighs, coordinated or noncompensated movements of the distal extremities will be limited. Therefore, during both pre- and postprosthetic phases, stretching and strengthening exercises for these areas of the body are essential. Stretching of the lower back and hip muscles can be performed using the single and double knee-to-chest stretches, lower trunk rotation stretch, and hip flexor, quadriceps, and hamstring stretches. Trunk and hip stability and strength can be gained by performing partial abdominal curl-ups, pelvic tilt, straight leg raise, and any other core stability training exercise. Proprioception and balance training can be performed initially on a stable base, then progress to a moveable surface such as a dynadisk (i.e., wobble board) or theraball (i.e., big bouncy >Swiss= ball). Exercises can also incorporate devices such as elastic tubing, medicine balls, or manual resistance movements with the therapist. Excellent resources that describe balance, agility, coordination, endurance, stretching, and strengthening exercises for LE amputees are found in the following three texts: *Stretching and Strengthening for Lower Extremity Amputees* (11); *Balance, Agility, Coordination and Endurance for Lower Extremity Amputees* (12); and *Home Exercise Guide for Lower Extremity Amputees* (13). Therapeutic exercises of this type may appear easy, but to the LE amputee recovering from trauma/surgery, they can be very fatiguing. Therefore, sufficient recovery time should be included between daily exercise sessions.

Coordinated movement of the arms for the UE amputee is dependent on the shoulder girdle. These joints include the sternoclavicular joint, acromioclavicular joint, scapulothoracic joint, and the glenohumeral joint. With the exception of a shoulder disarticulation amputation, all four of these joints remain intact with most upper-extremity amputations. Initially, full active range of motion must be provided through stretching exercises for all the joints listed to ensure adequate excursion of the prosthetic equipment. Exercises to increase strength of the muscles surrounding these joints include rows, shrugs, overhead press, bench press, and dips. Rotator cuff exercises with elastic tubing can include shoulder abduction, flexion, extension, and internal and external rotation. These exercises can be performed in straight-plane patterns or diagonal patterns. The diagonal pattern will help increase neuromuscular timing and coordination. Common exercises for muscles of the elbow for below-elbow, UE amputees include elbow curls and elbow extensions. As with all of the above exercises, they can initially begin as isometrics, progressing to isotonic strengthening.

PHARMACOLOGY

A large majority of LE amputations are a direct result of peripheral vascular disease and diabetes, and many amputees take drugs specific to these diseases. The kinds of medication usually taken and the effect these medications have on exercise capacity is covered in another text (14) and will not be addressed in this chapter.

Most amputees experience the phenomenons called "phantom pain" (i.e., pain emitting from their amputated limb) and "phantom limb" (i.e., the feeling that the amputated limb is still present). Phantom pain is covered in the "Education and Counseling" section of this chapter. Phantom pain from phantom limbs can range from an inconvenience to excruciating in nature. Amputees often obtain relief from this pain by using drugs that are also given to counteract epilepsy or depression, but will have little or no effect on their response to exercise. Some amputees find that their phantom pain is eased by a combination of antidepressants and narcotics (such as methadone). An amputee who is taking a narcotic for this phenomenon should consult with his/her physician before beginning an exercise program.

PHYSICAL EXAMINATIONS

In the words of the orthopedic surgeon, D.H. O'Donoghue, "let the patient tell the story"(15). Prior to conducting a physical examination, a thorough medical history, employment history, physical activities, and leisure time activities should be noted.

The physical examination should start by observing the stump. Observation of the skin can reveal superficial problems such as contact dermatitis, eczema, epidermal cysts, bacterial and fungal infections, discoloration, scarring, or drainage.

Second, different sensations should be tested over dermatone regions. This evaluation should be performed with the patient's eyes closed. A light sweep of the examiner's hands across the skin of the involved limb will determine if the individual can feel light sensation. Vials of hot and cold water should be used to determine temperature sensation, and tactile sensation to a sharp object can be assessed with a paper clip or pinwheel.

Third, the active and passive range of motion of the residual limb should be assessed with special consideration of the proximal joints (which are critical to optimal function of the limb) using a goniometer. Active range of motion gives the examiner an indication of the muscles' ability to move the joint, the range of motion of that joint, and the patient's willingness to move the extremity. During passive range of motion, the examiner moves the extremity through the available range of motion while the patient is relaxed. Passive range of motion assesses inert structures such as ligaments, bursa capsules, and cartilage.

Flexibility of the muscles should also be examined because flexibility measurements do differ from range-of-motion measurements. Flexibility measurements place the extremity in specific patterns of movement in an attempt to stretch a specific muscle. These measurements are important, for instance, for a lower-extremity amputee who is at risk of developing contracture of the anterior hip musculature, which results in the hip remaining in a slightly flexed position at all times.

And last, manual muscle testing should be assessed to determine the relative strength of the residual limb and the proximal joint. Generally, the manual muscle testing is performed in a static position so that inert tissues will not be involved. Manual muscle testing is usually graded with a 5/5 indicating full strength to 0/5 indicating no strength at all (16).

MEDICAL AND SURGICAL TREATMENTS

The recommended resource for this section is *Atlas of Limb Prosthetics: Surgical, Prosthetic and Rehabilitation Principles* (17).

DIAGNOSTIC TECHNIQUES

Diagnostic techniques pertain to amputees with vascular, hematological, or metabolic (i.e., diabetes) conditions, and not necessarily to the amputation. Therefore, this is not within the scope of this chapter.

EXERCISE/FITNESS/FUNCTIONAL TESTING

The basic principles for exercise testing stated in *ACSM's Guidelines for Exercise Testing and Prescription* (18) provide the foundation for this section and section 8, "Exercise prescription and programing." When not otherwise stated, these principles will apply. Special situations created by amputation will be covered in this section.

Lower-Extremity Amputation

Cardiovascular

Ergometer modifications for lower-extremity amputees in cardiovascular testing and training were addressed by Bostom et al. (19).

Unilateral above- or below-knee amputations, bilateral amputations involving both legs below-knee, and bilateral amputations involving one leg above-knee and one leg below-knee are all recommended to use an ergometer that involves both upper- and lower-body musculature as a mode of testing to determine aerobic fitness. The Schwinn Air-Dyne ergometer would be an example of such a mode. Depending on comfort, above-knee amputees can perform the test with their prosthesis on or off.

The amputee should first practice at work levels of 25 W (150 kpm) and 50 W (300 kpm) for 2 minutes at each level, or until the amputee feels comfortable with the movement. Amputees with peripheral vascular disease, diabetes, deconditioning, or other secondary conditions should start their initial workload at 25 W for 2 minutes, then increase incrementally 12.5 W every minute until volitional exhaustion. Younger and/or older physically fit amputees can begin at 50 W for 2 minutes and increase incrementally 25 W every minute until volitional exhaustion.

The recommended mode of testing for bilateral, above-knee amputees is the arm crank ergometer (ACE). The ACE should be positioned so that the pedal shaft is level with the amputee's acromioclavicular joint and the ergometer is placed far enough from the patient to allow slight flexion of the elbow at the farthest point of the pedal stroke. If the amputee is deconditioned (i.e., due to a sedentary lifestyle), initial workload should start at 0 W at a constant cadence of 50 rpm for 2 minutes (warm-up) with increases of 5 W every 2 minutes until volitional exhaustion. Younger and/or more active bilateral above-knee amputees should begin at 5 W for 2 minutes with increases of 5 W every two minutes until volitional exhaustion.

Strength, Range-of-Motion, and Endurance Testing

Most upper-body measurement techniques, used to assess range of motion, and upper-body strength and endurance test protocols, used to evaluate able-bodied individuals, can be performed by LE amputees. It is suggested that the LE amputee be seated or lie on a bench to allow the amputee to concentrate on his/her performance without concern of maintaining balance while standing. Variations for LE testing protocols depend on the level of amputation and leg involvement. For instance, a unilateral amputee could perform most test protocols used to evaluate able-bodied individuals. Knee flexion and extension tests can be measured for most below-knee amputations (i.e., depending on the length of stump), but not above-knee. Except for complete hip disarticulation, hemipelvectomy, or shortness of stump, most hip measurements (e.g., flexion, extension, adduction, abduction) used to evaluate able-bodied individuals can also be used for LE amputees. For upper-body measurements, the amputee should be sitting (as in knee or hip flexion and extension measurements) or prone (as in leg press) in order to maintain balance. Standing test measurements, like a squat, should be performed with caution for unilateral amputees and are contraindicated for bilateral amputees.

Upper-Extremity Amputation

Cardiovascular

As with able-bodied individuals, the treadmill and bicycle protocols outlined in ACSM's Guidelines (18) are applicable to UE amputees.

Strength, Range-of-Motion, and Endurance Testing

A UE amputation presents the opposite situation compared to an LE amputation. Most range-of-motion measurements and strength and endurance tests that are used to evaluate able-bodied individuals can be used for UE amputees. The same considerations and limitations are applied to UE amputees for upper extremities as are applied to LE amputees with one exception. The feet and legs for the UE amputee are paramount for balance and stability when performing upper-extremity measurements. Therefore, UE amputees should perform upper-extremity measurements while standing and, if sitting, allow their feet to be in contact with the floor.

EXERCISE PRESCRIPTION AND PROGRAMING

Lower-Extremity Amputations

Few studies have been published concerning the effects of exercise for LE amputees, but those few do report positive results. James (20) reported that for healthy male unilateral above-knee amputees, one-legged (noninvolved leg) bicycle ergometry training improved cardiovascular fitness of the participants. Improvement in cardiovascular fitness was also seen for healthy unilateral below- and above-knee amputees, and bilateral below- and above-knee amputees using a Schwinn Air-Dyne ergometer (21). Additionally, following a treadmill training program, a 63-year-old bilateral below-knee amputee with Class IV cardiac and restrictive-obstructive pulmonary disease improved cardiovascular fitness, improved cardiac Class IV to Class II, and therapeutically improved from Class E (bed rest) to Class C (moderate exercise restriction). This suggests that amputees, healthy or suffering from secondary disabilities, can improve their fitness levels with exercise using different modes of exercise.

An essential resource for any professional involved in training LE amputees for sport or health is the publication by the Department of Veterans Affairs, *Physical Fitness: A Guide for Individuals with Lower Limb Loss* (22). The publication represents a guide for prescribing exercises that will improve all aspects of physical fitness, including cardiovascular, flexibility, muscular strength and endurance, and motor skills. The publication includes illustrations for calisthenics, stretching exercises, as well as specific muscle strength and endurance exercises for arms, shoulders, legs, abdominals, chest, and back. It also includes training programs for walking, running, aerobic dance, swimming, cycling, rowing, cross-country skiing, and a variety of sports (e.g., basketball, hockey, soccer, squash). Another good resource for sports and recreation for those with LE amputation is the publication by Kegel (23).

The prescribed number of sets and repetitions for muscle strengthening should be adjusted to the needs of the amputee. The proper frequency, duration, and intensity of cardiovascular exercises should follow those prescribed by ACSM Guidelines (18).

It is important that an amputee have a comfortable prosthetic limb that is suited for the activity/exercise. Activities/exercises such as walking, bicycling, rowing, StairMaster, Body Trec, and other aerobic machines do not require special adaptations to standard artifical limbs. Such activities/exercises such as running, sprinting, and swimming do require special adaptations, and these special adaptations are addressed in the text by Burgess and Rappoport (22). It is recommended that the amputee work with their prosthetist to obtain any adaptation needed for his/her prosthetic device.

Upper-Extremity Amputation

Upper-extremity amputees, because of their intact lower extremities, are not as limited to modes of exercise as LE amputees. All activities and exercises involving the lower extremities that can be performed by able-bodied individuals are applicable to UE amputees.

EDUCATION AND COUNSELING

The issue of ***phantom pain/discomfort*** from "phantom limbs" has many times been inaccurately addressed by medical professionals. The publication by Bowler and Michael (17) warns medical professionals to **not** assume there is any pain in the residual area that is phantom in nature and, in fact, states that phantom pain is quite rare, and that the stump pain can easily mimic phantom pain. Phantom pain is **not rare.** Study designs using retrospect surveys have reported that the majority of amputees suffer from this phenomenon whether the amputation was due to trauma, surgery, or congenital limb deficiency (24–27). Phantom pain is a part of the luggage that comes with amputation for most amputees. Amputees know the difference between pain emitting from the stump (i.e., residual pain) and phantom pain. Pain from the stump usually occurs due to hair follicle infections, skin/scar tissue breakdown or from excessive pressure from the prosthetic device. Pain from the stump is recognized by the sensory cerebral hemisphere as pain **from the stump,** not from that portion of the anatomy that has been amputated. Indeed, the sensory cerebral hemisphere recognizes phantom pain as actually originating from the amputated areas of the limb (28).

Even though the cause of phantom pain remains an enigma for the amputee, the phenomenon is very real, and it is more common in LE amputations than in UE amputations and more common in proximal than in distal amputations (24). Amputees have identified exercise, objects approaching the stump, and cold weather as the primary triggers of phantom sensation (26). For instance, LE amputees are more likely to suffer phantom pain on days when the amputee has used his/her prothesis (e.g., standing, walking, mowing the lawn) for long periods of time. These activities might also intensify phantom pain. However, aerobic exercises using such non–weight-bearing exercise modes as swimming, stationary bicycle ergometry, and rowing ergometry should not cause or intensify phantom pain (author's [KHP] personal experience). If weight-bearing modes of exercise (jogging, fast walking, Stair-Stepper, etc) are increasing the incidence of phantom pain, it is suggested to substitute non–weight-bearing modes of exercise in their place. Of importance is the need for the LE amputee to not use phantom pain as a reason for eliminating exercise from his/her lifestyle.

Depression has been related to a higher incidence of phantom pain and, therefore, can be a potential barrier to exercise. In a study by Lindesay (29), it was found that many of the amputees with long-standing phantom pain were more depressed when compared to a group of amputees that did not report problems with phantom pain.

Skin breakdowns (blisters) or hair follicle infections can significantly affect the activity level of any amputee. Practicing good hygiene for not only the residual limb (stump) but also the inside lining of the prosthetic limb will help prevent skin problems. Stump socks should be changed daily, and determining the right size and number of stump socks for proper fit is essential to prevent skin irritations and blisters. Amputees have found that the use of nylon sheaths can significantly reduce friction between the skin and the wool/cotton stump sock. Socks should always be changed when damp or wet.

Managing body weight is also important to minimize stress on stump and weight-bearing surfaces.

CASE STUDY

Jessica C. Roberts

The following patient was referred for exercise testing for functional assessment and evaluation for a prosthesis. He is a 15-year-old male who was diagnosed with osteogenic sarcoma. He underwent a left-arm, above-the-elbow amputation 6 months prior to the assessment. He is currently receiving chemotherapy and radiation treatments. His stump is still healing, and he has had continuous phantom pains since the operation. He frequently complains of fatigue, has a poor appetite, and spends most of his time in his room watching TV or sleeping.

Throughout his childhood and adolescent years, he participated in organized baseball and basketball and had, prior to his diagnosis and operation, been looking forward to playing for his high school baseball and basketball teams.

RESTING DATA

ECG showed normal sinus rhythm with a heart rate of 72 bpm and a blood pressure of 118/76 mm Hg.

EXERCISE RESPONSE

The patient performed a modified Bruce Protocol (2-min stages), and the test was terminated after 9 minutes, 13 seconds when the patient reported fatigue and wanted to stop.

The maximal heart rate was 160 bpm and maximal blood pressure was 150/82 mm Hg with normal sinus rhythm.

INTERPRETATION

Although the treadmill test did not identify any cardiac anomalies, the patient is experiencing significant adjustment issues following his diagnosis, amputation, and cancer treatment. The patient has lost 10 pounds, his hair has fallen out, and he has become increasingly withdrawn from his family and friends. It has been determined by his medical staff that the patient has several psychosocial issues to resolve secondary to his amputation. The patient expresses little interest in being fitted for a prosthetic arm because he is concerned how his friends would respond to the prosthetic device (i.e., altered body image). The patient continues to keep his stump covered in public and in the presence of his family, even though it has healed. He has expressed concerns that people look at him as a "freak" when he is in public because he feels that everyone stares at his amputated arm.

Clinical Implications

The patient's clinical presentation suggests several areas that should be addressed. The patient is experiencing significant grief and loss issues secondary to his amputation and may be clinically depressed. Referral to a pediatric psychologist to work on these adjustment issues is indicated. The patient's difficulties with changed body image place him at risk of rejecting the use of an artificial limb. It is recommended that his physical therapist help him accept his changed body image by allowing the patient to unwrap and manipulate his stump during physical therapy sessions. This will increase his exposure to and acceptance of his changed physical appearance. The physical therapist will also play a crucial role in educating him concerning the importance of maintaining upper-body strength/range of motion by prescribing a "training schedule" that will maintain the muscle tone, muscle strength, and flexibility of: 1) the shoulder and upper arm to prevent flexion contracture of the shoulder; and 2) the hip on his involved side to maintain posture and upper-body control. Also, the "training schedule" should incorporate balance exercises designed to help him reestablish his center of gravity.

The patient's adjustment to his amputation can be facilitated by introducing him to other adolescents and young adult amputees. Support groups, sports specific for amputees (e.g., paralympics), and written or visual materials about the many options that amputees have in life could help lay the groundwork for a positive transition to prosthetic use. All of these will help the patient come to a realistic evaluation of his situation and will provide him with role models in coping with the challenges in the areas of sports and vocation.

References

1. Kerstein MD, Zimmer H, Dugdale FE. Amputation of the lower extemity: a study of 194 cases. *Arch Phys Med Rehabil* 1974; 55:454–459.
2. Brashear RH, Raney RB. *Handbook of orthopaedic surgery.* St Louis, MO: C.V. Mosby, 1978:296–322.

3. Huang C-T, Jackson JR, Moore NB, et al. Amputation: energy cost of ambulation. *Arch Phys Med Rehabil* 1979;60:18–24.
4. Ganguli W, Datta SR, Chatterjee BB, et al. Performance evaluation of an amputee prosthesis system in below-knee amputees. *Ergonomics* 1973;16:797–810.
5. Pagliarulo MA, Waters R, Hislop HS. Energy cost of walking of below-knee amputees having no vascular disease. *Phys Ther* 1979;59:538–542.
6. Waters RL, Perry J, Antonelli D, et al. Energy cost of walking of amputees: the influence of level of amputation. *J Bone Joint Surg Am* 1976;58:42–52.
7. Macfarlane PA, Nielsen DH, Shurr DG, et al. Perception of walking difficulty by below-knee amputees using a conventional foot versus the flex-foot. *J Prosthet Orthop* 1991;3(31): 114–119.
8. Hrubec Z, Ryder RA. Traumatic limb amputation and subsequent mortality from cardiovascular disease and other causes. *J Chronic Dis* 1978;33:239–250.
9. Rose HC, Schweitzer P, Charoenkul V, et al. Cardiovascular disease risk factors in combat veterans after traumatic leg amputation. *Arch Phys Med Rehabil* 1987;68:20–23.
10. Braune W, Fischer O. *On the center of gravity of the human body.* Berlin, Germany: Springer-Verlag, 1984.
11. Gailey RS, Gailey AM. *Stretching and strengthening for lower extremity amputees.* Miami, FL: Advanced Rehabilitation Therapy, Inc., 1994. (Correspondence: Advanced Rehabilitation Therapy, Inc., 7641 SW 126th Street, Miami, FL 33156.)
12. Gailey RS, Gailey AM. *Balance, agility, coordination and endurance for lower extremity amputees.* Miami, FL: Advanced Rehabilitation Therapy, Inc., 1994.
13. Gailey RS, Gailey AM, Sendelbach SJ. *Home exercise guide for lower extremity amputees.* Miami, FL: Advanced Rehabilitation Therapy, Inc., 1995.
14. American College of Sports Medicine. *ACSM's exercise management for persons with chronic diseases and disabilities.* Champaign, IL: Human Kinetics, 1997.
15. O'Donoghue DH. Treatment of acute ligament injuries of the knee. *Orthop Clin* 1973;4:617–645.
16. Kendall FP, McCreary EK, Provance PG. *Muscles: testing and function.* 4th ed. Baltimore, MD: Williams & Wilkins, 1993.
17. Bowler JH, Michael JW. *Atlas of limb prosthetics: Surgical, prosthetic and rehabilitation principles. American Academy of Orthopaedic Surgeons.* St. Louis, MO: Mosby-Year Book, 1992.
18. American College of Sports Medicine. *ACSM's guidelines for exercise testing and prescription.* 6th ed. Philadelphia: Lippincott Williams & Wilkins, 2000.
19. Bostom AG, Bates E, Mazzeralla N, et al. Ergometer modifications for combined arm-leg use by lower extremity amputees in cardiovascular testing and training. *Arch Phys Med Rehabil* 1987;68:244–247.
20. James U. Effect of physical training in healthy male unilateral above-knee amputees. *Scand J Rehabil Med* 1973;5:88–101.
21. Pitetti KH, Snell PG, Stray-Gunderson J, et al. Aerobic training exercise for individuals who had amputation of the lower limb. *J Bone Joint Surg* 1987;69:914–921.
22. Burgess EM, Rappoport A. *Physical fitness: a guide for individuals with lower limb loss.* Washington, DC: Department of Veterans Affairs. (Correspondence: Editor, Scientific and Technical Publications, Rehabilitation Research and Development Service, 103 S Gay Street, Baltimore, MD 21202-4051.)
23. Kegel B. Physical fitness: sports and recreation for those with lower limb amputation or impairment. *J Rehabil Res Dev Clin Suppl* 1985;(1):1–125.
24. Melzack R. Phantom Limbs. *Sci Am* 1992; April; 120–126.
25. Machin P, de C Williams AC. Stiff upper lip: coping strategies of World War II veterans with phantom limb pain. *Clin J Pain* 1998;14(4):290–294.
26. Wilkins KL, McGrath PJ, Finley GA, et al. Phantom limb sensations and phantom limb pain in child and adolescent amputees. *Pain* 1998;78(1):7–12.
27. Wartan SW, Hamann W, Wedley JR, et al. Phantom pain and sensation among British veterans amputees. *Br J Anaesth* 1997;78(6):652–659.
28. Schmid HJ. Phantom limb after amputation—overview and new knowledge. *Schweiz Rundsch Med Prax* 2000;89(3): 87–94.
29. Lindesay JE. Multiple pain complaints in amputees. *J R Soc Med* 1985;78(6):452–455.

SECTION THREE

Neoplastic, Immunologic, and Hematologic Conditions

SECTION EDITOR: *David C. Nieman*

CHAPTER **15**

NEOPLASMS

Kerry S. Courneya, John R. Mackey, and H. Arthur Quinney

PATHOPHYSIOLOGY AND EPIDEMIOLOGY

Cells that grow out of control and form a mass are called a tumor or neoplasm (i.e., "new growth"). Some tumors, referred to as benign, grow and enlarge only at the site where they began. Other tumors, called malignant or cancerous, have the potential to invade and destroy the normal tissue around them and to spread throughout the body. Cancer is not a single disease but rather a collection of many different diseases. What cancer cells typically share, however, is changes in the genes that regulate cell division, programmed cell death, and cell mobility. These genetic changes lead to the characteristic features of cancer, namely: (a) accumulation of abnormal cells, (b) invasion of nearby tissues, and (c) spread to distant sites. Cancers are classified into several groups depending on the kind of normal cell from which they arise. The most common cancers develop from epithelial cells that line the body's surfaces. These cancers are called carcinomas and include prostate, breast, colon, lung, and cervical cancers. Cancers can also arise from the cells of the blood (i.e., leukemias), the immune system (i.e., lymphomas), and bone and connective tissues (i.e., sarcomas).

Since 1990, approximately 12 million Americans have been diagnosed with some form of invasive cancer (1). Moreover, cancer is the second leading cause of death in the United States behind heart disease, with more than 563,000 deaths due to cancer expected in 1999 alone (1). Over their lifetime, Americans have about a 41% probability of developing cancer and about a 25% probability of dying from cancer (1). Prostate, breast, colorectal, and lung cancer account for more than 50% of all cancer cases and deaths (Table 15.1). In terms of demographics, the probability of developing cancer increases dramatically with age, making it a disease that primarily affects older persons (Table 15.2).

Fortunately, early detection and improved treatments for cancer have resulted in increased survival rates over the last few decades (1). The current 5-year relative survival rate (adjusted for normal life expectancy) is estimated to be about 60%, although this figure varies considerably depending on the type of cancer and extent of the disease at diagnosis (Table 15.3). Increased incidence rates, combined with improved survival rates, have resulted in more than 8.2 million Americans being alive today who have been through the cancer experience (1). Consequently, fitness professionals can expect to serve a large and increasing number of cancer survivors (i.e., persons who have completed medical treatment and are considered cured) and a smaller but likewise growing number of cancer patients (i.e., persons who are currently receiving medical treatment).

ETIOLOGY AND RISK FACTORS

Although the causes and risk factors for human cancer are diverse—ranging from genetics, to behavior, to the environment—lifestyle factors appear to be paramount. The Harvard Report on Cancer Prevention (2) concluded that nearly two-thirds of cancer mortality in the U.S. can be linked to tobacco use, poor diet, and lack of exercise (Table 15.4) (2). Moreover, only 5–10% of most types of cancer are caused by defects in single genes that run in families, and only a similar small percentage are because of occupational and environmental exposures.

Physical inactivity as a risk factor for cancer has received increased research attention based on a number of plausible biological mechanisms (3). Over the past decade, mounting evidence has indicated that physical activity may significantly reduce the risk of some cancers. The strongest evidence comes from research on colon cancer, where physical activity has been shown to reduce the risk by up to 50% (4). In terms of impact, Colditz et al. (4) estimate that increasing the amount of physical activity in the U.S. population by 3 hours of walking per week would result in 17% fewer cases of colon cancer. Moreover, evidence is also available to suggest that physical activity may have a protective effect against prostate cancer (5), lung cancer (6, 7), breast cancer (8), and other estrogen-dependent cancers in women (9), although definitive conclusions cannot be made at this time. Evidence for other cancers (e.g., pancreas, testicular, stomach) is currently too sparse to make even tentative conclusions.

Table 15.1. Estimated New Cancer Cases and Deaths Overall and by Sex and for the Major Cancer Sites

	Estimated New Cases			Estimated New Deaths		
Site	Total	Male	Female	Total	Male	Female
All Sites	1,221,800	623,800	598,000	563,100	291,100	272,000
Prostate	179,300	179,300	—	37,000	37,000	—
Breast	176,300	1,300	175,000	43,700	400	43,300
Colorectal	129,400	62,400	67,000	56,600	27,800	28,800
Lung	171,600	94,000	77,600	158,900	90,900	68,000

Excludes basal and squamous cell skin cancers and in situ carcinomas except urinary bladder. Adapted from Cancer Facts and Figures: 1999. Atlanta: American Cancer Society, 1999.

PRIMARY PREVENTION GUIDELINES

Given that the majority of cancer deaths are believed to be attributable to lifestyle/behavioral factors, cancer is largely a preventable disease. In light of this fact, the Harvard Center for Cancer Prevention (2, 10) has proposed guidelines for cancer prevention that consist of seven major recommendations: (a) stop smoking, (b) eat a healthy diet, (c) maintain a healthy body weight, (d) exercise regularly, (e) limit alcohol consumption, (f) practice safe sex, and (g) limit sun exposure. The specific guidelines for each lifestyle change, including exercise, are summarized in Table 15.5.

COMMON SIGNS AND SYMPTOMS

Because cancer is not one disease, the common signs and symptoms of cancer are not generic but rather cancer specific. Unfortunately, most of the signs and symptoms of cancer are similar to those of other medical conditions, and so their presence is not necessarily indicative of cancer. Nevertheless, when these symptoms do occur, it is important to have them checked by a physician. Table 15.6 summarizes the major signs and symptoms for the most common cancer sites.

Table 15.2. Percentage of the Population Developing the Most Common Invasive Cancers by Certain Ages

Site		Birth–39	40–59	60–79	Birth–Death
All Sites	—Male	1.65	8.25	34.94	44.66
	—Female	1.95	9.14	22.33	38.03
Prostate	—Male	<0.01	1.83	14.79	17.00
Breast	—Female	0.43	4.00	6.88	12.50
Colorectal	—Male	0.06	0.87	4.05	5.69
	—Female	0.05	0.67	3.14	5.62
Lung	—Male	0.04	1.34	6.55	8.27
	—Female	0.03	0.97	3.95	5.64

Excludes basal and squamous cell skin cancers and in situ carcinomas except urinary bladder. Adapted from Cancer Facts and Figures: 1999. Atlanta: American Cancer Society, 1999.

SCREENING AND DIAGNOSIS

A key to improving survival rates from cancer is early detection of the disease. Screening is the process of identifying disease in people who are asymptomatic. The major advantage of screening is that it can identify abnormalities that may be cancer at an early stage before physical signs and symptoms develop. Screening tests are available for many of the most common types of cancer, including breast, colorectal, prostate, and uterine. Unfortunately, there are no effective screening tests for lung cancer at this time. The recommended screening procedures for cancer in general and for the most common cancers in particular are provided in Table 15.7.

Screening tests for breast cancer include mammography, clinical breast examination (CBE), and breast self-examination (BSE). The most definitive test, called mammography, is a special type of x-ray procedure. Figure 15.1 shows the results of a mammogram comparing a normal breast to one with a tumor. Screening tests for colorectal cancer include digital rectal examination (DRE), fecal occult blood (stool blood) test, flexible sigmoidoscopy, double contrast barium enema, and colonoscopy. The most definitive test for colorectal cancer is a colonoscopy, which involves visualizing the internal surface of the rectum and large bowel using a flexible fiberoptic tube. Screening tests for prostate cancer include DRE and prostate-specific antigen (PSA) testing. PSA is a substance produced only by the prostate and is measured by a blood test. PSA values below 4.0 ng/mL are considered normal, values between 4.0

Table 15.3. 5-Year Relative Survival Rates for the Major Cancers by Stage at Diagnosis

Site	All Stages (%)	Local (%)	Regional (%)	Distant (%)
Prostate	93	100	99	33
Breast	85	97	77	22
Colorectal	62	91	66	9
Lung	14	50	20	2

Rates are adjusted for normal life expectancy and are based on cases diagnosed from 1989–1994 followed through 1995. Adapted from Cancer Facts and Figures: 1999. Atlanta: American Cancer Society, 1999.

Table 15.4. Estimated Percentage of Total Cancer Deaths Attributable to Established Causes of Cancer

Risk Factor	Percentage
Tobacco	30%
Adult dietary/obesity	30%
Sedentary lifestyle	5%
Occupational factors	5%
Family history of cancer	5%
Viruses/other biologic agents	5%
Perinatal factors/growth	5%
Reproductive factors	3%
Alcohol	3%
Socioeconomic status	3%
Environmental pollution	2%
Ionizing/ultraviolet radiation	2%
Prescription drugs/medical procedures	1%
Salt/other food additives/contaminants	1%

Reprinted with permission from Harvard Report on Cancer Prevention. Volume I: causes of human cancer. *Cancer Causes Control* 1996;7:S3–S59.

ng/mL and 10.0 ng/mL are considered borderline, and values greater than 10.0 ng/mL are considered high and suggest the possibility of prostate cancer. PSA testing is considered a more definitive screening tool for prostate cancer than a DRE.

Screening tests are only suggestive of cancer; they do not diagnose it. An actual diagnosis of cancer requires analysis of a tissue sample. By examining cells under the microscope, a trained pathologist can almost always distinguish malignant cells from their benign (i.e., nonmalignant) counterparts. The pathologist looks for cells that are frequently dividing, are invading normal surrounding tissue, or have unusual cellular features such as large and disorganized nuclei. Increasingly, it is possible to prove that suspicious cells are truly malignant by identifying cancer-related genetic mutations using the techniques of molecular biology.

Table 15.5. The Harvard Center for Cancer Prevention's Recommendations for the Primary Prevention of Cancer

Risk Factor	Recommendation
Smoking	Stop smoking or never start.
Dietary Factors	Eat a varied diet; reduce consumption of red meat to once a week or less; increase vegetable and fruit intake to at least five servings per day; do not blacken or char red meat, chicken, or fish.
Obesity	Maintain a healthy body weight (<135% of ideal weight) through proper diet and exercise.
Physical Activity	Participate in 30 minutes or more of moderate-intensity physical activity on most, preferably all, days of the week.
Alcohol	Consume no more than one alcoholic drink per day.
Sexual Activity	Protect yourself and your partner from sexually transmitted infections by practicing abstinence or safe sex.
Sun Exposure	Protect yourself from too much sun by limiting the amount of time spent in the sun (especially between 10:00 am and 4:00 pm) and using sun protection methods (e.g., hats, shirts, sunscreens ≥ 15 SPF.)

Adapted from Harvard Report on Cancer Prevention. Volume I: causes of human cancer. *Cancer Causes Control* 1996;7:S3-S59 and Harvard Report on Cancer Prevention. Volume II: prevention of human cancer. *Cancer Causes Control* 1997;8.

Table 15.6. Signs and Symptoms for the Most Common Cancers

Cancer Site	Signs and Symptoms
Breast	Breast lump, thickening, swelling, distortion, or tenderness; skin irritation or dimpling; nipple pain or retraction (turning inward), scaliness, unusual bleeding or discharge.
Colorectal	Rectal bleeding, blood in the stool, a change in bowel habits (persistent constipation or diarrhea), cramping or steady abdominal pain, a feeling that you need to have a bowel movement that is not relieved by doing so, decreased appetite, weakness and fatigue, jaundice (yellow-green discoloration of the skin and white part of the eyes).
Lung	Persistent cough, bloody or rust-colored sputum (spit or phlegm), chest pain aggravated by deep breathing, shortness of breath, new onset of wheezing, hoarseness, weight loss and loss of appetite, recurring pneumonia or bronchitis, and fever without a known reason.
Prostate	Weak or interrupted urine flow; inability to urinate, or difficulty starting or stopping the urine flow; the need to urinate frequently, especially at night; blood in the urine; pain or burning on urination; continuing pain in lower back, pelvis, or upper thighs; difficulty having an erection.

Adapted from the American Cancer Society: Hope, Progress, Answers. www.cancer.org.

STAGING

After the initial diagnosis, it is important to learn the extent to which the disease has progressed (i.e., stage). Cancer staging is essential in determining the choice of therapy and assessing prognosis. Cancer stage is determined by patient history, physical examination, laboratory testing, and/or diagnostic imaging (e.g., chest radiography, computed tomography, magnetic resonance imaging). A number of different staging systems are currently used to classify tumors, but the most common is the Tumor (T), Node (N), Metastasis (M) system (11). The TNM system stage's cancer based on the size of the primary tumor (T), the involvement of regional lymph nodes (N), and the presence or absence of distant metastases (M). Once the T, N, and M are determined, a "stage" of I (least advanced) through IV (most advanced) is assigned. In general, regionally confined cancers are stage I and II, locally advanced cancers are stage III, and cancers with overt distant metastases are stage IV.

MEDICAL AND SURGICAL TREATMENTS

Cancer treatments may be used to cure cancer, to prolong life when a cure is not possible, or to improve qual-

Table 15.7. The American Cancer Society's Recommendations for the Early Detection of Cancer in Asymptomatic People

SITE	RECOMMENDATION
General	A cancer-related checkup is recommended every 3 years for people ages 20–40 and every year for people ages 40 and older. This exam should include health counseling and, depending on a person's age, might include examinations for cancers of the thyroid, oral cavity, skin, lymph nodes, testes, and ovaries, as well as for some nonmalignant diseases.
Breast	Women 40 and older should have an annual mammogram, an annual clinical breast exam (CBE) performed by a health-care professional, and should perform monthly breast self-examination. The CBE should be conducted close to the scheduled mammogram. Women ages 20–39 should have a clinical breast exam performed by a health-care professional every 3 years and should perform monthly breast self-examination.
Colorectal	Men and women age 50 and older should undertake one of two courses of action in consultation with their physician: 1) an annual fecal occult blood (stool blood) test, together with a flexible sigmoidoscopy and digital rectal exam (DRE) every 5 years or 2) a total colon exam, either by colonoscopy with DRE every 10 years, or by double contrast barium enema with DRE every 5–10 years. People with any of the following colorectal cancer risk factors should begin colorectal cancer screening earlier and/or undergo screening more often: a personal history of colorectal cancer or adenomatous polyps, a strong family history of colorectal cancer or polyps (cancer or polyps in a first-degree relative younger than 60 or in two first-degree relatives of any age), a personal history of chronic inflammatory bowel disease, or families with hereditary colorectal cancer syndromes.
Prostate	An annual digital rectal exam (DRE) of the prostate gland and an annual prostate-specific antigen (PSA) blood test are recommended for men 50 and older, for men who have at least a 10-year life expectancy, and for younger men who are at high risk (those with two or more affected first-degree relatives or who are African Americans).
Uterus	Cervix: All women who are or have been sexually active or who are 18 and older should have an annual Pap test and pelvic examination. After three or more consecutive satisfactory examinations with normal findings, the Pap test may be performed less frequently. Discuss the matter with your physician. Endometrium: Women at high risk for cancer of the uterus should have a sample of endometrial tissue examined when menopause begins.

Adapted from the American Cancer Society: Hope, Progress, Answers. www.cancer.org.

ity of life (i.e., symptom relief). The three primary cancer treatment modalities are surgery, radiation therapy, and systemic therapy. Surgery is the oldest and most frequently used modality in cancer therapy and is the treatment of choice for most localized carcinomas and sarcomas. Cancer operations can be classified as either radical or conservative. Radical resections attempt to encompass all gross and microscopic tumor in a single operation and are performed with curative intent. These operations commonly involve excision of tumor and draining regional lymph nodes as a single specimen. Conservative surgeries are usually performed to minimize the volume of tissue removed and preserve organ function. In general, conservative surgeries require additional nonsurgical treatment with radiotherapy and/or systemic therapy to eradicate residual cancer cells. Some common cancer operations and their sequelae are described in Table 15.8.

Radiation therapy is the treatment of cancer using ionizing radiation. It is considered a local-regional treatment, with the goal to irradiate the known tumor volume while sparing adjacent radiation-sensitive tissues. Several types of radiation are used in the clinic, but the majority of radiotherapy treatments are external beams of high-energy photons produced by linear accelerators or from the decay of cobalt^{60} (Figure 15.2). These photons penetrate into tissue and produce ionized (electrically charged) particles that damage DNA. This DNA damage usually inhibits cell replication and often leads to cell death. Radiation therapy is delivered in repeated small doses over an extended period of time in order to kill cancer cells without undue damage to normal cells. A total dose of 60 grays (Gy), for example, may be "fractionated" into 2 Gy every weekday for 6 weeks in the treatment of breast cancer. A full course of external beam radiotherapy can range from 8 weeks of low-fraction therapy administered each weekday (given with curative intent) to a single high-dose treatment (given to palliate a patient with a painful bone metastasis). Although malignant cells are typically more radiosensitive than normal cells, normal tissue toxicity does occur and is entirely dependent on what part of the body is irradiated (Table 15.9).

Because cancer cells frequently metastasize beyond the primary site and regional lymph nodes, systemic therapy or chemotherapy (i.e., drugs) is prescribed for many advanced solid tumors. Moreover, systemic therapy is the mainstay of curative treatment for leukemia and lymphoma, where cancer cells are only rarely regionally confined. Cancer chemotherapy exploits biological differences between normal and malignant cells to preferentially kill malignant cells. Most of the currently used chemotherapy drugs have been selected to be toxic to proliferating cells (Table 15.10). However, newer anticancer drugs are being developed for their abilities to kill more slowly growing tumors. Increasingly, it is being realized that anticancer drugs trigger apoptosis—programmed cell death—and that cancer cells may be more susceptible to these triggers than normal tissues.

In general, curative chemotherapy requires combinations of several chemotherapy drugs, given in repeated courses or cycles 2–4 weeks apart, for 3–6 months. Adult cancers routinely cured by chemotherapy include acute leukemias, Hodgkin's disease, some lymphomas, and testicular cancers. Because the goal of treatment is cure, most patients are willing to accept the multiple side effects of systemic treatment (see Table 15.10). If these particular cancers recur after standard chemotherapy, treatment with high-dose chemotherapy (requiring bone marrow or stem cell transplantation to restore the blood-forming system) can provide long-term survival.

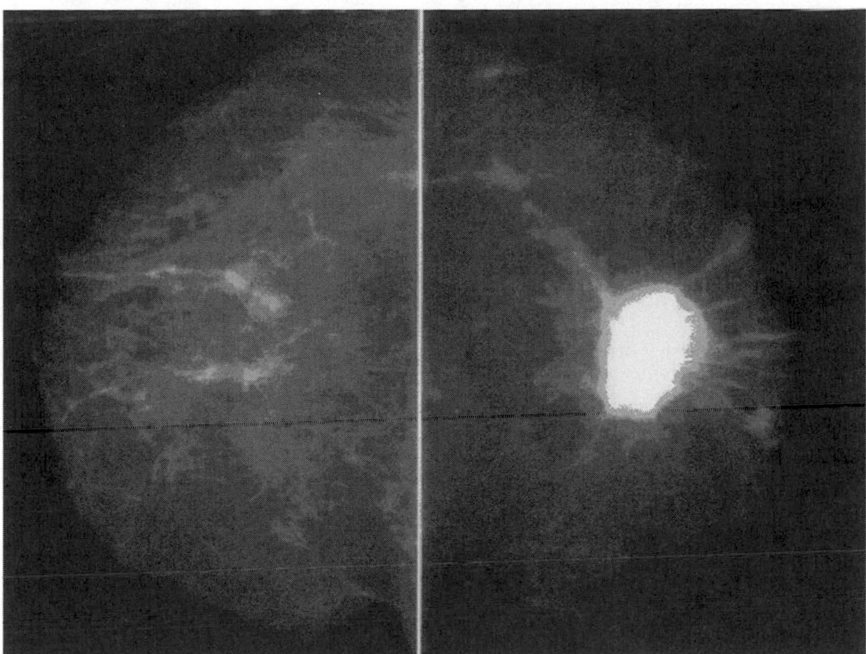

Figure 15.1. Radiographs of the breast using low doses of radiation reveal normal breast tissue (left) and a 2-cm breast carcinoma (right).

About 20% of cancers in males and about 40% in females arise in hormone-sensitive organs—prostate, breast, and uterus. The hormonal environment of the body can directly stimulate the growth of established cancers. Depriving an established prostate, breast, or uterine cancer of its sustaining hormones can not only halt growth but may also actually induce regression of the tumor. For example, a patient with metastatic breast cancer treated with an antiestrogen may have partial or complete disappearance of the metastatic lesions. Similarly, patients with advanced prostate cancer derive substantial benefit from depletion of testosterone. Although surgical removal of the ovaries or testes will, respectively, deplete estrogen or testosterone, drug treatment with luteinizing hormone releasing hormone (LHRH) agonists also stops sex hormone production without the need for surgery.

Glucocorticoid agents are cytotoxic to some leukemic and lymphoma cells and are used at high doses for these

Table 15.8. Common Cancer Operations and Their Sequelae

Operation	Description	Sequelae	Type
Pulmonary lobectomy	Removal of one lobe of one lung	Reduced lung capacity and function, dyspnea, deconditioning	Conservative
Pneumonectomy	Removal of one entire lung	Reduced lung capacity and function, dyspnea, deconditioning	Radical
Radical neck dissection	Removal of cervical lymphatics	Reduced neck ROM and muscle strength, occasional CN XI palsy	Radical
Mastectomy and axillary node dissection	Removal of entire breast and draining lymphatics	Chest wall pain, reduced arm ROM, occasionally arm lymphedema	Radical
Lumpectomy and axillary node dissection	Removal of breast tumor and sparing remaining breast	Reduced arm ROM, occasional arm lymphedema	Conservative
Radical prostatectomy	Removal of prostate, seminal vesicles, and ampullae of vasa deferentia	Urinary incontinence, erectile dysfunction are common, deconditioning	Radical
Abdominoperineal resection	Removal of rectum and draining lymphatics	Patient may require ostomy, deconditioning	Radical
Hemicolectomy	Removal of involved colon and draining lymphatics	Patient occasionally requires ostomy, deconditioning, diarrhea	Radical
Limb amputation	Removal of tumor with margin of normal tissue	Occasional chronic pain syndromes, deconditioning	Radical
Limb-sparing surgery	Removal of tumor and reattachment of distal limb	Postoperative casing leads to decreased joint ROM and muscle atrophy, occasional chronic pain syndromes, deconditioning	Conservative

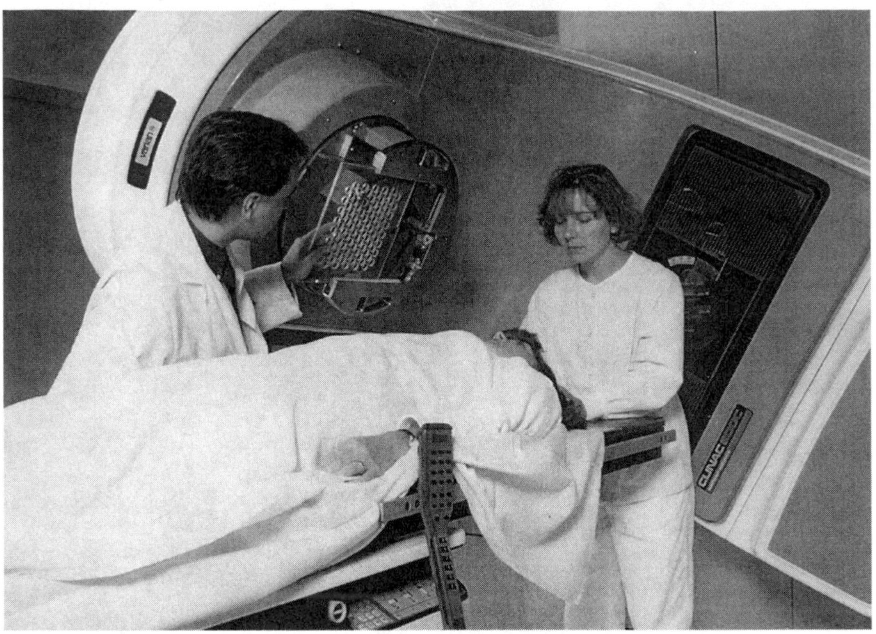

Figure 15.2. Radiation technologists position a patient on a linear accelerator table prior to receiving radiation therapy.

cancers. Additionally, glucocorticoids are commonly given to prevent and treat chemotherapy-induced nausea, reduce cancer-related pain and anorexia, and to treat and prevent allergic reactions from chemotherapy drugs. Unfortunately, use of these agents causes muscle loss, proximal muscle weakness, fat accumulation in the trunk and face, osteoporosis, and an increased susceptibility to infection.

Increasingly, combinations of the main cancer treatment modalities (surgery, radiotherapy, and systemic therapy) are being used to treat cancer. The major advantages of combined modality treatment include: (a) disease missed by locoregional therapy may be treated by systemic therapy, (b) tumor shrinkage by radiotherapy or systemic therapy can allow conservative surgery and thereby preserve organ function, and (c) tumors may respond more dramatically to combined therapy. Combined modality therapy is now the standard of care for high-risk or locally advanced solid tumors, including breast, lung, colon, rectal, cervical, ovarian, prostate, and esophageal carcinomas, as well as many sarcomas. Hodgkin's disease and aggressive lymphomas are commonly treated with combination chemotherapy and radiotherapy.

EFFECTS OF THE CANCER EXPERIENCE ON QUALITY OF LIFE

Not surprisingly, cancer and its treatments often result in significant reductions in quality of life (QOL). Some of the more common psychologic and emotional sequelae of the cancer experience include depression, anxiety, stress, body image concerns, decreased self-esteem, and loss of a sense of control (12–14). The physical and functional effects of the cancer experience may include asthenia, ataxia, cachexia, reduced cardiovascular and pulmonary function, muscle weakness and atrophy, weight change, difficulty sleeping, fatigue, nausea, vomiting, and pain (15–19). Although the side effects tend to peak during treatment, therapy-related symptoms may persist months or even years following treatment (14).

BENEFITS OF PHYSICAL EXERCISE FOLLOWING CANCER DIAGNOSIS

Currently, there are a number of QOL interventions available to assist cancer patients in coping with their dis-

Table 15.9. Common Adverse Effects of Radiation Therapy

Radiation Site	Common Cancers	Common Adverse Effects
Skin	All cancers	Redness, pain, blistering, and reduced elasticity
Brain	Brain cancers and metastases	Nausea and vomiting, fatigue
Pharynx	Upper-respiratory cancers	Mouth ulceration
Salivary gland	Upper-respiratory cancers	Xerostomia (dry mouth)
Thorax or	Breast, lung, lymphoma	Some degree of irreversible lung fibrosis; heart *may* receive radiation, causing pericardial inflammation fibrosis; premature atherosclerosis; cardiomyopathy
Abdomen	Pancreas, stomach, lymphoma	Vomiting and/or diarrhea
Pelvis	Prostate, uterine cervix	Diarrhea, pelvic pain, bladder scarring, and occasionally incontinence and sexual dysfunction
Joints	Sarcomas, bone metastases	Connective tissue and joint capsule fibrosis; may decrease range of motion

Table 15.10. Classes of Systemic Therapy for Cancer and Their Common Adverse Effects

Class	Examples	Common Adverse Effects
Antimetabolite chemotherapy (intravenous)	Methotrexate, fluorouracil, gemcitabine	Fatigue, anorexia, nausea, anemia, neutropenia, thrombocytopenia
Antitubulin chemotherapy (intravenous)	Taxol, taxotere, vinorelbine, vincristine	Fatigue, muscle pain, sensory and motor peripheral neuropathy, ataxia, anemia, neutropenia, thrombocytopenia
Alkylator chemotherapy	Cyclophosphamide, chlorambucil	Fatigue, anorexia, nausea, anemia, neutropenia, thrombocytopenia
Anthracycline chemotherapy (intravenous)	Doxorubicin (Adriamycin), mitoxantrone	Fatigue, cardiotoxicity (cardiac failure in <5% of patients), nausea, vomiting, anemia, neutropenia, thrombocytopenia
Platinum salt chemotherapy (intravenous)	Cisplatin, carboplatin	Fatigue, nausea, sensory and motor peripheral neuropathy, anemia neutropenia, thrombocytopenia
High-dose chemotherapy with bone marrow/stem cell transplantation	Combinations of 2–4 chemotherapy drugs in maximally tolerated doses	Loss of muscle mass, deconditioning, nausea, vomiting, neuropathy, anemia, neutropenia, thrombocytopenia, infection
Glucocorticoid hormonal therapy (oral)	Dexamethasone (Decadron), prednisone	Fat redistribution (truncal and facial obesity); proximal muscle weakness, osteoporosis, edema, infection
Antiestrogen hormonal therapy (oral)	Tamoxifen	Weight gain, fatigue, hot flashes
Antiandrogen hormonal therapy (oral)	Flutamide	Weight gain, fatigue, loss of muscle mass, hot flashes, osteoporosis
Luteinizing hormone releasing hormone agonists (subcutaneous injection)	Goserelin, buserelin	Weight gain, fatigue, hot flashes, osteoporosis

ease and treatments including cognitive-behavioral therapies, informational and educational strategies, individual and group psychotherapy, and other alternative treatments (20–21). Importantly, these interventions are largely psychologic in nature and not likely to address the physical and functional problems encountered by cancer patients (22). Physical exercise has well-documented links to physical, functional, and psychosocial well-being in healthy older persons (23) and older persons with other chronic diseases (24). Until recently, however, physical exercise has not been considered an important, or even appropriate, QOL intervention for cancer patients or survivors.

From a clinical perspective, some of the major concerns raised over prescribing exercise to cancer patients have included: (a) the potential immunosuppressive effects of vigorous exercise, (b) the increased likelihood of pathologic bone fractures arising from compromised bone integrity, (c) possible exacerbation of cardiotoxicity from chemotherapy and/or radiotherapy, (d) severe pain, nausea, and fatigue, which may be exacerbated by physical exercise, and (e) the inability and/or unwillingness of cancer patients to tolerate physical exercise given their weakened physical condition. Recent research, however, is beginning to dispel many of the myths and early fears over the safety, efficacy, and feasibility of exercise as a QOL intervention following cancer diagnosis.

Recent reviews have identified 36 studies that have examined the relationship between physical exercise and QOL following cancer diagnosis (22, 25). These studies have consistently demonstrated that exercise has beneficial effects on a wide variety of QOL outcomes (e.g., cardiovascular and muscular fitness, self-concept, mood states, fatigue) regardless of the exercise prescription (i.e., type, duration, frequency, intensity), cancer site, cancer treatment, or timing of the intervention, during or following treatment. Although these studies are not without limitations and many important questions remain to be answered (22), additional research is not likely to overturn the fundamental conclusion that physical exercise is a safe, efficacious, and feasible QOL intervention for most cancer patients and survivors. The issue of whether postdiagnosis exercise may influence tumor growth, disease progression, recurrence, and/or survival is still an open question. Consequently, fitness professionals should promote exercise following cancer diagnosis for its QOL benefits and not as a means of fighting cancer or improving survival. Table 15.11 lists some of the benefits that cancer patients and survivors can reasonably expect from a regular program of exercise.

SPECIAL PRECAUTIONS AND CONSIDERATIONS FOR EXERCISE TESTING FOLLOWING CANCER DIAGNOSIS

Exercise testing following cancer diagnosis may be used to (a) quantify the functional effects of the disease and its treatments, (b) identify comorbid conditions that may preclude exercise (e.g., cardiovascular disease), (c) develop an appropriate exercise prescription to assist patients in coping with and/or recovering from cancer and its treatments, and (d) determine the functional benefits of the prescribed exercise program. Not surprisingly, exer-

Table 15.11. Potential Benefits of Exercise Following Cancer Diagnosis

PSYCHOLOGICAL	PHYSIOLOGICAL
Reduced anxiety	Improved functional capacity
Less depression	Increased muscular strength
Increased vigor	Greater flexibility
Improved physical competence	Better body composition/weight control
Improved self-concept/esteem	Shorter durations of neutropenia and thrombocytopenia
Greater sense of control	Higher hemoglobin levels
Better general quality of life	Increased natural killer cell activity
Higher satisfaction with life	Reduced fatigue
	Less nausea and vomiting
	Greater pain control
	Less diarrhea

cise testing in cancer patients and survivors requires special precautions and considerations (Table 15.12) in addition to those recommended for healthy, asymptomatic middle-aged and older adults (23, 26). These special precautions arise from the significant morbidity experienced by cancer patients during and following individual or combined modality therapies.

Prior to exercise testing, it is important to have cancer patients and survivors complete a cancer history questionnaire in addition to other exercise and medical history questionnaires that may be indicated (e.g., Revised PAR-Q). The cancer history questionnaire should assess information on important diagnostic and treatment variables such as time since diagnosis, type and stage of disease, type of surgery and adjuvant therapy, and known or suspected side effects of treatment (e.g., ataxia, cardiomyopathy, pulmonary complications, orthopedic conditions). The patient's oncology team may need to be consulted to provide complete and accurate information. A sample cancer history questionnaire is provided in Figure 15.3.

Because cancer and its treatments may affect all aspects of physical functioning in cancer patients (i.e., cardiorespiratory endurance, muscular strength and endurance, flexibility, anthropometry and body composition, gait and balance), a comprehensive fitness test assessing all such parameters is warranted. In principle, the exercise tests should stress the patient to at least the level that will be experienced during the exercise program so that any symptoms that might be experienced are identified under the more controlled environment of an exercise test. Moreover, it is desirable to stress the patient as close to maximum capacity as is safely possible to provide better diagnostic information about cardiorespiratory function and to serve as a more accurate and reliable basis for exercise prescription. Notwithstanding the special precautions and considerations highlighted in Table 15.12, most otherwise healthy cancer survivors and early-stage cancer patients with good prognosis can safely perform symptom-limited maximal testing.

The decision concerning what exercise tests to use will depend on the specific limitations imposed by the cancer and its treatments, which, unfortunately, are too numerous to list and discuss individually. Some simple examples may provide the general idea. Cancer patients who have recently undergone rectal or prostate surgery, as one example, may prefer a treadmill test to assess functional capacity as opposed to a cycle ergometer test. Similarly, cancer patients presenting with specific limitations in range of movement in the upper extremities (e.g., breast, head, neck) following surgery or radiation therapy will likely be unable to perform tests involving upper-body movements (e.g., arm ergometer tests, bench press). Moreover, patients who have neurological complications

Table 15.12. Special Precautions/Considerations When Exercise Testing Cancer Patients/Survivors

COMPLICATION	PRECAUTION
Complete blood counts	
Hemoglobin level <8.0 g/dL	Avoid tests that require significant oxygen transport (i.e., maximal aerobic tests).
Absolute neutrophil count $\leq 0.5 \times 10^9$/L	Ensure proper sterilization of equipment and avoid maximal tests.
Platelet count $<50 \times 10^9$/L	Avoid tests that increase risk of bleeding (e.g., high-impact exercises).
Fever >38°C	May indicate systemic infection and should be investigated. Avoid exercise testing.
Ataxia/dizziness/peripheral sensory neuropathy	Avoid tests that require significant balance and coordination (e.g., treadmill, free weights).
Severe cachexia (loss of >35% of premorbid weight)	Loss of muscle mass usually limits exercise to mild intensity depending on degree of cachexia. Avoid exercise testing altogether.
Mouth sores/ulcerations	Avoid mouthpieces for aerobic tests. Use face masks.
Dyspnea	Avoid maximal tests.
Bone pain	Avoid tests that increase risk of fracture (e.g., high-impact/stress tests such as treadmill and 1 RM).
Severe nausea/vomiting	Avoid maximal tests.
Extreme fatigue/weakness	Begin tests at lower power output, use smaller incremental increases, and avoid maximal tests.
Surgical wounds/tenderness	Select a test that avoids pressure/trauma to the surgical site.
Poor functional status	Avoid exercise testing altogether if Karnofsky Performance Status (KPS) score ≤ 60%.

Modified from Courneya KS, Mackey JR, Jones LW. Coping with the cancer experience: can physical exercise help? *Physician Sports Med* In press, 2001.

1. Date of cancer diagnosis (day/month/year): ______________________.
2. Type of cancer (e.g., breast, colon): ______________________.
3. Stage of cancer at diagnosis (i.e., I, II, III, IV): ______________________.
4. Did/will treatment include surgery (please circle)? Yes No

If yes: (a) Type of surgery: ______________________.

(b) Date of surgery (day/month/year): ______________________.

(c) Limitations imposed by surgery: ______________________.

5. Did/will treatment include radiation therapy (please circle)? Yes No

If yes: (a) Beginning and end dates (day/month/year) ______________________.

(b) Treatment schedule: ______________________.

(c) Sites of the body irradiated: ______________________.

(d) Acute/chronic side effects: ______________________.

6. Did/will treatment include drugs/medications (please circle)? Yes No

If yes: (a) Beginning and end dates (day/month/year): ______________________.

(b) Treatment schedule: ______________________.

(c) Class/type of drugs: ______________________.

(d) Acute/chronic side effects: ______________________.

Anything else about your cancer diagnosis or treatment that we missed? Please add it here.

Figure 15.3. Sample cancer history questionnaire.

affecting coordination or balance (i.e., ataxia) will require stable tests (e.g., cycle ergometer) as opposed to less stable tests (e.g., treadmill test or step test). Finally, some cancer patients will experience severe sickness and fatigue at certain times during chemotherapy and/or radiation therapy and will not likely tolerate maximal testing. Consequently, submaximal tests should be used with lower initial power outputs and smaller incremental increases.

SPECIAL PRECAUTIONS AND CONSIDERATIONS FOR PRESCRIBING EXERCISE FOLLOWING CANCER DIAGNOSIS

To date, 26 of the 36 studies on exercise following cancer diagnosis have prescribed interventions. Unfortunately, all 26 studies have compared a single exercise prescription to a "no-exercise" condition and, thus, there is no direct evidence concerning the optimal type, frequency, duration, intensity, or progression of exercise for this population. Moreover, all studies have focused on either cancer survivors or cancer patients who had early-stage disease and good prognoses. No research to date has included cancer patients with extensive disease or who were receiving palliative care (i.e., curative treatment was discontinued). Clearly, determining the optimal exercise prescription for cancer survivors and patients at various stages of the disease trajectory is an important direction for future research. Nevertheless, some general guidelines can be drawn from the exercise and cancer literature (27–30), as well as from the literature on exercise in healthy older adults (23) and in older adults with other chronic diseases (24). A general summary of these guidelines is provided in Table 15.13.

With respect to exercise mode or type, the majority of studies on cancer patients and survivors have prescribed walking or cycle ergometer programs. Walking has been prescribed for the home-based programs and is the preferred and most common exercise in cancer patients. Its prescription takes advantage of this natural choice and also has direct implications for activities of daily living. Most studies prescribing cycle ergometry have been laboratory based, and the most likely reason for prescribing this type of exercise is the availability of the equipment and the particular cancer patients studied (i.e., breast). The advantages of cycle ergometry include a sitting position with leg exercises that minimize the effects of ataxia (i.e., coordination and balance problems) and limitations in upper-extremity movement. Other cancer patients, however, may not be able to perform cycle ergometry (e.g., following rectal or prostate surgery).

The key point when prescribing activity mode in cancer

Table 15.13. General Aerobic Exercise Recommendations for Otherwise Healthy Cancer Survivors and Early-Stage Cancer Patients

PARAMETER	GUIDELINE/COMMENT
Mode	Most exercises involving large muscle groups are appropriate, but walking and cycling are especially recommended. Key is to modify exercise mode based on acute/chronic treatment effects from surgery, chemotherapy, and/or radiation therapy.
Frequency	At least 3–5 times per week, but daily exercise may be optimal for deconditioned cancer patients performing lighter-intensity/shorter-duration exercises.
Intensity	Moderate intensity depending on current fitness level and severity of side effects from treatments. Guidelines include 50–75% VO_{2max} or $HR_{reserve}$, 60–80% HR_{max}, or 11–14 RPE. $HR_{reserve}$ is best guideline if HR_{max} is estimated rather than measured.[1]
Duration	At least 20–30 continuous minutes, but this goal may have to be achieved through multiple intermittent shorter bouts (e.g., 5–10 minutes) with rest intervals in deconditioned patients or those experiencing severe side effects of treatment.
Progression	Initial progression should be in frequency and duration, and only when these goals are met should intensity be increased. Progression should be slower and more gradual for deconditioned patients or those experiencing severe side effects of treatment.

[1]$HR_{reserve}$ = maximal heart rate (HR_{max}) minus standing resting heart rate (HR_{rest}). Multiply $HR_{reserve}$ by 0.60 and 0.80. Add each of these values to HR_{rest} to obtain the target heart rate range. HR_{max} can be estimated as 220 – age (years). Reprinted with permission from Courneya KS, Mackey JR, Jones LW. Coping with the cancer experience: can physical exercise help? *Physician Sports Med* In press, 2001.

patients and survivors is to take into account any acute or chronic physical impairments that may have resulted from medical treatment. Presently, there is no evidence that one type of aerobic exercise is superior to another for the general rehabilitation of cancer patients and survivors. As with all older, chronic disease populations, safety must be the primary issue (23, 24). Swimming should be avoided by those patients with nephrostomy tubes, nonindwelling central venous access catheters, and urinary bladder catheters. Swimming is not contraindicated for patients with continent urinary diversions, uterotomies, or colostomies, but patients should wait 8 weeks postsurgery and avoid open-ended pouch appliances. High-impact exercises or contact sports should be avoided in cancer patients or palliative care patients with primary or metastatic bone cancer. From a clinical perspective, it is probably safest to prescribe walking or cycle ergometry. Although evidence for the efficacy of weight training is only beginning to emerge, the optimal rehabilitation program for older persons with chronic diseases, including cancer, will likely combine aerobic and weight training (24).

The volume of exercise (i.e., frequency, intensity, and duration) prescribed for cancer patients has closely followed the American College of Sport Medicine's (26) guidelines. Most studies have prescribed moderate-intensity exercise performed 3–5 days per week for 20–30 minutes per session. This prescription appears appropriate for most cancer patients and survivors (28–31) but may need to be modified based on current medical treatments, comorbid conditions, and fitness level. Many cancer patients will not feel like exercising at certain times during their chemotherapy cycles. These so-called "down days" are different for each patient and may even vary from cycle to cycle. The key point is to build flexibility into the exercise prescription so that cancer patients are able to modify the frequency, intensity, or duration of their exercise depending on how well they tolerate treatment.

High-intensity exercise should be avoided during cancer treatment because of the potential immunosuppressive effects (32) but is not contraindicated in cancer survivors. From a duration perspective, it is likely that many cancer patients will not be able to tolerate 30 minutes of continuous exercise at the start of their treatments, especially if they were previously sedentary. Many researchers have used intermittent or interval training (i.e., alternating short bouts of exercise and rest) for patients during chemotherapy treatment (33, 34) or immediately following bone marrow transplantation (35, 36) as a way of accumulating the 30 minutes. This approach is recommended for older deconditioned persons with chronic diseases (23, 24) and may also be optimal for cancer patients who have been sedentary or who are receiving palliative care (30, 31).

It is also important to recognize that cancer patients exercise as much for psychological health as for physiological health (37–39). Consequently, it is important to take psychological benefits into account when prescribing exercise for cancer patients. As a general guideline, fitness professionals should prescribe exercise that is enjoyable, builds confidence, facilitates perceptions of control, develops new skills, incorporates social interaction, and takes place in an environment that engages the mind and spirit.

Although physical exercise may be an effective QOL intervention for many cancer patients and survivors, it is important to recognize that there may be mitigating factors that make it unwise or even dangerous for some cancer patients to exercise. Besides the general contraindications that are relevant for any older population (23), there are additional contraindications that apply to cancer patients (Table 15.14). This cautionary note is not meant to imply that cancer patients with such conditions could not benefit from an appropriately designed and supervised exercise program, but only that the risk/benefit ratio may be higher and close medical supervision may be required. Appropriately, early research took a cautious approach to exercise in cancer patients consistent with the physician's rule "First, do no harm." There are now reports in the literature of exercise tests/programs for more than 700 cancer patients undergoing various treatments with no reported major adverse events linked to exercise. In our own lab, we have tested

Table 15.14. Special Precautions/Considerations When Prescribing Exercise for Cancer Patients/Survivors

COMPLICATION	PRECAUTION
Complete blood counts	
Hemoglobin level <8.0 g/dL	Avoid activities that require significant oxygen transport (i.e., high intensity).
Absolute neutrophil count ≤0.5 × 10^9/L	Avoid activities that may increase risk of bacterial infection (e.g., swimming).
Platelet count <50 × 10^9/L	Avoid activities that increase risk of bleeding (e.g., contact sports or high-impact exercises).
Fever >38°C	May indicate systemic infection and should be investigated. Avoid high-intensity exercise.
Ataxia/dizziness/peripheral/sensory neuropathy	Avoid activities that require significant balance and coordination (e.g., treadmill).
Severe cachexia (loss of >35% of premorbid weight)	Loss of muscle mass usually limits exercise to mild intensity depending on degree of cachexia.
Dyspnea	Investigate etiology. Exercise to tolerance.
Bone pain	Avoid activities that increase risk of fracture (e.g., contact sports or high-impact exercises).
Severe nausea	Investigate etiology. Exercise to tolerance.
Extreme fatigue/muscle weakness	Exercise to tolerance.
Dehydration	Ensure adequate hydration.

Modified from Courneya KS, Mackey JR, Jones LW. Coping with the cancer experience: can physical exercise help? *Physician Sports Med* In press, 2001.

more than 300 cancer patients, many on chemotherapy, radiation therapy, or hormone therapy, and also have encountered no major adverse events. Consequently, there is evidence that exercise is safe and feasible for most cancer patients and survivors, if they are given an appropriate exercise prescription.

EXERCISE MOTIVATION AND ADHERENCE FOLLOWING CANCER DIAGNOSIS

The effectiveness of physical exercise as a QOL intervention following cancer diagnosis will depend to a large extent on the motivation and adherence of participants to such a program. Exercise adherence is a major challenge for health professionals regardless of the demographic profile of the group or the purpose of the exercise (40). The significant morbidity caused by cancer and its treatments makes it likely that exercise adherence is even more difficult following cancer diagnosis. Not surprisingly, research has documented that there is a significant decline in the volume of physical exercise performed by cancer patients that is not recovered even years after treatment is completed (41–43). Nevertheless, cancer patients are quite receptive to health-promotion programs, including exercise, and desire information soon after diagnosis (44).

Fortunately, research has started to examine the major incentives and barriers to exercise in cancer patients and survivors (37–39, 45–48). Although some general conclusions can be made, the specific incentives and barriers are likely to vary depending on the type of cancer, extent of disease, type of medical treatment, existence of other comorbid conditions, whether exercise is performed during or following treatment, and other personal factors (37–39). Table 15.15 lists the common incentives and barriers to exercise during treatment of breast and colorectal cancer, which are the only two cancers that have been examined at this time. These data may not generalize to other cancer patients. Not surprisingly, some of the incentives and barriers are unique to the cancer experience, whereas others are common to the general population. The key point for fitness professionals is that cancer patients will present with unique incentives and barriers to exercise that need to be understood and addressed. Creative exercise programming and adherence strategies for this population will be required.

SUMMARY AND CONCLUSION

More than 8 million Americans who have been through the cancer experience are alive today, and this number is increasing. Moreover, cancer treatments are intensive and cause significant morbidity that results in acute and chronic reductions in QOL. Good evidence exists for promoting physical exercise to enhance QOL in cancer patients and survivors. Currently, there are 36 studies that have addressed this issue using primarily intervention designs. Despite limitations in the studies, the evidence suggests that physical exercise will improve a broad array of QOL parameters both during and following cancer treatment. Exercise testing and prescription following cancer diagnosis must take into account the morbidity caused by treatments. Guidelines for exercise prescription in this population include moderate-intensity exercise performed 3–5 times per week for 30–60 minutes in an environment that optimizes psychosocial

Table 15.15. Common Exercise Incentives and Barriers for Cancer Patients

INCENTIVES	BARRIERS
Maintain a normal lifestyle	Bad weather
Recover from surgery and treatment	Fatigue/tiredness
Gain control over cancer and life	Concurrent medical condition
Cope with the stress of cancer and treatment	Lack of time/too busy
	Nausea
Get mind off cancer and treatment	Diarrhea
Feel better and improve well-being	Family responsibilities
General health benefits	Pain/soreness
Social aspects	Lack of support for exercise
Enjoy weather/outdoors	Lack of counseling for exercise

health. Finally, facilitating exercise adherence among cancer patients and survivors will require a good understanding of the unique incentives and barriers in this population and the application of creative behavior change strategies.

Acknowledgment: Dr. Courneya's research program is supported by the National Cancer Institute of Canada (NCIC) with funds from the Canadian Cancer Society (CCS) and the CCS/NCIC Sociobehavioral Cancer Research Network. Dr. Mackey's research program is supported by the NCIC and the Alberta Cancer Board.

References

1. Cancer Facts and Figures: 1999. Atlanta: American Cancer Society, 1999.
2. Harvard Report on Cancer Prevention. Volume I: causes of human cancer. *Cancer Causes Control* 1996;7:S3–S59.
3. Shephard RJ, Shek PN. Associations between physical activity and susceptibility to cancer. *Sports Med* 1998;26:293–315.
4. Colditz GA, Cannusico CC, Frazier AL. Physical activity and reduced risk of colon cancer: implications for prevention. *Cancer Causes Control* 1997;8:649–667.
5. Oliveria SA, Lee I-M. Is exercise beneficial in the prevention of prostate cancer? *Sports Med* 1997;23:271–278.
6. Lee I-M, Sesso HD, Paffenbarger RS. Physical activity and risk of lung cancer. *Int J Epidemiol* 1999;28:620–625.
7. Thune I, Lund E. The influence of physical activity on lung cancer risk. *Int J Cancer* 1997;70:57–62.
8. Friedenreich CM, Thune I, Brinton LA, et al. Epidemiologic issues related to the association between physical activity and breast cancer. *Cancer* 1998;83:600–610.
9. Kramer MM, Wells CL. Does physical activity reduce risk of estrogen-dependent cancer in women? *Med Sci Sports Exerc* 1996;28:322–334.
10. Harvard Report on Cancer Prevention. Volume II: prevention of human cancer. *Cancer Causes Control* 1997.
11. American Joint Committee on Cancer Staging Manual. AJCC Cancer Staging Manual. 5th Ed. Philadelphia: Lippincott-Raven Publishers, 1998.
12. Glanz K. Psychosocial impact of breast cancer. A critical review. *Ann Behav Med* 1992;14:202–212.
13. Grassi L, Rosti G, Albertazzi L, et al. Psychological stress symptoms before and after autologous bone marrow transplantation in patients with solid tumors. *Bone Marrow Transplant* 1996;17:843–847.
14. Spiegel D. Psychosocial aspects of breast cancer treatments. *Semin Oncol* 1997;24:S1–S36, S1–S47.
15. Ferrell BR. The impact of pain on quality of life: a decade of research. *Nurs Clin North Am* 1995;30:609–624.
16. Jenney ME, Faragher EB, Morris-Jones PH, et al. Lung function and exercise capacity in survivors of childhood leukemia. *Med Pediatr Oncol* 1995;24:222–230.
17. Morrow GR, Dobkin PL. Anticipatory nausea and vomiting in cancer patients undergoing chemotherapy treatment: prevalence, etiology, and behavioral interventions. *Clin Psychol Rev* 1988;8:517–556.
18. Pelletier C, Lapointe L, LeBlanc P. Effects of lung resection on pulmonary function and exercise capacity. *Thorax* 1990; 45:497–502.
19. Winningham MLNLM, Burke MB, Brophy L, et al. Fatigue and the cancer experience: the state of the knowledge. *Oncol Nurs Forum* 1994;21:23–36.
20. Fawzy FI, Fawzy NW. Psycho-social aspects of cancer: diagnosis and management of cancer. Menlo Park, CA: Addison-Welsey Publishing Co, 1995.
21. Meyer TJ, Mark MM. Effects of psychosocial interventions with adult cancer patients: a meta-analysis of randomised experiments. *Health Psychol* 1995;14:101–108.
22. Courneya KS, Friedenrich CM. Physical exercise and quality of life following cancer diagnosis. *Ann Behav Med* 1999;21: 171–179.
23. American College of Sports Medicine. Position stand on exercise and physical activity for older adults. *Med Sci Sports Exerc* 1998;30:992–1008.
24. Petrella RJ. Exercise for older patients with chronic disease. *Physician Sports Med* 1999;27:79–102.
25. Courneya KS, Mackey JR, Jones LW. Coping with the cancer experience: can physical exercise help? *Phys Sports Med* In press, 2001.
26. American College of Sports Medicine. Position stand on the recommended quantity and quality of exercise for developing and maintaining cardiorespiratory and muscular fitness, and flexibility in healthy adults. *Med Sci Sports Exerc* 1998; 30:975–991.
27. Hicks JE. Exercise for cancer patients. In: Basmajian JV, Wolf SL. Therapeutic Exercise. Baltimore: Williams & Wilkins, 1990.
28. Mock V. The benefits of exercise in women with breast cancer. In: Dow KH. Contemporary issues in breast cancer. Sudbury: Jones & Bartlett, 1996.
29. Winningham M, MacVicar M, Burke C. Exercise for cancer patients: guidelines and precautions. *Phys Sports Med* 1986; 14:125–134.
30. Winningham M. Walking programs for people with cancer: getting started. *Cancer Nurs* 1991;14:270–276.
31. Winningham M. Exercise and cancer. In: Goldberg L, Elliot DL. Exercise for prevention and treatment of illness. Philadelphia: Davis Company, 1994.
32. Shephard RJ, Shek PN. Exercise, immunity, and susceptibility to infection: a J-shaped relationship? *Phys Sports Med* 1999; 27:47–71.
33. MacVicar MG, Winningham ML. Response of cancer patients on chemotherapy to a supervised exercise program. *Cancer Bull* 1986;13:265–274.
34. Mock V, Burke MB, Sheehan P, et al. A nursing rehabilitation program for women with breast cancer receiving adjuvant chemotherapy. *Oncol Nurs Forum* 1994;21:899–907.
35. Dimeo FC, Stieglitz RD, Fischer-Novelli U, et al. Effects of physical activity on the fatigue and psychologic status of cancer patients during chemotherapy. *Cancer* 1999;85:2273–2277.
36. Dimeo F, Tilmann MHM, Bertz H, et al. Aerobic exercise in the rehabilitation of cancer patients after high dose chemotherapy and autologous peripheral stem cell transplantation. *Cancer* 1997;79:1717–1722.
37. Courneya KS, Friedenrich CM. Determinants of exercise during colorectal cancer treatment: an application of the theory of planned behavior. *Oncol Nurs Forum* 1997; 24: 1715–1732.
38. Courneya KS, Friedenrich CM. Utility of the theory of planned behavior for understanding exercise during breast cancer treatment. *Psychooncology* 1999;8:112–122.
39. Courneya KS, Friedenrich CM, Arthur K, et al. Understanding exercise motivation in colorectal cancer patients: a

prospective study using the theory of planned behavior. *Rehabil Psychol* 1999;44:68–84.

40. Robison JI, Rogers MA. Adherence to exercise programs: recommendations. *Sports Med* 1994;17:39–52.
41. Courneya KS, Freidenrich CM. Relationship between exercise during cancer treatment and current quality of life in survivors of breast cancer. *J Psychosoc Oncol* 1997;5:120–127.
42. Courneya KS, Friedenrich CM. Relationship between exercise pattern across the cancer experience and current quality of life in colorectal cancer survivors. *J Altern Complement Med* 1997;3:215–226.
43. Keats MR, Courneya KS, Danielson S, et al. Leisure-time physical activity and psychosocial well-being in adolescents after cancer diagnosis. *J Pediatr Oncol Nurs* 1999;16:180–188.
44. Demark-Wahnefried W, Peterson B, McBride C, et al. Current health behaviors and readiness to pursue life-style changes among men and women diagnosed with early stage prostate and breast carcinomas. *Cancer* 2000;88:674–684.
45. Cooper H. The role of physical activity in the recovery from breast cancer. *Melpomene J* 1995;14:18–20.
46. Courneya KS, Keats MR, Turner AR. Social cognitive determinants of physical exercise in cancer patients following high dose chemotherapy and autologous bone marrow transplantation. *Int J Behav Med* In press, 2001.
47. Leddy SK. Incentives and barriers to exercise in women with a history of breast cancer. *Oncol Nurs Forum* 1997;24: 885–890.
48. Nelson JP. Perceived health, self-esteem, health habits, and perceived benefits and barriers to exercise in women who have had and who have not experienced stage I breast cancer. *Oncol Nurs Forum* 1991;18:1191–1211.

CHAPTER **16**

Physical Activity, Diet, and the Immune System

Laurel T. Mackinnon

Recent interest in the effects of exercise on immune function arises from several directions (1). First, athletes and coaches believe that athletes experience frequent illness while training intensely. Recent epidemiological evidence supports this perception that athletes are susceptible to upper respiratory tract infection (URTI; e.g., common cold, "flu") during prolonged periods of intense training and after major competition. Second, regular physical activity is recommended in prevention of a number of diseases with significant lifestyle-associated factors such as cardiovascular disease, osteoporosis, or non-insulin-dependent diabetes. There is interest in whether regular exercise may also help prevent other diseases with lifestyle-associated risk factors such as cancer; epidemiological evidence suggests that physical activity lowers the risk of some types of cancer, in particular colon cancer and possibly reproductive system cancers. Third, exercise has become an integral part of treatment or management of several diseases with significant immune system involvement, such as HIV/AIDS, rheumatoid arthritis, and cancer. Although exercise is often an adjunct therapy to alleviate debilitating symptoms of disease or treatment (e.g., muscle wasting in HIV/AIDS, nausea in cancer patients), it is also useful to understand the immune system response to exercise in healthy individuals and patients. Such information is important to determine whether exercise has any positive or adverse effects on the disease process, and to best tailor exercise prescription for particular patients. Finally, it is well-known that there is close interaction between the neuroendocrine and immune systems, which share many messenger molecules and hormones. Physical and psychological stressors are known to influence immunity to disease. Studying the immune response to a quantifiable physical stress such as exercise leads to further understanding of the overall regulation of immune function.

RELEVANCE OF EXERCISE IMMUNOLOGY TO CLINICAL EXERCISE PHYSIOLOGY

The clinical exercise physiologist may encounter clients with diseases or conditions directly affecting immune function or in which treatment may influence the immune system. These clients may range from high-performance athletes to elderly clients to those with diseases involving the immune system. Athletes may seek advice about avoiding frequent illness during intense training and competition, or when to resume training after viral illness; healthy active individuals may also seek advice about exercising during mild illness (e.g., common cold or flu). The clinical exercise physiologist may be involved in exercise testing or programming of patients for whom the disease and/or treatment(s) affect or involve the immune system. For example, in the cancer patient, radiation and chemotherapy can significantly reduce immune cell number and function, as well as blood electrolyte levels (discussed in the preceding chapter). Transplant patients will be taking immunosuppressive drugs to prevent rejection of transplanted tissue; these drugs may influence immune function (see Table 16.1). As described in Chapters 17 and 18 of this section, HIV infection and chronic fatigue syndrome involve immune system dysfunction. It can be questioned, for example, whether intense exercise is to be recommended for HIV-positive individuals, based on observations that intense exercise may suppress immune function. Individuals with autoimmune diseases, such as myasthenia gravis or multiple sclerosis, may be taking drugs with immunosuppressive activity. When selecting appropriate exercise test protocols and exercise prescription, the clinical exercise physiologist will need to consider the effects of these diseases and/or treatments on exercise capacity and, in turn, the effects of exercise on immunity in these patients.

OVERVIEW OF THE IMMUNE SYSTEM

The immune system most likely evolved as a means of self-identification, as a way for the body to distinguish its own cells from those originating outside the body. In theory, the immune system is capable of defending the host against infinite environmental challenges, including foreign cells, proteins, and microorganisms such as viruses, bacteria, or parasites. To accomplish such a formidable task, the

Table 16.1 Diseases, Conditions, and Medications That May Alter Immune Function

DISEASES	CONDITIONS	MEDICATIONS OR TREATMENT
Some bacterial infections (e.g., staphylococcus)	*Malnutrition*	*Corticosteroids*
Some viral infections (e.g., measles virus, HIV)	*Physical stress* (e.g., intense exercise)	*Cytotoxic drugs*
Anemia	*Psychological stress* (e.g., bereavement)	*Radiation therapy*
Inherited *immunodeficiency*	*Trauma, burns*	*Surgery*
Acquired *immunodeficiency* syndrome (AIDS)		Tissue/organ transplantation
Autoimmune diseases (e.g., insulin-dependent diabetes, rheumatoid arthritis)		

Compiled from Janeway CA, Travers P, Walport M, et al. *Immunobiology: the immune system in health and disease*. 4th ed. New York: Elsevier Science Ltd., 1999. Items in *italics* indicate that immunosuppression may result.

immune system has evolved as a complex system that incorporates complementary and overlapping functions.

One of the most important functions (although not the only one) of the immune system is to prevent or combat infection by pathogenic microorganisms. The immune system works at several levels to prevent infection: physical barriers such as the skin and mucous membranes, and chemical barriers provided by substances contained in saliva, tears, and other body fluids, maintain the body's structural integrity to prevent entry by most pathogens. If these defenses are breached, several different cellular mechanisms may be activated to counteract the pathogen: cells engulf and degrade the pathogen (a process called phagocytosis), other cells directly kill the pathogen or infected cells (cytotoxicity), yet other cells produce antibodies that may neutralize the foreign agent, and many types of cells produce soluble factors that may assist in killing the pathogen. In most instances, this combined effort is sufficient to eventually overcome infection, although there are times when the body's response is ineffective or inappropriate.

General Summary of the Immune Response

A simplified scheme of the immune response to a pathogen, such as a virus or bacterium, is depicted in Figure 16.1. The immune response is initiated when a pathogen penetrates the chemical and physical barriers, and is engulfed by phagocytic cells, which degrade the foreign proteins (called antigens). Once degraded, parts of these antigens are displayed on the phagocyte's surface, along with special self-recognition proteins (termed major histocompatibility complex or MHC proteins). Upon presentation of the foreign antigens, specialized immune cells called T lymphocytes are activated to produce factors that stimulate other immune cells to divide and produce substances to further combat the pathogen: B lymphocytes produce antibody to the foreign proteins, other T lymphocytes may directly kill the foreign cells or infected cells, natural killer (NK) cells may directly kill infected cells, and various cells produce soluble factors that assist in killing or neutralizing the pathogen. During the initial encounter with the pathogen, spe-

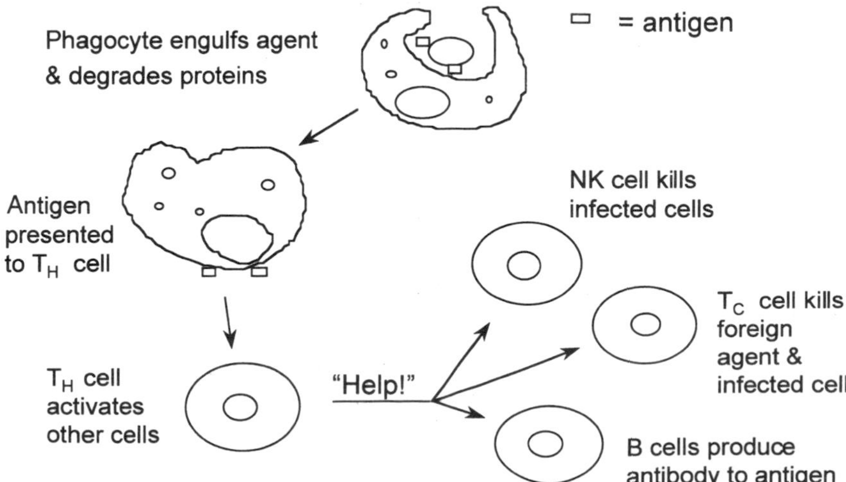

Figure 16.1. General scheme of the immune response. T_H = helper (CD4) T lymphocyte; T_C = cytotoxic (CD8) lymphocyte; NK = natural killer cell. Reproduced with permission from Mackinnon LT. *Advances in exercise immunology*. Champaign, IL: Human Kinetics, 1999.

cial "memory" T and B cells are produced; these respond rapidly to subsequent infection by the same agent (the basis of immunization). Obviously, such a complex response requires close communication between the various effectors of immune function (immune cells and messenger molecules).

Cells of the Immune System

Leukocytes, called white blood cells in the blood, are immune cells produced by several lymphoid tissues. Leukocytes originate from a common stem cell found in the bone marrow, and then differentiate into specific immune cells in various lymphoid tissues. Immature and differentiated cells migrate throughout the body via the blood and lymph circulations. At any given time, only about 1–2% of the body's total leukocytes are found in the blood. This point should be remembered when reviewing the literature on exercise and human immune function; because of obvious ethical limitations in research on humans, cells can be obtained only from the peripheral blood circulation.

Table 16.2 presents a summary of the major types of leukocytes found in the blood. Leukocyte subsets are identified by a unique combination of proteins expressed on the cell surface. Because proteins are antigenic (i.e., an antibody can be raised to them), these cell-surface proteins can be identified and quantified using commercially available monoclonal antibodies. By international consensus, these cell-surface proteins and the cells they identify are now designated by the prefix CD, which stands for clusters of differentiation. For example, helper/inflammatory T lymphocytes are defined as CD3+CD4+ cells, that is, they are identified by the CD3 and CD4 antigens expressed on the cell surface. Table 16.3 summarizes the major CD antigens used in the exercise immunology literature.

Table 16.3 CD Antigens Used to Identify Leukocytes in the Exercise Immunology Literature

CD Antigen	Predominant Cell Type Identified
CD2	T, NK cells
CD3	T cells
CD4	Helper, inflammatory T cells
CD8	Cytotoxic T cells
CD14	Monocytes
CD16	NK cells, neutrophils
CD19	B cells
CD25	Activated T, B, NK cells
CD45	Leukocytes
CD45RO	Activated T, B cells
CD45RA	Naïve T, B cells
CD56	NK cells
CD69	Activated T, B, NK cells
CD122	NK cells, subset of T cells

Compiled from Janeway CA, Travers P, Walport M, et al. *Immunobiology: the immune system in health and disease*. 4th ed. New York: Elsevier Science Ltd., 1999.

Enumeration of leukocyte and various subset concentrations in the blood is important to clinical diagnosis and monitoring of treatment for many conditions. Cell counts may be disturbed by a number of factors, including trauma (e.g., burns, surgery), medication (e.g., corticosteroids), bacterial infection, hematological disorders (e.g., leukemia, infectious mononucleosis), immune disorders (e.g., HIV infection), treatment (e.g., chemotherapy), inflammation, and allergy (see Table 16.1). Monitoring leukocyte and subset numbers may also be useful in assessing the patient's response to treatment (e.g., chemotherapy) or prognosis in immune disorders (e.g., HIV infection). Moreover, acute or chronic stress may also influence circulating immune cell number. As will be discussed later in this chapter, circulating leukocyte number and the ratio of various subsets are dramatically altered during and for up to several hours after intense exercise.

Leukocyte Subsets

Polymorphonuclear leukocytes, or granulocytes, are large (10–20 μm) leukocytes containing granules that can be seen with a light microscope. These cells are among the first to react to infection or inflammation. Neutrophils, the most prevalent granulocyte, are phagocytic cells important to early defense against bacterial and viral infection. Neutrophils live only a few days, but are quickly mobilized to

Table 16.2 Description and Normal Values for Major Types of Circulating Leukocytes

Cell Type	Percentage of Cells	Reference Norm	Major Function(s)
Granulocyte, mainly neutrophil	60–70%	3.0–6.0	Phagocytosis, chemotactic factors
Monocyte	10–15%	0.15–0.60	Phagocytosis, antigen presentation, cytokine secretion
Lymphocyte	20–25%	1.0–2.5	Antigen recognition, antibody production, cytokine secretion, memory
T cell	60–75% of lymphocytes	1.0–2.5	Antibody production, memory
CD4 T cell	60–70% of T cells	0.5–1.6	
CD8 T cell	30–40% of T cells	0.3–0.9	
B cell	5–15% of lymphocytes	0.3	
Natural killer cell	10–20%	0.1–0.5	Cytotoxicity, cytokine secretion

Percentage of cells = percentage of total circulating leukocytes unless otherwise stated. Cell concentrations are expressed as number of cells $\times 10^9$ per liter of blood.
Compiled from Janeway CA, Travers P, Walport M, et al. *Immunobiology: the immune system in health and disease*. 4th ed. New York: Elsevier Science Ltd., 1999.

sites of infection or inflammation (e.g., damaged tissues). It is thought that neutrophils may play a role in degradation and repair of tissues such as skeletal muscle injured during exercise. Monocytes (in blood) and macrophages (monocytes localized to tissues) are relatively large phagocytic cells crucial to the early response to infection. Monocyte/macrophage activities include ingesting and killing microorganisms (phagocytosis), presenting antigen to and thus stimulating T cells, and secreting cytokines (regulatory molecules) that further stimulate activity of other immune cells.

Lymphocytes are comprised of several subsets with specialized functions. B lymphocytes (or B cells) are small cells (6–10 μm) that produce antibody. Memory B cells rapidly produce antibody in response to previously encountered pathogens. T cells (CD3+) are small (6–10 μm) cells involved in initiating and modulating virtually all aspects of the immune response. T-cell functions include stimulating B cells to differentiate and produce antibody; directly killing some pathogens, tumor cells, and virally infected cells; and secreting cytokines that regulate the activity of many other types of immune cells. There are two main subsets of T cells, called helper/inflammatory T cells and cytotoxic T cells (identified by the CD4 and CD8 antigens, respectively). CD4 T cells are central to regulation of immune function, as shown by the devastating effect on immunity by HIV-infection, which destroys these cells. CD4 helper cells stimulate B cells to produce antibody; CD4 inflammatory T cells stimulate monocyte/macrophage antibacterial activity. Both types of CD4 cells produce several types of cytokines. CD8 T cells help combat viral infection by killing infected cells.

NK cells may represent a distinct cell lineage. NK cells are defined as non–T cells (CD3-) that express NK-specific markers CD16 and CD56. Because NK cells are capable of recognizing and killing certain tumor and virally infected cells, it is believed that these cells function in the early defense against tumor growth and viral infection. NK cells also release some cytokines.

Soluble Factors

Soluble factors are found in blood and other body fluids, and act as mediators of a wide range of immune functions. These factors may act directly, for example by killing or neutralizing pathogens, or indirectly, as chemical messengers between different types of immune cells. The major classes of soluble factors relevant to exercise immunology include cytokines, immunoglobulin and antibody, acute-phase proteins, and complement; their major functions are listed in Table 16.4.

Cytokines

Cytokines are polypeptide messenger molecules central to cellular communication and immune regulation. Primarily growth and regulatory factors, cytokines are produced mainly but not exclusively by immune cells. There are also naturally occurring factors that inhibit and thus help regulate cytokine activity. The major types of cytokines examined in the exercise immunology literature are the interleukins (IL-), interferons (IFN-), and tumor-necrosis factor (TNF). Interleukins, numbered IL-1 through IL-18 (at present) (2), are unrelated cytokines produced primarily by T cells, monocytes, and NK cells and are mainly involved in regulation of lymphocyte activation and proliferation. Interferons (α, β, and γ), produced mainly by T and NK cells, exert antiviral activity and stimulate NK cell and macrophage cytotoxicity. TNFα, produced by macrophages, NK

Table 16.4 Sources and Major Functions of Soluble Factors

Factor	Produced by	Major Functions
Immunoglobulin and Antibody	Resting and mature B lymphocytes	Antigen binding Complement activation Inhibition of pathogen entry into the body Neutralization of bacterial toxins Passive immunity in newborn
Cytokines	Various leukocytes and other cells (e.g., fibroblasts, endothelial cells)	Immune system regulation Cellular communication Activation of immune cells to proliferate and differentiate Antiviral activity Cytotoxicity (cell killing) Chemotaxis (attracting cells to sites of inflammation/infection)
Acute Phase Proteins	Liver	Binding to bacteria Binding serum metals, thus limiting bacterial growth Complement activation Stimulation of phagocytosis Chemotaxis
Complement		Direct killing of bacteria Stimulation of phagocytosis Chemotaxis

Compiled from Janeway CA, Travers P, Walport M, et al. *Immunobiology: the immune system in health and disease*. 4th ed. New York: Elsevier Science Ltd., 1999.

cells, and T cells, is an important mediator of defense against viral infection and tumor growth.

Several cytokines, in particular IL-1, IL-6, and TNFα, act as mediators of inflammation. Besides involvement in general inflammation such as in soft-tissue or joint injury, these inflammatory cytokines are also linked to atherosclerosis. It is thought that leukocytes localized to atherosclerotic plaques may release inflammatory cytokines, which act as mediators of damage to the arterial wall. Some anti-inflammatory cytokines, such as IL-4 and IL-10, may be protective against atherosclerosis. As discussed later in this chapter, prolonged weight-bearing exercise induces release of some of these cytokines, which may reflect inflammation within damaged skeletal muscle.

Immunoglobulin and Antibody

Immunoglobulin (Ig) is a class of glycoproteins produced by resting and mature B lymphocytes. Ig is expressed on the B-cell surface and is also found in serum and other body fluids such as tears and saliva. Because of the unique structure of the Ig molecule, it is able to bind specifically to various foreign proteins or antigens. Antibody is an Ig molecule that binds specifically to a particular antigen; each antibody binds specifically to only one type of antigen. All antibodies are Ig molecules, but not all Igs exhibit antibody activity. Antigen-antibody binding initiates further immune responses by other lymphocytes and cytotoxic cells. Antibody acts in many ways, both directly to inhibit pathogens from entering the body and indirectly by stimulating phagocytosis and cytotoxicity by other immune cells.

There are five classes of Ig: IgA, IgD, IgG, IgE, and IgM, each with different complex structures and functions. IgG is most prevalent in serum, while IgA is the major Ig in mucosal fluids such as saliva and tears. IgA in mucosal secretions plays a major role in preventing infection by viruses that gain entry via mucosal surfaces of the mouth, eye, nose, and respiratory, genitourinary, and gastrointestinal tracts.

Acute Phase Proteins

Acute phase proteins (APPs) are unrelated glycoproteins released from the liver in response to infection or inflammation. Pro-inflammatory cytokines IL-1, IL-6, and TNFα stimulate release of APPs. The concentration of APPs increases in the blood following trauma such as bacterial infection, surgery, and myocardial infarction, and during chronic inflammation. Some APPs stimulate immunity by binding to bacteria and activating complement and phagocytosis. Others lower serum iron and copper concentrations, inhibiting bacterial growth by limiting availability of these metals. Still other APPs act to inhibit protein degradation in skeletal muscle and to neutralize free radicals.

Complement

Complement represents a complex group of diverse plasma proteins produced in response to infection and inflammation. Complement acts in three main ways: by recruiting immune cells to the site of infection or inflammation, by binding to pathogens and thus stimulating phagocytes to kill the pathogens, and by directly killing pathogens such as bacteria.

METHODS TO ASSESS OR QUANTIFY IMMUNE FUNCTION

Because of the immune system's complexity, there is no single measure of "immune function," and many different types of assays are used to assess particular immune parameters. Only those most commonly used in the exercise immunology literature will be briefly described in this chapter. Assays can be simplistically classified as those quantifying the concentration of a particular factor (e.g., antibody concentration, cell number in the blood) and those measuring the functional status of particular cells (e.g., neutrophil antibacterial activity, lymphocyte proliferation). In humans, most functional assays are performed in vitro, because of ethical issues and to specifically measure one parameter independent of the effects of others. Obviously, there are some limitations to extension of data from in vitro experiments to in vivo function.

Measuring Cell Counts

In the human, leukocytes can be isolated from peripheral blood using density centrifugation. Whole blood is layered over a gradient and centrifuged, which separates the peripheral blood mononuclear cells (PBMCs) from red blood cells and granulocytes. PBMCs include lymphocytes and monocytes. Lymphocytes can be further separated from monocytes by incubating PBMCs in plastic culture dishes; monocytes adhere to the plastic, and the lymphocytes are removed in the culture medium. Cells obtained from peripheral blood may then be used to quantify cell number or function (discussed further below). Leukocytes may also be isolated from sites of inflammation by aspiration (e.g., synovial fluid in rheumatoid arthritis) or, less frequently, by biopsy or surgery. (Animal models are not limited by mode of cell sampling as in the human, and cells may be obtained from various lymphoid tissues.)

Automated electronic cell counters are used to assess blood leukocyte and subset number. In the electronic counter, a stream of blood is passed through a narrow orifice one cell at a time, triggering an electronic signal for each cell. A leukocyte "differential" count gives the number of total leukocytes, as well as neutrophils, lymphocytes, monocytes, basophils, and eosinophils per volume of blood; clinical reference norms for these cell concentrations in blood are given in Table 16.2.

Lymphocyte subsets can be identified and quantified using flow cytometry. In this technique, fluorescently labeled antibodies to specific cell-surface markers (e.g., CD antigens discussed above) are incubated with whole blood or isolated cells, allowing the labeled antibody to bind specifically to the cells via cell-surface proteins. The sample is then passed in front of a special laser that excites the fluorescent dye. The signals are sent to a computer, which calculates a number of variables, cell subset number and proportion relative to other subsets (based on the number of positively stained cells), cell size (based on how cells scatter light), and the density of cell-surface marker per cell (based on the intensity of fluorescent dye bound to the cells). Recent advances allow the detection of up to four different dyes simultaneously; this permits recognition of cell subsets identified by multiple surface markers.

Measuring the Concentration of Soluble Factors

Techniques to quantify concentration of soluble factors can be broadly divided into those directly assessing concentration and those indirectly assessing concentration via the biological activity of the substance of interest (called a bioassay). Immunoassays are widely used to measure the concentration of immunoglobulin, cytokines, hormones, peptides, and many other proteins. Two commonly used immunoassays are the radioimmunoassay (RIA) and enzyme-linked immunosorbent assay (ELISA). In these assays, the molecule of interest (antigen) is incubated with an antibody directed against it. The antibody binds the antigen in a specific and quantifiable way. In the RIA, a radioactively (^{125}I) labeled antibody is used, and the amount of labeled antibody is detected by counting radioactivity. In the ELISA, an enzyme is attached to the antibody, which develops color when incubated with an appropriate substrate. The amount of radioactivity (RIA) or color developed (ELISA) is directly proportional to the amount of antibody bound to antigen, which in turn is proportional to the concentration of the molecule of interest.

Since the introduction of specific and sensitive immunoassays, bioassays are used less frequently to assess the concentration of soluble factors. In a bioassay, concentration of the substance of interest is assessed in vitro by incubating that substance with a cell line that requires it for cell growth. Cell growth is then quantified, and the amount or activity of the substance of interest is inferred from the amount of cell growth. The sensitivity of a bioassay may be limited by other growth or inhibitory factors in the sample, which may alternately stimulate or inhibit cell growth.

Cytokine gene expression may be assessed by a new technique called reverse transcriptase-polymerase chain reaction (RT-PCR). Because cytokines may act only locally and are rapidly removed from the circulation, measuring levels in blood may not give an accurate measure of cytokine production. In RT-PCR, messenger RNA (mRNA) is isolated from cells of interest (e.g., lymphocytes, skeletal muscle) and reverse transcription used to make multiple copies of complementary DNA (cDNA) to the mRNA. The cDNA is then amplified chemically and quantified. The amount of cDNA is proportional to the amount of mRNA, which gives a measure of cytokine gene expression. This technique has been applied in studies trying to determine the source of cytokines appearing after exercise (discussed below).

Measuring Lymphocyte Proliferation

Once activated by an encounter with a pathogen, the lymphocyte proliferates to produce more cells to combat the infection. This process can be simulated in vitro by incubating whole blood or isolated lymphocytes with substances that induce proliferation. These substances are called "mitogens" because of their ability to induce mitosis in lymphocytes. When studying human cells, the most commonly used mitogens include phytohemagglutinin (PHA) and concanavalin A (conA), which stimulate T-cell proliferation, and pokeweed mitogen (PWM), which stimulates T-cell–dependent B-cell proliferation. After incubation with the mitogen for a given period of time, DNA synthesis is measured either via assessing uptake of radioactively labeled thymidine (used to synthesize DNA) or, more recently, via dyes that bind to newly synthesized DNA that can be detected using colorimetry or fluorometry.

Because lymphocytes are first activated before proliferating, cell proliferation may also be assessed by expression of activation markers on the cell surface. Monoclonal antibodies to these activation markers are incubated with whole blood or lymphocytes and flow cytometry used to quantify the number of cells expressing the activation marker.

Measuring Cell-Mediated Cytotoxic Activity

NK cells and cytotoxic T cells can directly kill certain tumor and virally infected cells. Cytotoxic (killing) activity of these cells can be assessed by two general methods. In the standard ^{51}Cr release assay, target cells (those killed by the cytotoxic cells, usually a tumor cell line) are first incubated with radioactively labeled chromium, which is taken up and retained by the target cells. The labeled target cells are then incubated with whole blood or isolated effector cells, during which time the effector cells of interest (either NK or cytotoxic T cells) will kill a number of target cells. Upon death of target cells, ^{51}Cr is released into the fluid medium. Radioactivity in the fluid medium is proportional to the number of target cells killed, which gives a measure of cytotoxic activity.

Cytotoxicity can also be assessed using flow cytometry. Target and effector cells are incubated together, and dead target cells are identified with a fluorescently labeled dye that distinguishes dead from live target cells.

Measuring Monocyte and Neutrophil Function

Monocytes and neutrophils exhibit a wide range of functions, including phagocytosis and killing of pathogens such as bacteria and viruses. Phagocytosis is a complex process involving several steps, each of which may be assessed independently. The ability of phagocytes to ingest microbes can be assessed in vitro by incubating cells with fluorescently labeled beads (e.g., latex) and then quantifying the amount of internalized beads histologically or with flow cytometry. Once activated or "primed" to kill, phagocytes exhibit an oxidative burst that can be quantified in vitro as production of reactive oxygen or nitrogen species (which are toxic to microbes), or as an increase in respiratory rate. Neutrophil activation can also be assessed by the appearance of proteolytic enzymes released into the incubation medium, such as myeloperoxidase, or by expression of certain cell-surface markers, such as the complement receptor CD11b.

Using In Vivo Assays in Humans

Whereas in vitro assays are important in studying particular immune parameters, there is sometimes a limited ability to extrapolate these data to understanding immune competence in the intact body. On the other hand, ethical considerations limit the types of in vivo tests that may be applied in humans. In vivo tests of immune function commonly used in humans involve exposure to a particular antigen and then measuring the response. An antigen may be injected (as in immunization) and the amount of antibody produced to that antigen measured in the blood. Alternatively, the antigen may be applied to the skin (as in the tuberculin test), and the size of the skin reaction gives an indication of T-cell function; this is called delayed-type hypersensitivity.

EXERCISE AND THE IMMUNE SYSTEM

The exercise immunology literature has focused on the effects of exercise on illness, as well as the responses of key components of immunity, such as cell number and function, levels of soluble mediators, and other factors that may influence immunity. As mentioned above, the immune system is very complex, and a physical stress such as exercise may influence immune function at any number of points. Moreover, as will be discussed below, responses may vary between different immune parameters, between acute and chronic exercise, and between trained and untrained individuals.

Effects of Exercise on Risk for Upper Respiratory Tract Infection

Athletes and coaches have long perceived an association between intense exercise and increased risk of upper respiratory tract infection (URTI; e.g., common cold, sore throat). This perception is supported by several epidemiological studies on distance runners, which show increased risk of URTI during the 2 weeks after major competition such as a marathon or ultramarathon (3–5). As many as 50–70% of runners may experience URTI symptoms after a race (3–5). Moreover, the risk of URTI has been related to competition pace (4) and average training distance (3, 6).

There appears to be a threshold of exercise below which risk of URTI does not increase. For example, the risk of URTI was not elevated in those participating in "fun runs" of 21 km or less (7). Similarly, moderate exercise training (e.g., brisk walking) does not increase, and may even reduce, the incidence of URTI (8). Based on these data, a "J-curve" model has been proposed that suggests that the risk of URTI is reduced by regular moderate exercise, but increased by intense exercise (9). It is not known whether this relationship holds true for other types of athletes, such as sprinters or power athletes, or for the general public. The minimum and optimum amounts of exercise needed to enhance resistance to infectious illness are also currently unknown. From the public health and clinical perspective, however, there is no evidence that, at least in healthy individuals, resistance to infectious illness is compromised by regular moderate exercise as recommended for long-term health.

Aerobic exercise capacity and muscular strength decline during febrile viral illness, suggesting that physical performance may be temporarily impaired during illness with fever (10). The athlete is not advised to continue intense exercise training during the active stages of viral infection, since this has been associated with an increased risk of developing viral myocarditis (10) or chronic fatigue syndrome (11). On the other hand, moderate exercise training (e.g., 40 min at 70% heart rate reserve, 3 sessions per week) did not influence the severity of mild, experimentally induced URTI (12). Athletes are advised to follow the "above the neck" rule—if illness is mild, without fever, and affects only the mouth, nose, and throat, as in a common cold, then exercise training is permitted, perhaps with slightly reduced intensity or duration. In contrast, systemic illness (e.g., swollen glands) or illness involving fever, should be evaluated by a physician before any intense exercise is performed. All individuals should resume normal physical activity patterns gradually after illness.

Effects of Exercise on Peripheral Blood Leukocyte Number

Acute exercise causes dramatic changes in the number and relative distribution of circulating leukocyte subsets (reviewed by 1). Changes in cell number are primarily mediated by stress hormones, such as cortisol and epinephrine. The magnitude of change is a function of exercise intensity, duration, and mode, and the time of blood sampling after exercise (Table 16.5).

Leukocytes, neutrophils, monocytes, and lymphocytes all increase in concentration during and immediately after exercise. These increases are larger and persist for longer after intense or prolonged compared with moderate exercise. Exercise with an eccentric bias (e.g., downhill running) causes greater perturbation of cell number compared with level running, even at the same metabolic cost (13), suggesting some form of communication between skeletal muscle and immune cells.

Leukocyte and neutrophil numbers may increase threefold immediately after prolonged exercise and continue to increase further for several hours. After brief, intense exer-

Table 16.5 Summary of Acute and Chronic Exercise Responses of Selected Immune Parameters

	Acute Response		
Immune Parameter	*Postexercise*	*1–5 hr postexercise*	Chronic Response
Cell number			
Leukocyte	↑↑	↑↑	— or may ↓
Neutrophil	↑↑	↑↑	—
Lymphocyte	↑	↓	—
NK cell	↑↑	↓	— or may ↑
Cell function			
Neutrophil activity	↑	↑	↓
NK-cell cytotoxic activity	↑	↓	— or may ↑
Lymphocyte proliferation	↓	↓	—

Postexercise = immediately postexercise, 1–5 hr postexercise = 1–5 hr postexercise. Acute response = after intense prolonged exercise, Chronic response = resting values in athletes compared with nonathletes or clinical norms. ↑ = increase; ↑↑ = large increase, more than double resting values; ↓ = decrease; — = no change.
Compiled from various sources.

cise, however, there is a biphasic response, in that cell number returns to resting levels by 1 hour postexercise, but then increases again 1–3 hours postexercise. Lymphocytes also exhibit a biphasic response, but of a different pattern. Lymphocyte number increases during and immediately after exercise, but declines and remains below baseline levels between 1 and 5 hours postexercise. T-, B-, and NK-cell counts follow a similar pattern. Normal cell counts are generally restored by 24 hours postexercise.

The postexercise increase in the number of leukocytes does not result from synthesis of new cells, but rather reflects redistribution of cells between the circulation and other sites (recall that, at any given time, only 1–2% of all immune cells are in the circulation). Increased cardiac output, release of cells from marginated pools in underperfused tissues (e.g., lungs), and the spleen are all sources of cells appearing in the circulation after exercise. It is not currently known where cells go after leaving the circulation, when normal blood levels are restored during recovery after exercise.

There appear to be few chronic effects of exercise training on circulating leukocyte number, since athletes generally exhibit clinically normal cell counts at rest. There are two possible exceptions: total leukocyte and NK-cell numbers may decline during prolonged periods of very intense exercise training. Leukocyte number was reported to decrease to clinically low levels after 4 weeks of intensified training in distance runners (14). NK-cell number declined after 7 months of swim training in elite swimmers despite no changes in other cell counts (15). It is not known whether these changes reflect increased cell turnover or migration of cells out of the circulation, nor whether there are any long-term implications.

Clinicians who treat physically active patients should be aware of both acute and chronic exercise-induced changes in circulating immune cell counts, since these data are often used in diagnosis or to make decisions about treatment. If an accurate leukocyte differential count is needed for clinical purposes, physically active patients should refrain from exercise for at least 24 hours before blood sampling.

Effects of Exercise on Leukocyte Function

Despite only transient perturbation in circulating leukocyte number, there is good evidence to show both acute and chronic effects of exercise on immune cell function. Neutrophil and monocyte functions, NK-cell cytotoxicity, and lymphocyte proliferation are all affected by intense exercise.

Effects of Exercise on NK-Cell Function

NK-cell cytotoxic activity (NKCA) increases during and immediately after moderate and intense exercise; the magnitude of change is directly related to exercise intensity and duration. NKCA returns to resting levels soon after moderate exercise, but declines below baseline values between 1 and 6 hours after intense prolonged exercise. The mechanisms responsible for these changes in NKCA during and after exercise are complex. The increase in NKCA immediately after exercise appears to result from the rise in NK-cell number in the blood. The reasons for the delayed decrease in NKCA have been debated (reviewed by 1), and it is beyond the scope of this chapter to fully discuss this issue. Briefly, it appears that this delayed decline in NKCA reflects both decreased number and suppressed killing activity of NK cells in the blood. Given the role of NK cells in defense against viruses, it has been suggested that prolonged suppression of NKCA after intense exercise may provide an "open window," during which the athlete may be susceptible to infection (16).

Despite this apparent suppression of NKCA acutely after intense exercise, NKCA does not appear to be adversely affected by intense exercise training over the long term, since resting NKCA is normal in athletes. Moderate exercise training may enhance NKCA. For example, resting NKCA was higher in moderately trained distance runners compared with matched nonrunners (17). In an animal model, exercised mice exhibited higher NKCA and less tumor retention compared with sedentary controls (18).

Effects of Exercise on Neutrophil Function

Acute intense, but not moderate, exercise stimulates several aspects of neutrophil function, including migration, activation, degranulation, phagocytosis, and antimicrobial activity. Stimulation may last for several hours after prolonged exercise. Recruitment of younger, more active neutrophils into the circulation is thought to be responsible. While enhanced neutrophil activity may boost immunity to bacteria and viruses, it is believed that frequent activation may also elicit adverse effects in athletes (19). After exercise, neutrophils have been shown to infiltrate tissues such as nasal mucosa and skeletal muscle

(20), and this has been suggested to cause local inflammation by release of reactive oxygen species and chemotactic factors, which attract inflammatory cells (21).

Although neutrophil function is stimulated by acute exercise, chronic exercise appears to downregulate this response. Athletes undergoing intense training exhibit lower resting and postexercise neutrophil function compared with nonathletes and their own values obtained during moderate training (22, 23). It has been suggested that this apparent downregulation of neutrophil function may be protective by limiting neutrophil involvement in inflammation associated with daily intense exercise (1, 19). It is possible that mild downregulation of an important immune function such as neutrophil activity may be an adaptive compromise to limit chronic inflammation (1). Whether such downregulation of neutrophil activity increases susceptibility to illness is not known. One report found no association between depressed neutrophil function and the incidence of URTI in elite swimmers (23). Moderate exercise training appears to have little effect on neutrophil function.

Effects of Exercise on Lymphocyte Proliferation

Lymphocyte proliferation is sensitive to exercise intensity and duration. Acute moderate exercise has little or a slight stimulating effect on proliferation. In contrast, intense exercise appears to suppress proliferation for up to 3 hours after exercise. The mechanism responsible is not fully known and is likely to be complex. Some, but not all, of the suppression can be attributed to increased catecholamine levels and fewer lymphocytes in the blood during recovery after exercise (24). Exercise training, regardless of intensity, has little effect on resting lymphocyte proliferation, indicating that any effects are transitory, and perhaps of limited clinical significance. Exercise training has been associated with increased expression of lymphocyte activation markers, suggesting that chronic exercise may enhance the ability of these cells to respond to immune challenges.

Effects of Exercise on Soluble Mediators of Immune Function

The exercise immunology literature has explored the effects of exercise on diverse soluble mediators of immune function, focusing mainly on cytokines, immunoglobulin, and antibody, and to a lesser extent on complement and acute phase proteins.

Effects of Exercise on Cytokines

Intense, prolonged exercise induces release of several cytokines. Exercise increases concentration of inflammatory cytokines, such as interleukin-1 (IL-1), IL-6, and tumor-necrosis factor-α (TNFα), and those with antiviral activity, such as interferon-α/β (IFN-α/β) (25). Cytokines are generally released only after prolonged load-bearing exercise (e.g., distance running) or after exercise requiring a large eccentric component (e.g., downhill running), suggesting that release is related to tissue damage. The time course of cytokine release differs between cytokines. Early release of inflammatory cytokines, such as IL-1, IL-6, and TNFα after distance running is balanced by later release of other cytokines, such as IL-10, that inhibit the inflammatory cytokines (26).

Release of cytokines is not always apparent from blood samples, because cytokines act locally and are rapidly removed from circulation. However, their appearance in urine for up to several days after prolonged exercise provides evidence for their release (27). The source of cytokines released during exercise is unclear at present, because many different types of cells are capable of producing cytokines. Recent evidence suggests that skeletal muscle damaged by eccentric exercise may be one source of inflammatory cytokines such as IL-6. For example, in a recent study using RT-PCR technology, IL-6 mRNA expression was detected in skeletal muscle biopsies obtained after marathon running (28). Cytokines released from skeletal muscle damaged during eccentric exercise may act to recruit leukocytes to sites of tissue damage, where they may participate in the removal of degraded proteins.

Exercise training may alter the amount and pattern of cytokine release, possibly via downregulation of inflammatory processes. In individuals at risk of ischemic heart disease, 6 months' moderate exercise training resulted in lower production of inflammatory and higher production of anti-inflammatory cytokines in PBMC (29). As mentioned above, inflammatory cytokines are involved in the process of atherosclerosis. It is possible that training-induced alterations in the ratio of inflammatory to anti-inflammatory cytokines may be protective against heart disease. It is not clear whether acute or chronic exercise-induced changes in cytokine levels influence immune function.

Effects of Exercise on Immunoglobulin (Ig) and Antibody

Serum and mucosal Ig serve different functions and are independently regulated; exercise appears to affect serum and mucosal Ig differently (reviewed by 1). Serum Ig levels remain relatively unchanged after both acute and chronic exercise, although clinically low levels of some IgG subclasses were observed in elite athletes undergoing months of intense training (15). However, the ability to mount a specific antibody response (i.e., to a specific antigenic challenge or immunization) is normal in athletes (30, 31); it is not clear whether there are clinical implications of the low levels of serum IgG subclasses in athletes.

Mucosal IgA is a major effector of host defense against viruses causing URTI. Low mucosal IgA concentration has been observed in some athletes (reviewed by 1), and low levels may be predictive of risk for URTI (32, 33). Mucosal IgA concentration declines after brief or prolonged intense exercise but is unaffected by moderate exercise (reviewed by 1). These observations are consistent with the "J-curve" model (discussed above), in which the risk of

URTI increases with exercise intensity or volume, and may at least partially explain the elevated risk of URTI in endurance athletes.

Are Athletes Immunocompromised?

As mentioned above, athletes experience high rates of URTI during intense training and after major competition. Viral URTI appears to be the only illness to which athletes are at increased risk, suggesting that, from a clinical perspective, any suppression of immune function is relatively mild. On the other hand, the occurrence of URTI at a particular time in the athlete's training cycle or competition may be critical to the athlete's career.

Thus, although athletes are not considered clinically immune deficient, recent evidence discussed above suggests that mild suppression of several immune parameters occurs during intense training. It is possible that, in athletes, the combined effects of small changes in several immune parameters may compromise resistance to minor infectious agents. In contrast, moderate exercise training appears to have either no effect, or to slightly enhance resistance to upper respiratory infection, possibly by stimulating immune function. Although competitive athletes must train intensely on a regular basis, monitoring athletes' adaptation to training, allowing adequate recovery between sessions and after major competition, and attention to other factors such as proper nutrition and stress management may help athletes avoid immune suppression and associated illness (Table 16.6).

DIET, EXERCISE, AND IMMUNE FUNCTION

Proper nutrition is essential to a competent immune system. Malnutrition is the most common cause of immune suppression throughout the world, primarily in less-developed countries (2). In developed countries, where malnutrition is less of an issue, nutrition has relevance to immune function in various groups, including athletes, the elderly, and obese individuals attempting to lose weight.

Table 16.6 Practical Advice for Athletes Wishing to Avoid Immune Suppression

Avoid overtraining
- Schedule rest days
- Include periodization and recovery training
- Allow adequate rest after competition
- Avoid too frequent competition

Limit exposure to potential sources of illness
- Limit exposure to crowds during and after competition
- Avoid extended air travel immediately before and after competition

Ensure adequate nutrition
- Total energy, protein, carbohydrates
- Iron, vitamin C
- Avoid rapid weight loss (e.g., wrestlers, lightweight rowers)

Rest or only light exercise during systemic viral illness
- Seek medical advice for all but simple head cold
- Avoid exercise when febrile
- Return to training/competition only when asymptomatic

Optimal immune function depends on adequate intake of a number of factors. Deficiency in immune function may result from inadequate intake of total energy, protein, minerals such as zinc or iron, vitamins such as vitamin C or E, and other antioxidants. On the other hand, it is questionable whether supplementation with any of these substances enhances immune function in the absence of deficiency. It is beyond the scope of this chapter to fully present the relationship between diet, exercise, and immune function, and only a brief discussion of some relevant aspects is included.

Physical work capacity may be compromised by inadequate diet. It is well-known that athletes may have special dietary needs: dietary carbohydrate supplementation either before or during prolonged exercise may delay the onset of fatigue, endurance exercise performance is compromised in iron-deficient athletes, and endurance and power athletes require additional protein intake compared with the sedentary population. Athletes are avid consumers of a range of dietary products purported to enhance physical performance or immunity to infection, such as vitamins, minerals, antioxidants, carbohydrate or protein supplements, and glutamine.

Dietary Carbohydrate (CHO)

During prolonged exercise, depletion of muscle glycogen and blood glucose contributes to the onset of fatigue. Consumption of a high CHO diet in the days before, or CHO-containing fluids (e.g., sports drink) during prolonged exercise helps maintain blood glucose levels and may delay the onset of fatigue. Maintaining blood glucose levels through dietary CHO manipulation also attenuates some of the exercise-induced changes in immune parameters. This is thought to occur by preventing the rise in stress hormones such as catecholamines and cortisol during exercise.

CHO ingestion during prolonged exercise attenuates the perturbation from resting levels of blood leukocyte and lymphocyte counts and of inflammatory cytokines (reviewed by 34). On the other hand, CHO supplementation has no effect on NK-cell cytotoxic activity. It has been suggested that, during prolonged exercise, maintaining blood glucose levels through CHO supplementation reduces the overall stress response (34). Further research is needed to determine whether there are clinical implications of altering the immune system response to exercise in athletes or other groups.

Iron

Iron and other minerals (e.g., zinc, selenium) are required for normal immune function. Iron deficiency has been associated with impaired lymphocyte proliferation, NK-cell cytotoxic activity, and phagocytic function (35, 36).

Iron is lost from the body during exercise via sweat and destruction of red blood cells; endurance athletes may have increased iron requirements because of increased turnover of red blood cells. Menstruating female endurance athletes may be especially susceptible to iron deficiency due to additional losses each cycle. The prevalence of iron deficiency among athletes of either gender is not known, since the expansion of plasma volume due to endurance training (a positive adaptive response) may lead to artificially low blood hemoglobin levels ("pseudoanemia"). This topic is discussed in detail in Chapter 19.

The relationship between iron status and immune function has not been extensively studied in athletes. A preliminary report noted lower NKCA in female runners with low compared with normal serum ferritin levels (37). However, in this study, 8 weeks' iron supplementation (100 mg elemental iron/d) had no effect on NKCA in the low ferritin runners, despite increasing serum ferritin toward normal levels. It is possible that 8 weeks' supplementation was insufficient to alter NKCA.

Various diseases or treatments may influence iron status. For example, cancer therapy may induce anemia and low red blood cell counts (discussed further in Chapters 15 and 19). It is possible that immune suppression may result, although these patients will be taking other medications that may also contribute to impaired immunity (e.g., cytotoxic drugs). Certainly, the clinical exercise physiologist should consider, among other factors, the possible adverse effect of iron status on immune function when prescribing exercise for such patients.

Antioxidant Vitamins

A diet rich in antioxidants is thought to protect against cancer, although it is unclear whether such protection directly involves the immune system. Immune cells are susceptible to damage by oxidants such as free radicals produced in oxidative metabolism and normal leukocyte function (21). Neutrophils release reactive oxygen and nitrogen species, which are toxic to pathogens but may also cause inflammation and damage within normal cells. Increased oxidative metabolism (as occurs in prolonged exercise) produces reactive oxygen species. This suggests that free-radical–induced damage to leukocytes may be one mechanism by which prolonged exercise may impair immune function. Indeed, recent evidence suggests that programmed cell death (apoptosis) occurs in lymphocytes after intense exercise (38). If this hypothesis is correct, then it is possible that antioxidant supplementation may prevent or limit exercise-induced immune suppression.

One antioxidant vitamin, vitamin C, has long been purported to be prophylactic against the common cold. Despite years of scrutiny, however, the evidence is still equivocal in normal populations, and it appears that any effect of supplementation may occur by reduction of the duration and severity of symptoms rather than reduction in the incidence (39). On the other hand, there is evidence to suggest that vitamin C may prevent the common cold in certain conditions such as physical stress (39). For example, in a double-blind study, 84 distance runners and 73 nonrunners consumed either 600 mg/d of vitamin C or placebo for 3 weeks before a 90-km ultramarathon race (5). In the 2 weeks after the race, the incidence of URTI symptoms was reduced by more than half in supplemented runners compared with those consuming placebo. In contrast, vitamin C supplementation had no effect on the incidence of symptoms in nonrunners. Vitamins A and E had no effect on URTI incidence after an ultramarathon (40). The mechanisms by which vitamin C may protect against URTI are unknown, but it has been suggested that any effects may relate to the vitamin's antioxidant activity and protection against reactive oxygen species produced by activated neutrophils (40). At present, there are few data to support a role of other antioxidants in enhancement of immune function in athletes (reviewed by 36).

Glutamine

Glutamine is the most abundant amino acid in the body; skeletal muscle provides the largest source of glutamine. Proliferating lymphocytes require glutamine as an energy source and for nucleotide synthesis. A decrease in glutamine levels during physiological stress such as surgery, burns, and trauma has been associated with immunosuppression. Glutamine supplementation helps restore immunity in these conditions (reviewed by 41).

Plasma glutamine concentration declines acutely and remains low for up to several hours after prolonged exercise. Levels also decline during intense exercise training and are lower in overtrained compared with well-trained athletes (reviewed by 41). It has been suggested that low plasma glutamine levels may compromise lymphocyte function, and thus impair immunity to infection (41). A brief report suggests the possibility that glutamine supplementation may prevent URTI after endurance competition (distance running) (42). However, there are also data that do not support a role of glutamine in prevention of immune suppression after exercise. For example, despite significantly lower plasma glutamine concentration in overtrained compared with well-trained swimmers, glutamine levels did not differ between athletes who developed URTI and those who did not during 4 weeks of intensified training (43). Moreover, glutamine supplementation to maintain plasma glutamine levels had no effect on exercise-induced changes in leukocyte numbers, lymphocyte proliferation, or NK-cell function after prolonged exercise (reviewed by 41). Thus, at present, there is insufficient evidence to support a role of glutamine in maintenance of immune competence in athletes.

Diet, Exercise, and Immune Function in the Elderly

Aging is associated with declines in several aspects of immune function, especially lymphocyte proliferation, T-cell function, antibody production, IL-2 production, and macrophage and NK-cell responsiveness (44, 45). It is unclear, however, whether such changes are inevitable or result from diseases that increase in prevalence with aging, such as cardiovascular disease and cancer, or other factors, such as increased body fat or inactivity. One viewpoint is that, in the absence of disease, age-related changes in immune function are relatively small, as shown in studies of healthy centenarians (people ≥100 years old). It has been suggested that a "continuous remodeling" of the immune system occurs from birth, during which some immune variables change while others are maintained during senescence (46).

The immune response to exercise is qualitatively similar in older and younger subjects, although there are quantitative differences between ages (44, 45). Both young and older adult subjects exhibit leukocytosis after maximal exercise, but the magnitude of leukocytosis is attenuated and persists for longer in older subjects (44). Lymphocyte proliferation and NK-cell responsiveness to cytokines may be lower in older compared with younger subjects (45). It has been suggested that quantitative differences between ages may be related to differences in the stress hormone response to maximal exercise. It is not clear whether there are long-term consequences of relatively modest differences between older and younger individuals in the immune system response to exercise. Six months of moderate exercise training in the elderly produced few changes in immune parameters (47).

Whereas the aging process may be responsible for changes in immune function in the elderly, poor nutrition may also play a role; for a number of reasons including economic, the elderly are often mildly deficient in protein and key vitamins and minerals (48). Daily supplementation of micronutrients may improve immune function in the healthy elderly. For example, 17 weeks of dietary supplements with or without regular exercise increased blood indicators of nutritional status (e.g., vitamin, ferritin levels) in elderly subjects (48).

Effects of Weight Loss on Immune Function

Obesity is associated with a higher incidence of infection and cancer, suggesting impairment of immune function, although it is not clear whether this results directly from obesity or indirectly from other factors such as a sedentary lifestyle or nutritional imbalance. Obesity has been linked with high circulating leukocyte concentrations (primarily neutrophils and monocytes), reduced T- and B-lymphocyte proliferation, and lower NK-cell activity (8, 49). It would seem logical, then, that weight loss may enhance immune function in the obese, although evidence for this view is equivocal. Some studies have shown enhanced immune parameters after weight loss in obese subjects, whereas others have shown the opposite.

It appears that the model of weight loss and immune parameters assessed influence the results of these studies. For example, in a recent study on 22 healthy obese women, diet alone (900 kcal/d liquid diet for 8 weeks) resulted in significant declines in NKCA and IL-2 receptor expression by PBMC (49). In contrast, in the same study, a combined diet plus exercise regime (same diet plus mild aerobic and resistance exercise 3 times/wk) prevented the decreases in NKCA and IL-2 receptor expression, despite similar loss of body mass in both regimes (11–12 kg). In another recent study of 91 obese women, lymphocyte proliferation declined similarly after weight loss regardless of the method, (12-week diet alone, exercise alone, or diet plus exercise) compared with controls who did not lose weight (8). However, other immune parameters such as NKCA and phagocytosis did not change with weight loss. Compared with the former study (49), the latter study (8) induced less energy restriction (1200 vs 900 kcal/d), more gradual weight loss (2–8 kg over 12 weeks vs 11–12 kg over 8 weeks), and more exercise (5 vs 3 d/wk), which may partially explain the different results.

The mechanisms responsible for changes in immune function after weight loss are unknown at present. It is unclear which factors associated with weight loss influence the immune system: energy deficit, changes in body composition, changes in metabolism, or some combination of factors. At present, it would appear that gradual weight loss induced by moderate dietary restriction and exercise, as generally recommended for good health, may avoid or attenuate any adverse effects on immune function. Certainly, there are compelling health reasons for weight reduction in the obese and overweight (e.g., reduced risk of cardiovascular and metabolic diseases), and any possible mild impairment of immune function does not negate the general recommendation for all individuals to maintain a healthy body weight.

SUMMARY AND CONCLUSIONS

The human immune system is a complex system with overlapping and complementary functions requiring extensive communication and coordination between its various effector cells and messenger molecules. Immune function may be altered by a variety of conditions, including disease, medication, surgery, trauma, dietary imbalance, and physical or psychological stress. Physical stress such as strenuous exercise causes an influx of immune cells into the peripheral circulation and may induce changes in immune cell function; most effects are transitory, and normal levels are generally restored within 24 hours. Long-term moderate exercise training appears to have little effect on, and may slightly enhance, immune function. In contrast, prolonged periods of intense exercise training may induce mild suppression of several immune parameters. While athletes are not considered clinically immune deficient, this mild suppression of immunity may contribute to the high incidence of upper respiratory tract infection in endurance athletes. Inadequate nutrition, obesity, and rapid weight loss may also compromise immunity. Dietary supplementation may be of value in some individuals such as the elderly or in those with specific deficiencies. Moderate exercise training attenuates adverse effects on immune function resulting from weight loss in obese individuals. The clinical exercise physiologist should be aware of the immune response to exercise in healthy individuals and those with diseases affecting immune function in order to safely prescribe exercise for these individuals. Given the suppressive effects of intense exercise on immune function in healthy individuals, it would be prudent to prescribe moderate physical activity for patients with immune system dysfunction, regardless of whether such dysfunction is caused directly by disease or is secondary to treatment.

References

1. Mackinnon LT. *Advances in exercise immunology*. Champaign, IL: Human Kinetics, 1999.
2. Janeway CA, Travers P, Walport M, et al. *Immunobiology: the immune system in health and disease*. 4th ed. New York: Elsevier Science Ltd. 1999.
3. Nieman DC, Johanssen LM, Lee JW, et al. Infectious episodes in runners before and after the Los Angeles Marathon. *J Sports Med Phys Fitness* 1990;30:316–328.
4. Peters EM, Bateman ED. Ultramarathon running and upper respiratory tract infections. *S Afr J Sports Med* 1983;64:582–584.
5. Peters EM, Goetzsche JM, Grobbelaar B, et al. Vitamin C supplementation reduces the incidence of postrace symptoms of upper respiratory tract infection in ultramarathon runners. *Am J Clin Nutr* 1993;57:170–174.
6. Heath GW, Ford ES, Craven TE, et al. Exercise and the incidence of upper respiratory tract infections. *Med Sci Sports Exerc* 1991;23:152–157.
7. Nieman DC, Johanssen LM, Lee JW. Infectious episodes in runners before and after a roadrace. *J Sports Med Phys Fitness* 1989;29:289–296.
8. Nieman DC, Nehlsen-Cannarella SL, Henson DA, et al. Immune responses to exercise training and/or energy restriction in obese women. *Med Sci Sports Exerc* 1998;30:679–686.
9. Nieman DC, Nehlsen-Cannarella SL. Exercise and infection. In: Watson RR, Eisinger M, eds. *Exercise and disease*. Boca Raton, FL: CRC Press, 1992.
10. Friman G, Ilback N-G. Acute infection: metabolic responses, effects on performance, interaction with exercise, and myocarditis. *Int J Sports Med* 1998;19:S172–S182.
11. Parker S, Brukner PD, Rosier M. Chronic fatigue syndrome and the athlete. *Sports Med Training Rehab* 1996;6:269–278.
12. Weidner TG, Cranston T, Schurr T, et al. The effect of exercise training on the severity and duration of a viral respiratory illness. *Med Sci Sports Exerc* 1998;30:1578–1583.
13. Pizza FX, Mitchell JB, Davis BH, et al. Exercise-induced muscle damage: effect on circulating leukocyte and lymphocyte subsets. *Med Sci Sports Exerc* 1995;27:363–370.
14. Lehmann M, Mann H, Gastmann U, et al. Unaccustomed high-mileage vs intensity training-related changes in performance and serum amino acid levels. *Int J Sports Med* 1996; 17:187–192.
15. Gleeson M, McDonald WA, Cripps AW, et al. The effect on immunity of long-term intensive training in elite swimmers. *Clin Exp Immunol* 1995;102:210–216.
16. Pedersen BK, Ullum H. NK cell response to physical activity: possible mechanisms of action. *Med Sci Sports Exerc* 1994; 26:140–146.
17. Nieman DC, Buckley KS, Henson DA, et al. Immune function in marathon runners vs sedentary controls. *Med Sci Sports Exerc* 1995;27:986–992.
18. MacNeil B, Hoffman-Goetz L. Chronic exercise enhances *in vivo* and *in vitro* cytotoxic mechanisms of natural immunity in mice. *J Appl Physiol* 1993;74:388–395.
19. Smith JA. Neutrophils, host defense and inflammation: a double-edged sword. *J Leukocyte Biol* 1994;56:672–686.
20. Belcastro AN, Arthur GD, Albisser RA, et al. Heart, liver, and skeletal muscle myeloperoxidase activity during exercise. *J Appl Physiol* 1996;80:1331–1335.
21. Niess AM, Dickhuth HH, Northoff H, et al. Free radicals and oxidative stress in exercise—immunological aspects. *Exerc Immunol Rev* 1999;5:22–56.
22. Hack B, Strobel G, Weiss M, et al. PMN cell counts and phagocytic activity of highly trained athletes depending on training period. *J Appl Physiol* 1994;77:1731–1735.
23. Pyne DB, Baker MS, Fricker PA, et al. Effects of an intensive 12 week training program by elite swimmers on neutrophil oxidative activity. *Med Sci Sports Exerc* 1995;27:536–542.
24. Hinton JR, Rowbottom DG, Keast D, et al. Acute intensive interval training and *in vitro* T lymphocyte function. *Int J Sports Med* 1997;18:132–137.
25. Pedersen BK, Ostrowski K, Rohde T, et al. The cytokine response to strenuous exercise. *Can J Physiol Pharmacol* 1998; 76:505–511.
26. Ostrowski K, Rohde T, Asp S, et al. Pro- and anti-inflammatory cytokine balance in strenuous exercise. *J Physiol* 1999;515: 287–291.
27. Sprenger H, Jacobs C, Nain N, et al. Enhanced release of cytokines, interleukin-2 receptors, and neopterin after long-distance running. *Clin Immunol Immunopathol* 1992;53: 188–195.
28. Ostrowski K, Rohde T, Zacho M, et al. Evidence that interleukin-6 is produced in human skeletal muscle during prolonged running. *J Physiol* 1998;508.3:949–953.
29. Smith JK, Dykes R, Douglas RE, et al. Long-term exercise and atherogenic activity of blood mononuclear cells in persons at risk of developing ischemic heart disease. *JAMA* 1999;281: 1722–1727.
30. Bruunsgaard H, Hartkopp A, Mohr T, et al. *In vivo* cell-mediated immunity and vaccination response following prolonged, intense exercise. *Med Sci Sports Exerc* 1997;29: 1176–1181.
31. Gleeson M, Pyne DB, McDonald WA, et al. Pneumococcal antibody responses in elite swimmers. *Clin Exp Immunol* 1996;105:238–244.
32. Gleeson M, McDonald WA, Pyne DB, et al. Salivary IgA levels and infection risk in elite swimmers. *Med Sci Sports Exerc* 1999;31:67–73.
33. Mackinnon LT, Ginn EM, Seymour GJ. Temporal relationship between exercise-induced decreases in salivary IgA and subsequent appearance of upper respiratory tract infection in elite athletes. *Aust J Sci Med Sport* 1993;25:94–99.
34. Nieman DC. Influence of carbohydrate on the immune response to intensive, prolonged exercise. *Exerc Immunol Rev* 1998;4:64–76.
35. Konig D, Weinstock C, Keul J, et al. Zinc, iron, and magne-

sium status in athletes—influence on the regulation of exercise-induced stress and immune function. *Exerc Immunol Rev* 1998;4:2–21.
36. Shephard RJ, Shek PN. Immunological hazards from nutritional imbalance in athletes. *Exerc Immunol Rev* 1998;4:48.
37. Flynn MG, Mackinnon LT, Gedge V, et al. Iron status and cell-mediated immune function in female distance runners. *Med Sci Sports Exerc* 1996;28:S90.
38. Mars M, Govender A, Weston A, et al. High intensity exercise: a cause of lymphocyte apoptosis? *Biochem Biophys Res Comm* 1998;249:366–370.
39. Hemila H. Vitamin C and common cold incidence: a review of studies with subjects under heavy physical stress. *Int J Sports Med* 1996;17:379–383.
40. Peters EM. Exercise, immunology, and upper respiratory tract infections. *Int J Sports Med* 1997;18:S69–S77.
41. Rohde T, Kryzwkowski K, Pedersen BK. Glutamine, exercise, and the immune system—is there a link? *Exerc Immunol Rev* 1998;4:49–63.
42. Castell LM, Newsholme EA, Poortmans JR. Does glutamine have a role in reducing infection in athletes? *Eur J Appl Physiol* 1996;73:488–490.
43. Mackinnon LT, Hooper SL. Plasma glutamine concentration and upper respiratory tract infection during over-training in elite swimmers. *Med Sci Sports Exerc* 1996;28:285–290.
44. Ceddia MA, Price EA, Kohlmeier CK, et al. Differential leukocytosis and lymphocyte mitogenic response to acute maximal exercise in the young and old. *Med Sci Sports Exerc* 1999;31:829–836.
45. Woods JA, Evans JK, Wolters BW, et al. Effects of maximal exercise on natural killer (NK) cell cytotoxicity and responsiveness to interferon-alpha in the young and old. *J Gerontol* 1998;53:B430–B437.
46. Franceschi C, Monti D, Sansoni P, et al. The immunology of exceptional individuals: the lesson in centenarians. *Immunol Today* 1995;16:12–16.
47. Woods JA, Ceddia MA, Wolters BW, et al. Effects of 6 months of moderate aerobic exercise training on immune function in the elderly. *Mech Ageing Dev* 1999;109:1–19.
48. deJong N, Paw MJ, deGroot LC, et al. Functional biochemical and nutrient indices in frail elderly people are partly affected by dietary supplements but not by exercise. *J Nutr* 1999;129:2028–2036.
49. Scanga CB, Verde TJ, Paolone AM, et al. Effects of weight loss and exercise training on natural killer cell activity in obese women. *Med Sci Sports Exerc* 1998;30:1666–1671.

CHAPTER **17**

Exercise and HIV Infection

Heather R. Schmitz, Jennifer E. Layne, and Ronenn Roubenoff

INTRODUCTION

Infection with human immunodeficiency virus (HIV) has dramatically changed social conditions in the developed world, altered the very fabric of society in Africa, and killed millions of people over the past 2 decades. HIV infection begins with a primary infection phase, which generally feels like a bad case of influenza. This phase usually lasts several weeks and is then followed by a long asymptomatic period during which the infected patient feels well. The asymptomatic phase usually lasts many years—10 years on average. However, during this time, HIV is replicating in lymphoid tissue and slowly destroying CD4 positive T-helper cells, the main targets of the virus. During this time, the patient is infectious and can spread the disease through sexual contact or blood borne transmission in shared intravenous drug paraphernalia. As the T-helper cell count falls, the patient becomes susceptible to more infections and eventually develops an infection with one or more of a list of defined opportunistic organisms, which would not cause disease if the immune system were normal. This is the hallmark of clinical AIDS (acquired immunodeficiency syndrome). Once an AIDS-defining condition has been diagnosed, a person is said to have AIDS, even if they later recover completely from that condition. AIDS can also be defined by developing unusual cancers (Kaposi's sarcoma, some types of lymphoma, and cervical cancer in women), or by developing wasting (unintentional loss of more than 10% of usual weight), or a persistent CD4 count less than 200 cells/mm^3. Until 1996, once AIDS occurred, survival was usually about 2 years.

With the advent of highly active antiretroviral therapy (HAART), however, survival has improved dramatically, so that mortality rates in 1999 were 85% lower than in 1995, opportunistic infections are much less common, and T-helper cell counts often increase enough to prevent life-threatening infections (*www.cdc.gov/hiv*). However, in Africa and Asia, where HAART is not available, mortality remains extremely high. In advance of the 2000 International HIV Meeting, the United Nations estimated that 19 million adults have died of AIDS since the epidemic began (*www.us.unaids.org*).

It is for treatment (and prevention) of body composition and metabolic changes that most exercise physiologists will come into contact with HIV-positive patients. Rehabilitating patients with HIV infection to the point that their muscle mass and strength are normal requires an integrated anabolic approach using diet, exercise, and pharmacologic agents when indicated. In patients with AIDS, wasting is an independent risk factor for death, disability, and loss of independence; thus, this integrated approach is essential. In addition, as patients live longer with HIV infection, a new problem of increased abdominal mass and loss of subcutaneous fat on the face, arms, and legs has been described. Here, too, it is likely that the exercise professional can offer unique and valuable treatment options for these patients.

In this chapter, we review the major impact of HIV infection on fitness and body composition and discuss the effect of exercise for treatment of this life-threatening condition. Current research provides evidence that exercise is important, beneficial, and may increase quality of life in both healthy and HIV-infected populations.

EPIDEMIOLOGY AND PATHOPHYSIOLOGY

Wasting was recognized as a life-threatening complication of HIV infection quite early in the history of the epidemic (2). Wasting causes weakness, loss of functional capacity, and loss of important protein reserves needed for times of acute illness. These changes can be opposed by high-intensity resistance training, which can overcome the catabolic effects of AIDS wasting in many cases and lead to improved strength, functioning, and muscle mass.

The Centers for Disease Control and Prevention desig-

Supported by USDA Cooperative Agreement 58–1950-9–001 and NIH Grant DK45734.

The contents of this publication do not necessarily reflect the views or policies of the U.S. Department of Agriculture, nor does mention of trade names, commercial products, or organizations imply endorsement by the U.S. government.

nated unintentional weight loss of ≥10% of usual body weight as a definition of wasting and as one of several AIDS-defining conditions. This has been in general use since the mid-1980s (1). However, it has subsequently been shown that even a 5% weight loss has a significant impact on mortality in patients with HIV infection, so that a biologically plausible case can be made for using the latter definition (3). Although AIDS wasting is less aggressive and less common in countries where HAART is available, it remains a major cause of morbidity and mortality in Africa, Asia, and other countries where such treatment is not available. Even in the United States, weight loss and especially loss of muscle continue to commonly occur. Recent data from the greater Boston area indicate that 18% of patients have evidence of wasting despite taking HAART (Wanke C, Gorbach SL, et al.: unpublished observations).

Lipodystrophy, or fat-redistribution syndrome, is a more recently recognized metabolic complication of HIV infection whose etiology, prevalence, and even definition are still being determined. The terms refer to a loss of subcutaneous fat in the arms, legs, and face, coupled with an increase in abdominal fat that occurs primarily in the visceral fat compartment (Figure 17.1). Along with these changes, it is common to also see increased dorsocervical fat deposition (clinically called a "buffalo hump"), breast enlargement in women, and increased visibility of arm and leg veins. Lipodystrophy was originally reported in patients taking the protease inhibitor class of antiretroviral drugs but has since been demonstrated in patients taking all classes of medications and also in treatment-naïve individuals (4). The prevalence of lipodystrophy occurring in HIV-infected individuals has varied from 10–85%, depending on the series of medications (5, 6). Because lipodystrophy has been associated with elevated serum glucose levels and was first identified in patients taking protease inhibitors, an early hypothesis has been that the drugs themselves cause insulin resistance and accumulation of abdominal fat (4). In support of this theory, Walli et al. showed that treatment with protease inhibitors is associated with peripheral insulin resistance (7), suggesting that the drugs themselves may be involved in the pathogenesis of lipodystrophy, or at least in magnifying the condition to the level of a clinically relevant problem.

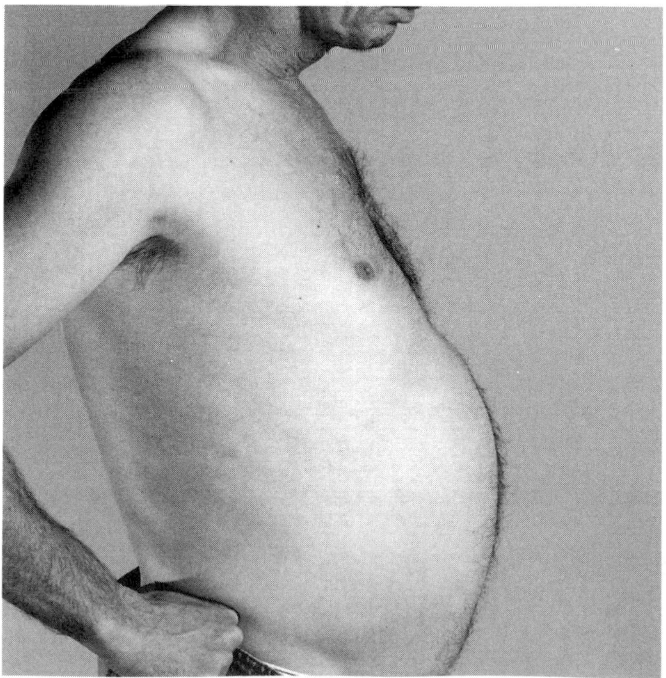

Figure 17.1. Typical example of abdominal fat gain and arm fat loss in a patient with HIV-associated fat redistribution (lipodystrophy).

Regardless of etiology, lipodystrophy is associated with insulin resistance, low high-density lipoprotein-cholesterol, and central obesity. In addition to the cosmetic, social, and self-esteem problems caused by the loss of peripheral fat, the gain in central fat causes concern about long-term complications, including vascular disease, stroke, and heart disease. At the moment, it appears that exercise therapy can be used to mitigate the central fat gain of lipodystrophy, but it is not likely to have an effect on the peripheral fat loss.

CLINICAL EXERCISE PHYSIOLOGY

It is important for the clinical exercise professional to keep in mind that patients with HIV infection run the gamut from asymptomatic to critically ill, and it is a cardinal error to try and lump them all together. Patients must be evaluated on an individual basis to assess the effects of the infection. There are a number of physiological and psychological changes that occur during the course of HIV infection. Loss of strength, skeletal muscle mass, and functional status are some of the changes associated with the disease. Many possible causes for these abnormal manifestations are hypothesized, but the exact mechanism is unknown. In addition to the disease itself, decreases in physical activity and psychological well-being may contribute to this muscle atrophy, weakness, and fatigue (8). Nonetheless, there is evidence supporting using exercise interventions to treat or attenuate the loss of muscle size, strength, and functional capacity.

An increasing number of health professionals are recommending exercise interventions to prevent disease or to mitigate the symptoms caused by chronic disease states. Exercise and other nonpharmacologic interventions have the potential to significantly enhance traditional medical treatment and patient outcome. The mode of exercise prescribed for HIV-infected individuals may be endurance, resistance, or a combination of both. The goal is to enhance cardiopulmonary and musculoskeletal system function and improve overall health and quality of life (9). However, when working with HIV-infected patients, the primary consideration of an exercise physiologist must be not to worsen the patient's condition, or lead to immunosuppression in those individuals who are already immunocompromised.

Embarking on an exercise program has been shown to improve aerobic fitness, mood, immune indices, and chronic disease incidence in non–HIV-infected adults (10). It has also been shown that exercise significantly increases strength, decreases resting heart rate, and increases endurance, which are all important attributes to potentially reverse the deleterious body composition changes and nervous system disorders commonly associated with HIV infection (11). These patients should benefit from the physiological (i.e., increase in muscle mass) and psychological (i.e., increase in functional status) effects of an exercise regimen.

Thus, HIV-positive status should not be a deterrent to begin an exercise program; rather, it should be the reason to do so. The goals and prescriptions of exercise may vary by the metabolic problem being addressed—wasting, lipodystrophy, both, or neither (health maintenance in asymptomatic HIV-positive persons). Those already experiencing wasting should be encouraged to participate in activities designed to promote preservation of muscle mass, such as progressive resistance training (PRT). Those experiencing lipodystrophy should be prescribed a program tailored to provide a combination of aerobic and PRT exercises. These recommendations should be incorporated while the individual is asymptomatic. It has been suggested that PRT may be a method of increasing body protein stores before the onset of acute illness (12). Even during a secondary opportunistic infection, exercise of some sort should still be sustained, although tapering may be necessary with consideration of current physical limitations. The goal is to remain physically active to the extent that the illness allows. This implies that if the patient has the energy to be mobile throughout the day, he should be encouraged to do so. Maintaining even a low level of activity will also benefit patients during recovery from the illness and make it easier for them to return to their exercise regimen when they feel better. Any type of physical activity may lessen the severity of the disease and promote quicker recovery both physically and mentally.

Exhaustive exercise has profound effects on the immune system, with activation of humeral and cellular immunity that parallels the level of muscle injury caused by so-called "acute" exercise (see references 13 and 14 for review). However, the relevance of this to exercise training is limited because the level of injury and exhaustion during routine training at moderate intensity are generally less than that associated with acute intense exercise. Nevertheless, there has been concern that the damaged immune system of patients with HIV infection could lead to abnormal exercise-induced immune responses and could even increase circulating HIV burden.

To assess this question, Roubenoff et al. studied HIV viral loads in patients before and after a 15-minute bout of moderately intense exercise (Fig. 17.2) (15). Participants stepped up and down a 60-cm step at a cadence of 15 steps per minute, so that patients raised and lowered their body weight 225 times in 15 minutes. The exercise caused a mild acute phase response with a rise in circulating neutrophil counts, serum creatine kinase concentration, and urinary 3-methylhistidine. Nevertheless, there was no increase in plasma viral load, as measured by reverse transcriptase-polymerase chain reaction (RT-PCR). We concluded that exercise is likely to be safe in patients with HIV infection. Thus, prescription of an aerobic or resistance training program should not be avoided in these patients because of concern about increased HIV viremia.

Illness of any sort easily leads to reduced physical activity, deconditioning, and loss of both aerobic capacity and muscle strength, which has also been observed for HIV infection. Johnson et al. (16) demonstrated poor aerobic capacity in 32 male patients with HIV infection but without AIDS who were extensively evaluated for the presence of pulmonary disease. In 32 patients in whom pulmonary tests were normal, the authors found significantly lower workload (195 ±30 vs. 227 ±31 W, $p < 0.001$), anaerobic threshold (49.2 ±13 vs. 61.9 ±9.1% of predicted oxygen consumption, $p < 0.001$), and maximal oxygen utilization (VO_{2max} 69.9 ±11.2 vs. 95.9 ±17.5% of predicted) compared to an age-matched control group.

Endurance Training in HIV Infection

MacArthur et al. (17) demonstrated the reversibility of such deconditioning with aerobic training. In this study, the investigators sought to compare low-intensity exercise

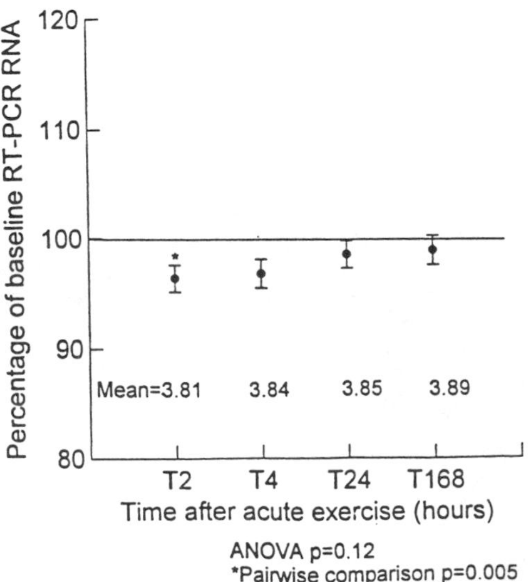

Figure 17.2. Change in blood HIV viral load (RNA) after a 15-minute bout of exercise. Points indicate % of baseline (pre-exercise) HIV RNA. Error bars indicate one standard error. Numbers under the points indicate the mean log concentration of HIV RNA at each time point. Reprinted from Roubenoff et al. (15) with permission.

(4×10 minute intervals at 50–60% VO_{2max}), and high-intensity exercise (6×4 minute intervals at 75–85% VO_{2max}) cardiovascular training three times per week for 24 weeks. Unfortunately, only 6 of the 32 patients recruited for the study were compliant with the protocol, apparently because of a combination of advanced disease, transportation problems, and difficulty with the exercise protocol. There was a correlation between CD4 count and noncompliance, with poorest compliance in patients with the lowest CD4 counts. Nevertheless, in the six compliant patients, there was a significant improvement in cardiopulmonary fitness. There was a tendency toward more improvement in the high-intensity group than the low-intensity group, but the small sample size and the absence of a control group precluded a definitive conclusion on this point.

Rigsby et al. (11) examined the effect of combined aerobic and strengthening exercise on immune parameters in 37 HIV-positive and 8 HIV-negative men. The subjects were randomly allocated to exercise training or counseling. Subjects in the exercise group trained for 12 weeks, 3 times per week, for 1 hour each session. They performed 20 minutes of stationary bicycling at 60–80% of age-predicted maximal heart rate. They then performed strength training on an isokinetic weight-training machine for 20–25 minutes. The resistance was increased progressively across three sets, with the subject performing the maximum number of repetitions he could do in 30 seconds for each set. There was a 26% improvement in mean chest press strength, and a 31% increase in leg-extension strength. No significant effect was found on CD4, CD8, or total lymphocyte counts with exercise. The authors concluded that exercise training of this sort did not have an important effect on lymphocyte subsets.

In contrast, LaPerriere et al. (18) examined the effect of a 10-week aerobic training program on lymphocyte subsets and mood in a group of homosexual men awaiting the results of HIV testing, and thus under considerable psychological stress. Subjects were randomly assigned to aerobic training on a stationary bicycle for 45 minutes per session at 70–80% maximal heart rate three times a week, or a control group; the nature of the control intervention was not described. There were 12 seronegative and 10 seropositive men in the training group, and 11 seronegative and 6 seropositive men in the control group. Aerobic fitness improved in the training group but not in the control group, as estimated by submaximal bicycle protocol. Seronegative subjects who exercised showed an increase in their CD4 cell count of 220 cells/mm^3, while seropositive subjects had an increase of 115 cells/mm^3. However, the results for the control group were not reported, and no statistical test was performed.

Resistance Training in HIV Infection

Spence et al. (8) studied 24 men who had recently recovered from *Pneumocystis carinii* pneumonia (PCP) infection. They were all taking zidovudine (AZT), and were randomly assigned to training or control (usual activity) intervention for 6 weeks. The subjects in the intervention group were trained three times a week for 6 weeks using an isokinetic resistance training program to train the knee, shoulders, and chest in extension and flexion. There were significant improvements in power and torque production in the knee and shoulder with training, compared to moderate deteriorations in the control groups. In addition, there was a mean weight loss of 1.9 kg in the control group compared to a gain of 1.7 kg in the training group ($p < 0.0001$). There was also a significant improvement in combined midarm and midthigh circumference in the training group compared to a decline in the control group ($p < 0.003$).

These data, while encouraging, are difficult to interpret in the modern era of HAART for several reasons. First, the study is limited to men, so its relevance to women is unclear. Second, these men were recovering from PCP at a time (1987–1988) when this condition, although treatable, was often associated with poor long-term survival. Thus, the decline seen in the control group is more severe than would be expected if the study were replicated today. Third, the recent acute illness experienced by these men probably left them with acutely suppressed protein status and lean body mass, so that they should have been "primed" to show an improvement in lean mass with any anabolic intervention. Thus, the degree of training applied to these subjects may not have as dramatic an effect in a more stable population.

More recently, Roubenoff et al. completed a short-term (8 weeks of training 3 times per week for about 1 hour per day) study of intense (80% of 1-repetition max) PRT in patients with HIV infection with and without wasting. All the volunteers successfully increased strength, lean body mass, and functional status (12). The mean increase in lean mass in our study was 1.94 kg, while fat mass declined 0.9 kg. This is comparable to the effect size obtained with pharmacologic treatment such as growth hormone or anabolic steroids (19–21). In addition, the gains were maintained over an additional 8-week follow-up period of usual activity. Subjects with HIV wasting had a larger gain in lean mass (2.8 vs. 1.4 kg, $p < 0.06$) after 8 weeks, which persisted at follow-up, measured at 16 weeks after starting the training (Fig. 17.3). Physical function, measured using the Medical Outcomes Study SF-36 instrument (22), increased significantly in the wasted subjects (up 6 points, $p < 0.02$), but not in the nonwasted subjects, so that at 16 weeks the wasted subjects functioned at a higher level than the nonwasted patients ($p < 0.05$). Both increase in LBM ($p < 0.001$) and in strength ($p < 0.001$) were significantly and independently associated with increase in physical function. Thus, it appears that wasting in HIV infection is reversible with PRT.

Exercise Training in Lipodystrophy

We recently examined whether exercise training could reduce trunk fat in men with fat redistribution (23). In an open-label pilot study, 10 men with increasing abdominal

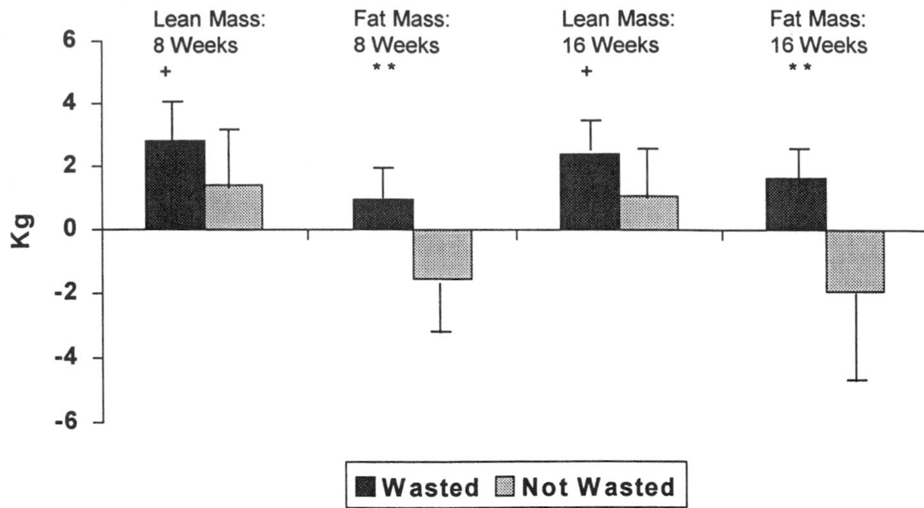

Figure 17.3. Change from baseline in lean body mass and fat mass at the end of 8 weeks of resistance training and after an additional 8 weeks of usual activity in subjects with (dark bars) or without (light bars) AIDS wasting. Error bars indicate one standard deviation. From Roubenoff et al. (12) with permission.

girth trained in a community health club three times per week for 16 weeks. Total body lean and fat mass, and trunk fat mass, were assessed by dual-energy x-ray absorptiometry (DEXA). After 16 weeks of exercise, strength increased for three of the four exercises tested (leg press + 13% [p <0.02], leg extension + 19% [p <0.03], seated row + 7% [p <0.13], chest press + 18% [p <0.005]). There was a significant decline in total body fat by 1.5 kg (E= 2.1 percentage points, p <0.01); most of the decline in body fat occurred in trunk fat, which decreased by 1.1 kg (p <0.03). Weight, lean mass (+1.1 ±2.6 kg, p = 0.23), and bone mineral density measured by DEXA did not change. No adverse effects were seen from the training. These data suggest that exercise training may reduce trunk fat mass in HIV-positive men with fat redistribution. Controlled trials of this approach are warranted.

PHARMACOLOGY

Treatment of HIV infection and AIDS has become a distinct subspecialty of internal medicine, and a full discussion of the treatment options is beyond the scope of this chapter. Current therapy of HIV infection requires a combination of 2–5 medications, collectively known as HAART, each requiring 1–4 doses per day, often with strict restrictions in terms of eating or drinking within an hour or two of taking the medication. Many patients report that taking their medications becomes a full-time job. Although there is a bewildering array of medications used for treatment of HIV itself, as well as for complications of HIV, HAART medicines fall into three categories: nucleoside reverse-transcriptase inhibitors (NRTIs, such as AZT), nonnucleoside reverse-transcriptase inhibitors (NNRTIs, such as nevirapine), and protease inhibitors (PIs, such as indinavir). Table 17.1 lists the antiretroviral drugs commonly used to treat HIV, along with common side effects and nutritional/food recommendations.

Today, the goal of therapy is to reduce blood HIV levels to undetectable. Single-drug regimens clearly do not do this and do not prevent wasting. Combination therapy (HAART) can do both. Since the advent of HAART, the problem of lipodystrophy has developed; however, it is unclear whether this occurs because of the drugs themselves, or just because they improve survival to the point that lipodystrophy—caused by other factors—can manifest itself.

Often, patients also take adjunctive therapy to prevent secondary infections such as trimethoprim-sulfamethoxazole (Bactrim) or antifungal medications for thrush. In addition, patients may be taking appetite stimulants such as megestrol acetate (Megace) or Dronabinol, testosterone or a synthetic steroid such as oxandrolone or nandrolone, and possibly growth hormone.

Exercise and Anabolic Pharmacotherapy

At least two studies have shown that exercise is synergistic with anabolic steroids. Sattler et al. (24) found that the combination of strength training with nandrolone decanoate, a synthetic androgen, increased lean mass by 5.2 ±5.7 kg vs. 3.9 ±2.3 kg for nandrolone alone (p <0.03). Strawford et al. (25) found similar results with resistance training plus oxandrolone 6.9 ±1.7 kg lean mass vs. 3.8 ±2.9 kg with oxandrolone alone (p <0.005). Thus, clinicians should consider pharmacologic and exercise interventions in persons with HIV wasting as complementary, rather than mutually exclusive, approaches.

Table 17.1. Antiretroviral Drugs Commonly Used to Treat HIV, along with Common Side Effects and Nutritional/Food Recommendations

Drug type	Generic name (Trade name)	Also known as:	Side effects	Nutritional/food recommendations
Nucleoside Reverse-Transcriptase Inhibitors (NRTIs)	Abacavir (Ziagen)		Fatal hypersensitivity, lactic acidosis	
	Zidovudine/Lamivudine (Combivir)	Combines ZDV and 3TC		
	Didanosine (Videx)	ddI	Pancreatitis	
	Lamivudine (Epivir)	3TC		
	Stavudine (Zerit)	d4T	Neuropathy	
	Zalcitabine (Hivid)	ddC, dideoxycytidine	Neuropathy	
	Zidovudine (Retrovir)	AZT, ZDV	Granulocytopenia	
NonNucleoside Reverse-Transcriptase Inhibitors (NNRTIs)	Delavirdine (Rescriptor)	DLV		
	Efavirenz (Sustiva)	DMP-266		
	Nevirapine (Viramune)	BI-RG-587, NVP	Skin reactions, hepatotoxicity	
Protease Inhibitors (PIs)	Amprenavir (Agenerase)	APV, 141W94		
	Indinavir (Crixivan)	IDV		Take on an empty stomach or with low-fat, light meal. No food restriction if administered with Ritonavir
	Nelfinavir (Viracept)	NFV		Administer with meal or light snack
	Ritonavir (Norvir)	RTV		Take with meals
	Saquinavir (Fortovase)	SQV		Take within 2 hours after a full meal

PHYSICAL EXAMINATION

The general and musculoskeletal examinations are paramount in diagnosing HIV-related wasting and lipodystrophy. It is important to look for muscle wasting in the temporal region, glutei, and quadriceps to determine whether there is abdominal obesity; to assess gluteal fatness; to examine the skin of the arms, legs, and face for evidence of subcutaneous fat atrophy; and to ask about functional status, activities of daily living, and difficulty with daily tasks. The waist circumference should be measured at the level of the lowest rib; the hip circumference should be measured at the level of the most protuberant point on the gluteus maximus. These bony landmarks facilitate precise follow-up measures. Skinfolds should be measured using a caliper at the triceps, subscapular area, and thigh, at the very least (see Diagnostic Techniques, below). Strength should be examined in arms and legs, including the ability to rise from a chair. It is also important to assess whether peripheral neuropathy, a common complication of both HIV infection and several of the medications used to treat it, is present. Both sensory and motor testing should be performed. Patients who have a normal examination and do not have evidence of either wasting or lipodystrophy will still benefit from regular exercise for all the reasons that all persons do. However, their exercise prescription should be targeted at any other comorbid conditions and not necessarily altered by their HIV status.

MEDICAL AND SURGICAL TREATMENTS

Treatment for HIV-related wasting consists of providing adequate dietary intake of energy, protein, micronutrients, and fluid. If this cannot be done by mouth, tube feedings or even parenteral nutrition can be used. However, even if adequate energy and protein are available, getting these nutrients into muscle is often slow or absent without an anabolic stimulus to the muscles. That stimulus is the proper role of resistance training (see below). If patients are hypogonadal, then replacement doses of testosterone in men, or estrogen and sometimes testosterone in women, should be given (26). Appetite can be stimulated with megestrol acetate, but it tends to cause fat accretion rather than increased lean mass (27). Growth hormone can be used if other methods fail and if the expense can be borne.

Treatment of lipodystrophy remains unclear. Certainly, successful HIV suppression with HAART should not be stopped only to treat lipodystrophy, as the results may be catastrophic in terms of viral resistance and uncontrolled AIDS. Weight gain beyond the healthy range should be prevented using judicious dieting, combined with a mixed aerobic-resistance training program. At this time, little can be done to reverse peripheral fat atrophy, but it is hoped that diet plus exercise can prevent the consequences of abdominal obesity.

DIAGNOSTIC TECHNIQUES

Body Mass and Composition

The best way to diagnose wasting is to document a 5% or greater weight loss using the same scale over time. Self-reported weights vary in their accuracy, especially when fear of wasting, or desire for secondary gain, can be at issue. Hence, objective measurement of weight is ideal. If the clinical exercise specialist is seeing the patient for the first time, it is worth trying to document change in weight by calling the patient's clinic or primary caregiver. Equally important is to document the patient's current weight and to weigh the patient at regular intervals over time to determine the effectiveness of therapy.

The role of body composition measurements is more controversial (28). Many of the methods available to measure body composition are too imprecise to apply with confidence to a single individual (e.g., bioelectrical impedance), are expensive and hard to obtain (in many cases DEXA), or are best used for longitudinal follow-up over time if a single trained observer is available to perform the measurements at each time point (e.g., anthropometry) (29). These methods are useful in research settings, but in the one-on-one situation of treating a patient with wasting, close measurements of body weight are generally adequate. It is more important to assess functional status and strength, frankly, than to commit limited resources to complex body composition measures.

In the case of lipodystrophy, however, body composition measurements are crucial. Because lipodystrophy is a *redistribution* of fat, with little change in *total* fat, weight alone is misleading. It is much more important to document change in abdominal girth over time, and perhaps to also measure triceps, subscapular, abdominal, and calf or thigh skinfolds in lipodystrophy than it is in wasting. Because CT or MRI measures of visceral fat mass are not generally available in the clinical setting, measuring waist circumference or the waist-to-hip ratio is the preferred alternative.

Functional Status

It is crucial to assess functional capacity using an objective test such as timed chair stands, stair climbing, or walking for a fixed distance or time (50 feet or 6 minutes). In addition, validated questionnaires of functional status such as the MOS-HIV should be used to follow patients' self-reported function in their home environments (30, 31). Questionnaires examining functional status focus on several levels: high-intensity activities (running, lifting heavy objects, climbing stairs, walking more than a mile), intermediate-level–intensity activities (walking one block, shopping, preparing meals or doing laundry), and basic activities of daily living (bathing and dressing, getting around in the home, or eating.) While testing in the gym or clinic is more objective and precise, it is also less relevant to how the patient perceives his situation: the clinical setting eliminates obstacles such as stairs, darkness, fear, and motivation and does not record how the patient functions in the real world. Since measuring real world function is impractical in the clinical situation, questionnaires offer a reasonable alternative.

EXERCISE/FITNESS/FUNCTIONAL TESTING

Assessment of Physical Fitness and Functional Status

Baseline assessment of physical fitness and functional status are recommended, in addition to medical history and physical examination, to evaluate the patient to determine the appropriate exercise prescription. Baseline assessment values are also useful to evaluate the patient's response to the exercise program and for comparison in subsequent assessment and evaluation. Selection of the appropriate assessment tools should be based upon the patient's current disease status and the fitness component of interest. For patients starting an exercise program, disease status can be categorized into three groups according to the following guidelines: 1) recovering from an intercurrent illness or medical event, 2) medically stable and sedentary, or 3) medically stable and active. Fitness components, including cardiorespiratory endurance, body composition, flexibility, muscle endurance, muscle strength, and physical function need to be evaluated using different protocols and modes based on the patient's status. Table 17.2 summarizes recommendations for assessment of physical fitness and function in the HIV population based on the criteria described in this section.

Protocols for assessments are described in detail in the ACSM Guidelines for Exercise Testing and Prescription. Research-based protocols for estimating cardiovascular endurance, functional status, and muscular endurance are also appropriate. These protocols, the 6-minute walk distance, 10–chair-stand time, and the modified 60-second sit-up test, require minimal equipment, are easy to administer, and are highly reproducible (32–34).

The 6-minute walk distance provides a measure of cardiovascular endurance (32). This protocol can be administered using two methods. Patients may walk back and forth in an unobstructed flat area such as a long corridor or follow a circular path along a corridor for 6 minutes. Patients are instructed to walk as fast as possible for 6 minutes, with verbal encouragement given every 30 seconds. The tester rolls a measuring wheel that records distance to the nearest meter just behind the subject during the test (Redi Measure, Redington, Windsor, CT). This assessment may also be conducted along a course of known distance, e.g., a track or measured path of corridors. The tester can

Table 17.2. Assessment of Physical Fitness and Function by Disease Status

FITNESS COMPONENT	PATIENT DISEASE STATUS		
	RECOVERING	STABLE/SEDENTARY	STABLE/ACTIVE
Cardiorespiratory Endurance	6-minute walk	6-minute walk Submaximal exercise[1] Maximal exercise[1]	Submaximal exercise[1] Maximal exercise[1]
Body Composition	Triceps Skinfold Midarm Circumference Thigh Circum. Waist-hip ratio	Triceps Skinfold Midarm Circumference Thigh Circum. Waist-hip ratio	Triceps Skinfold Midarm Circumference Thigh Circum. Waist-hip ratio
Flexibility	Sit-and-reach test[1]	Sit-and-reach test[1]	Sit-and-reach test[1]
Muscular Endurance	6-minute walk	Modified 1-minute sit-up test	1-minute sit-up test[1]
Muscular Strength	1-RM[1]	1-RM[1]	1-RM[1]
Physical Function	10-chair-stand time	10-chair-stand time	Submaximal exercise[1] Maximal exercise[1]

[1]American College of Sports Medicine. ACSM's guidelines for exercise testing and prescription. 5th ed. Baltimore: Williams & Wilkins, 1995.

calculate the distance walked in 6 minutes based on the number of cycles and/or partial cycles of the course completed by the patient.

The 10–chair-stand time, performance of rapid chair rising, incorporates strength, balance power, and mobility skills and has been shown to be associated with self-reported disability and future institutionalization in older adults (33). This protocol is performed with a sturdy chair (standard seat height of 17 inches from the floor) placed against the wall to prevent movement during the test. The patient begins the assessment in the seated position with feet shoulder width apart and upper back against the chair pad, arms crossed over the chest. On the command "ready, go," the patient leans forward slightly and stands as quickly as possible from the seated position to full knee extension and returns to the starting position. This sequence is repeated for 10 repetitions, as fast as possible, with the 10th repetition counted in the standing position. Two trials separated by 5 minutes' rest may be performed to account for a learning effect, and the fastest time is used as the assessment value. It is beneficial for the tester to demonstrate the proper chair-stand technique to the patient and allow the patient to perform one chair stand prior to the timed test.

A modified 1-minute sit-up test has been developed to measure muscular endurance in the HIV patient population (34). The standard protocol has been adapted so that the patient performs abdominal crunches instead of full sit-ups to accommodate the physical limitations of the sedentary HIV patient. The patient begins the assessment in the supine position with the arms crossed over the chest and the fingertips touching the shoulders, with knees bent and feet flat on the exercise mat, with the tester holding the patient's ankles. The patient flexes his trunk, moving his chest toward his thighs until his elbows touch his thighs. One sit-up is counted each time the patient returns to the supine (starting) position with his shoulder blades in complete contact with the exercise mat. The patient performs as many modified sit-ups as possible during 1 minute, with verbal encouragement from the tester.

Periodic assessments should be performed to evaluate the efficacy of the exercise prescription and to facilitate individualized exercise programming on an on-going basis. In a clinical setting, it may be appropriate to perform assessment of physical fitness frequently, e.g., 3–4 times per year. In a fitness center or community health setting, it may only be feasible to perform these measures biannually or annually.

EXERCISE PRESCRIPTION AND PROGRAMMING

The optimal exercise prescription for the individual is based on many factors that include the medical history, current health status, fitness history, current fitness participation, and health-related fitness goals. As noted earlier, it is critical that each HIV patient be evaluated on an individualized basis. The patient, physician, and other healthcare professionals involved must carefully select and monitor the mode, intensity, and volume of the exercise prescription to optimize the patient's outcome. Research supports the following general exercise prescription that focuses on two modalities: PRT and cardiovascular endurance training.

PRT develops muscular strength and size with little or no increase in cardiovascular endurance. PRT is based on the overload principle of placing progressively greater-than-normal demands on the exercising musculature over time. The greatest gains in strength occur when muscle actions generate force against a near-maximal level of resistance. For example, muscle actions that generate force against resistance that causes fatigue after only a few contractions, approximately 80% 1-RM or greater or 5–8 contractions, result in increased muscle strength (35).

PRT has also been shown to induce muscle hypertrophy in both diseased and healthy subjects (8, 12). This increase in muscle size correlates with an increase in contractile protein content. Previous research has shown that HIV-infected individuals are able to increase protein synthetic rate and reverse the loss of muscle protein after participating in a strength-training exercise program (4).

PRT Prescription

A basic PRT prescription for patients with HIV infection, wasting, and lipodystrophy is described in Table 17.3. This periodized program is 1 year in duration and consists of three unique phases. Each phase is 4 months in duration and includes a unique exercise prescription. Six exercises targeting the large muscle groups of the entire body have been selected, with special consideration given to balancing strength between opposing muscle groups. Exercises for the lower extremity are emphasized due to the relatively higher proportion of muscle mass and functional significance. Exercises are performed in an order that alternates between the lower and upper body. This approach allows for adequate intraexercise session rest and may contribute to improved muscle strength and endurance.

The frequency of training is fixed at three times per week for approximately 45 minutes per session throughout the duration of the study. Exercise sessions should be separated by a minimum of 48 hours' rest. The resistance training session should be preceded by a 5-minute warm-up period using an aerobic mode, e.g., walking, stationary bicycle, stair stepper, treadmill, or rowing ergometer.

All resistance exercises can be performed using resistance machines, free weights, and/or body weight. Proper exercise technique is defined as movement in a controlled manner, using a two-count concentric movement and a four-count eccentric movement, to ensure proper and effective overload of the muscle. During each phase, the initial exercise intensity is low, 60–65% 1-RM, and will be based on

Table 17.3. One-Year PRT Prescription for Patients with HIV Wasting and Lipodystrophy

Mode:	Resistance machines, free weights, body weight			
Frequency:	Three times per week			
Intensity:	60–80% 1-RM			
Duration:	1 year, three phases			
Time:	45 minutes			
Exercise:	Selection varies by phase			
Phase I	Leg extension, chest press, knee flexion, seated row, leg press, pelvic tilt			
	Week 1	Week 2	Week 3	Week 4
Month 1	1 set × 8 reps 60–65% 1-RM	2 sets × 8 reps 60–65% 1-RM	3 sets × 8 reps 65–70% 1-RM	3 sets × 8 reps 65–70% 1-RM
Month 2	3 sets × 8 reps 70–75% 1-RM	3 sets × 8 reps 70–75% 1-RM	3 sets × 8 reps 75–80% 1-RM	2 sets × 8 reps 65–70% 1-RM
Month 3	3 sets × 8 reps 75–80% 1-RM	3 sets × 8 reps 75–80% 1-RM	3 sets × 8 reps 75–80% 1-RM	3 sets × 8 reps 75–80% 1-RM
Month 4	2 sets × 8 reps 65–70% 1-RM	3 sets × 8 reps 75–80% 1-RM	3 sets × 8 reps 75–80% 1-RM	3 sets × 8 reps 75–80% 1-RM
Active Rest	1 week			
Phase II	Squat, incline chest press, step-up, assisted pull-up, assisted dip, abdominal crunch			
	Week 1	Week 2	Week 3	Week 4
Month 1	1 set × 8 reps 60–65% 1-RM	2 sets × 8 reps 60–65% 1-RM	3 sets × 8 reps 65–70% 1-RM	3 sets × 8 reps 65–70% 1-RM
Month 2	3 sets × 8 reps 70–75% 1-RM	3 sets × 8 reps 70–75% 1-RM	3 sets × 8 reps 75–80% 1-RM	2 sets × 8 reps 65–70% 1-RM
Month 3	3 sets × 8 reps 75–80% 1-RM	3 sets × 8 reps 75–80% 1-RM	3 sets × 8 reps 75–80% 1-RM	3 sets × 8 reps 75–80% 1-RM
Month 4	2 sets × 8 reps 65–70% 1-RM	3 sets × 8 reps 75–80% 1-RM	3 sets × 8 reps 75–80% 1-RM	3 sets × 8 reps 75–80% 1-RM
Active Rest	1 week			
Phase III	Leg press, chest fly, knee extension, lat pull-down, knee flexion, lateral abdominal flexion			
	Week 1	Week 2	Week 3	Week 4
Month 1	1 set × 10 reps 60–65% 1-RM	2 sets × 10 reps 60–65% 1-RM	3 sets × 10 reps 65–70% 1-RM	3 sets × 10 reps 65–70% 1-RM
Month 2	3 sets × 10 reps 70–75% 1-RM	3 sets × 10 reps 70–75% 1-RM	3 sets × 10 reps 75–80% 1-RM	2 sets × 10 reps 65–70% 1-RM
Month 3	3 sets × 10 reps 75–80% 1-RM	3 sets × 10 reps 75–80% 1-RM	3 sets × 10 reps 75–80% 1-RM	3 sets × 10 reps 75–80% 1-RM
Month 4	2 sets × 10 reps 65–70% 1-RM	3 sets × 10 reps 75–80% 1-RM	3 sets × 10 reps 75–80% 1-RM	3 sets × 10 reps 75–80% 1-RM

the individual's maximal strength test results and training experience. During month two, exercise intensity should progress from moderate to high, 70–80% 1-RM. Intensity will remain relatively high, between 75–80% 1-RM for the remainder of the phase. Two weeks of reduced intensity and volume are incorporated at weeks 8 and 13 to minimize the risk of injury and overtraining that has been shown to increase infection and worsen immune indices in humans (10). Each resistance training session ends with a 5-minute cool-down period consisting of stretching and flexibility exercises. The three resistance training phases will be separated by 1 week of active rest. The patients will not perform any resistance training during this time but are instructed to maintain an active lifestyle.

It is recommended that physiologists and trainers perform periodic assessment of 1-RM to evaluate the patient's progress and provide feedback. With adequate adherence, strength will increase over time. One-RM strength must be reevaluated to ensure that the correct maximum load is used to calculate training intensity and maintain adequate intensity of the training stimulus. For example, if a patient's baseline 1-RM for a given exercise is 100 lb and training intensity is at 80% 1-RM, the training load will be 80 lb. After the patient completes 4 months of PRT, his/her 1-RM may increase to 125 lb or a training load of 100 lb at 80% 1-RM. Between 1-RM retests, the Relative Perceived Exertion (RPE) scale should be used to maintain the intensity of exercise in the desired range. Depending on where in the cycle the person is, the goal is an RPE of 15–18 out of 20 at the end of each set.

Aerobic Training Prescription

Aerobic exercise is defined as muscle contraction against little or no resistance, which can be performed for an extended period of time (35). The data indicate that aerobic exercise can decrease fat mass, especially when combined with a hypocaloric diet. Increase in aerobic endurance depends on the frequency, intensity, and duration of an exercise regimen (35). A basic aerobic training prescription for patients with lipodystrophy is described in Table 17.4. This periodized program is 1 year in duration and consists of three unique phases, each 4 months in duration. The frequency of training will remain fixed at three times per week over the course of the year. The patient's preferred mode of exercise, e.g., stationary bike, treadmill, stair stepper, or rowing ergometer, may be used throughout the year, or he/she may vary the exercise mode by phase. The amount of time required for the aerobic training protocol increases from 15 to 25 minutes over each phase. The intensity of training also increases from 65% to 85% of heart rate reserve (HRR) as each phase progresses. Patients should use heart rate monitors to ensure that they exercise at the prescribed target heart rate. The aerobic training protocol may be performed before or after the resistance training protocol or on alternate days of the week. The combined PRT and aerobic training prescriptions can be completed in approximately 1 hour to 1 hour and 15 minutes. Periodic assessment of cardiorespiratory function may be performed to evaluate the patient's progress and provide feedback and updated information for calculating training intensity.

Table 17.4. Cardiovascular Training Program for HIV Lipodystrophy

Mode:	Bicycle, treadmill walking or running, stair-stepper machine, elliptical machine, rowing ergometer			
Frequency:	Three times per week			
Intensity:	65–85% HRR			
Duration:	1 year, three phases			
Time:	15–25 minutes			
Phase I	Bicycle, treadmill walking or running, stair-stepper machine, elliptical machine, rowing ergometer			
	Total time	Warm-up	Target HRR	Cool-down
Month 1	15 min.	5 min.	5 min. at target 65–70% HRR	5 min.
Month 2	20 min.	5 min.	10 min. at target 70–75% HRR	5 min.
Month 3	25 min.	5 min.	15 min. at target 75–80% HRR	5 min.
Month 4	25 min.	5 min.	15 min. at target 80–85% HRR	5 min.
Active Rest	1 week			
Phase II	Bicycle, treadmill walking or running, stair-stepper machine, elliptical machine, rowing ergometer			
	Total time	Warm-up	Target HRR	Cool-down
Month 1	15 min.	5 min.	5 min. at target 65–70% HRR	5 min.
Month 2	20 min.	5 min.	10 min. at target 70–75% HRR	5 min.
Month 3	25 min.	5 min.	15 min. at target 75–80% HRR	5 min.
Month 4	25 min.	5 min.	15 min. at target 80–85% HRR	5 min.
Active Rest	1 week			
Phase III	Bicycle, treadmill walking or running, stair-stepper machine, elliptical machine, rowing ergometer			
	Total time	Warm-up	Target HRR	Cool-down
Month 1	15 min.	5 min.	5 min. at target 65–70% HRR	5 min.
Month 2	20 min.	5 min.	10 min. at target 70–75% HRR	5 min.
Month 3	25 min.	5 min.	15 min. at target 75–80% HRR	5 min.
Month 4	25 min.	5 min.	15 min. at target 80–85% HRR	5 min.

HIV Wasting

The primary goal of exercise interventions for patients with HIV wasting is to maintain or increase body weight, lean body mass, muscle strength, and functional status. Based upon the current level of research in the HIV-infected population, PRT is the preferred modality and the only nonpharmacologic, physiologic way to increase protein rate of synthesis, muscle mass, and strength to offset the loss of muscle mass that occurs with wasting (12). It is important to maintain energy balance in patients with wasting. The energy expended through exercise should be accompanied by increased energy intake to prevent negative energy balance and further wasting.

Patients should be seen by a dietitian to ensure that their dietary intake is adequate. In general, protein intake should be 12–18% of total energy (1.0–1.5 g/kg protein/day), and 25–30% of calories should come from fat, with 8–9% each from saturated, monounsaturated, and polyunsaturated fats. If the goal is weight gain, total energy intake can be increased by increasing fat content in the diet to 35% of calories. The remaining calories should come from complex carbohydrates, with high intake of fiber, fruits, and vegetables as recommended for all adults (36).

Lipodystrophy

The primary goal of an exercise intervention for patients with lipodystrophy is to optimize body composition and offset the potential deleterious health effects associated with central adiposity. A combination of PRT and cardiovascular endurance training is recommended for patients with lipodystrophy. PRT has been shown to decrease fat mass in HIV-infected individuals, in addition to the benefits of increasing muscle mass, strength, and functional status as described with HIV wasting (12).

Aerobic training is incorporated in the exercise program to help decrease abdominal fat mass and may potentially improve immune function. Previous research has shown aerobic exercise to increase insulin sensitivity and muscle glucose transporter (GLUT-4) levels, which may be important to patients experiencing fat redistribution. There has been some epidemiological evidence that suggests that cardiorespiratory fitness is positively associated with increased immune status and survival time in HIV-infected men (11). However, it is important to consider that research has shown that HIV-infected subjects exercise to a lower peak workload and have lower minute ventilation and maximal oxygen consumption versus controls (HIV seronegative) (17). Thus, incorporating aerobic and resistance training should optimize the fat-reducing and muscle-enhancing benefits of both, thus having the maximal impact on the lipid and glucose disorders at the heart of lipodystrophy.

Promoting Exercise Adherence

Despite the numerous benefits of exercise in both health and disease such as HIV infection, long-term adherence to an exercise program is often difficult to achieve. Several factors must be taken into consideration to effectively promote adoption and adherence to an exercise program in HIV-infected individuals, including the influence of prior behavioral, social, and psychological factors. Research has shown that continued substance abuse, fear of treatment side effects, practical inconvenience, and depression may be potential factors increasing noncompliance to exercise interventions in this population (37). Strategies to enhance compliance include involvement of the entire healthcare team to incorporate counseling, education, and behavior modification techniques that stress the benefits of partaking in an exercise program. It is imperative that the exercise physiologist provide encouragement, promote proper exercise technique, and assist with both the intensity level and progression of the regimen (12). Ongoing assessments should be made by all members of the healthcare team to better understand and document each individual's progress.

Exercise logs should be used to assess each individual's compliance with the exercise intervention. During each training session, individuals should record all exercise completed, the weight lifted, the number of repetitions and sets, and if applicable, the number of minutes of aerobic exercise completed. Each week, the trainer should review the log of each individual and discuss the progress of the training program with each individual.

Precautions

As HIV infection progresses, the number and functional effects of CD4+ T lymphocytes decreases. Opportunistic infections are likely to develop due to low levels of these T-helper cells (38, 39). The immune system becomes more compromised over time, and patients develop fevers, lymphadenopathy, fatigue, and weight loss. They are also extremely susceptible to many secondary infections such as PCP, mycobacterium avium-intracellulare, lymphoma, and Kaposi's sarcoma, any of which may be fatal. These, along with other HIV-associated illnesses and symptoms, lead to a decrease in physical activity and deconditioning, and loss of both aerobic capacity and muscle strength, resulting in a need for an exercise intervention to reverse this downward spiral.

Some subjects may have concerns about participating in an exercise program because of low CD4+ cell counts. MacArthur et al. found a positive correlation between CD4 cell count and compliance with an exercise intervention (17). Those subjects with the highest CD4 cell count had the highest compliance with the training protocol. There was also an increase in VO_2 in those HIV-infected subjects who completed the 24-week training protocol. The mechanism by which exercise directly affects CD4 cell counts is unknown, but it is likely that at the time of MacArthur et al.'s study, low CD4 cell count was a surrogate for poor health status. The same is not necessarily true today, but low CD4 cell counts should be an indicator to the exercise professional that the patient may be relatively frail and exercise intensity should be adjusted accordingly. Some studies found that aerobic plus resistance exercise had no effect on CD4 or total lymphocyte counts, while others found that aerobic exercise conditioning caused an increase in CD4 cell counts (15, 39). A proposed mechanism for the changes in immunologic status includes hormonal effects such as changes in cortisol and adrenaline levels (39).

In the case of intercurrent illness, the entire healthcare team's recommendations should be considered when deciding to discontinue or restart exercise regimens. It should be stressed that exercise training should begin as soon as the patient's health status allows. However, it is of equal importance to balance the exercise intensity so it is low enough to avoid injury, but high enough to stimulate the muscles, heart, and lungs and improve overall function.

Aside from a low CD4 cell count as a possible precaution to exercise, programs and testing should not be performed when the patient has a fever higher than 100 degrees or any acute symptom such as nausea, vomiting, uncontrolled diarrhea, or dehydration. The involvement of the entire healthcare team is essential to each individual's success.

EDUCATION AND COUNSELING

The initiation of an exercise program must take into account the significant alteration of an individual's routine, along with health status and general limitations. One must consider that many people with HIV may have had no prior exercise training and this will be a significant lifestyle change. For this population, some common barriers to adhering to an exercise program include lack of transportation, motivation, drug/alcohol abuse, family matters, and economic difficulties. In addition, some HIV-infected individuals may be reluctant due to confidentiality or unwillingness to disclose of their disease status, or they may be uncomfortable with their body image if lipodystrophy or wasting has occurred.

Unfortunately, some healthcare practitioners are only recommending minimal exercise, if any at all, despite evidence that clearly shows its physiological and psychological benefits. A goal for all those in the healthcare field should be education regarding the use of both aerobic exercise and PRT as therapies in primary healthcare promotion for HIV-infected individuals.

CONCLUSIONS

It appears that exercise interventions are safe and beneficial for patients with HIV infection. The current scientific research provides compelling evidence that exercise is important and beneficial, may increase quality of life, and should be an integral part of treatment for patients in all phases of HIV infection. To reiterate, HIV-positive status should not be a deterrent to begin an exercise program; rather, it should be reason to do so. As stated earlier, the key to the optimal exercise prescription is balancing energy expenditure and intensity with each individual's current condition, and periodic assessments are crucial to maintain an appropriate regimen.

With body composition changes (i.e., wasting, lipodystrophy) becoming more pronounced as pharmacological treatments evolve, exercise prescription should be seen as an integral aspect to this lifelong therapy of combating HIV. However, there needs to be more clinical research to further understand these body composition changes associated with current medications. Recommending PRT for individuals with wasting and PRT plus aerobic training for individuals with lipodystrophy remains appropriate; however, as this topic is further explored, more data may lead to further modifications in exercise prescription.

Moreover, if health professionals can encourage patients to exercise while asymptomatic, patients may be able to maintain a stronger, more infection-resistant immune system and maintain their strength and protein reserves during an illness. This in turn may assist recovery from secondary opportunistic infections. The benefits of exercise for those infected with HIV are extremely promising, but much work remains before they can truly be applied to the entire population of HIV-infected adults.

References

1. Centers for Disease Control and Prevention. 1993 revised classification system for HIV infection and expanded surveillance case definition for AIDS among adolescents and adults. *MMWR* 1993;41:1–19.
2. Kotler DP, Tierney AR, Pierson RN. Magnitude of body cell mass depletion and the timing of death from wasting in AIDS. *Am J Clin Nutr* 1989;50:444–447.
3. Guenter P, Muurahainen N, Simons G. Relationships among nutritional status, disease progression, and survival in HIV infection. *J Acquir Immune Defic Syndr Hum Retrovirol* 1993;6: 1130–1138.
4. Carr A, Samaras K, Chisholm DJ, et al. Pathogenesis of HIV-1-protease inhibitor-associated peripheral lipodystrophy, hyperlipidemia, and insulin resistance. *Lancet* 1998;352:1881–1883.
5. Carr A, Samaras K, Thorisdottir A, et al. Diagnosis, prediction, and natural course of HIV-1 protease-inhibitor-associated lipodystrophy, hyperlipidemia, and diabetes mellitus: a cohort study. *Lancet* 1999;353:2093–2099.
6. Engelson ES, Kotler DP, Tan YX, et al. Fat distribution in HIV-infected patients reporting truncal enlargement quantified by whole-body magnetic resonance imaging. *Am J Clin Nutr* 1999;69:1162–1169.
7. Walli R, Herfort O, Michl GM, et al. Treatment with protease inhibitors associated with peripheral insulin resistance and impaired oral glucose tolerance in HIV-1–infected patients. *AIDS* 1998;12:F167–F173.
8. Spence DW, Galantino ML, Mossberg KA, et al. Progressive resistance exercise: effect on muscle function and anthropometry of a select AIDS population. *Arch Phys Med Rehabil* 1990;71:644–648.
9. Roubenoff R. Exercise and HIV infection. In: Miller TL,

Gorbach SL, eds. *Nutritional aspects of HIV infection*. London: Arnold, 1999.

10. Stringer WW, Berezovskaya M, O'Brien WA, et al. The effect of exercise training on aerobic fitness, immune indices, and quality of life in HIV+ patients. *Med Sci Sports Exerc* 1998;30: 11–16.
11. Rigsby LW, Dishman RK, Jackson AW, et al. Effects of exercise training on men seropositive for the human immunodeficiency virus-1. *Med Sci Sports Exerc* 1992;24:6–12.
12. Roubenoff R, McDermott A, Weiss L, et al. Short-term progressive resistance training increases strength and lean body mass in adults infected with human immunodeficiency virus. *AIDS* 1999;13:231–239.
13. Nieman DC. Immune response to heavy exertion. *J Appl Physiol* 1997;82:1385–1394.
14. Cannon JG. Exercise and resistance to infection. *J Appl Physiol* 1993;74:973–981.
15. Roubenoff R, Skolnik PR, Shevitz AH, et al. The effect of a single bout of acute exercise on plasma human immunodeficiency virus RNA levels. *J Appl Physiol* 1999;86:1197–1201.
16. Johnson JE, Anders GT, Blanton HM, et al. Exercise dysfunction in patients seropositive for the human immunodeficiency virus. *Am Rev Resp Dis* 1990;141:618–622.
17. MacArthur RD, Levine SD, Birk TJ. Supervised exercise training improves cardiopulmonary fitness in HIV-infected persons. *Med Sci Sports Exerc* 1993;25:684–688.
18. LaPerriere A, Fletcher MA, Antoni MH, et al. Aerobic exercise training in an AIDS risk group. *Int J Sports Med* 1991;12: S53–S57.
19. Schambelan M, Mulligan K, Grunfeld C, et al. Recombinant human growth hormone in patients with HIV-associated wasting. *Ann Intern Med* 1996;125:873–882.
20. Grinspoon S, Corcoran C, Askari H, et al. Effects of androgen administration in men with the AIDS wasting syndrome: a randomized, double-blind, placebo-controlled trial. *Ann Intern Med* 1998;129:18–26.
21. Gold J, High HA, Li Y, et al. Safety and efficacy of nandrolone decanoate for treatment of wasting in patients with HIV infection. *AIDS* 1996;10:745–752.
22. Ware JE, Kosinski M, Gandek B. *The SF-36 health survey: manual and interpretation guide*. Boston: The Health Institute, New England Medical Center, 1993.
23. Roubenoff R, Weiss L, McDermott A, et al. A pilot study of exercise training to reduce trunk fat in adults with HIV-associated fat redistribution. *AIDS* 1999;13:1373–1375.
24. Sattler FR, Jaque SV, Schroeder ET, et al. Effects of pharmacological doses of nandrolone decanoate and progressive resistance training in immunodeficient patients infected with human immunodeficiency virus. *J Clin Endocrinol Metab* 1999;84:1268–1276.
25. Strawford A, Barbieri T, van Loan M, et al. Resistance exercise and supraphysiologic androgen therapy in eugonadal men with HIV-related weight loss. A randomized controlled trial. *JAMA* 1999;281:1282–1290.
26. Corcoran C, Grinspoon S. Treatments for wasting in patients with the acquired immunodeficiency syndrome. *N Engl J Med* 1999;340:1740–1748.
27. Von Roenn JH, Armstrong D, Kotler DP, et al. Megestrol acetate in patients with AIDS-related cachexia. *Ann Intern Med* 1994;121:393–399.
28. Roubenoff R. Applications of bioelectrical impedance analysis for body composition to epidemiologic studies. *Am J Clin Nutr* 1996;64:459S–462S.
29. Earthman CP, Matthie JR, Reid PM, et al. A comparison of bioimpedance methods for detection of body cell mass change in HIV infection. *J Appl Physiol* 2000;88:944–956.
30. Wu AW, Hays RD, Kelly S, et al. Applications of the Medical Outcomes Study health-related quality of life measures to HIV/AIDS. *Qual Life Res* 1997;6:531–554.
31. Wu AW, Revicki DA, Jacobson D, et al. Evidence for reliability, validity, and usefulness of the Medical Outcomes Study HIV Health Survey (MOS-HIV). *Qual Life Res* 1997;6:481–493.
32. Lipkin D, Scriven A, Crake T, et al. Six minute walking test for assessing exercise capacity in chronic heart failure. *Br Med J* 1986;292:653–655.
33. Guralnik J. Epese short physical performance battery. *Geri Notes* 1998;5:18–19.
34. *ACSM's guidelines for exercise testing and prescription*. 6th edition. Philadelphia: Lippincott Williams & Wilkins, 2000.
35. Fleck SJ, Kraemer WJ. *Designing resistance training programs*. 2nd ed. Champaign, IL: Human Kinetics Press, 1997.
36. USDA, USDHHS. *Nutrition and your health: dietary guidelines for Americans*. 3rd ed. Washington, DC: U.S. Government Printing Office, 1990.
37. Perna FM, LaPerriere AR, Klimas N, et al. Cardiopulmonary and CD4 cell changes in response to exercise training in early symptomatic HIV+ patients. *Med Sci Sports Exerc* 1999; 31:973–979.
38. Roubenoff R, Rall LC. Cytokine mediators of metabolic changes in HIV infection. In: Miller TL, Gorbach SL, eds. *Nutritional aspects of HIV infection*. London: Arnold, 1999.
39. Eichner ER, Calabrese LH. Immunology and exercise: physiology, pathophysiology, and implications for HIV infection. *Sports Med* 1994;78:377–388.

CHAPTER **18**

Chronic Fatigue Syndrome

John J. LaManca and Sue Ann Sisto

EPIDEMIOLOGY AND PATHOPHYSIOLOGY

A cluster of symptoms and signs of abnormal functioning that have no discernible medical cause define chronic fatigue syndrome (CFS). The major patient-reported symptom is a prolonged and debilitating feeling of fatigue that is not improved with rest and is often worsened after even minimal mental or physical stress.

The source of the term CFS arose out of four reports in the first half of the 1980s concerning patients suffering from a chronic and recurring complex of symptoms of unknown origin that included severe fatigue, fever, tender lymph nodes, sore throat, decreased memory, confusion, and depression (1–4). Preliminary clinical serological investigation revealed that many patients exhibited antibody profiles consistent with mononucleosis-associated Epstein-Barr virus (EBV) infection. This illness came to be called the chronic EBV syndrome or the chronic mononucleosis-like syndrome. Data from two subsequent scientific investigations cast doubt on EBV as the syndrome's etiology by indicating that these patients would be just as likely to have serological profiles consistent with infections by cytomegalovirus, herpes simplex virus types 1 and 2, or the measles virus (5, 6).

Case Definition of CFS

In 1988, researchers and physicians were assembled by the U.S. Centers for Disease Control and Prevention (CDC) to formulate a working case definition for the syndrome discussed above. To prevent premature association with a particular etiology, they named it the chronic fatigue syndrome. According to this definition, a diagnosis of CFS can be made if a patient exhibits a new onset of severe fatigue that has persisted or relapsed for at least 6 months, caused at least a 50% reduction in premorbid activity, and cannot be attributed to known medical conditions. The patient must also exhibit eight or more of the following symptoms: mild fever, sore throat, painful lymph nodes, muscle weakness, myalgia, severe fatigue after mild exercise, headaches, migratory arthralgia, neuropsychological complaints, sleep disturbance, and sudden onset of symptoms. This case definition excluded diagnosis of CFS if there was any present or history of psychiatric disease or personality disorder (7).

This working case definition was established to help identify the illness and to provide guidelines for investigators concerned with its possible etiology and pathology. Case definitions were also developed in Britain (8) and Australia (9) that are similar but do differ somewhat from the 1988 CDC definition. The British or, as it is often referred to, the Oxford definition does not put as much emphasis on a list of specific symptoms that must accompany the fatigue but instead emphasizes the possible presence of both mental and physical fatigue (8). They realized that in many patients, psychological symptoms such as depression, anxiety, and loss of interest cannot explain the severe fatigue reported and may actually have developed as a result of the chronic illness. Therefore, unlike the CDC 1988 case definition, the Oxford guidelines do not exclude for many psychological conditions (8).

In 1991, the National Institutes of Health (NIH) convened a workshop to examine the state of CFS research and to evaluate the effectiveness of the case definition. They concluded that revisions should be made in the CDC guidelines to accommodate for the premorbid and comorbid presence of certain psychiatric disorders, diseases, or syndromes. Also, they recommended specific laboratory and psychological tests to help rule out for known causes of fatigue (10).

An international working group including representatives from the CDC, NIH, United States, Britain, and Australia convened in 1994 to amend the CDC case definition and research guidelines. The result was the most recent CDC case definition (11). Here, a diagnosis of CFS is established " . . . *by the presence of the following: 1) clinically evaluated, unexplained, persistent or relapsing chronic fatigue that is of new or definite onset (has not been lifelong); is not the result of ongoing exertion; is not substantially alleviated by rest; and results in substantial reduction in previous levels of occupational, educational, social, or personal activities; and 2) the concurrent occurrence of four or more of the following symptoms, all of which must have persisted or recurred during 6 or more consecutive months of illness and must not have predated the fatigue: self-reported impairment in short-term memory or concentration severe enough to cause substantial reduction in previous levels of occupational, educational, social, or personal activities; sore throat; tender cervical or axially lymph nodes; muscle pain, multi joint pain without joint swelling or redness; headaches of a new type, pattern, or severity; unrefreshing sleep; and postexertional malaise lasting more than 24 hours"* (11; page 956).

Theories of Etiology and Pathophysiology

All of the above CFS case definitions still appear in the scientific literature, and since their formulations, volumes of data from research studies investigating possible etiologies of CFS have been published, but a definitive cause or marker has not been identified. Therefore, it is somewhat difficult to separate the etiology and pathophysiology of this illness.

As discussed earlier, the first suspected etiology of CFS was a viral or bacterial infection. This theory originated from patients reporting that fatigue symptoms started suddenly after a "flu-like" illness that included a low-grade fever and swollen glands. Many other viruses have been suspected, such as human herpesvirus-6 (HHV-6), which often becomes latent after early infection, can be reactivated, and affects a number of body systems. Recently, both multiple sclerosis (70%) and CFS (57%) patients were found to have higher HHV-6 blood antibody levels when compared to healthy controls (16%) (12). Also, retroviruses and enteroviruses have been implicated within subsets of CFS patients. However, there has been no evidence presented for these infectious agents that shows an association with CFS (13, 14). A multitude of viruses and bacteria have been investigated, but positive findings in this area remain isolated. To date, no single infectious organism has been found consistently in CFS patients such that it would be considered a marker for the illness.

Because so many different viral agents have been implicated in CFS and patients seem to have an exaggerated response to infections, many theorize that an abnormal immune system may be the origin of CFS. There are data that support a possible chronic immune activation (15) and/or an insufficient immune response in CFS patients (16). Many researchers contend that the evidence of chronic immune abnormalities in CFS patients that is based upon lymphocyte cell surface markers is relatively consistent (17). Most often reported are abnormal CD8+ cytotoxic T-cell activation (15) and a depression of natural killer cell activity (16). However, others have reported no abnormal blood concentration or activation of lymphocyte cell surface markers in CFS (18).

Evidence of cytokine abnormalities in CFS patients has been even more conflicting. Several authors have reported immune activation associated with interleukins (i.e., IL-1, IL-2, IL-4, and IL-6) and tumor-necrosis factor, as well as other cytokines (17). However, others have not been able to find a difference in the cytokine levels in CFS patients when compared to healthy control subjects (19). Data have been presented that support an upregulation of the pathways involved in the antiviral activity of interferon, specifically the 2–5A synthetase/ribonuclease L pathway in CFS patients. Some have suggested that the presence of a low-molecular-weight protein in this pathway may be a possible marker for CFS (20). Still, many researchers feel that the etiological evidence for an immune irregularity in CFS has been just as nonspecific as that which has been presented for an infectious agent. They suggest that CFS is a disease arising out of what may be many etiological agents (19).

Neuroendocrine abnormalities have also been implicated in the etiology of CFS. The research here has centered primarily around the hypothalamic-pituitary-adrenal axis (HPA). The HPA is considered the primary axis in response to both physical and psychological stress. Deficiency of glucocorticoids released by the adrenal gland can result in fatigue, and evidence has been presented of low glucocorticoid levels in the blood and urine of CFS patients (21). Also, adrenal glands in CFS patients have been shown to have low secretory reserve when stimulated with exogenous doses of adrenocorticotrophic hormone (ACTH) and to be reduced in size (22). Furthermore, data have shown a blunted release of ACTH from the anterior pituitary when stimulated with doses of corticotrophin-releasing hormone (CRH), which seems to indicate that the hyporesponsiveness of the HPA is central in origin (21). However, as with other theorized etiologies of CFS, the data here are inconsistent because there are many reports of no HPA hypoactivity in CFS patients (23).

Because the symptoms of CFS are so heterogeneous and the illness seems to affect numerous body functions, many speculate that the neural system must be involved either as a primary or secondary cause. Magnetic resonance imaging (MRI) has shown significantly more abnormalities in the cerebral white matter of CFS patients when compared to healthy subjects (24). Single-photon-emission computed tomography (SPECT) studies have demonstrated brain-stem hypoperfusion and decreased regional cerebral blood flow in CFS patients (25). The exact significance and origin of these MRI and SPECT abnormalities are subject for debate. Peripherally decreased motor evoked potentials have been reported in CFS following exercise (26), and gait abnormalities have been seen in CFS patients (27).

Investigations of the autonomic nervous system have revealed both parasympathetic and sympathetic abnormalities in CFS patients, while others have reported normal autonomic activity. Prominent in this area are reports indicating a high percentage (90%) of CFS patients who exhibit neurally mediated hypotension (NMH) during tilt-table testing (28). These reports have triggered major treatment trials for NMH in CFS. However, data have shown that the percentage of CFS patients with orthostatic intolerance during tilt-table testing was not significantly higher when compared to a group of healthy but physically inactive control subjects (29). Furthermore, even when NMH is treated, CFS patients may indicate that they are somewhat better but not back to a premorbid level of functioning (30).

Psychological factors are significantly involved in the etiology or pathophysiology of many CFS cases. Some physicians feel that CFS patients are suffering from primary psychiatric disorders or psycho-physiological reactions. Suggested psychological causes of chronic fatigue include depression, anxiety disorder, somatization disorder, and dysthymia and grief (31). A high premorbid and comorbid incidence of these disorders is associated with CFS. For example, comorbid major depression has been indicated in 50% of CFS patients (31). In some investigations, 66% have been found to have a history of major depression at sometime during their lives (31). This may not be unusual due to significant lifestyle disruption. One can argue that comorbid presence of symptoms of depression does not necessarily indicate a cause for fatigue, since these symptoms can be a result of being chronically ill and physically compromised. Also, it has been pointed out that the biological abnormalities found in depression are different from those found in CFS. Furthermore, a significant number of CFS patients have no indication of psychopathology (32).

The proposed etiologies and pathologies discussed above are just a sample of the many reported in the medical and scientific literature concerned with CFS. Also, several unifying theories of the origins of CFS have been suggested, but to date, none are supported by enough clinical evidence to be validated as the true etiology.

Prevalence and Incidence

Because there is no definitive marker for CFS, estimates of incidence in the general population are difficult to make and must be approached with caution. Physicians in four U.S. cities were asked to refer patients complaining of severe unexplained fatigue persisting for 6 months to a CDC surveillance system; 26% of these patients met criteria for the case definition of CFS (33). The estimated rate of CFS in the general population of the four cities ranged between 4.6 to 11.3 per 100,000. The overall prevalence rate was estimated to be 7.6 per 100,000. The rate for nonwhite was much smaller, at 1 per 100,000. Cases were predominately women (80%). The mean age at disease onset was 30.2 years, and the average duration of illness was 7.4 years. Compared to the general population, CFS patients had more education (13.8 vs. 12.7 years) and yearly income ($41,250 vs. $34,500). This study involved physician referral and may have underestimated the prevalence of CFS in socioeconomic groups that do not seek medical help for fatigue or that do not have medical help available (33). Therefore, an examination of a community-based population may give a clearer epidemiological picture of CFS.

A community-based study in San Francisco found that chronic fatigue was very rare in the <18 years of age group but was reported by 2.0% of the adult population, with 0.2% satisfying criteria for CFS (34). Contrary to data from clinical populations, this study found that chronic fatigue occurred in all socioeconomic groups and was most prevalent in women, persons with lower income, and blacks. It was least common among Asians. Also, the data showed that unexplained chronic fatigue did not cluster by household, thus indicating that it may not be contagious. Similar results were estimated from a randomly selected sample of the general Chicago population, where the highest levels of CFS were among women, minority groups, and the less educated (35). However, in this study, the prevalence rate for CFS was higher (0.42%) (35).

Risk Factors

No health organization such as the NIH or CDC has published or endorsed a list of risk factors for CFS. However, one risk factor that seems to be consistently reported is female sex, for which the relative risk has been estimated to be between 1.3 to 1.7 per 100,000 (36). Other factors such as severe infection, premorbid depression, stress, and a combination of negative life events and infection have been suggested to predispose an individual to develop a case of CFS (37). A recent case control study of individuals making insurance claims as a result of a CFS diagnosis revealed that these patients reported significantly more illness for several years prior to their diagnosis when compared to claimants with other diagnoses (38).

Functional Consequences

Data concerned with the degree of disability in CFS are biased by the fact that one of the primary criteria for diagnosis is a substantial reduction in daily activity. However, even when compared to patients with multiple sclerosis and depression, CFS patients report spending more days in bed and a decreased ability to carry out activities of daily living (39). On the Medical Outcomes Study Short-Form General Health Survey (SF-36) (40) when compared to individuals with chronic fatigue, major depression, acute infectious mononucleosis, and healthy controls, CFS patients scored lowest on physical functioning, role functioning, social functioning, general health, and body pain subscales (41). Unemployment has been reported to be approximately 37% in CFS patients and 51% in those diagnosed with both CFS and fibromyalgia (42). An epidemiological study indicated that 43% of CFS patients could not work or go to school (9).

Two studies have used electronic activity monitors to acquire more objective assessments of the daily activity levels in CFS patients. The first found the activity levels of CFS patients to be comparable to those of patients with multiple sclerosis and significantly less (~30%) when compared to healthy subjects (43). In the second study, daily activity levels of CFS patients were approximately 15% less than the levels found for healthy sedentary subjects (44).

Prognosis

There is no indication that CFS is a fatal condition, but the prognosis for patients is not very promising in terms of complete recovery (45). However, during the progression of the illness, CFS patients will often have periods where symptoms will get better and then relapse. Patient follow-up studies ranging from approximately 1–6 years from the time of first diagnosis reveal that <10% of CFS patients return to premorbid functioning levels and that even those indicating some improvement are still quite impaired (45). Data show that time can be of some help, since the longer the period of follow-up, the higher the percentage of subjects who indicate improvement. However, 10–20% of CFS patients indicate that their symptoms have worsened at the time of follow-up (45). The factors related to a poor prognosis have been reported to be older age, chronic illness prior to diagnosis of CFS, comorbid psychiatric disorders, and holding to a belief that there is a physical cause of their illness (45).

DIAGNOSTIC TECHNIQUES

To date, there are no diagnostic tests to definitively establish the presence of CFS. Therefore, establishing if the 1994 CDC case definition given above applies to an individual patient and ruling out any definable medical cause of the fatigue must be done in order to make a diagnosis of CFS. A flow chart of the suggested diagnostic steps to take when evaluating a patient and further subgrouping for research purposes is presented in Figure 18.1 (11).

Since many patients presenting themselves to a clinic express fatigue as a symptom, the first diagnostic step is to make a distinction between prolonged fatigue lasting for at least 1 month and chronic fatigue lasting or relapsing for at least 6 months. Next, specific clinical and laboratory tests are recommended when attempting to rule out medically definable causes of the fatigue (see Figure 18.1) (11).

A diagnosis of CFS is excluded if a patient has a clinically defined and treatable illness that is known to cause fatigue. These include recent or current substance abuse, untreated hypothyroidism, sleep disturbances, and side effects from medications. Also, an unresolved case of such illnesses as treated malignancies and hepatitis B or C virus infection is exclusion for a CFS diagnosis. Finally, while the new criteria allows for psychological conditions such as anxiety or panic disorders when diagnosing CFS, such illnesses as major depressive disorders, bipolar affective disorders, schizophrenia, delusional disorders, dementia, anorexia nervosa, and bulimia nervosa are exclusions (11).

Other medical conditions that cannot be conclusively diagnosed but have fatigue as a significant part of a symptom complex are not exclusions for a diagnosis of CFS (see Table 18.1). Furthermore, a condition such as hypothyroidism, where treatment is such that all related symptoms have been resolved, is not exclusion for the diagnosis of CFS. Finally, any slightly positive clinical test result that is not normally associated with chronic fatigue or is of insufficient magnitude to definitively indicate a specific illness should not exclude a diagnosis of CFS (11).

If the 1994 case definition criteria are met, the diagnosis of CFS is made. If the medically unexplained fatigue has persisted or relapsed for at least 6 months but all of the criteria for CFS are not met, the diagnosis is idiopathic chronic fatigue (see Figure 18.1). For research purposes, it is suggested that subgrouping CFS patients on the basis of such factors as psychological status, gradual or sudden "flu-like" illness onset, fatigue severity ratings, or functional status may help in ascertaining disease etiology (11). The Composite International Diagnostic Instrument (46), National Institute of Mental Health Diagnostic Interview Schedule (47), and the Structured Clinical Interview for DSM-III(R) (48) are some of the psychological tests recommended for diagnoses or subgrouping purposes (11). Such instruments as the SF-36 (40) and the Sickness Impact Profile (49) are recommended to assess functional status (11).

PHYSICAL EXAMINATION

Along with severe fatigue, the CFS patient could express any number of symptoms. From the symptoms listed in the case definition, the most frequent complaints, secondary to fatigue, are sleep disturbances, impaired memory or concentration, and postexertional fatigue (34). Muscle and joint pain are often major complaints, and many CFS patients can also meet the diagnostic criteria for fibromyalgia (34). Additional symptoms that are not a part of the case definition but have a high incidence in CFS include general weakness and depression (34). The significance here is that much variability exists in symptoms expressed. Therefore, it is important to attempt to individualize the treatment and/or disease management of the patient.

Defining symptoms and ruling out medical conditions play such major roles in this illness that most physical examinations of the patient will be basically uneventful. Often, after the initial diagnosis of CFS, actual physical presentation may be overlooked. In this syndrome of unknown origin, the presence of physical evidence instead of subjective complaints could be an indication of sickness "flare-up" and should be investigated. For example, many individuals complain of frequent fevers; however, when a true increase in body temperature is measured (>100.4°) this could be a sign of acute infection. In such cases, limiting physical activity and rest could be indicated until the infection is treated and the fever is resolved (50).

Also, many of these chronically ill patients are extremely inactive and have long periods of bed rest. The result of this inactivity may be extreme muscle weakness, muscle wasting, orthostatic intolerance, and loss of balance. It is suggested that one should test for these conditions and perhaps prescribe physical rehabilitation (50).

A significant majority of CFS patients will exhibit at

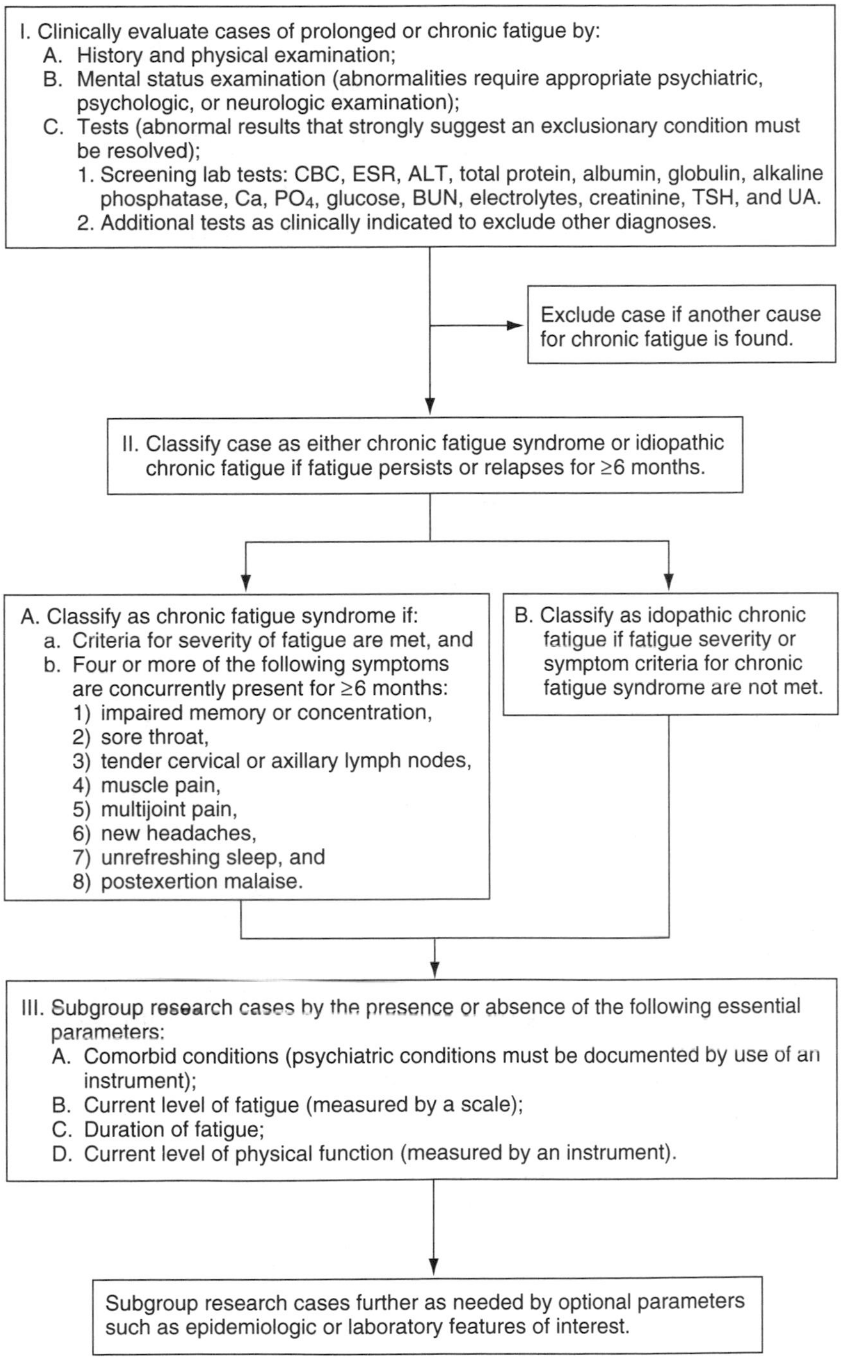

I. Clinically evaluate cases of prolonged or chronic fatigue by:
  A. History and physical examination;
  B. Mental status examination (abnormalities require appropriate psychiatric, psychologic, or neurologic examination);
  C. Tests (abnormal results that strongly suggest an exclusionary condition must be resolved);
    1. Screening lab tests: CBC, ESR, ALT, total protein, albumin, globulin, alkaline phosphatase, Ca, PO_4, glucose, BUN, electrolytes, creatinine, TSH, and UA.
    2. Additional tests as clinically indicated to exclude other diagnoses.

→ Exclude case if another cause for chronic fatigue is found.

II. Classify case as either chronic fatigue syndrome or idiopathic chronic fatigue if fatigue persists or relapses for ≥6 months.

A. Classify as chronic fatigue syndrome if:
  a. Criteria for severity of fatigue are met, and
  b. Four or more of the following symptoms are concurrently present for ≥6 months:
    1) impaired memory or concentration,
    2) sore throat,
    3) tender cervical or axillary lymph nodes,
    4) muscle pain,
    5) multijoint pain,
    6) new headaches,
    7) unrefreshing sleep, and
    8) postexertion malaise.

B. Classify as idopathic chronic fatigue if fatigue severity or symptom criteria for chronic fatigue syndrome are not met.

III. Subgroup research cases by the presence or absence of the following essential parameters:
  A. Comorbid conditions (psychiatric conditions must be documented by use of an instrument);
  B. Current level of fatigue (measured by a scale);
  C. Duration of fatigue;
  D. Current level of physical function (measured by an instrument).

Subgroup research cases further as needed by optional parameters such as epidemiologic or laboratory features of interest.

Figure 18.1. Evaluation and classification of unexplained chronic fatigue. ALT = alanine aminotransferase; BUN = blood urea nitrogen; CBC = complete blood count; ESR = erythrocyte sedimentation rate; PO_4 = phosphorus; TSH = thyroid-stimulating hormone; UA = urinalysis. Reprinted with permission from Fukuda et al. The chronic fatigue syndrome: a comprehensive approach to its definition and study. *Ann Intern Med* 1994;121:953–959, the American College of Physicians—American Society of Internal Medicine.

least one comorbid psychiatric disorder (75–78%) (51). In one study, approximately 75% of CFS patients had some type of mood disorder such as depression or dysthymia, while 30% of these CFS patients had some form of anxiety disorder such as panic disorder, and 28% were diagnosed with somatization disorder (52).

PHARMACOLOGY

No universal pharmacological regimen is prescribed nor recommended for CFS. However, the American Association for Chronic Fatigue Syndrome (AACFS) has made some recommendations for the management of CFS symptoms (53). Low doses of antidepressants are widely prescribed for the relief of associated symptoms such as depression, myalgia, and sleep disorders. Common prescriptions include tricyclic antidepressants (TCAs), such as amitriptyline (Elavil), desipramine (Norpramin), doxepin (Sinequan), and nortriptyline (Pamelor), and selective serotonin reuptake inhibitors (SSRIs), such as fluoxetine hydrochloride (Prozac) and sertraline (Zoloft) (53). A regimen of low doses of an SRRI in the morning and a TCA at bedtime is often suggested (31, 53).

Additional drugs commonly prescribed or utilized by

Table 18.1. Exclusions and Inclusions for a Diagnosis of Chronic Fatigue Syndrome (CFS)

Exclusive		Inclusive	
Medical Condition	**Examples**	**Medical Condition**	**Examples**
Active or untreated	Hypothyroidism, sleep apnea, narcolepsy, iatrogenic conditions	Symptom defined	Fibromyalgia, anxiety disorders, somatoform disorders, mild depression, neurasthenia, multiple chemical sensitivity
Unresolved premorbid CFS	Malignancies, hepatitis B or C virus infection	Treated and symptom elevated	Hypothyroidism, asthma
Major psychological	Major depression, bipolar affective disorders, schizophrenia, delusional, dementias, anorexia or bulimia nervosa	Resolved premorbid CFS	Lyme disease, syphilis
Alcohol and substance abuse		Isolated and unexplained clinical finding	Insignificant elevated antinuclear antibody titer
Severe obesity (BMI ≥45)			

these patients include nonsteroidal anti-inflammatory drugs (NSAIDs) or acetaminophen to relieve pain. The AACFS suggests that quinine sulfate (Quinine), carisoprodol (Soma), or cyclobenzaprine (Flexeril) may help relieve muscle spasms and myalgia (53). Also, nonsedating antihistamines such as astemizole (Hismanal) and loratadine (Claritin) may be given to reduce allergic symptoms. In some cases, CFS patients may be taking anxiolytic medication to treat panic disorder or anxiety. These can include alprazolam (Xanax), clonazepam (Klonopin), and lorazepam (Ativan) (31, 53).

Many pharmacological therapies that are based on the different theories of the etiology of CFS have been investigated with mixed results (54). These include immunological therapy with intravenous immunoglobulin G and interferon-alpha. Some improvements in CFS patients using Ampligen, an antiviral and immunomodulatory drug, have been reported. Another antiviral drug, Acyclovir, has been investigated, but no beneficial effects were seen. Based on data indicating a decreased activity in the HPA, low-dose hydrocortisone therapy has been tried, but the results are not very promising. Finally, because of the reports of a high incidence of NMH in CFS, fludrocortisone (Florinef) treatment or in some cases beta blockers such as atenolol (Tenormin) may be prescribed to CFS patients who demonstrate orthostatic intolerance during a tilt-table test.

Due to the heterogeneity of CFS complaints and the fact that pharmacological treatment of CFS is based on relieving specific symptoms expressed by the patient, a thorough medication list should be obtained prior to exercise testing or prescription. In most cases, the dose of antidepressants prescribed for CFS patients is small and may have no effect on exercise performance. However, in therapeutic doses, some antidepressants, especially TCAs, can increase heart rate, decrease blood pressure, and cause ECG changes (55). Quinidine sulfate is an antiarrhythmic agent and can cause increased heart rate and ECG changes during rest or exercise. Carisoprodol or cyclobenzaprine can reduce blood pressure and cause dizziness (56). Anxiolytic medication can reduce heart rate and blood pressure but does not significantly affect exercise ECG (55, 56). Alprazolam and lorazepam can also cause muscular in-coordination (56). Most CFS patients with suspected or demonstrated NMH are prescribed fludrocortisone or increased salt intake for treatment. However, a few of these patients may be given beta blockers that can affect exercise by decreasing heart rate and blood pressure, reducing exercise capacity in patients without angina (55).

MEDICAL AND SURGICAL TREATMENTS

There are no medical treatments for CFS that have been found to be universally effective, and no therapy can be endorsed on the basis of sound clinical research. With the exception of the pharmacological management of symptoms discussed, no specific treatment of CFS is advanced by physicians, researchers, or health organizations. For instance, the position statement of the Vancouver Chronic Fatigue Syndrome Consensus Group recommended that treatment of CFS should be directed toward symptom relief and reducing the patient's functional disability (57).

Also, this group stated that the treatment should include helping the patient avoid harmful situations that could possibly worsen his/her condition. The patient needs help in understanding the vast amounts of information published about the nature, prognosis, and effective treatments of CFS. Unproven treatments that are advocated by clinicians or groups who have their own theories of the CFS etiology can delay appropriate care, be costly, and do harm (57).

The Vancouver Group and others suggest that a multidisciplinary approach such as cognitive behavioral therapy (CBT) and physical rehabilitation may be helpful (57). Some evidence has shown that a combination of CBT and exercise resulted in improvement in CFS symptoms, but this has not been supported in all cases (54, 57). There is not enough evidence to say that these therapies will cure CFS, but they may help improve a patient's functional capacity and counteract the synergistic negative effects of inactivity on their symptom complex. Also, if administered cautiously and competently, the risk of doing harm with these therapies can be minimized.

CLINICAL EXERCISE PHYSIOLOGY

Physiological Responses to Activity/Exercise

A number of studies have investigated the aerobic capacity and cardiopulmonary functioning of CFS patients during a graded exercise test to exhaustion. Most have found CFS patients to have low normal VO_{2peak} values with basically routine cardiopulmonary responses (58–60). In these studies, the average peak oxygen consumption for the CFS groups ranged between 23 and 32 mL/kg/min. However, Montague et al. (61) found that when compared to healthy control subjects, chronically fatigued patients had slow heart rate acceleration as workloads increased during supine ergometry. There are some concerns about this conclusion, since the slow heart rate acceleration was not found to be significant until after 12 minutes of exercise, but only 10 of their 41 patients exercised for this amount of time (61).

Mullis and associates (60) concluded that their data supported those of Montague et al. (61), since the group of CFS patients they tested only achieved 77% of age-related predicted maximal heart rate. On close inspection, the data do not seem to indicate heart chronotropic problems in CFS patients as much as they indicate an early voluntary termination of the maximal test, since the average respiratory exchange ratio was only 0.95, with no one achieving greater than 0.97 (60). The significance here may be in mode of exercise, since both Mullis et al. (60) and Montague et al. (61) used cycle ergometry. Perhaps leg fatigue rather than cardiopulmonary insufficiencies caused CFS patients to terminate the test early. During a graded exercise test utilizing a treadmill walking protocol, 80% of CFS patients achieved higher than 90% of age-related predicted maximal heart rate, and there was no evidence of an abnormal heart rate to VO_2 relationship in these patients (62).

Most studies of aerobic capacity report a significantly higher rating of perceived exertion (RPE) at every workload by CFS patients when compared to healthy controls (59, 63). The conclusion here is that the limiting factors in the exercise capacity of CFS patients may be central in origin as opposed to peripheral. However, it has been reported that when an RPE at a relative percentage of peak oxygen uptake is compared, CFS patients and sedentary healthy controls do not indicate a difference in perception of effort (58).

Limitations in muscle strength and endurance have not been observed by Lloyd and associates (64), who tested isometric strength of elbow flexors during maximal voluntary contraction in 20 CFS patients compared to controls. Stokes and associates (65) found maximal muscle strength of the quadriceps of most CFS patients to be within normal range and muscle endurance under ischemic and nonischemic conditions to also be normal. In general, clinical tests of static muscle strength do not reveal significant weakness.

Some studies report limitations in muscle endurance (66); however, many of these did not normalize exercise levels to maximal strength. Kent-Braun and associates (67) found increased fatigue in muscles with superimposed electrical twitches and explained this phenomenon as a drop in neural activation rather than a change in muscle function. Stokes and associates (65) found that maximal quadricep strength in CFS patients was generally normal, with only a subgroup out of the normal range when compared to healthy controls.

Magnetic resonance spectroscopy (MRS) studies suggest that a subpopulation of CFS patients have muscle metabolic abnormalities such as abnormally high or low ADP levels during steady exercise, which represents the degree of mitochondrial activation (68). Additional MRS studies show that some CFS patients have abnormal phosphocreatine (PCr) recovery rates after exercise, which are related to increased muscle acidification (69). One study utilizing both MRS and near-infrared spectroscopy revealed a reduced muscle oxygen delivery capacity in CFS patients (70). However, all of these exercise-related abnormalities have been associated with deconditioning in healthy volunteers, which suggests that many of the deficiencies seen in the muscle functioning of CFS patients could be a result of deconditioning. The occurrence of muscle pathology is rare (71) and therefore does not play a significant role in CFS.

Clapp and associates (72) determined that 30 minutes of light-intensity, intermittent exercise did not exacerbate symptoms in CFS subjects up to 7 days after exercise. There was no abnormality in oxygen consumption, minute ventilation, heart rate, or respiratory exchange ratio. Improvements were noted in self-reported reduction of tension and depression. It is important to note that there was no worsening of health and well-being scores.

Supervision and Monitoring

A heart rate monitor allows for independent monitoring of the prescribed target heart rate range during exercise sessions. Also, it is important to monitor heart rate during recovery from exercise. The typical response of a slow return to resting heart rate due to deconditioning is not always the case. Some individuals with CFS demonstrate abnormally rapid decline in heart rate and should be instructed to continue low-level exercise to lower the heart rate more gradually. Blood pressure monitoring can be used for those individuals who demonstrate postural hypotension. In this case, blood pressure monitoring provides the practitioner and the patient with feedback about what postures produce undesirable responses. For example, exercises may have to be done in supine, progressing to semireclining, sitting, standing, and finally walking while monitoring blood pressure. Blood pressure responses help to determine when exercises can be progressed or if the patient needs to return to a reclined position.

Early on during exercise intervention, monitoring should occur every other day or twice a week, but as the patient begins to learn the management of his/her symptoms, exercise supervision could be more protracted. If individuals with CFS demonstrate serious cognitive difficulties, more frequent supervision may be needed to correct exercise errors. Providing written and pictorial exercise reminders is extremely important in this case.

EXERCISE/FITNESS/FUNCTIONAL TESTING

As a group, CFS patients tolerate standard cardiopulmonary and strength testing fairly well and without signs of muscle damage (69), compromised immune system (65), or severe signs of a worsened disease state (60). However, patient complaints of fatigue are increased for several days after testing (58), and there are some signs of decreased cognitive abilities. It is recommended that the patient adjust his/her daily affairs so that he/she does very little physical activity prior to testing and has time to rest afterward. Also, it would be helpful for the patient to be accompanied by someone to assist in postexercise testing.

Because of the heterogeneity of symptoms, the variety of prescribed medications, and the fluctuation of illness severity, the history and physical prior to testing is very important. Cardiopulmonary testing with metabolic measurements is often used to help rule out known causes of the fatigue. However, one should not assume that heart disease has been specifically ruled out, and the American College of Sports Medicine Guidelines for Exercise Testing and Prescription (55) should be applied. Although many physicians doubt the existence of a distinct illness of chronic fatigue and the syndrome's etiology is unknown, these patients are ill and express symptoms. Medical clearance and clinical exercise tests are recommended prior to participating in an exercise program.

Standard protocols can be utilized when measuring aerobic power on either a cycle ergometer or a treadmill. Workload increments are typically 20–25 watts or 1–2 METS. A ramping protocol may be appropriate. Interpretation of gas exchange data and measurement of aerobic power can reveal signs of possible underlying vascular, metabolic, and/or muscle disease. Additional specialized diagnostic testing may then be recommended. Because one of the primary goals of an exercise program in CFS would be to increase the patient's functional capacity, tests of daily activities such as the continuous-scale physical functional performance test (73) could be employed to evaluate a patient's progress. Also, questionnaires such as the SF-36 (40) can be used to evaluate the subjective effects of the prescribed exercise program.

EXERCISE PRESCRIPTION AND PROGRAMMING

Multidisciplinary Treatment Intervention

The first principle that must be applied to most patients with CFS is that exercise training must be very-light to light and progress extremely gradually. Probably the greatest error that occurs when providing an exercise regimen for individuals with CFS is the viewpoint that this is a case of simple deconditioning. This conclusion leads to the erroneous approach that a standard strengthening and conditioning program will return the patient to healthy functioning. This is most definitely not the case.

Individuals with the diagnosis of CFS have been chronically ill for at least 6 months and often longer. They have most likely attempted to return to their previous level of exercise either on their own or with assistance from healthcare professionals or personal trainers. These efforts have met with little success and often with detrimental results. The negative effects of approaching CFS patients with a standard strengthening and reconditioning program include an exacerbation of flu-like symptoms, severe fatigue for days to weeks, and cognitive dysfunction.

This is not to imply that no type of exercise is of any benefit to the patient with CFS; quite the contrary. Fulcher and White (74) evaluated aerobic exercise versus flexibility and relaxation exercise. Nearly twice as many patients reported feeling better from the aerobic exercise than from the flexibility/relaxation exercises. These authors subscribe to the benefits of graded aerobic exercise in the management of CFS.

It is important to recognize that CFS is a multifactorial illness, and consequently, the treatment intervention should be multidisciplinary. Patients with CFS can have anxiety or affective disorders, sleep disorders, pharmacological management requirements, difficulties in pacing activity, and family difficulties as a result of the illness. Therefore, exercise alone will not usually help the patient manage the overall illness. Communication with other professionals like psychologists, physical and occupational therapists, vocational counselors, and physicians is essential. Marlin and associates (75) reported a significant number of patients returned to work or functioned at a level equivalent to gainful employment when a multidisciplinary intervention was applied. This entailed optimal medical management; pharmacological treatment of the affective, anxiety, or sleep disorder; activity management; and "coping" techniques.

Program Guidelines and Initial Exercise Prescription

Establishing Goals

Goals should be patient-focused in the areas of self-care; productivity such as school or work, whether it is in-house or out of the house; and leisure activity. Basic self-care goals may include activities like morning hygiene, walking within the house, and meal preparation. Intermediate self-care goals may include activities such as stair climbing, walking longer distances, and out-of-the-house activities such as running errands. As early as possible, it is advisable for the patient to make a regular weekly commitment. This could include a social activity such as visiting a friend, an educational activity such as attending a lecture, or a leisure activity such as dancing or playing golf.

Breathing/ Relaxation Exercises

Patients with CFS often have an apical breathing pattern and are prone to hyperventilation (71, 76). Therefore, proper diaphragmatic breathing exercises coupled with relaxation techniques may help to reduce these problems. Some individuals with CFS also have concomitant history of panic attacks. Teaching proper breathing and relaxation exercises is extremely successful in reducing panic attacks and giving the individual a sense of control over his/her condition. Breathing/relaxation exercises are recommended during any time of stress, even during challenging exercises. In particular, they should be recommended at night to promote sleep.

Stretching/Flexibility Exercises

Individuals with CFS have been sedentary and often experience significant muscle aches and pains over months to years. Posture is usually faulty and cannot be corrected without prior stretching. Stretching exercises usually require a focus on the anterior chest wall and neck region. Gentle stretching of the anterior and posterior neck region can provide great relief for common headache complaints. Stretching exercises should be done daily, particularly upon waking. This allows for an improved sense of mobility and vitality when the day begins.

Strengthening Exercises

Strengthening should address active motion with gravity-only resistance first. Weight training should be reserved for later. These exercises should first focus on trunk stability, followed by extremity-strengthening exercises. Typically, only when the individual can perform three sets of 15 repetitions are weights added. Sometimes, individuals fatigue and relapse if these are done in one bout, in which case they should be encouraged to split the tasks between morning and afternoon. Depending on the patient's response to exercise, a recommendation to alternate days of strengthening with submaximal aerobic exercise is advisable.

Submaximal Aerobic Exercise

These exercises should begin at a low level and increase in duration before intensity. This decision is often based on the subject's current level of activity. For example, if an individual is bedridden or extremely sedentary, walking on a treadmill may, at the start, be limited to 1 minute or less. Conversely, if daily activities are more plentiful, treadmill walking may start at 5 or 10 minutes. It is important for the individual to monitor the heart rate and stay within the prescribed range. If individuals are extremely ill and fatigued most of the time, working at 50% of the age-predicted maximal heart rate is not unreasonable. Exercise intensity is usually increased to 55%, 60%, and 65% of maximal heart rate. The higher-functioning patients will be able to be progressed to 70–85%. Patients should be reminded to breathe during all exercise and to avoid exercise if there are other significant duties to be conducted that day.

Exercise Progression

Most importantly, after an initial level of exercise intensity is decided, best results are most often achieved if there is no increase in intensity sooner than once a week. This duration allows for possible unexpected exacerbation requiring a downgrade of intensity. If an exercise program is progressed every session, it becomes unclear which intensity was too extreme or whether the exacerbation was due to the cumulative effect of the exercise program increase. During this initial period, it is important to point out to the patient that the other daily activities should not be significantly altered, confusing the impact of the exercise regimen with that of an increase in home or social activity. After submaximal aerobic exercise reaches 15–20 minutes, patients are most likely ready to increase exercise intensity. Initially, supervised exercise is best administered approximately twice per week. Clapp and associates (72) determined that approximately 15 minutes of discontinuous treadmill exercise was the upper limit, based on subjects' self-report of fatigue and fear of exacerbation.

Exercise Considerations and Symptom Relapse

Patients with CFS must understand that there will continue to be periods of worsening of symptoms but should be informed that with graded exercise and energy-conservation techniques, these should occur less frequently and be less severe. Smith (77) described the course of recovery, indicating that in the progression of the illness, the symptom severity decreases and periods of symptom exacerbation become more predictable. This knowledge, surprisingly, has a psychological benefit to the patient because it demonstrates the practitioner's understanding of the recovery trajectory and gives hope of eventual recovery to an improved state. It is very important that patients with CFS learn how to manage their activity during this period of relapse, recognizing that rest is needed and excess mental or physical exertion can cause further deterioration. Some simple exercises can be performed based on the individual's symptoms. These can include breathing, relaxation, and stretching exercises. If symptoms are worsening, simple strengthening exercises with which the patient is already familiar should be done but with less intensity, frequency, and/or duration than usual.

Strategies for Promoting Adherence

Education about the need to interrupt the continuous downward cycle of exercise, relapse, rest, and deconditioning is usually enough to promote exercise adherence provided the patient is given a manageable program that does not result in relapses. Most CFS patients want to feel better and welcome guidance as to how best to encourage recovery. It is important for the patient to learn self-management of symptoms to avoid frustration. For example, if severe headaches limit activity, teaching relaxation, breathing, and neck-stretching exercises to reduce pain will lead to the sense of control over the illness. This improvement in control is reinforcing, and patients most often are quite willing to proceed with exercise maintenance and progression. It is advisable to remind patients that as they begin to feel better, it is common to overdo other activities, as they may not be defined as exercise. In fact, all the activities of the day must be taken into account to plan how strenuous the exercise should be. In some cases where there are significant activities such as attending a family function, exercise might be skipped altogether for that day. Giving patients similar scenarios allows them to take control of their activity planning and gives permission for lapses in exercise due to other real-life activities or responsibilities.

Precautions

CFS patients often report a relapse of severe symptoms following acute and even mild exercise for hours (59, 78) to days (44, 58). Furthermore, there appears to be no clear warning of the point at which too much exercise will trigger a relapse (76). In other words, by the time the individual reports that he/she feels tired enough to stop exercising, it is likely to be too late to avoid exacerbation of symptoms. Using only the patient's response as an end limit to exercise bouts is likely to prove unsuccessful. Therefore, a structured mild and gradually progressed exercise regimen avoids most severe relapsing.

EDUCATION AND COUNSELING

Patients with CFS should be instructed about fitness as a lifetime goal, but that increases in the fitness regimen should be taken on gradually. Patients should stay on track and avoid the tendency to overdo the workout because of the immediate sense of well-being, a common problem resulting in significant frustration. Patients should be instructed not to increase the intensity and duration of fitness exercises any faster than once a week. Also, the frequency should always allow a rest day in between exercise sessions. For example, an individual could begin an independent outdoor exercise program by walking one block every other day and monitoring the time needed to complete the walk. This could be increased to longer distances and consequently longer time. Generally, when 15–20 minutes are achieved, then patients can be instructed to modify their walking pace to a faster speed, thereby covering a greater distance in the same amount of time. Patients should be instructed to increase such a program as tolerated, but energy should be saved for other activities such as leisure, social, and work activities.

Patients should be counseled in a manner to self-manage symptoms while continually but gradually progressing levels of exercise intensity. These instructions can be in the form of home exercise programs. When designing these exercise programs for the home, it is important to realize that they should be simple because CFS patients sometimes have difficulty understanding complex multitask instructions, especially during periods of symptom exacerbation. The home exercise program should also include relaxation, stretching, strengthening, and aerobic exercises. It is advisable for the material to be written and include pictures to facilitate compliance.

Patients with CFS can experience barriers to exercise. Sometimes, these individuals can demonstrate avoidance of exercise due to somatic complaint (79). This is most likely because of learned behavior from when exercise attempts have failed and resulted in serious exacerbation. Cognitive limitations can preclude CFS patients from completing tasks according to the exercise guidelines recommended. Therefore, individuals may not comply due to inability to recall and follow instructions. When patients are limited by serious exacerbation, they should be encouraged to rest and reminded that in time, the exacerbation will become less severe and shorter. Many patients also must attend a significant number of medical visits that require energy consumption and may result in an inability to comply with an exercise regimen. Patients should be reminded to set aside a few minutes for gentle exercises on such days to avoid getting out of the habit of regular exercise.

CASE STUDIES

The examples illustrate the management of a severe and a moderate-to-mild case of CFS. The cases do not represent the only mechanism for management of CFS but are an attempt to illustrate the complexity and uniqueness of exercise prescription.

CASE 1

A 35-year-old woman complains of severe fatigue for 2 years. The onset time was after suffering a week-long bout with the flu. The fatigue from the flu only partially subsided. Fatigue and cognitive problems are her primary complaints. She reports a history of seeing a variety of doctors and psychologists who were unable to make an affirmative diagnosis until 6 months ago, when she received the diagnosis of chronic fatigue syndrome (CFS) by an immunologist.

Since her initial illness, she has become extremely weak and unable to sustain everyday activities for longer than 15 minutes at a time, less if there is a significant cognitive demand. Her strength tests within the normal range; however, she complains of lack of vigor and inability to complete more than one repetition of antigravity limb exercises. She complains the greatest difficulty is carrying heavy objects, especially up a flight of stairs.

She is able to walk within her house for short intervals and avoids out-of-house activities altogether. She requires the assistance of friends and relatives to do her shopping and errands. She has become depressed due to inability to participate in even minimal activities socially.

Prior to her illness, she was a competitive jogger, and she has attempted exercising on her own several times since. Each time she exerted herself even at a minimal intensity, she would suffer from worsening fatigue a day or two later. This was true even though she did not experience any deleterious effects during the exercise. This exacerbation of fatigue would often last several days, during which most of the time was spent in bed. Because of her long bouts of rest during the day, her dietary and hydration habits were poor. Medications caused significant weight gain and resulted in dry mouth and eyes.

S: Easy fatigability with minimal exertion

O: Range of motion and strength when tested statically were within normal limits. Unable to repeat antigravity limb exercises more than once. Heart rate was 80 bpm at rest and increased to 100 during standing activities. Able to walk on a treadmill at 1 mph for 5 minutes, however, this resulted in worsening fatigue reported at the next visit. Peak VO_2 is 20 mL/kg/min. Blood pressure was 120/80 mm Hg in sitting and lying but dropped to 100/60 initially upon standing. Medications include Florinef to improve postural hypotension and Paxil to reduce anxiety. Occasionally, Halcyon is taken at bedtime if sleep is difficult.

A: Low endurance and conditioning; hypotension upon standing

P: 1. Gentle antigravity exercise strengthening and conditioning

2. Gentle aerobic conditioning

Exercise Program

Goal: Increase antigravity exercise endurance repetitions for trunk and limbs.

Mode: Antigravity exercise without weights, treadmill and sitting or supine cycle ergometry, calf strengthening, and/or elastic stockings to promote venous return during standing activities; may have to exercise initially in sitting or lying.

Intensity: Active exercise without weights with arms, legs, and trunk to tolerance to establish initial repetition level i.e., 3–5 repetitions for each muscle; treadmill or cycle ergometry at 0.5 to 1 mph.

Frequency: Every other day; reevaluate weekly to determine if repetitions should be decreased or increased

Duration: 20 minutes of active exercise; 5 minutes on treadmill or cycle ergometry on alternate days from active exercise days, monitoring exercise and recovery heart rate.

Time course of supervised exercise: 3 months

Note: Exercise intensity should be evaluated weekly to determine if there is any exacerbation of symptoms of fatigue or flu-like symptoms. If symptoms are present, intensity should be reduced and/or exercise bouts should be more spaced. If there are no symptoms, exercise intensity should be increased slightly and reevaluated again each week.

CASE 2

A 30-year-old woman complains of severe fatigue for 2 years. The onset time was after suffering a week-long bout with the flu. The fatigue from the flu only partially subsided. Her primary complaints are fatigue and cognitive problems. She claims that she has seen a variety of doctors who were unable to make an affirmative diagnosis until 6 months ago when she received the diagnosis of chronic fatigue syndrome (CFS) by a neurologist. She was previously a regular exerciser and jogged three times per week to total approximately 15 miles per week.

She is able to work her full-time job, but when she comes home and on weekends, she is unable to do anything but sleep until the next morning. Her strength tests within the normal range; however, she complains of lack of vigor and inability to concentrate on mental tasks during complex multisequencing tasks. She complains of difficulty carrying heavy objects. She requires the assistance of friends and relatives to do her shopping and errands. She has become depressed due to inability to participate in even minimal activities socially outside of work.

She has attempted exercising on her own several times since, prior to her illness, she was a competitive jogger. Each time she exerted herself at what she considered a minimal amount, she would still suffer from worsening fatigue a day or two later, even though she did not experience any deleterious effects during that exercise. This exacerbation of fatigue would often last several hours.

S: Easy fatigability with minimal exertion

O: Range of motion and strength when tested statically were within normal limits. She was unable to repeat antigravity limb exercises more than 10 times. Heart rate was 70 bpm at rest, and she was able to walk on a treadmill at 2.5 mph for 15 minutes; however, this resulted in worsening fatigue reported at the next visit. Her peak VO_2 is 33 mL/kg/min. Blood pressure was 120/80 mm Hg in sitting and standing. Medications include Paxil to reduce anxiety and Flexeril for muscle pain.

A: Low endurance and conditioning

P: 1. Gentle strengthening and conditioning

2. Gentle aerobic conditioning

Exercise Program

Goal: Increase antigravity exercise endurance repetitions for trunk and limbs

Mode: Antigravity exercise without weights, treadmill and sitting or supine cycle ergometry
Intensity: Active exercise without weights with arms, legs, and trunk to tolerance to establish initial repetition level i.e., 10–15 repetitions for each muscle; treadmill or cycle ergometry at an intensity of 2.5 to 3 METS.
Frequency: Every other day; reevaluate weekly to determine if repetitions should be decreased or increased.
Duration: 20 minutes of active exercise; 15 minutes on treadmill or cycle ergometry on alternate days from active exercise days, monitoring exercise and recovery heart rate.
Time course of supervised exercise: 1.5 months
Note: Exercise intensity should be evaluated weekly to determine if there is any exacerbation of symptoms of fatigue or flu-like symptoms. If symptoms are present, intensity should be reduced and/or exercise bouts should be more spaced. If there are no symptoms, exercise intensity should be increased slightly and reevaluated again each week.

References

1. Tobi M, Morag A, Ravid Z, et al. Prolonged atypical illness associated with serological evidence of persistent Epstein-Barr virus infection. *Lancet* 1982;1:61–64.
2. Straus SE, Tosato G, Armstrong G, et al. Persisting illness and fatigue in adults with evidence of Epstein-Barr virus infection. *Ann Intern Med* 1985;102(1):7–16.
3. Jones JF, Ray CG, Minnich LL, et al. Evidence for active Epstein-Barr virus infection in patients with persistent, unexplained illnesses: elevated anti-early antigen antibodies. *Ann Intern Med* 1985;102:1–6.
4. DuBois RE, Seeley JK, Brus I, et al. Chronic mononucleosis syndrome. *South Med J* 1984;77(11):1376–1382.
5. Holmes GP, Kaplan JE, Stewart JA, et al. A cluster of patients with a chronic mononucleosis-like syndrome: is Epstein-Barr virus the cause? *JAMA* 1987;257(17):2297–2302.
6. Buchwald D, Sullivan JL, Komaroff AL. Frequency of 'chronic active Epstein-Barr virus infection' in a general medical practice. *JAMA* 1987;257(17):2303–2307.
7. Holmes GP, Kaplan JE, Gantz NM, et al. Chronic fatigue syndrome: a working case definition. *Ann Intern Med* 1988;108(3):387–389.
8. Sharpe MC, Archard LC, Banatvala JE, et al. A report—chronic fatigue syndrome: guidelines for research. *J R Soc Med* 1991;84(2):118–121.
9. Lloyd AR, Hickie I, Boughton CR, et al. Prevalence of chronic fatigue syndrome in an Australian population. *Med J Aust* 1990;153:522–528.
10. Schluederberg A, Straus SE, Peterson P, et al. Chronic fatigue syndrome research definition and medical outcome assessment. *Ann Intern Med* 1992;117(4):325–331.
11. Fukuda K, Straus SE, Hickie I, et al. The chronic fatigue syndrome: a comprehensive approach to its definition and study. *Ann Intern Med* 1994;121(12):954–959.
12. Ablashi DV, Eastman HB, Owen CB, et al. Frequent HHV-6 reactivation in multiple sclerosis (MS) and chronic fatigue syndrome (CFS) patients. *J Clin Virol* 2000;15(3):179–191.
13. Wallace HL 2nd, Natelson B, Gause W, et al. Human herpesviruses in chronic fatigue syndrome. *Clin Diag Lab Immunol* 1999;6(2):216–223.
14. Mawle AC, Reyes M, Schmid DS. Is chronic fatigue syndrome an infectious disease? *Infect Agents Dis* 1993;2(5):333–341.
15. Landay AL, Jessop C, Lennette ET, et al. Chronic fatigue syndrome: clinical condition associated with immune activation. *Lancet* 1991;338:707–712.
16. Barker E, Fujimura SF, Fadem MB, et al. Immunologic abnormalities associated with chronic fatigue syndrome. *Clin Infect Dis* 1994;18(Suppl 1):S136–S141.
17. Evengard B, Schacterle RS, Komaroff AL. Chronic fatigue syndrome: new and old ignorance. *J Intern Med* 1999;246:435–469.
18. Natelson BH, LaManca JJ, Denny TN, et al. Immunologic parameters in chronic fatigue syndrome, major depression, and multiple sclerosis. *Am J Med* 1998;105(3A):43S–49S.
19. Dickinson CJ. Chronic fatigue syndrome—etiological aspects. *Eur J Clin Invest* 1997;27:257–267.
20. Suhadolnik RJ, Peterson DL, O'Brien K, et al. Biochemical evidence for a novel low molecular weight 2–5A-dependent Rnase L in chronic fatigue syndrome. *J Interferon Cytokine Res* 1997;17:377–385.
21. Demitrack M, Dale J, Straus S, et al. Evidence for impaired activation of the hypothalamic-pituitary-adrenal axis in chronic fatigue syndrome. *J Clin Endocrinol Metab* 1991;73:1224–1234.
22. Scott LV, Teh J, Reznek R, et al. Small adrenal glands in chronic fatigue syndrome: a preliminary computer tomography study. *Psycho-neuroendocrinology* 1999;24(7):759–768.
23. Hudson M, Cleare AJ. The 1mug short Synacthen test in chronic fatigue syndrome. *Clin Endocrinol (Oxf)* 1999;51(5):625–630.
24. Natelson BH, Cohen JM, Brassloff I, et al. Controlled study of brain magnetic resonance imaging in patients with fatiguing illnesses. *J Neurol Sci* 1993;120:213–217.
25. Costa DC, Tannock C, Brostoff J. Brainstem profusion is impaired in chronic fatigue syndrome. *QJM* 1995;88:767–773.
26. Samii A, Wassermann EM, Ikoma K, et al. Decreased postexercise facilitation of motor evoked potentials in patients with chronic fatigue syndrome or depression. *Neurology* 1996;47(6):1410–1414.
27. Boda WL, Natelson BH, Sisto SA, et al. Gait abnormalities in chronic fatigue syndrome. *J Neurol Sci* 1995;131(2):156–161.
28. Bou-Holaigah I, Rowe PC, Kan J, et al. The relationship between neurally mediated hypotension and the chronic fatigue syndrome. *JAMA* 1995;274(12):961–967.
29. LaManca JJ, Peckerman A, Walker J, et al. Cardiovascular response during head-up tilt in chronic fatigue syndrome. *Clin Physiol* 1999;19(2):111–120.
30. De Lorenzo F, Hargreaves J, Kakkar VV. Pathogenesis and management of delayed orthostatic hypotension in patients with chronic fatigue syndrome. *Clin Auton Res* 1997;7:185–190.
31. Buchwald D. Fibromyalgia and chronic fatigue syndrome. *Rheum Dis Clin North Am* 1996;22(2):219–243.
32. Johnson SK, DeLuca J, Natelson BH. Chronic fatigue syndrome: reviewing the research findings. *Ann Behav Med* 1999;21(3):258–271.
33. Gunn WJ, Connell DB, Randall B. Epidemiology of chronic fatigue syndrome: the Centers for Disease Control Study. *Ciba Found Symp* 1993;173:83–93, discussion 93–101.
34. Steele L, Dobbins JG, Fukuda K, et al. The epidemiology of

chronic fatigue in San Francisco. *Am J Med* 1998;104(3A): 83S-90S.
35. Jason LA, Richman JA, Rademaker AW, et al. A community-based study of chronic fatigue syndrome. *Arch Intern Med* 1999;159:2129–2137.
36. Wessely S. The epidemiology of chronic fatigue syndrome. *Epidemiol Rev* 1995;17(1):139–151.
37. Levine PH. Epidemiologic advances in chronic fatigue syndrome. *J Psychiatr Res* 1997;31(1):7–18.
38. Hall GH, Hamilton WT, Round AP. Increased illness experience preceding chronic fatigue syndrome: a case control study. *J R Col Physicians Lond* 1998;32(1):44–48.
39. Natelson BH, Johnson SK, DeLuca J, et al. Reducing heterogeneity in chronic fatigue syndrome: a comparison with depression and multiple sclerosis. *Clin Infect Dis* 1995;21:1204–1210.
40. Ware JE, Sherbourne CD. The MOS 36-item Short-Form health survey (SF-36). I. Conceptual framework and item selection. *Med Care* 1992;30:473–483.
41. Buchwald D, Pearlman T, Umali J, et al. Functional status in patients with chronic fatigue syndrome, other fatiguing illnesses, and healthy individuals. *Am J Med* 1996;101(4):364–370.
42. Bombardier CH, Buchwald D. Chronic fatigue, chronic fatigue syndrome, and fibromyalgia. Disability and health care use. *Med Care* 1996;34:924–930.
43. Vercoulen JH, Bazelmans E, Swanink CM, et al. Physical activity in chronic fatigue syndrome: assessment and its role in fatigue. *J Psychiatr Res* 1997;31(6):661–673.
44. Sisto SA, Tapp WN, LaManca JJ, et al. Physical activity before and after exercise in women with chronic fatigue syndrome. *QJM* 1998;91(7):465–473.
45. Joyce J, Hotopf M, Wessely S. The prognosis of chronic fatigue and chronic fatigue syndrome: a systematic review. *QJM* 1997;90:223–233.
46. Robins LN, Wing J, Wittchen HU, et al. The Composite International Diagnostic Interview. An epidemiologic instrument suitable for use in conjunction with different diagnostic systems and in different cultures. *Arch Gen Psychiatry* 2988;45:1069–1077.
47. Robins LN, Helzer JE, Croughan J, et al. National Institute of Mental Health Diagnostic Interview Schedule. Its history, characteristics, and validity. *Arch Gen Psychiatry* 1981;38: 381–389.
48. Splizer RL, Williams JR, Gibbon M, et al. The Structured Clinical Interview for DSM-III-R (SCID). I: history, rationale, and description. *Arch Gen Psychiatry* 1992;49:624–629.
49. Bergner M, Bobbit RA, Carter WB, et al. The Sickness Impact Profile: development and final revision of a health status measure. *Med Care* 1981;19:787–805.
50. Sharpe M, Chalder T, Palmer I, et al. Chronic fatigue syndrome: a practical guide to assessment and management. *Gen Hosp Psychiatry* 1997;19(3):185–199.
51. Wessely S, Chalder T, Hirsch S, et al. Psychological symptoms, somatic symptoms, and psychiatric disorder in chronic fatigue and chronic fatigue syndrome: a prospective study in the primary care setting. *Am J Psychiatry* 1996;153(8):1050–1059.
52. Lane TJ, Manu P, Matthews DA. Depression and somatization in the chronic fatigue syndrome. *Am J Med* 1991;91(4): 335–344.
53. American Association for Chronic Fatigue Syndrome. A statement for the advisory board of The American Association for Chronic Fatigue Syndrome (AACFS), 2000.
54. Reid S, Chalder T, Cleare A, et al. Extracts from "clinical evidence" chronic fatigue syndrome. *BMJ* 2000;320:292–296.
55. American College of Sports Medicine. *ACSM's Guidelines for exercise testing and prescription*. 6th ed. Baltimore: Lippincott Williams & Wilkins, 2000.
56. Hodgson B, Kizior RJ. *Saunders nursing drug handbook 1999*. Philadelphia: W.B. Saunders Co., 1999.
57. Salit IE. The chronic fatigue syndrome: a position paper. *J Rheumat* 1996;23(3):540–544.
58. Sisto SA, LaManca JJ, Cordero DL, et al. Metabolic and cardiovascular effects of a progressive exercise test in patients with chronic fatigue syndrome. *Am J Med* 1996;100:634–640.
59. Gibson H, Carroll N, Clague JE, et al. Exercise performance and fatigability in patients with chronic fatigue syndrome. *J Neuro Neurosurg Psychiatry* 1993;56:993–998.
60. Mullis R, Campbell IT, Wearden AJ, et al. Prediction of peak oxygen uptake in chronic fatigue syndrome. *Br J Sports Med* 1999;33:352–356.
61. Montague TJ, Marrie TJ, Klassen GA, et al. Cardiac function at rest and with exercise in the chronic fatigue syndrome. *Chest* 1989;95:779–784.
62. LaManca JJ, Sisto SA, Zhou XD, et al. Immunological response in chronic fatigue syndrome following a graded exercise test to exhaustion. *J Clin Immunol* 1999;19(2):135–142.
63. Riley MS, O'Brien CJ, McCluskey DR, et al. Aerobic work capacity in patients with chronic fatigue syndrome. *BMJ* 1990; 301:953–956.
64. Lloyd AR, Gandevia SC, Hales JP. Muscle performance, voluntary activation, twitch properties, and perceived effort in normal subjects and patients with the chronic fatigue syndrome. *Brain* 1991;114:85–98.
65. Stokes MJ, Cooper RG, Edwards RH. Normal muscle strength and fatigability in patients with effort syndromes. *BMJ* 1988; 297:1014–1017.
66. Wong R, Lopachuk G, Zhu G, et al. Skeletal muscle metabolism in the chronic fatigue syndrome. In vivo assessment by P nuclear magnetic resonance spectroscopy. *Chest* 1992;102: 1716–1722.
67. Kent-Braun JA, Sharma KR, Weiner MW, et al. Central basis of muscle fatigue in chronic fatigue syndrome. *Neurology* 1993;43:125–131.
68. Barnes PR, Taylor DJ, Kemp GJ, et al. Skeletal muscle bioenergetics in the chronic fatigue syndrome. *J Neuro Neurosurg Psychiatry* 1993;56:679–683.
69. McCully KK, Natelson BH, Lotti S, et al. Reduced oxidative muscle metabolism in chronic fatigue syndrome. *Muscle Nerve* 1996;19:621–625.
70. McCully KK, Natelson BH. Impaired oxygen delivery to muscle in chronic fatigue syndrome. *Clin Sci* 1999;97:603–608.
71. Edwards RH, Gibson H, Clague JE, et al. Muscle histopathology and physiology in chronic fatigue syndrome. *Ciba Found Symp* 1993;173:102–17, discussion 117–131.
72. Clapp LL, Richardson MT, Smith JF, et al. Acute effects of thirty minutes of light-intensity, intermittent exercise on patients with chronic fatigue syndrome. *Phys Ther* 1999;79:749–756.
73. Cress ME, Buchner DM, Questad KA, et al. Continuous-scale physical functional performance in healthy older adults: a validation study. *Arch Phys Med Rehabil* 1996;77:1243–1250.
74. Fulcher KY, White PD. Randomized controlled trial of graded

exercise in patients with chronic fatigue syndrome. *BMJ* 1997;314:1647–1652.

75. Marlin RG, Anchel H, Gibson JC, et al. An evaluation of multidisciplinary intervention for chronic fatigue syndrome with long-term follow-up, and a comparison with untreated controls. *Am J Med* 1998;105(3A):110S–114S.
76. Sisto SA. Chronic fatigue syndrome: an overview and intervention guidelines. *Neurol Rep* 1993;17:30–34.
77. Smith DG. The management of postviral fatigue syndrome in general practice. In: Jenkins R, Mowbray J, eds. *Postviral fatigue syndrome.* John Wiley & Sons Ltd., 1991. NY.
78. Komaroff AL. Clinical presentation of chronic fatigue syndrome. *Ciba Found Symp* 1993;173:46–54, discussion 54–61.
79. Fischler B, Dendale P, Micheils V, et al. Physical fatigability and exercise capacity in chronic fatigue syndrome: association with disability, somatization, and psychopathology. *J Psychom Res* 1997;42(4):369–378.

CHAPTER **19**

Hematologic Disorders

Louise M. Burke and Robin Parisotto

IRON DEFICIENCY

EPIDEMIOLOGY AND PATHOPHYSIOLOGY

At a global level, iron-deficiency anemia is the most commonly occurring nutritional deficiency. In developing countries or among high-risk groups, iron deficiency can affect 30–40% of the population, whereas the prevalence of iron-deficiency anemia in the general community is typically 1–3%. Recently, athletes have come under scrutiny as one such high-risk group. During the 1970s, exercise scientists commented on some interesting differences in the hematological characteristics of long-distance runners. Endurance athletes were seen to have reduced plasma hemoglobin concentrations; a characteristic that seemed unfavorable for the performance of events reliant on the delivery of oxygen to working muscles (1). After study, this phenomenon was found to be a false or dilutional anemia, resulting from the acute increase in plasma volume that accompanies heavy aerobic training (2). Termed "sports anemia," it is not considered a pathology or disadvantage to performance, does not limit the production of red blood cells, and does not respond to iron-supplementation therapy (3). Some decades later, it might be argued that we are in a similar situation with our concern about the iron status of athletes; while we recognise that suboptimal iron status can reduce exercise performance, we are also likely to overdiagnose the true prevalence and problem among people who exercise.

The Role of Iron

About 3–5 g of iron is found in the body in three main pools: storage iron (ferritin and hemosiderin) found predominantly in the spleen, liver, and bone marrow; transport iron (transported through the plasma and extravascular fluids by the carrier, transferrin); and oxygen-transport iron (within the active centers of hemoglobin in the erythrocyte and myoglobin in the muscle). The majority of iron in the body is carefully recycled, with iron from destroyed erythrocytes being salvaged for storage or reincorporation into new reticulocytes. Iron status is a result of the balance between the small amounts of dietary iron that are absorbed each day and small iron losses from skin, sweat, and the gastrointestinal and urinary tracts. It should be noted that, apart from blood loss, there is no mechanism to remove excess iron from the body. Important functions of iron and iron-related compounds in the body are:

- Transport of oxygen in the blood (hemoglobin) and muscle (myoglobin)
- As a component of enzyme systems such as the electron transport chain, ribonucleotide reductase (required for the production of DNA), catalase, and succinate dehydrogenase
- As a catalyst in the production of free oxygen radical species

Whereas a small percentage of the population (usually male) suffers from hemochromatosis, or iron-overload disease, whereby excessive amounts of iron are absorbed and deposited in major organs, the more common problem with iron status is iron depletion. (For further reviews of iron metabolism, see Refs. 3–5.)

Iron drain is thought to progress through a number of stages with different functional and diagnostic criteria. These stages are summarized in Table 19.1. The end stage of iron-deficiency anemia is detected by blood iron status measures that are below population reference standards and also below the "normal or usual" concentrations for an individual. At this stage, there is inadequate iron available in the bone marrow for the normal manufacture of hemoglobin and erythrocytes, leading to the production of red blood cells that are small and pale. Interference with oxygen transport and enzyme function leads to clinical symptoms associated with the impairment of muscle metabolism, brain metabolism, immunity, and temperature control.

Causes of Iron Deficiency

Iron deficiency occurs in athletes and people who exercise for the same reason it occurs in sedentary populations:

Table 19.1 Stages of Iron Drain (3)

		General Diagnostic Criteria—Blood Measures		
Stage	Characteristics	Hemoglobin (g/100 mL)	Ferritin (ng/mL)	Transferrin Saturation (%)
Normal iron status	Iron status measurements within normal reference ranges, normal appearance of erythrocytes	>12.0 (F) >16.0 (M)	>30 (F) >110 (M)	20–40 (M, F)
Iron depletion	Normal hematocrit, normal hemoglobin, low serum ferritin, normal to high transferrin saturation	As above	<30 (M, F)	20–40 (M, F)
Iron deficiency	Low serum ferritin, low serum iron and serum transferrin, reduced transferrin saturation, normal hemoglobin	As above	<12 (M, F)	<16 (M, F)
Iron-deficiency anemia	Low hemoglobin, change in erythrocytes (microcytic, hypochromic, reduced mean corpuscular volume), low hematocrit, low serum iron, low serum transferrin and transferrin saturation	<12.0 (F) <14.0 (M)	<10 (M, F)	<6 (M, F)

iron requirements and/or losses exceed iron intake over a sufficient period of time. Iron requirements are increased during periods of growth, reflected by the higher recommended daily allowances for iron during adolescence and while pregnant (see Table 19.2). Iron needs are higher in females of reproductive age than in males to account for the monthly menstrual blood losses (Table 19.2).

Increased iron losses may also occur through conditions or problems that cause substantial or prolonged blood loss, such as tumors, gastrointestinal ulcers, surgery, or severe bruising. Given the individual characteristics of athletes, it is not possible to make general recommendations for iron requirements of people who exercise; however, there is a general appreciation that there is an increase in iron requirements and iron turnover in those who undertake prolonged and heavy training. It is believed that iron losses are greater in athletes because of increased iron losses through sweating (7), gastrointestinal blood loss (8), and mechanical trauma to red blood cells (9). Although these losses might seem small and inconsequential, over a prolonged period they may lead to iron drain unless there is a compensatory increase in iron intake. Although undetected blood losses are generally the cause of iron deficiency in older and male populations, at a global level, inadequate intake of available iron is the major cause of iron deficiency. This is probably also true in the sports world.

Iron is found in a range of plant and animal food sources, with the iron density of a mixed diet being 5–6 mg/1000 kcal. Dietary iron is found in two forms: as heme iron, found only in flesh or blood containing animal foods, and organic iron, which is found in both animal foods and plant foods (see Table 19.3). Whereas heme iron is relatively well absorbed from single foods and mixed meals (15–35% bioavailability), the absorption of nonheme iron from single plant sources is low and variable (2–8%) (11). The bioavailability of nonheme iron is affected by the presence of enhancing or inhibiting factors

Table 19.2 Recommended Daily Allowances for Iron (6)

Population		Iron RDA (mg/d)
Males	11–18 yr	12
	19–24 yr	10
	24–50 yr	10
	51+ yr	10
Females	11–18 yr	15
	19–24 yr	15
	24–50 yr	15
	51+ yr	10
	Pregnant	30
	Lactating	15

Table 19.3 Dietary Sources of Iron (10)

Food	Serving	Iron (mg)
ANIMAL SOURCES: containing both heme and nonheme iron		
Liver (beef, cooked)	3.5 oz (100 g)	8.8
Liver pâté	1 oz (30 g)	1.6
Lean cooked beef steak	3.5 oz (100 g)	4.0
Lean cooked roast lamb	3.5 oz (100 g)	3.2
Lean cooked chicken breast	3.5 oz (100 g)	1.1
Lean cooked chicken drumstick	(50 g)	1.4
Oysters	1/2 doz (100 g)	5.5
Canned tuna	6.5 oz (185 g)	2.1
Fish, white flesh	3.5 oz (100 g)	0.9
Sliced ham (lean)	1 oz (30 g)	0.3
PLANT SOURCES: containing nonheme iron		
Fortified oat flakes cereal	2/3 cup (30 g)	8.1
Nonfortified cornflakes	1 cup (30 g)	0.8
Porridge	3/4 cup (170 g)	1.2
Whole wheat bread	1 slice (24 g)	0.8
White bread	1 slice (24 g)	0.6
Baked beans in sauce	8 oz (225 g)	3.6
Lentils	2/3 cup (100 g)	2.1
Raisins	2/3 cup (100 g)	1.8
Almonds	1 oz (30 g)	1.4
Spinach (cooked)	1/2 cup (90 g)	2.0
Apple	small (140 g)	0.3

in foods eaten during the same meal. Enhancing factors include vitamin C (found in citrus, tropical and berry fruits, and some vegetables), peptides from meat/fish/chicken (often called the meat-enhancement factor), alcohol, and some foods with a low pH due to fermentation or the presence of citric or tartaric acids (3). Inhibiting factors include phytate (found in whole-grain cereals and soy protein), polyphenol (found in tea and red wine), calcium (found in milk and cheese), and peptides such as soy protein (found in plants) (3). Until recently, the absorption of heme iron was considered to be relatively unaffected by other dietary compounds; however, updated study techniques have shown that other meal components such as calcium and plant peptides may reduce heme iron bioavailability (12). The absorption of both heme and nonheme iron is increased as an adaptive response in people who are iron deficient or have increased iron requirements. It should be noted that iron bioavailability studies from which these observations have been made have not been undertaken on special groups such as athletes. However, it is generally assumed that the results can be applied across populations of healthy people.

In a mixed diet where lean meats are consumed regularly, heme iron may provide about half of the absorbable iron. However, in many Western countries such as the United States and Australia, cereal products such as bread and breakfast cereals are the single greatest source of total dietary iron because of the fortification of these products with additional iron and the frequency with which they are consumed (3). Assessment of total dietary iron intake is not necessarily a good predictor of iron status; the mixing and matching of foods at meals plays an important role by determining the bioavailability of dietary iron intake. For example, in two groups of female runners who reported similar intakes of total dietary iron, the group who reported regular intake of meat was estimated to have a greater intake of absorbable iron and showed higher iron status than a matched group of runners who were semivegetarian (13).

Prevalence of Iron Deficiency in Athletes

Finding the true prevalence of problematic iron deficiency in people who exercise is dependent on answering the following questions:

1. Can the reference standards for biochemical and hematological parameters used to diagnose the stages of iron deficiency in normal populations be applied to athletes?
2. At what stage of iron depletion are impairments to exercise performance observed?
3. What is optimal iron status for an athlete, particularly an endurance athlete?

Our current understanding of these issues will be discussed later in this chapter. However, when examining the literature related to iron deficiency in athletes, it should be noted that the prevalence was overstated in earlier times because of different interpretations of this information. According to the review by Haymes (14), the prevalence of anemia reported among groups of athletes ranges from 0–12.5%, whereas low ferritin levels might be expected in 0–44% of an athletic group. However, since many studies lack control groups for comparison and use different cut-off values to designate low or suboptimal levels, it is hard to gain an overview of the true problem. Fogelholm has also undertaken a sophisticated summary of the literature (15), in which only those studies that included control groups were evaluated. He concluded that the reported prevalence of iron-deficiency anemia is quite low (<3%) and similar between athletes and untrained individuals. Meanwhile, the pooled mean prevalence of low serum ferritin was 37% (range 13–50%) in male and female athletes and 23% (range 10–46%) in controls. The highest prevalence of low ferritin levels was seen in endurance sports, and among female and adolescent athletes, irrespective of the type of sport and intensity of training (15).

CLINICAL EXERCISE PHYSIOLOGY

Effect of Anemia on Exercise Performance

It is well known that anemia causes a reduction in exercise performance. In cases of severely reduced hemoglobin levels, individuals may be unable to carry out everyday activities and work tasks and may report a noticeable breathlessness on even the mildest exertion. The major effects result from impairment of oxygen transport in blood and muscle and impaired functioning of iron-related enzymes; however, reductions in cognition, temperature control, and immunity may also exacerbate the impaired exercise tolerance.

Although the effects of gradually reduced hemoglobin on performance have not been systematically studied, it is believed that even a small decline in hemoglobin levels (e.g., 1–2 mg/100 mL) will reduce the competition performance of athletes (4). Since the range of "normal" hemoglobin levels is reasonably wide, it is possible that an athlete may show a level that is within reference standards but is below the level that is "usual" for him/her, and below that required for his/her optimal performance. Although a low hemoglobin level may be relatively easy to detect, it is difficult to confirm optimal iron status from a single blood test. There is great value in establishing a history of iron status results from the individual athlete to establish a feel for what is normal for them, and how parameters may vary even when steps are taken to prevent or interpret these fluctuations (see below).

Athletes often believe that the "more is better" principal applies to hemoglobin levels per se. However, in the absence of hemoconcentration due to dehydration, very high hemoglobin levels are usually explained by genetic individuality or drug use (e.g., EPO) and are not possible for most athletes to achieve.

Effect of Reduced Iron Status Without Anemia on Exercise Performance

The most contentious and badly interpreted issue about the iron status of athletes lies with the effect of reduced iron status, in the absence of anemia, on performance. It is assumed that serum ferritin levels reflect the total storage of ferritin iron in the body. Low serum ferritin levels have become synonymous with reduced iron status, and the effect on performance has been investigated mostly by studying the effects of iron supplementation on the performance with low ferritin levels. Those who have studied this literature conclude that there is little evidence that iron depletion, in the absence of anemia, impairs the performance of a single exercise task, or that iron supplementation enhances the performance of athletes with moderately low serum ferritin but normal hemoglobin levels (3–5, 16). The two studies in which a performance improvement was seen after iron supplementation in subjects with low ferritin levels also show an increase in hemoglobin levels in response to the therapy, suggesting that the subjects had suboptimal hemoglobin levels prior to the supplementation (17, 18). It appears that there are various reasons for reduced ferritin levels, or dissociation between serum and total body ferritin levels that do not represent pathology or a detriment to exercise performance (4). However, there are many criticisms of the current studies of iron supplementation in iron-depleted groups. These include the failure to implement the recommended iron supplementation program, differences in the cut-off values considered as low and adequate for serum ferritin, and the mixing of subjects with varying levels of ferritin within treatment groups. Studies have also failed to address the complaint commonly made by athletes with reduced iron stores that they fail to recover between a series of competition or training sessions.

Therefore, at the present time there is no evidence to suggest that a moderately reduced ferritin level per se is detrimental to performance, or that endurance athletes should receive routine iron supplementation. However, since low ferritin levels may become progressively lower and eventually lead to problematic iron deficiency, there is merit in providing such athletes with routine assessment of their iron status, and on occasions, implementing therapy in individuals deemed to be at high risk of a further decline in iron stores.

DIAGNOSTIC TECHNIQUES

There is no single test or piece of information that can assess iron status adequately in all situations. Therefore, such an assessment should be made from a careful interpretation of information from a variety of sources.

Clinical Presentation

Frank anemia can usually be detected by a clinical presentation of pallor, breathlessness after mild exercise, and complaints of fatigue, lethargy, headaches, and an increase in illness. Of course, these symptoms are nonspecific and may be found as a result of overtraining or various infections. However, athletes are more likely to present at an early stage of iron depletion. Athletes who are iron deficient without anemia may complain of feeling "run down" or failing to recover between training or competition sessions. Sometimes, however, athletes present without symptoms but with concern about a low reading on a routine hematologic or biochemical screen for iron status.

Hematologic and Biochemical Tests

Parameters that are routinely measured to indicate iron status are summarized in Table 19.1, along with the reference standards that are used to denote the various stages of iron depletion in normal populations. These should be cautiously applied to athletic populations since various issues related to exercise can alter these parameters, both to falsely elevate and to decrease the measures. A summary of common changes to iron status measurements is presented in Table 19.4. In addition, most parameters are subject to diurnal fluctuations and other physiological variations. Blood tests should be collected in a way that minimizes interference from these issues (e.g., taken after a rest day to avoid increases in ferritin, which as an acute phase reactant may be elevated in response to a single bout of hard exercise, or after ensuring that the athlete is well hydrated). The results should also be interpreted with consideration of these issues. For example, in athletic populations, ferritin levels below 30–35 ng/mL (3, 5) are generally marked for further consideration or review. As previously mentioned, the comparison of results to the established iron status history of an individual can help to make a differential diagnosis, as can the assessment of risk factors likely to cause or explain iron drain.

Table 19.4 Reported Changes in Iron Status Parameters in Conditions Encountered by Exercise (adapted from 3)

	Hemoglobin	Transferrin Saturation (Saturation of Iron-Transport Proteins)	Serum Iron	Ferritin
Plasma volume expansion in response to aerobic training	↓	↓	↓	↓
Dehydration at the time of testing	↑	↑	↑	↑
Infection (URTI, flu, virus) or inflammation	↓	↓	↓	↑
After acute strenuous exercise (after 24 hr)	↓	↓	↓	↓

Other hematologic and biochemical tests are becoming available to add further clarity to the assessment of iron status. These include the measurement of serum transferrin receptors (which are increased in response to reduced iron status to assist in the transport of iron from the blood to tissues), and the characteristics of reticulocytes. These and other parameters are reviewed by Deakin (3). However, since these tests are not routinely available in all laboratories and need to be studied carefully in relation to iron status in athletes, at the present time they are not of general clinical utility.

Presence of Other Risk Factors

Support for an assessment of low iron status assessment, and in particular a substantial reduction in blood parameters of iron status, can often be found by looking for the presence of risk factors for iron drain or negative iron balance. Important risk factors are listed in Table 19.5.

PHARMACOLOGY

Iron Injections

A rapid reversal of iron depletion and an increase in iron stores can be achieved via intramuscular injections of iron. This is sometimes provided in cases of extreme iron depletion, which carry a significant penalty to the individual involved, or where oral iron intake is not tolerated.

Table 19.5. Risk Factors for Iron Drain or Negative Iron Balance

Predictors of increased iron requirements
- Recent growth spurt in adolescents
- Pregnancy (current or within the past year)

Predictors of increased iron losses or iron malabsorption
- Sudden increase in heavy training load, particularly involving running on hard surfaces
- Gastrointestinal malabsorption problems (e.g., Crohn's disease, ulcerative colitis, parasite infestation)
- Gastrointestinal bleeding due to chronic use of some anti-inflammatory drugs, ulcers, or other problems
- Heavy menstrual blood losses
- Excessive blood losses such as frequent nose bleeds, recent surgery, substantial contact injuries
- Frequent blood donation

Predictors of inadequate intake of bioavailable iron
- Chronic low energy intake (<2000 kcal/day)
- Vegetarian eating—especially poorly constructed diets in which alternative food sources of iron are ignored (e.g., legumes, nuts, seeds)
- Fad diets or erratic eating patterns
- Restricted variety of foods in diet and failure to promote mixing and matching of foods at meals (especially vitamin-C–containing fruit and vegetables)
- Heavy reliance on convenience foods and micronutrient-poor sports foods (high CHO powders, bars, and gels)
- Very high carbohydrate diet with high fiber content and infrequent intake of meats/fish/chicken
- Natural food diets: failure to consume iron-fortified cereal foods such as commercial breakfast cereals and bread

However, in some athletic circles, it has become popular as a more "high-tech" method of supplementation and is even known to be used in cases where iron deficiency has not been characterized. Iron injection does not provide a superior technique of iron repletion per se, particularly as a significant proportion of the iron remains in the buttock, unabsorbed. Because it carries a risk of anaphylactic shock as well as iron overload, it should not be regarded as the first choice of treatment or a benign therapy. Iron injections will not increase hemoglobin levels or other iron parameters in people who are not otherwise suboptimal in iron status (19).

Iron Supplements

Oral iron supplements provide part of the usual therapy recommended to treat iron deficiency and anemia. Most authorities recommend that such therapy should be prescribed on a case-by-case basis, as part of a treatment plan involving strategies to reduce or prevent unusual iron losses, and dietary counseling to maximize the intake of bioavailable iron (3, 5). The recognized therapy is a daily dose of 100 mg elemental iron (which may be equal to 500 mg of ferrous sulphate), taken on an empty stomach. Many people take a vitamin C supplement or juice with their supplement to enhance the absorption of this organic iron. A 3-month period of supplementation is needed to restore depleted iron stores (5). In some cases, when it is not possible to enhance dietary iron intake sufficiently, it may be necessary to continue iron supplementation at a lower dose, or as a 1–2/week intake to prevent ongoing iron drain.

Although iron supplements are available as over-the-counter medications, there are dangers in self-prescription as a tonic, or long-term supplementation in the absence of medical follow-up. Iron supplementation is not a replacement for medical and dietary assessment and therapy, since it fails to correct underlying problems that have caused iron drain. In many cases, a diet that is inadequate in iron will also fail to meet other sports nutrition goals. Chronic supplementation with high doses of iron carries a risk of iron overload, especially in males for whom the genetic traits for hemochromatosis are more prevalent. Iron supplements can also interfere with the absorption of other minerals such as zinc and copper. Some individuals suffer from gastrointestinal side effects arising from the use of iron supplements.

DIETARY PRESCRIPTION AND COUNSELING

The major goal of dietary counseling is to increase the person's intake of bioavailable iron, with eating patterns that are compatible with his/her other nutritional goals (e.g., achieving fuel requirements for sport, achieving desired physique). This is often a specialized task, requiring the expertise of a dietitian. Key dietary goals are summarized below:

- Consume enough energy to allow nutritional goals to be met. Avoid chronic periods of energy restriction and severe weight loss.
- Include small amounts of lean red meats in meals at least 3–4 times each week. Meat can be added to a high-carbohydrate meal to achieve overall sports nutrition goals (e.g., sandwich with roast beef, pasta with meat sauce, lamb kabobs with rice, beef stir fry with vegetables and noodles). The presence of meat enhances iron absorption from other foods at the meal.
- Add chicken and pork at other meals to provide a reasonable source of iron and to enhance iron absorption at the meal.
- Consider shellfish or liver (e.g., pâté) as an alternative to red meat.
- Make use of cereals that are iron fortified (e.g., many commercial breakfast cereals).
- Include iron-rich foods such as whole grains, dried fruit, legumes, eggs, nuts, and seeds in meals, and use the match with an iron-absorbing food (meat or vitamin-C–containing food) to enhance the bioavailability of iron. For example, combine parsley with an omelet, or tomato sauce with rice and lentils.
- Combine vitamin-C–containing foods at meals where whole-grain cereals are eaten (to counteract the iron-inhibiting phytate). For example, drink a glass of juice with breakfast cereal, or have fruit or salad vegetables with a whole-meal sandwich.
- If you are at risk of iron drain, drink tea and coffee between meals rather than at meals.

EXERCISE PRESCRIPTION

Exercise prescription for people with iron deficiency is dependent on the degree to which reduced iron status interferes with exercise capacity and the possibility that exercise is increasing the iron drain. Because fatigue is one of the principal symptoms of anemia and possibly also iron deficiency without anemia, it may reduce the ability to undertake or enjoy exercise. Therefore, it is prudent not to commence or increase an exercise regimen for the iron-deficient person. Rather, exercise prescription should achieve a level that is comfortable for the individual and his/her symptoms of fatigue. Depending on the individual, the duration, frequency, and/or intensity of exercise sessions should be considered. These factors may need to be reduced or modified until iron-replacement therapy has progressed sufficiently to abate the feelings of fatigue or poor recovery between sessions. This may be simple for the recreational exerciser but is likely to require careful planning in the case of the serious athlete, so that there is minimal compromise of long-term fitness and competition goals.

Exercise prescription should also consider the possibility that activity patterns can cause iron losses that are adding to the iron drain. In this case, it may be prudent to modify exercise patterns or associated activities to provide an opportunity for iron status to be improved. A sudden increase in exercise load, particularly involving foot strike damage or blood loss/contact injuries, may exacerbate iron drain in individuals with low iron intake and precarious iron balance. While iron-replacement treatment and improved iron intake are the cornerstones of therapy, it also makes sense to monitor exercise patterns to avoid excessive iron losses. Tactics may include choosing a slower rate of introducing or increasing a training program, finding softer surfaces to run on, replacing worn shoes with footwear that offers better cushioning, and avoiding activities with a high risk of blood loss or substantial bruising. Some activities associated with exercise, such as the use of certain nonsteroidal anti-inflammatory drugs to manage pain or overuse injuries may need to be examined for their possible role in causing gastrointestinal blood losses. Again, the modification of an exercise program may be simple in the case of the recreational exerciser, but compromise and creativity are often needed for the care of the serious or elite athlete.

CASE STUDIES

CASE 1

A female cross-country skier presented with moderate anemia. Ferritin and other parameters were normal, eliminating chronic iron-deficiency anemia but suggestive of acute blood loss. She began iron therapy, and her hemoglobin increased from 10.2–12.5 g/100 mL in 3 weeks. Symptoms of fatigue abated, leaving her ready to compete. It was subsequently found that she had suffered unusually heavy menstrual flow.

CASE 2

A female basketball player presented for a routine blood screen. Although her hemoglobin level was within the normal range, some of the reticulocyte parameters were abnormal. On questioning, she revealed symptoms of lethargy and poor recovery between training sessions. She reported that she had been following a strict weight-loss diet over the previous 3 months and was avoiding the intake of all meats, which were considered to be "too fatty." Further blood tests were taken on the suspicion of low iron status, which was confirmed by a low ferritin level. She was referred for dietary counseling to allow her to achieve body fat goals, while increasing her intake of well-absorbed iron. Simultaneously, she was started on a 3-month course of oral iron supplements. Review after 3 months showed an increase in ferritin levels from 16–42 ng/mL and improvement in well-being. Her hemoglobin concentration also rose, indicating that her initial reading, although within the normal range, was suboptimal for her. After assessment of high iron eating patterns, iron supplementation was ceased, and a further blood and dietary review was organized for 6 months.

CASE 3

A female swimmer was reviewed by a new doctor in the sports medicine clinic after her routine blood tests revealed a ferritin concentration of 28 ng/mL. She reported training well and performing well. She had been eating all her meals in an athlete dining hall for the previous year and reported eating a varied menu, including meat-containing meals at least 3 times a week. All other hematological and biochemical tests were normal. Her medical history showed that ferritin test results from the previous 2 years, during similar periods of training, were 29, 32, 27, and 35 ng/mL. It was concluded that the present results represented normal iron status for this swimmer, and no therapy was needed.

CASE 4

A male triathlete presented with tiredness and a history of mild to moderate diarrhea persisting over the previous month. The triathlete reported being under the care of a sports dietitian and was following a high-carbohydrate diet, with attention to a good intake of bioavailable iron. History revealed that the gastrointestinal problems had begun after completing a triathlon swim in a dam in an area where *Giardia lamblia* infestation was common. Cultures confirmed this problem, and a course of treatment was commenced. However, a blood screen also showed a ferritin level of 23 ng/mL, in comparison to his previous test results of 85 ng/mL. Hemoglobin levels were within the normal range. Iron supplementation was prescribed to replete iron stores, and a 3-month follow-up check was organized.

SICKLE-CELL ANEMIA

EPIDEMIOLOGY AND PATHOPHYSIOLOGY

The most common structural hemoglobinopathy, sickle-cell anemia, was first recorded by James Herrich of Chicago in 1910 (20). He described crescent-shaped "sickle cells" in a young black student from the West Indies. The greatest prevalence of sickle-cell anemia is in Africa; however, the gene is also common in northern Mediterranean countries; North, Central, and South America; the Middle East; and India. The heterozygous form (sickle-cell trait-HbAS) is found in up to 8–10% of American blacks, and in some regions of Africa, may reach as high as 40% (20). The prevalence of HbS in professional football players (21) and high school athletes (22) has been nearly identical to the prevalence in the corresponding general population. In a study conducted in the Ivory Coast, the incidence of the gene was 12% (23). The homozygous form (HbSS) has an incidence rate of up to 1.3% (20). It is of interest that the gene occurs most frequently in areas where malarial infections caused by the parasite *Plasmodium falciparum* is common. This suggests a selective advantage, and immunity to this form of malaria may exist in these individuals; consequently, the gene frequency has built up over time.

HbSS, which usually presents as a moderate to severe anemia, suggests that affected individuals cannot physiologically perform at a level consistent with elite competition due to the low total Hb mass. Conversely, heterozygous sickle-cell anemia (sickle-cell trait) with normal hemoglobin levels allows affected individuals to compete at the elite level. However, evidence collected since the early 1970s suggests that individuals with sickle-cell trait are at increased risk of exertional rhabdomyolysis and/or sudden death, after exercise (24–28). This is a significant issue, given the prevalence of the gene in the African-American population.

Hemoglobin S (HbS) is the mutant hemoglobin produced when nonpolar valine is substituted for polar glutamic acid in the beta chain. The solubility of HbS in the deoxygenated state (sickled cells) is markedly reduced, producing a tendency for deoxyhemoglobin S molecules to polymerize into rigid aggregates, causing occlusions in the capillaries. Exercise that can substantially influence temperature, hypoxia, acidosis, and dehydration in the body can potentially trigger changes in hemoglobin status of individuals with HbS, by promoting deoxygenation and the formation of HbS polymers. The hypoxic, acidotic, and hypertonic microenvironments of the kidney, spleen, and retina also promote HbS polymerization and sickling, and intense exercise may exacerbate this (20).

The concentration of hemoglobin also influences sickling. The more concentrated the HbS within the red blood cell, the greater the potential for HbS aggregates to form. Some have speculated that hydrating the cells can prevent sickling (20).

Polymerization of deoxyhemoglobin S begins when the oxygen saturation of hemoglobin falls below 85% and is complete at about 38% oxygen saturation. Altitude exposures for training and/or acclimatization purposes are important issues to consider in individuals with HbS (20).

The oxygen affinity of HbS may result in important physiological changes in vivo. HbS has decreased oxygen affinity. The 2,3-DPG levels of homozygote HbS are increased, and hence, the right shift in the oxygen dissociation curves means more oxygen is released to the tissues. This results in the increase in the concentration of deoxyhemoglobin S, promoting the formation of sickle cells. This may occur in the heterozygous state; however, the presence of HbA ensures that any polymers formed are weak (20).

CLINICAL EXERCISE PHYSIOLOGY

There is ample evidence suggesting that individuals with HbS can perform at levels normal or near normal in relation to exercise capacity and maximal oxygen uptake when compared to appropriate control individuals (26). In a half-marathon held in the Ivory Coast, there were no significant differences in the rankings of HbS individuals and normal individuals (23). One HbS individual finished second; however, it was later determined that he was a double heterozygote HbS/alpha thalassemia. The authors noted that of all the internationally ranked runners in the race, none had HbS, and that this may indicate that HbS is a limiting factor in endurance performance. They also made the point that a double heterozygote may be a performance-enhancing factor.

PHARMACOLOGY

There are no agents/drugs used to treat HbS because it is generally a benign condition. There are, however, pharmacologic agents that can reduce intracellular sickling in homozygous HbSS. Hydroxyurea and butyrate are drugs currently used to prevent sickling. These agents elevate fetal hemoglobin (HbF) levels, causing a decrease in intracellular polymerization of HbS.

MEDICAL TREATMENT

Aside from sudden collapse during exercise, other signs of exertional rhabdomyolysis include muscular weakness, muscle swelling, and/or cramping with darkened urine. In advanced cases of exertional rhabdomyolysis and sickling, appropriate emergency medical care is required to alleviate symptoms and prevent organ failure and/or possible death.

In acute cases of sickling, which may lead to morbidity and/or mortality, the most effective treatment regime to minimize organ damage is to remove the stimulus precipitating sickling, such as dehydration and/or altitude exposure.

PHYSICAL EXAMINATION

In homozygous HbSS individuals, a physical examination may reveal findings associated with sickling, such as anemia, splenomegaly, and dyspnea. In heterozygous HbS, the physical findings are not so obvious, and only an adequate history and appropriate blood tests would identify such individuals. Diagnostic tests include hemoglobin electrophoresis, where up to 35–45% of the total hemoglobin is made up of HbS; sickling test, where red blood cells are induced to sickle in the presence of a reducing agent such as sodium metabisulphite; and solubility test, in which HbS is deoxygenated with dithionite, increasing the opacity of the solution.

EXERCISE PRESCRIPTION

Between 1977 and 1981, the sudden, unexplained exercise-induced deaths of 62 recruits involved in basic training revealed that individuals with HbS were 28–40 times at greater risk (25). These sudden deaths could, however, be related to acute cardiac arrest of undefined mechanism, exertional heat stroke, or heat stress. In particular, exertional rhabdomyolysis, a syndrome characterized by skeletal muscle degeneration and muscle enzyme leakage (26), has been linked to at least 17 cases of sudden collapse and/or deaths in persons with HbS (24–28). There are also numerous cases of nonfatal exertional collapse (29). The mechanisms are not known; however, renal tubule damage can be caused by extreme physical exertion when myoglobin is released from working muscles. A metabolite of myoglobin breakdown, ferriheme, has been shown to be toxic to renal tubule epithelium in vitro (30). Another possible mechanism for such catastrophic events is the "sickling" of red blood cells. This sickling may occur for a number of reasons, and the end result is organ failure due to the polymerization of HbS, causing vaso-occlusion in the capillaries (20).

It is not known whether HbS itself predisposes these individuals to greater risk of exertional rhabdomyolysis and/or sudden death. It has been proposed that dehydration could result in the sickling of red blood cells in the muscle capillaries, or of their inability to concentrate their urine when deprived of water (31). This defect may result in the poor conservation of water in HbS individuals and increase the risks of dehydration. This could lead to the inevitable cascade of events resulting in organ failure and/or death.

There is sufficient evidence now to implicate HbS with exertional rhabdomyolysis and/or sudden postexercise death, although the mechanisms are still unclear. The significant risk in HbS individuals suffering from either of these is sobered by the fact that most cases still occur in athletes without sickle-cell trait. This should not, however, diminish the importance of implementing proper prevention strategies for those at risk. It is unlikely that the risks will deter athletes with HbS from competing. Any coach and/or athlete associated with or afflicted by HbS should at all times practice caution during training and/or competition. Primary risk factors such as extreme heat and humidity, high altitude, illness, and fatigue should be evaluated and addressed before each session of intense exercise. Attention to hydration status is particularly important, and strict compliance should be observed with fluid replacements in all athletes and not just those with HbS.

Ignoring such simple strategies could lead to fatal outcomes, which emphasizes the importance of HbS in the sporting context. Table 19.6 lists recommended measures for preventing exertional rhabdomyolysis in athletes with HbS (28).

CASE STUDIES

CASE 5

In 1991, a 22-year-old football player suddenly collapsed after completing an 800-m run. The athlete had been training intensively for 4 weeks and had passed a preevent physical. Despite aggressive and immediate treatment for exertional rhabdomyolysis, the athlete died 46 hours after his collapse. It was subsequently found that the athlete had HbS (32).

Table 19.6 Suggested Strategies for the Prevention of Exertional Rhabdomyolysis in Athletes with HbS (28)

1. Develop and implement conditioning programs prior to the resumption of intense training or competition.
2. Develop and implement aggressive hydration policies before, during, and after all activity.
3. Avoid the use of beverages that have diuretic effects (e.g., caffeine, alcohol).
4. Avoid strenuous exercise in hot, humid conditions and at altitudes of 2500 ft or more.
5. Modify activities during or following viral illness, particularly when vomiting and diarrhea has occurred.
6. Modify activities during periods of poor sleep or general fatigue.
7. Avoid stressful exercise routines such as time trials or repeated high-intensity interval sessions with brief recovery periods.

CASE 6

In a reported case of exertional rhabdomyolysis in a 20-year-old African-American football player with HbS, bilateral pain in the lower back, hamstrings, and calves after completing a timed 1–1.5-mile run resulted in his hospitalization. The diagnosis was exercise-induced asthma and rhabdomyolysis. Blood chemistries, excluding creatine kinase, were normal, and he was allowed to return to supervised training and within 2 weeks had returned to full practice except distance runs. He was "aggressively" hydrated before, during, and after all activity. Due to his exercise-induced asthma, supplemental oxygen was administered during all games. He completed the season with no other adverse health effects (29).

CASE 7

An African-American cross-country runner with HbS collapsed suddenly on two separate occasions. After the first incident, the athlete vomited and complained of shortness of breath, abdominal pain, nausea, and leg cramps. He also reported that he had taken a decongestant the previous evening. Although recovering without complications, he was advised to discontinue competitive running. He continued running until a second incident a year later. He collapsed and required mouth-to-mouth resuscitation and was transported to the local emergency facility. He was diagnosed with rhabdomyolysis and renal insufficiency. After regaining consciousness, he was disorientated and complained of severe leg cramps. He was discharged 1 month later with some residual renal damage, and he no longer runs competitively (28).

References

1. Brotherhood J, Brozovic B, Pugh LG. Haematological status of middle- and long-distance runners. *Clin Sci Mol Med* 1975;48:139–145.
2. Dill DB, Braithwaite K, Adams WC. Blood volume of middle-distance runners: effect of 2,300 m altitude and comparison with nonathletes. *Med Sci Sports Exerc* 1974;6:1–7.
3. Deakin V. Iron depletion in athletes. In: Burke L, Deakin V, eds. *Clinical sports nutrition.* 2nd ed. Sydney: McGraw Hill, 2000. In press.
4. Eichner ER. Minerals: iron. In: Maughan R, ed. *Nutrition in sport.* London: Blackwell Science, 2000.
5. Nielsen P, Nachtigall D. Iron supplementation in athletes: current recommendations. *Sports Med* 1998;26:207–216.
6. Food and Nutrition Board, National Academy of Sciences—National Research Council, *Recommended dietary allowances.* 10th ed. Washington: National Academy Press, 1989
7. Lamanca JJ, Haymes EM, Daly JA, et al. Sweat iron loss of male and female runners during exercise. *Int J Sports Med* 1988;9:52–55.
8. Rudzki SJ, Hazard H, Collinson D. Gastrointestinal blood loss in triathletes: its etiology and relationship to sports anemia. *Aust J Science Med* 1995;27:3–8.
9. Miller BJ, Pate RR, Burgess W. Foot impact force and intravascular hemolysis during distance running. *Int J Sports Med* 1988;9:56–60.
10. Pennington JA, Church HN. *Bowes and Church's food values of portions commonly used.* 14th ed. Philadelphia: JB Lippincott Company, 1985.
11. Monsen ER, Hallberg L, Layrisse M, et al. Estimation of available dietary iron. *Am J Clin Nutr* 1978;31:134–141.
12. Hallberg L, Hultén L, Gramatkovski E. Iron absorption from the whole diet in men: how effective is the regulation of iron absorption? *Am J Clin Nutr* 1978;66:347–356.
13. Snyder AC, Dvorak LL, Roepke JB. Influence of dietary iron source on measures of iron status among female runners. *Med Sci Sports Exerc* 1989;21:7–10.
14. Haymes EM. Trace minerals and exercise. In: Wolinsky I, ed. *Nutrition in exercise and sport.* 3rd ed. Boca Raton: CRC Press, 1998.
15. Fogelholm M. Indicators of vitamin and mineral status in athletes' blood: a review. *Int J Sports Nutr* 1995;5:267–284.
16. Garza D, Shrier I, Kohl HW, et al. The clinical value of serum ferritin tests in endurance athletes. *Clin J Sport Med* 1997;7:46–53.
17. Lamanca JJ, Haymes EM. Effects of iron repletion on VO_2max, endurance, and blood lactate in women. *Med Sci Sports Exerc* 1993;25:1386–1392.
18. Schoene RB, Escourrou P, Robertson HT, et al. Iron repletion decreases maximal exercise lactate concentration in female athletes with minimal iron-deficiency anemia. *J Lab Clin Med* 1983;102:306–312.
19. Ashenden MJ, Fricker PA, Ryan RK, et al. The haematological response to an iron injection amongst female athletes. *Int J Sports Med* 1998;19:474–478.
20. McKenzie SB. *Textbook of hematology.* Baltimore: Williams and Wilkins, 1996.
21. Murphy JR. Sickle cell hemoglobin (HbAS) in black football players. *JAMA* 1973;225:981–982.
22. Diggs L, Flowers E. High school students with sickle cell trait (HbA/S). *J Natl Med Assoc* 1976;68:492–493.
23. Le Gallais D, Prefaut C, Mercier J, et al. Sickle cell trait as a limiting factor for high level performance in a semi-marathon. *Int J Sports Med* 1994;15:309–402.
24. Eichner ER. Sickle cell trait, heroic exercise, and fatal collapse. *Phys Sports Med* 1993;21(7):51–64.
25. Kark JA, Posey DM, Schumacher HR, et al. Sickle cell trait as a risk factor for sudden death in physical training. *N Eng J Med* 1987;317:781–787.

26. Kark JA, Ward FT. Exercise and hemoglobin S. *Sem Hematol* 1994;31:181–225.
27. Shaskey D, Green G. *Sports hematology. Sports Med* 2000; 29:27–38.
28. Harrelson G, Fincher L, Robinson J. Acute exertional rhabdomyolysis and its relationship to sickle cell trait. *J Athl Training* 1995;30(4):309–312.
29. Browne RJ, Gillespie CA. Sickle cell trait: a risk factor for life-threatening rhabdomyolysis? *Phys Sports Med* 1993;21(6): 80–88.
30. Milne CJ. Rhabdomyolysis, myoglobinuria, and exercise. *Sports Med* 1988;6:93–106.
31. Sherry P. Sickle cell trait and rhabdomyolysis: a case report and review of the literature. *Milit Med* 1990;155:59–61.
32. Rosenthal MA, Parker DJ. Collapse of a young athlete. *Ann Emerg Med* 1992;21:1493–1498.

APPENDIX

ACSM's Registered Clinical Exercise Physiologist (RCEP) Knowledge, Skills, and Abilities (KSAs)

William Jay Gillespie, Reed Humphrey, William G. Herbert, and Leonard A. Kaminsky

Preface

This text was designed to help bridge the knowledge gap and better define the role of the clinical exercise physiologist working with patients with musculoskeletal, neuromuscular, and immunologic diseases and disorders. Guidelines for working with patients with cardiovascular, pulmonary, and metabolic diseases have been adequately covered in prior publications, such as *ACSM's Guidelines for Exercise Testing and Prescription* and *ACSM's Resource Manual for Exercise Testing and Prescription.* However, a text alone cannot cover all of the competencies required of a clinical exercise physiologist, given the wide variety of practice settings in which the clinical exercise physiologist works. Indeed, what has become clear is that while the clinical exercise physiologist has a core set of knowledge, skills, and abilities (KSAs), there is not a definitive set of competencies that will cover *all* clinical exercise physiologists in *all* practice settings. This is more a function of the adaptability of the clinical exercise physiologist as he/she carves out a niché in various practice settings and treatment domains.

Certainly, it is the hope of the editors, authors, and contributors to these KSAs that a consensus for the role of the clinical exercise physiologist will continue to evolve and become explicit over the course of the next several years. The KSAs that follow do not provide for a clear distinction of the role of the clinical exercise physiologist in performing specific tests, in prescribing exercise, or in delivering specific treatment plans for a variety of important outcome assessments. In clinical practice, specific tests and measures employed for most components of fitness are not uniform among the wide variety of practice settings and treatment domains, and only continual practice analysis will yield a consensus for subsequent versions of the KSAs. The nature and complexity of those assessments vary, but eventual clarification of specific knowledge, skills, and abilities is a mandate for all clinical exercise physiologists as they work with a variety of patient populations.

William Jay Gillespie

Scope of Practice. In 1996, the ACSM Board of Trustees approved a scope of practice for the Clinical Exercise Physiologist: "The Clinical Exercise Physiologist works in the application of exercise and physical activity for those clinical and pathological situations where it has been shown to provide therapeutic or functional benefit. Patients for whom services are appropriate may include, but not be limited to those with cardiovascular, pulmonary, metabolic, musculoskeletal, neuromuscular, neoplastic, immunologic, and hematologic diseases and conditions. This list will be modified as indications and procedures of application are further developed and mature. Furthermore, the Clinical Exercise Physiologist applies exercise principles to groups such as geriatric, pediatric, or obstetric populations, and to society as a whole in preventive activities. The Clinical Exercise Physiologist performs exercise evaluation, exercise prescription, exercise supervision, exercise education, and exercise outcome evaluation. The practice of Clinical Exercise Physiologists should be restricted to clients who are referred by and are under the continued care of a licensed physician."

Code of Ethics. The code of ethics of the Clinical Exercise Physiology Practice Board is intended to aid its members, individually and collectively, to maintain a high level of ethical and professional conduct. The code represents standards by which a member may determine the propriety of his/her conduct, relationship with colleagues, members of the medical profession, members of allied health professions, the public, and all persons with whom a professional relationship has been established. Members of the CEP Registry shall be dedicated to providing competent medical and health services within the scope of practice of the Clinical Exercise Physiologist and within the knowledge, skill, and abilities contained herein. These skills shall be provided with compassion and respect for human dignity.

Knowledge, Skills, and Abilities (KSAs). The KSAs for the Registered Clinical Exercise Physiologist (RCEP) were written to expand on the above scope of practice, to provide the framework for the National Registry examination, and to provide the foundations for academic and internship standards. These KSAs are based on the assumptions that candidates have completed the following: 1) a master's degree with a content focus in exercise physiology, exercise science, or physiology; and 2) 1200 hours of supervised clinical experience, representative of the areas that are defined by the RCEP's scope of practice. Furthermore, these KSAs are written to reflect required competencies that are specific to the major chronic diseases and conditions and needed to meet threshold requirements for providing service to patients with some level of professional independence. In addition, it is assumed that those who qualify for this Registry already possess broad educational background and competencies expected of physical fitness professionals prepared at the bachelor's degree level, equivalent to the KSAs for an ACSM Health Fitness Instructor.

Organization and Development of the KSAs. The KSAs are organized into a core and six major practice areas, each with 12 major content domains. The core contains KSAs common to each of the six practice areas. Whereas, each of the six practice areas contain KSAs that are unique to each practice area. These KSAs have been written by groups of expert clinicians and academicians within each of the six practice areas. Focus groups of 6–15 practicing clinical exercise physiologists within each practice area reviewed and rated the KSAs as either entry or advanced level. An entry-level KSA was defined as a competency that is expected of a graduate of a master's program in clinical exercise physiology or exercise science with the appropriate internship experiences. An advanced KSA was a competency that could only be achieved with on-the-job training beyond that of the internship. Only entry-level KSAs are included in this document.

The following are the major practice areas and content domains with approximate relative weightings reflected in the registry examination and in internship requirements:

Practice Areas	Approximate Relative Weighting
0.0 Core	Contained throughout each practice area
1.0 Cardiovascular	30%
2.0 Pulmonary	10%
3.0 Metabolic	20%
4.0 Orthopedic/ Musculoskeletal	20%
5.0 Neuromuscular	10%
6.0 Immunologic/ Hematologic	10%

Major Content Domains	Approximate Relative Weightings
0.1 Pathophysiology	10%
0.2 Clinical Exercise Physiology	22%
0.3 Pharmacology	5%
0.4 Physical Examination	5%
0.5 Medical and Surgical Treatments	4%
0.6 Diagnostic Techniques	8%
0.7 Exercise/Fitness/ Functional Testing	15%
0.8 Exercise Prescription and Programming	10%
0.9 Education and Counseling	10%
0.10 Emergency Procedures	3%
0.11 Quality Assurance, Outcome Assessment, and Discharge Planning	3%
0.12 Administration	5%

The following are the Knowledge, Skills, and Abilities of the Registered Clinical Exercise Physiologist (RCEP) listed by Practice Area with 12 content domains:

0.0 CORE KNOWLEDGE, SKILLS, AND ABILITIES

0.1 **Core Pathophysiology.** Basic knowledge of the epidemiology and pathophysiology common to the cardiovascular, pulmonary, metabolic, musculoskeletal, neuromuscular, and immunologic chronic and infectious diseases and disabilities cited in this document.

- 0.1.1 Basic knowledge of the findings of epidemiology used to establish risk factors for the chronic and infectious diseases and disabilities indicated above.
- 0.1.2 Basic knowledge of the pathophysiology of the chronic and infectious diseases and disabilities indicated above.

0.2 **Core Clinical Exercise Physiology.** Basic knowledge of the clinical applications of exercise physiology common to individuals with the cardiovascular, pulmonary, metabolic, musculoskeletal, neuromuscular, or immunologic chronic and infectious diseases and disabilities cited in this document.

- 0.2.1 Knowledge of the cardiovascular, hemodynamic, and musculoskeletal responses to postural changes before and after exercise.
- 0.2.2 Knowledge of the resting and exercise values associated with increasing workloads for heart rate, stroke volume, cardiac output, arteriovenous oxygen difference, systolic and diastolic blood pressure, rate-pressure product, minute ventilation, tidal volume, and breathing frequency.
- 0.2.3 Knowledge of the variables that may be directly assessed or predicted (calculated) during clinical exercise testing, such as maximal oxygen consumption (L/min, kcal, mL/kg/min, METS),

ventilation, respiratory exchange ratio, RPE, discomfort scales (e.g., chest pain, dyspnea), heart rate, blood pressure, rate-pressure product, ventilatory threshold, muscular strength, and muscular endurance.

0.2.4 Knowledge of the determinants of myocardial oxygen consumption ($MVO_2 = HR \times SBP \times$ contractility) and the usefulness of measuring the rate-pressure product ($RPP = SBP \times HR$).

0.2.5 Knowledge of the determinants of total body oxygen consumption ($VO_2 = HR \times SV \times$ a-v O_2 difference) and typical values at rest and submaximal and maximal exercise.

0.2.6 Knowledge of the determinants of mean arterial pressure ($MAP = DBp + [SBp - (DBp)/3]$) and values for rest and submaximal and maximal exercise.

0.2.7 Knowledge of the principle of specificity of training.

0.2.8 Knowledge of the principle of progressive overload as applied to resistance and cardiorespiratory endurance training.

0.2.9 Knowledge of approaches to resistance training to induce muscle force production and/or muscle endurance.

0.2.10 Knowledge of the use and relative value of continuous versus intermittent exercise training.

0.2.11 Knowledge of the benefits of resistance training and flexibility exercises.

0.2.12 Knowledge of the mechanisms of adaptation that lead to changes in submaximal and maximal physiologic responses following exercise training (e.g., decreases in submaximal exercise heart rate and systolic blood pressure, increases in ventilatory threshold and functional capacity, increases in muscular strength and endurance).

0.2.13 Knowledge of the physiologic effects of bed rest and appropriate physical activities, which may counteract these changes.

0.2.14 Knowledge of the effects of exercise training on the determinants of myocardial oxygen consumption (heart rate, contractility, preload, and postload) during submaximal and maximal exercise.

0.2.15 Knowledge of the effects of temperature, humidity, and altitude on the exercise responses.

0.2.16 Knowledge of the nutritional and fluid considerations of individuals with the above-listed chronic diseases and disabilities participating in regular exercise programs.

0.2.17 Knowledge of the effects of air pollutants and tobacco products (CO, nicotine) on response to exercise.

0.3 **Core Pharmacology.** Basic knowledge of the drug classifications commonly used in the treatment of individuals with the cardiovascular, pulmonary, metabolic, musculoskeletal, neuromuscular, or immunologic chronic and infectious diseases and disabilities cited in this document, including the purposes, indications, major side effects, and the major effects, if any, on the exercising individual. (See specific Pharmacology sections within each practice area.)

0.4 **Core Aspects of the Physical Examination.** Basic knowledge, skills, and abilities related to the physical exam of individuals with the cardiovascular, pulmonary, metabolic, musculoskeletal, neuromuscular, or immunologic chronic and infectious diseases and disabilities cited in this document. (See specific sections on Aspects of the Physical Examination within each practice area.)

0.5 **Core Medical and Surgical Treatments.** Basic knowledge of techniques and understanding of key findings in reports of medical and surgical treatments used in the management of individuals with the cardiovascular, pulmonary, metabolic, musculoskeletal, neuromuscular, and immunologic chronic and infectious diseases and disabilities cited in this document. (See specific Medical and Surgical Treatments sections within each practice area.)

0.6 **Core Diagnostic Techniques.** Basic knowledge of techniques and understanding of key findings in reports of diagnostic techniques and specific knowledge and abilities to administer certain techniques used in the management of individuals with the cardiovascular, pulmonary, metabolic, musculoskeletal, neuromuscular, and immunologic chronic and infectious diseases and disabilities cited in this document. (See specific sections on Diagnostic Techniques within each practice area.)

0.7 **Core Exercise/Fitness/Functional Testing.** Knowledge, skills, and abilities used in administering an exercise/fitness/functional test common to individuals with the cardiovascular, pulmonary, metabolic, musculoskeletal, neuromuscular, or immunologic chronic and infectious diseases and disabilities cited in this document.

0.7.1 Knowledge of and ability to identify indications and contraindications (absolute and relative) prior to testing.

0.7.2 Knowledge of and ability to identify individuals with disease for whom physician supervision is recommended during testing.

0.7.3 Knowledge of and ability to identify factors that may increase anxiety prior to or during testing, and ability to reduce anxiety in a patient prior to testing.

0.7.4 Knowledge of and ability to perform techniques used to calibrate a motor-driven treadmill, mechanical cycle ergometer and arm ergometer, electrocardiograph, aneroid and sphygmomanometer, spirometer, respiratory gas analyzer, and resistance equipment.

0.7.5 Knowledge of and ability to select the appropriate exercise modes (treadmill, leg and arm cycle ergometers, resistance equipment) and protocols (including starting level, increments of work, length of stages, and frequency of physiologic measures) for a variety of individuals with disease.

0.7.6 Ability to screen for pretest probability of comorbid disease.

0.7.7 Knowledge of and ability to administer pretest procedures, including obtaining informed consent, obtaining a focused medical history (including medications and symptoms), obtaining results of prior tests and physical exam, explaining test procedures to the patient, recognizing contraindications to testing, and presenting concise information to the physician, healthcare providers, and third-party payors.

0.7.8 Knowledge of and ability to identify probable end points for testing individuals with disease.

0.7.9 Knowledge of and ability to administer immediate postexercise procedures and various approaches to cool-down.

0.7.10 Knowledge of and ability to record, organize, and perform necessary calculations of test data for summary presentation.

0.7.11 Ability to minimize poor results from exercise testing attributable to lack of motivation, fear, low functional capacities, and balance/gait problems.

0.8 **Core Exercise Prescription and Programming.** Knowledge, skills, and abilities in prescribing and supervising exercise programs common to individuals with the cardiovascular, pulmonary, metabolic, musculoskeletal, neuromuscular, and immunologic chronic and infectious diseases and disabilities cited in this document.

0.8.1 Knowledge of the level of supervision and monitoring recommended for individuals with the diseases and disabilities indicated above based upon risk stratification.

0.8.2 Knowledge of contraindications to exercise as related to the current clinical status of participants in a rehabilitative exercise session.

0.8.3 Knowledge of and ability to conduct appropriate exercise prescriptions based on medical information and exercise test data, including modes, intensity, duration, frequency, progression, and precautions.

0.8.4 Knowledge of and ability to modify an exercise prescription or discontinue exercise based upon changes in symptoms, current clinical status, orthopedic limitations, and environmental considerations.

0.8.5 Knowledge of and ability to conduct appropriate warm-up and cool-down, including specific skills in modifying warm-up/cool-down secondary to fatigue, balance, and/or orthopedic limitations.

0.8.6 Knowledge of the differences in the physiologic training effects to arm and leg exercise and the ability to determine the appropriateness of use.

0.8.7 Knowledge of and ability to determine possible adverse responses to exercise and precautions that may be taken to prevent them.

0.8.8 Knowledge of and ability to identify characteristics associated with poor compliance to exercise programs and discuss methods of overcoming these barriers to adherence.

0.9 **Core Education and Counseling.** Knowledge, skills, and abilities for conducting education and counseling programs for individuals with the cardiovascular, pulmonary, metabolic, musculoskeletal, neuromuscular, and immunologic chronic and infectious diseases and disabilities cited in this document.

0.9.1 Knowledge of and ability to apply basic theories and contemporary techniques of behavior change to promote healthful physical activity habits, e.g., social cognitive theory, self-efficacy analysis, relapse prevention, health belief model.

0.9.2 Knowledge of and ability to deliver appropriate lecture topics for individuals and small groups of individuals.

0.9.3 Knowledge of an appropriate referral system for individuals with specific disease states requiring nutrition, stress management, weight management, and psychosocial support.

0.9.4 Ability to instruct and reinforce behavioral strategies for risk factor intervention and behavior modification for primary and secondary prevention.

0.9.5 Ability to recommend proper precautions and contraindications to exercise.

0.9.6 Knowledge of the basic behavioral psychology of crisis management, coping, and lifestyle modification.

0.9.7 Knowledge of and ability to identify signs and symptoms of maladjustment/failure to cope during illness crisis, personal adjustment crisis (e.g., job loss), and/or acute and chronic illness behaviors.

0.9.8 Knowledge of the psychologic issues associated with an acute event vs. those associated with chronic conditions, such as depression, social isolation, aggression, and suicidal ideation.

0.9.9 Ability to refer to appropriate healthcare professional as indicated.

0.9.10 Ability to work as a team with other healthcare professionals.

0.10 **Core Emergency Procedures.** Basic knowledge, skills, and abilities to respond with appropriate emergency procedures for use prior to, during, or after administration of an exercise test or therapeutic exercise sessions for individuals with the cardiovascular, pulmonary, metabolic, musculoskeletal, neuromuscular, or immunologic chronic and infectious diseases and disabilities cited in this document.

- 0.10.1 Basic knowledge of certain emergency equipment and drugs present in an exercise testing laboratory and therapeutic exercise session.
- 0.10.2 Basic knowledge of and ability to verify operating status of emergency equipment.
- 0.10.3 Basic knowledge of emergency procedures for responding to cardiac arrest, tachycardia, bradycardias, severe myocardial ischemia, hypoglycemia, syncope, hypotension, bronchospasm, respiratory fatigue and arrest, autonomic hyperreflexia, grand mal or partial seizure, sprains and strains, and falls and fractures of spine or hip.
- 0.10.4 Knowledge of and ability to administer Basic First Aid and Basic Cardiac Life Support techniques and possess current certification.

0.11 **Core Quality Assurance, Outcome Assessment, and Discharge Planning.** Knowledge, skills, and abilities in quality assurance, outcome assessment, and discharge planning common to individuals with the cardiovascular, pulmonary, metabolic, musculoskeletal, neuromuscular, or immunologic chronic and infectious diseases and disabilities cited in this document.

- 0.11.1 Knowledge of continuous quality improvement and performance improvement plans.
- 0.11.2 Knowledge of and ability to identify sources of technical error, including measurement unreliability, that may affect interpretation of tests.
- 0.11.3 Ability to evaluate patient (client) outcomes from serial exercise testing and training data collected before and after application of specific clinical treatments.
- 0.11.4 Ability to document and report relevant treatment outcomes using results of: exercise tests; physical work simulations; laboratory tests of physiologic status important to specific chronic diseases or disabilities; and surveys of physical functioning and health-related quality of life.

0.12 **Core Administration of Testing and Rehabilitation Programs.** Knowledge, skills, and abilities used in the management of rehabilitation programs and exercise testing laboratories in the areas of cardiovascular, pulmonary, metabolic, musculoskeletal, neuromuscular, or immunologic rehabilitation.

- 0.12.1 Knowledge of appropriate staffing for rehabilitation programs and exercise testing laboratories.
- 0.12.2 Knowledge of and ability to identify and describe the role of various allied health professionals and the indications and procedures for referral in a multidisciplinary rehabilitation program.
- 0.12.3 Knowledge of appropriate equipment and supplies for rehabilitation programs and exercise testing laboratories.
- 0.12.4 Knowledge of appropriate marketing and public relations strategies for rehabilitation programs.
- 0.12.5 Knowledge of reimbursement issues in rehabilitation programs and exercise testing laboratories.
- 0.12.6 Knowledge of content of typical annual budgets in terms of sources for expenses and revenue for rehabilitation programs and exercise testing laboratories.
- 0.12.7 Knowledge of basic legal issues pertinent to health care delivery by licensed and non-licensed providers, tort and contract law, negligence and malpractice, and legal risk management techniques affecting rehabilitation programs and exercise testing laboratories.

1.0 CARDIOVASCULAR PRACE AREA

1.1 **Pathophysiology of Cardiovascular Diseases.** Basic knowledge of the epidemiology and pathophysiology of cardiovascular diseases and disabilities, *including:* atherosclerosis, coronary artery disease (CAD), angina, myocardial infarction (MI), hypertension (HTN), congestive heart failure (CHF), valvular heart disease, and peripheral vascular disease (PVD).

- 1.1.1 Knowledge of the risk factors for atherosclerosis and the efficacy of reducing these with respect to cardiovascular disease prevention and intervention.
- 1.1.2 Knowledge of the current hypotheses regarding the etiology and rate of progression of atherosclerosis, including the specific role of certain risk factors in endothelial function/dysfunction.
- 1.1.3 Knowledge of the lipoprotein classifications and the relationship of these to the rate of progression of atherosclerosis.
- 1.1.4 Knowledge of the Joint National Commission's classification scheme for rating blood pressure and the relationship of these classes to cardiovascular disease risk.
- 1.1.5 Knowledge of the effects of myocardial ischemia on diastolic and systolic ventricular dysfunction at rest and during exercise.
- 1.1.6 Knowledge of the differences between classic and vasospastic angina, typical and atypical angina.
- 1.1.7 Knowledge of the pathophysiology of the healing myocardium following infarction and

the potential complications (remodeling, extension, expansion, and aneurysm).

1.1.8 Knowledge of the pathophysiology of congestive heart failure.

1.1.9 Knowledge of the pathophysiology of valvular heart disease.

1.1.10 Knowledge of the pathophysiology of peripheral vascular disease.

1.1.11 Knowledge of the pathophysiology of coronary artery bypass and cardiac transplant surgeries.

1.1.12 Knowledge of the risk stratification schemes for classifying patients following myocardial infarction (e.g., American Heart Association, American College of Cardiology, American Association of Cardiovascular and Pulmonary Rehabilitation).

1.2 **Clinical Exercise Physiology Applied to Cardiovascular Diseases.** Basic knowledge of the clinical applications of exercise physiology as applied to individuals with cardiovascular diseases and following various cardiovascular surgeries and procedures.

1.2.1 Knowledge of the abnormal cardiac chronotropic and inotropic responses to acute exercise in individuals with myocardial ischemia, chest pain syndromes, myocardial infarction, valvular disease, and ventricular dysfunction.

1.2.2 Knowledge of the acute cardiovascular responses to and potential hazards of resistance training and isometric exercise in individuals with cardiovascular diseases and disabilities.

1.2.3 Knowledge of the hemodynamic responses of arm vs. leg and static vs. dynamic exercise in individuals with cardiovascular diseases.

1.2.4 Knowledge of the hemodynamic responses of pharmacologic and pacing stress testing in individuals with cardiovascular diseases.

1.2.5 Knowledge of the classification schemes for and interpretation of maximal oxygen consumption values for individuals with cardiovascular diseases.

1.2.6 Knowledge of the beneficial effects of exercise training on the risk factors for coronary artery disease.

1.2.7 Knowledge of the effects of exercise training on the determinants of total body oxygen consumption during submaximal and maximal exercise in individuals with cardiovascular diseases.

1.2.8 Knowledge of the effects of temperature, humidity, and altitude on the exercise responses of individuals with cardiovascular diseases.

1.3 **Cardiovascular Pharmacology.** Basic knowledge of the drug classifications commonly used in the treatment of individuals with cardiovascular diseases and disabilities, including the purposes, indications, major side effects, and the effects, if any, on the exercising individual.

1.3.1 Antiarrhythmics

1.3.2 Anticoagulants and antiplatelets

1.3.3 Antihyperlipidemic agents

1.3.4 Beta-adrenergic blocking agents

1.3.5 Calcium channel blocking agents

1.3.6 Digitalis glycosides

1.3.7 Diuretics

1.3.8 Peripheral vasodilators

1.3.8.1 Angiotensin converting enzyme (ACE) Inibitors

1.3.8.2 Alpha-adrenergic blocking agents

1.3.8.3 Anti-adrenergic agents without selective receptor blockade

1.3.8.4 Nitrates and nitroglycerin

1.3.9 Psychotropics (antianxiety, antidepressants, and antipsychotics)

1.3.10 Sympathomimetic agents

1.4 **Cardiovascular Aspects of the Physical Examination.** Basic knowledge, skills, and abilities related to the cardiovascular physical exam of individuals with cardiovascular diseases and disabilities.

1.4.1 Basic knowledge of and ability to understand the results of a cardiovascular physical examination, including blood pressure, peripheral pulses, and heart and lung sounds.

1.4.2 Basic skills and abilities to measure blood pressure, heart and lung sounds, and peripheral pulses for the purpose of identifying contraindications prior to an exercise test or therapeutic exercise session.

1.4.3 Basic knowledge of and ability to identify the signs and symptoms of cardiovascular diseases and disorders, including typical and atypical angina; *nonanginal,* peripheral vascular disease; congestive heart failure; and arrhythmias.

1.5 **Cardiovascular Medical and Surgical Treatments.** Basic knowledge of techniques and understanding of key findings in reports of medical and surgical treatments used in the management of individuals with cardiovascular diseases and disabilities.

1.5.1 Basic knowledge of techniques and ability to understand key findings in reports of treatments using various thrombolytic agents.

1.5.2 Basic knowledge of techniques and ability to understand key findings in reports of treatments using percutaneous transluminal coronary angioplasty (PTCA), including the use of stents.

1.5.3 Basic knowledge of techniques and ability to understand key findings in reports of coronary artery bypass surgery (CABG).

1.5.4 Basic knowledge of techniques and ability to understand key findings in reports of pacemaker and implantable cardiac defibrillator (ICD) treatments.

1.5.5 Basic knowledge of techniques and ability to understand key findings in reports of cardiac transplant surgery.

1.5.6 Basic knowledge of techniques and ability to understand key findings in reports of angioplasty and the use of stents in peripheral vascular disease.

1.6 **Cardiovascular Diagnostic Techniques.** Basic knowledge of techniques and understanding of key findings in reports of diagnostic techniques and specific knowledge and abilities to administer certain specific techniques currently used in cardiovascular disease.

1.6.1 Basic knowledge of techniques and ability to understand key findings in a 24/48 hr ECG (Holter monitor) report.

1.6.2 Basic knowledge of techniques and ability to understand key findings in reports of various laboratory tests used in the diagnosis of cardiovascular disease, including CBC, hematocrit, hemoglobin, cardiac enzymes, and electrolytes.

1.6.3 Basic knowledge of techniques and ability to understand key findings in reports of radionuclide imaging tests for cardiovascular function.

1.6.4 Basic knowledge of techniques and ability to understand key findings in reports of tests of rest and stress echocardiography.

1.6.5 Basic knowledge of techniques and ability to understand key findings in reports of pharmacologic stress testing.

1.6.6 Basic knowledge of techniques and ability to understand key findings in reports of coronary angiography.

1.6.7 **Electrocardiography**. Knowledge, skills, and abilities in clinical electrocardiography (ECG), including determination of rate, rhythm, axis, hypertrophy, ischemia, and infarction, and additional factors altering the electrocardiogram in individuals with cardiovascular disease.

1.6.7.1 Knowledge of the normal and abnormal responses for each of the following in individuals with coronary artery disease (CAD): function of the myocardium, generation and propagation of the action potential, repolarization, and major variants in pathways of electrical activity.

1.6.7.2 Ability to determine ventricular rate from rhythm strip and 12-lead ECG.

1.6.7.3 Ability to identify sinus, atrial, junctional, and ventricular dysrhythmias from a rhythm strip, 12-lead ECG, and/or monitor and knowledge of the clinical significance for each.

1.6.7.4 Ability to identify SA, AV, and bundle branch blocks from a rhythm strip, 12-lead ECG, and monitor and knowledge of the clinical significance for each.

1.6.7.5 Ability to determine normal axis, left axis deviation, and right axis deviation from a 12-lead ECG and knowledge of the clinical significance for each.

1.6.7.6 Ability to determine right and left atrial and ventricular enlargement and hypertrophy from a 12-lead ECG and knowledge of clinical significance for each.

1.6.7.7 Ability to determine ECG changes associated with subendocardial and transmural ischemia, injury, and infarction and knowledge of the clinical significance for each.

1.6.7.8 Ability to determine the lead sets that correspond to the general areas of the myocardium for ischemia, injury, or infarction.

1.6.7.9 Ability to identify ECG changes that typically occur due to hyperventilation, electrolyte abnormalities, and cardiovascular drug therapies.

1.7 **Cardiovascular Exercise/Fitness/Functional Testing.** Knowledge, skills, and abilities used in administration of cardiopulmonary exercise, pharmacologic stress, and functional capacity tests for individuals with cardiovascular diseases and disabilities.

1.7.1 Knowledge of and ability to employ appropriate techniques for measurement of the ECG, blood pressure, RPE, symptoms, and expired gases at appropriate intervals during the exercise test.

1.7.2 Knowledge of and ability to employ techniques used to minimize ECG artifact.

1.7.3 Knowledge of and ability to use single-lead and multiple-lead ECG systems in exercise testing.

1.7.4 Knowledge of and ability to perform routine tasks prior to exercise testing, including obtaining appropriate standard and exercise 12-lead EKGs; accurately recording right and left arm blood pressure; and instructing the test participant in the use of rating of perceived exertion (RPE) scale and other appropriate subjective scales (e.g., dyspnea and angina scales).

1.7.5 Knowledge of the probable effects of angina, myocardial infarction, PTCA, CABG, and CHF on exercise performance, hemodynamics, functional capacity, and safety.

1.7.6 Knowledge of and ability to determine pretest probability of angina and coronary artery disease in patients.
1.7.7 Ability to administer appropriate test protocols and procedures for exercise tests that involve radionuclide or echocardiographic imaging.
1.7.8 Basic knowledge of and ability to assist with pharmacologic stress testing.

1.8 **Cardiovascular Exercise Prescription and Programming.** Knowledge, skills, and abilities in prescribing and supervising exercise programs for individuals with cardiovascular diseases and disabilities.
1.8.1 Knowledge of the appropriate use of static and dynamic resistance exercise for individuals with cardiovascular disease.
1.8.2 Knowledge of and ability to design a strength training program for individuals who are post-MI, post-CABG, post-PTCA, post-PTCA with stents, postatherectomies, and postcardiac transplant.
1.8.3 Ability to supervise exercise programs for outpatients hospitalized for MI, PTCA, CABG, and angina for the immediate posthospital recovery period, as well as the 3 months following hospitalization.

1.9 **Cardiovascular Education and Counseling**. Knowledge, skills, and abilities in conducting education programs and counseling individuals with cardiovascular diseases and disabilities. (See Core Education and Counseling.)

1.10 **Cardiovascular Emergency Procedures.** Basic knowledge, skills, and abilities to respond with appropriate emergency procedures for use prior to, during, or after administration of an exercise test or therapeutic exercise sessions for individuals with cardiovascular diseases and disabilities. (See Core Emergency Procedures.)

1.11 **Cardiovascular Quality Assurance, Outcome Assessment, and Discharge Planning.** Knowledge, skills, and abilities in quality assurance, outcome assessment, and discharge planning for programs for individuals with cardiovascular diseases and disabilities. (See Core Quality Assurance, Outcome Assessment, and Discharge Planning.)

1.12 **Cardiovascular Administration of Testing and Rehabilitation Programs.** Knowledge, skills, and abilities used in the management of rehabilitation programs and exercise testing laboratories in the areas of cardiovascular rehabilitation. (See Core Administration of Testing and Rehabilitation Programs.)

2.0 PULMONARY PRACE AREA

2.1 **Pathophysiology of Pulmonary Diseases.** Basic Knowledge of the epidemiology and pathophysiology of pulmonary diseases, *including:* obstructive lung diseases (emphysema, chronic bronchitis, asthma, bronchiectasis, cystic fibrosis), restrictive lung diseases (interstitial pulmonary fibrosis, neuromuscular diseases, thoracic cage abnormalities), vascular lung disease (pulmonary hypertension—primary or thromboembolitic), and right heart failure.
2.1.1 Knowledge of the risk factors for chronic lung disease (CLD—emphysema, chronic bronchitis, and asthma) and the efficacy of reducing these with respect to pulmonary disease prevention and intervention.
2.1.2 Knowledge of the pathophysiology of emphysema, chronic bronchitis, and asthma. Knowledge of the pathophysiologic mechanisms of hypoxemia, hypercapnea, and dyspnea. Basic knowledge of the pathophysiology of restrictive lung diseases.
2.1.3 Basic knowledge of the pathophysiology of vascular lung disease and right heart failure.

2.2 **Clinical Exercise Physiology Applied to Pulmonary Diseases.** Basic knowledge of the clinical applications of exercise physiology as applied to individuals with pulmonary diseases and disabilities.
2.2.1 Knowledge of the limitations (ventilatory, cardiac, muscular, psychologic) to exercise for individuals with chronic pulmonary disease.
2.2.2 Knowledge of the influence of posture and body position (ex. use of breathing support) on exercise performance in individuals with chronic pulmonary disease.
2.2.3 Knowledge of the implications of low functional capacity in individuals with chronic pulmonary disease.
2.2.4 Knowledge of the effects of exercise scheduling relative to meals for dyspnea control secondary to mechanical distention of the abdomen and limitations on diaphragmatic excursion for individuals with chronic pulmonary disease.
2.2.5 Knowledge of the effects of fat and carbohydrate metabolism on carbon dioxide production and the exercise response in individuals with chronic pulmonary disease.

2.3 **Pulmonary Pharmacology.** Basic knowledge of the drug classifications commonly used in the treatment of individuals with pulmonary diseases and disabilities, including the purpose, indications, major side effects, and the major effects, if any, on the exercising individual:
2.3.1 Anticholinergic agents
2.3.2 Antibiotics
2.3.3 Antihistamine agents
2.3.4 Antitussive agents
2.3.5 Anti-inflammatory agents
2.3.6 Beta-agonists
2.3.7 Corticosteriods
2.3.8 Cromolyn sodium

2.3.9 Decongestants
2.3.10 Expectorants
2.3.11 Metered dose inhalers
2.3.12 Mucolytic agents
2.3.13 Oxygen
2.3.14 Theophyllines

2.4 **Pulmonary Aspects of the Physical Examination.** Basic knowledge, skills, and abilities related to the pulmonary physical exam in individuals with chronic pulmonary diseases and disabilities.

2.4.1 Basic knowledge of and ability to understand the results of a pulmonary physical examination, including lung sounds.

2.4.2 Basic skills in and abilities to obtain measures of respiratory rate, oxygen saturation, dyspnea ratings, and lung sounds for the purpose of identifying the associated contraindications to an exercise test or therapeutic exercise session.

2.4.3 Basic knowledge of and ability to identify signs and symptoms of various chronic pulmonary diseases, including hypoxemia and hypercapnea, bronchospasm, and right-sided congestive heart failure.

2.5 **Pulmonary Medical and Surgical Treatments.** Basic knowledge of techniques and understanding of key findings in reports of medical and surgical treatments used in the management of individuals with chronic pulmonary diseases and disabilities.

2.5.1 Basic knowledge of the techniques and ability to understand the key findings associated with the administration of various types of bronchodilator therapy (e.g. beta-agonist, anti-inflammatory agents).

2.5.2 Basic knowledge of techniques and ability to understand key findings in reports of bronchoscopy (diagnostic and laser) treatment.

2.5.3 Basic knowledge of techniques and ability to understand key findings in reports of bronchial provocation therapy.

2.5.4 Basic knowledge of techniques and ability to understand key findings in reports of lung surgery, including volume reduction, resection, and transplantation.

2.6 **Pulmonary Diagnostic Techniques.** Basic knowledge of techniques and understanding of key findings in reports of diagnostic techniques and specific knowledge and abilities to administer certain techniques used in the management of individuals with pulmonary diseases and disabilities.

2.6.1 Basic knowledge of techniques and ability to understand key findings in reports of bronchial provocation tests, arterial blood gases, and pulse oximetry.

2.6.2 Basic knowledge of techniques and ability to understand key findings in reports of laboratory tests used in the diagnosis of pulmonary disease, including CBC, hematocrit, hemoglobin, and electrolytes.

2.6.3 Basic knowledge of techniques and ability to understand key findings in reports of imaging modalities (scan, radionuclide, ventilation-perfusion scans, etc.)

2.6.4 **Pulmonary Function Testing.** Knowledge, skills, and abilities in pulmonary function testing of individuals with chronic pulmonary disease.

2.6.4.1 Knowledge of lung volumes and capacities (tidal volume, residual volume, inspiratory volume, expiratory volume, total lung capacity, vital capacity, and functional residual capacity).

2.6.4.2 Ability to understand and explain key findings from reports of the results of the above tests.

2.7 **Pulmonary Exercise/Fitness/Functional Testing.** Knowledge, skills, and abilities used in administering cardiopulmonary exercise tests for individuals with chronic pulmonary disease.

2.7.1 Knowledge of and ability to employ appropriate techniques for measurement of oxyhemoglobin saturation, arterial blood gases when appropriate, and expired gases at appropriate intervals during the exercise test.

2.7.2 Knowledge of and ability to identify probable end points for testing individuals with chronic pulmonary diseases and disabilities

2.7.3 Knowledge of, and ability to administer basic pulmonary function tests (forced vital capacity and forced expiratory volumes) in the context of cardiopulmonary exercise testing.

2.8 **Pulmonary Exercise Prescription and Programming.** Knowledge, skills, and abilities in prescribing and supervising exercise programs for individuals with chronic pulmonary diseases and disabilities.

2.8.1 Knowledge of and ability to design an aerobic and strength training program for individuals with chronic pulmonary diseases, including lung resection, transplantation surgery, and lung volume reduction surgery.

2.8.2 Ability to supervise exercise programs for patients following an acute exacerbation of underlying chronic lung disease, including lung resection, transplantation surgery, and lung volume reduction surgery

2.8.3 Ability to supervise outpatient exercise programs for individuals with chronic pulmonary disease.

2.9 **Pulmonary Education and Counseling.** Knowledge, skills, and abilities in conducting education programs and counseling individuals with pulmonary diseases and disabilities. (See Core Education and Counseling.)

2.10 **Pulmonary Emergency Procedures.** Basic knowledge, skills, and abilities to respond with appropriate emergency procedures for use prior to, during, or after administration of an exercise test or therapeutic exercise sessions for individuals with pulmonary diseases and disabilities. (See Core Emergency Procedures.)

2.11 **Pulmonary Quality Assurance, Outcome Assessment, and Discharge Planning.** Knowledge, skills, and abilities in quality assurance, outcome assessment, and discharge planning for programs for individuals with pulmonary diseases and disabilities. (See Core Quality Assurance, Outcome Assessment, and Discharge Planning.)

2.12 **Pulmonary Administration of Testing and Rehabilitation Programs.** Knowledge, skills, and abilities used in the management of rehabilitation programs and exercise testing laboratories in the areas of pulmonary rehabilitation. (See Core Administration of Testing and Rehabilitation Programs.)

3.0 METABOLIC PRACE AREA

3.1 **Pathophysiology of Metabolic Diseases.** Basic knowledge of the epidemiology and pathophysiology of metabolic diseases and disorders, *including:* diabetes mellitus, obesity, end-stage renal disease (ESRD), and hyperlipidemia.

- 3.1.1 Knowledge of diabetes mellitus, specifically normal and abnormal pancreatic endocrine function during rest and exercise, type 1 and type 2 diabetes, complications of diabetes, and risk factors for developing diabetes.
- 3.1.2 Knowledge of obesity, specifically, the interaction between environment and genetics and the mechanisms of diet and physical inactivity.
- 3.1.3 Knowledge of mechanisms by which upper- and lower-body obesity increases the risk and severity of diabetes, coronary heart disease, hypertension, dyslipidemia, musculoskeletal injuries, respiratory complications, psychological disturbances, and cancer.
- 3.1.4 Basic knowledge of the etiology and progression of renal failure (e.g., loss of glomerular function, uremia).
- 3.1.5 Knowledge of the consequences of renal failure, including hypertension, congestive heart failure, muscle weakness, renal osteodystrophy, cardiac disease, and anemia.
- 3.1.6 Knowledge of the mechanisms of dyslipidemia.

3.2 **Clinical Exercise Physiology Applied to Metabolic Diseases.** Basic knowledge of the clinical applications of exercise physiology as applied to individuals with various metabolic diseases and disorders.

- 3.2.1 Knowledge of metabolic responses to exercise according to the timing and administration of different types of insulin in type 1 diabetes.
- 3.2.2 Knowledge of the heart rate and blood pressure responses to submaximal and maximal exercise in diabetes, obesity, and renal failure.
- 3.2.3 Knowledge of and ability to recognize abnormal signs and symptoms during exercise in individuals with diabetes, obesity, and renal failure.
- 3.2.4 Knowledge of limitations in functional capacity in diabetes, obesity, and renal failure.
- 3.2.5 Knowledge of the energy cost of various forms of physical activity for obese vs. lean adults.
- 3.2.6 Knowledge of factors that may affect the acute and chronic responses to exercise, including fluid intake, adequacy of dialysis, timing of dialysis, dietary compliance, comorbidities, and medical compliance in individuals with renal failure.
- 3.2.7 Knowledge of the acute and chronic effects of exercise on blood lipids and lipoproteins in individuals with dyslipidemia.
- 3.2.8 Knowledge of the effects of exercise training and weight reduction on blood glucose control in type 1 and type 2 diabetes.
- 3.2.9 Knowledge of the effects of exercise training in the prevention and treatment of type 2 diabetes and obesity.
- 3.2.10 Knowledge of the risks of chronic exercise for obese adults.
- 3.2.11 Knowledge that the goal of training for many patients with ESRD may be to maintain function, without significant improvement.
- 3.2.12 Knowledge of the precautions that the diabetic must make prior to, during, and following exercise, specifically: footwear, foot care, carbohydrate snacks, fluid replacement, and insulin management.
- 3.2.13 Knowledge of the major issues surrounding physical activity in the treatment of obesity (i.e., lean mass preservation, spot reduction, changes in basal and resting metabolic rate, appetite control, and weight maintenance).
- 3.2.14 Knowledge of basic precautions during exercise in individuals with renal failure.

3.3 **Metabolic Pharmacology.** Basic knowledge of the drug classifications commonly used in the treatment of individuals with various diseases, including the purposes, indications, major side effects, and the effects, if any, on the exercising individual:

- 3.3.1 Antibiotics.
- 3.3.2 Antihyperlipidemics.
- 3.3.3 Antihypertensive agents.
- 3.3.4 Appetite suppressants and digestive inhibitors.
- 3.3.5 Oral hypoglycemic agents (first and second generation).
- 3.3.6 Human recombinant erythropoeitin (EPO).
- 3.3.7 Inotropic agents.

3.3.8 Insulin (animal and human) and means of administration.

3.3.9 Iron supplementation.

3.3.10 Phosphate binders/calcium supplementation.

3.3.11 Vitamin supplementation (vitamin D in particular).

3.4 **Metabolic Aspects of the Physical Examination.** Basic knowledge, skills, and abilities related to the physical examination of individuals with metabolic diseases and disabilities.

3.4.1 Basic knowledge of and ability to understand the results of a physical exam in individuals with diabetes, obesity, and renal failure.

3.4.2 Basic knowledge of and ability to understand the signs and symptoms of individuals with diabetes, obesity, and renal failure, including hypo/hyperglycemia, ketoacidosis, retinal changes, peripheral neuropathies, and orthopedic problems (i.e., Charcot's joint, ulcers).

3.4.3 Ability to recognize signs and symptoms in individuals with renal disease, including fluid overload, loss of appetite, leg weakness, fatigue, lightheadedness/dizziness, low hematocrit, elevated creatinine, hypertension, and hypotension.

3.5 **Metabolic Medical and Surgical Treatments.** Basic knowledge of techniques and understanding of key findings in reports of medical and surgical treatments used in the management of individuals with metabolic diseases.

3.5.1 Basic knowledge of techniques and understanding of key findings in reports of insulin pump implant, pancreas transplant, retinal laser repair, cardiovascular surgeries for secondary cardiovascular complications, amputation, vascular surgeries, and dialysis for secondary renal failure.

3.5.2 Basic knowledge of techniques and understanding of key findings in reports of medical and surgical procedures used in the management of obesity (i.e., stomach stapling, jejunoileal bypass, starvation/modified fast diets, gastroplasties, jaw wiring, intragastric balloons, fat excision, and antiobesity medications).

3.5.3 Basic knowledge of techniques and understanding of key findings in reports of treatment options for renal disease, including pre–end-stage dietary intervention, hemodialysis, peritoneal dialysis (cycle and ambulatory), and kidney transplantation.

3.5.4 Basic knowledge of the following dialysis access sites, including fistula/grafts for hemodialysis, subclavian catheter for temporary access, and peritoneal dialysis catheter.

3.5.5 Basic knowledge of techniques and understanding of key findings in reports of amputation; laser surgery, cardiac-disease–related surgery, vascular surgeries, and graft surgery/declotting procedures.

3.6 **Metabolic Diagnostic Techniques.** Basic knowledge of the techniques and understanding of key findings in reports of diagnostic techniques and specific knowledge and abilities in certain techniques currently used in the management of individuals with metabolic diseases.

3.6.1 Basic knowledge of techniques and understanding of key findings in reports of routine diagnostic tests for individuals with diabetes and renal disease.

3.6.2 Specific knowledge of techniques and ability to determine blood glucose using monitoring instruments and techniques used in assessment of individuals with diabetes.

3.6.3 Basic knowledge of techniques and understanding of key findings in reports of tests for glomerular filtration rate (GFR), blood urea nitrogen (BUN), creatinine/dialysis adequacy (kT/v or urea reduction rate), and hematocrit.

3.6.4 **Body Composition Testing.** Knowledge, skills, and abilities in administering body composition tests for individuals with metabolic diseases.

3.6.4.1 Knowledge of the theories and limitations of measurement of body composition by various methods.

3.6.4.2 Knowledge of and skills and abilities in body densitometry techniques (i.e., body pod and hydrostatic weighing).

3.6.4.3 Knowledge of and skills and abilities in various anthropometric techniques (i.e., skinfold, height/weight, body mass index [BMI], and body circumference measurements).

3.6.4.4 Knowledge of radiometry techniques (i.e., CT, MRI, and DEXA).

3.6.4.5 Knowledge of and skills and abilities in bioelectrical impedance techniques.

3.6.4.6 Ability to choose the appropriate method to evaluate body composition for particular individuals with metabolic disease.

3.6.4.7 Ability to interpret the results of various body composition tests and to provide appropriate goals for the individual with various metabolic diseases and disabilities.

3.7 **Metabolic Exercise/Fitness/Functional Testing.** Knowledge, skills, and abilities used in administering exercise, fitness, work simulation, and/or functional tests for individuals with metabolic diseases.

3.7.1 Knowledge of the probable effects of hypo/hyperglycemia, obesity, and ESRD on exercise performance, functional capacity, and safety.

3.7.2 Knowledge of differences in test protocol and procedures when testing involves individuals who are amputees or have peripheral vascular disease, neuropathy, orthopedic limitations, or vision impairments.

3.7.3 Ability to perform appropriate techniques for measurement of glucose monitoring prior to exercise testing.

3.7.4 Ability to identify probable end points for testing a variety of individuals with metabolic disease.

3.8 **Metabolic Exercise Prescription and Programming.** Knowledge, skills, and abilities in prescribing and supervising exercise programs for individuals with metabolic diseases and disabilities.

3.8.1 Ability to supervise exercise programs for individuals with diabetes, obesity, and renal failure.

3.8.2 Ability to adapt exercise prescriptions for complications of metabolic diseases such as amputations, retinopathy, autonomic neuropathies, vision impairment, during hemodialysis treatments, leg fistula, blunted heart rate response, and abnormal blood pressure responses (both hypertension and hypotension).

3.8.3 Ability to instruct an individual with metabolic diseases in techniques for performing physical activities safely and effectively in an unsupervised exercise setting.

3.8.4 Knowledge of the stresses and the time requirements associated with the various treatment options for individuals with renal disease.

3.9 **Metabolic Education and Counseling.** Knowledge, skills, and abilities in conducting education programs and counseling individuals with metabolic diseases and disabilities. (Also see Core Education and Counseling.)

3.9.1 Knowledge and understanding of the detection and treatment guidelines for obesity as stated in the 1998 NIH "Clinical Guidelines on the Identification, Evaluation and Treatment of Overweight and Obesity in Adults" (NHLBI 1998).

3.9.2 Knowledge and understanding of the screening and treatment guidelines for dyslipidemia as stated in the National Cholesterol Education Program (NCEP).

3.9.3 Knowledge and understanding of the diagnosis, classification, and treatment guidelines for diabetes as summarized by the American Diabetes Association (1997).

3.9.4 Knowledge and understanding of counseling and education of patients with renal failure.

3.10 **Metabolic Emergency Procedures.** Basic knowledge, skills, and abilities to respond with appropriate emergency procedures for use prior to, during, or after administration of an exercise test or therapeutic exercise sessions for individuals with metabolic diseases and disabilities. (See Core Emergency Procedures.)

3.11 **Metabolic Quality Assurance, Outcome Assessment, and Discharge Planning.** Knowledge, skills, and abilities in quality assurance, outcome assessment, and discharge planning for programs for individuals with metabolic diseases and disabilities. (See Core Quality Assurance, Outcome Assessment, and Discharge Planning.)

3.12 **Metabolic Administration of Testing and Rehabilitation Programs.** Knowledge, skills, and abilities used in the management of rehabilitation programs and exercise testing laboratories in the areas of metabolic rehabilitation. (See Core Administration of Testing and Rehabilitation Programs.)

4.0 MUSCULOSKELETAL PRACE AREA

4.1 **Pathophysiology of Musculoskeletal Diseases.** Basic knowledge of the epidemiology and pathophysiology of musculoskeletal diseases and disabilities, *including:* osteo- and rheumatoid-arthritis, back pain, osteoporosis, cumulative trauma disorders, joint sprains and strains, fractures, and status post–orthopedic surgeries.

4.1.1 Knowledge of the classification of spinal disorders, including spinal stenosis and spondylosis, spondylolysis, spondylolysthesis, herniated nucleus pulposus, and degenerative disk disease.

4.1.2 Knowledge the pathophysiology of osteo- and rheumatoid arthritis.

4.1.3 Knowledge of the pathophysiology and risk factors associated with osteoporosis.

4.1.4 Knowledge of the risk factors associated with repetitive motion/cumulative trauma disorders.

4.1.5 Basic knowledge of recovery factors associated with bone fractures, amputations, joint sprains and strains, and orthopedic surgery.

4.2 **Clinical Exercise Physiology Applied to Musculoskeletal Diseases.** Basic knowledge of the clinical applications of exercise physiology to individuals the musculoskeletal diseases and disabilities listed above.

4.2.1 Knowledge of the appropriate use of rest and avoidance of physical activity in patients with back pain and cumulative trauma disorders.

4.2.2 Knowledge of the use of spinal extension versus flexion exercises as they relate to directional symptom preference in patients with back pain.

4.2.3 Knowledge of the principle of specificity of training as applied to work simulation.

4.2.4 Knowledge of isometric, isotonic and isokinetic exercise in individuals with the musculoskeletal diseases and disabilities listed above.

4.2.5 Knowledge of cardiovascular training in persons with back pain.

4.2.6 Knowledge of functional anatomy and biomechanics.

4.2.6.1 Knowledge of directional and movement terminology, joint actions, and primary and secondary movers.

4.2.6.2 Knowledge of spinal anatomy, including the ability to describe degenerative spinal changes.

4.2.6.3 Knowledge of the spinal curves and how imbalances affect posture.

4.2.6.4 Knowledge of the effects of cyclical loading.

4.2.6.5 Ability to identify the interrelationships among center of gravity, base of support, balance, and stability with lifting.

4.2.6.6 Knowledge of the biomechanical differences between open- and closed-chain exercises.

4.2.6.7 Knowledge of the use of spinal extension in patients with osteoporosis.

4.3 **Musculoskeletal Pharmacology.** Basic knowledge of the drug classifications commonly used in the treatment of individuals with musculoskeletal diseases and disabilities, including the purposes, indications, major side effects, and the effects, if any, on the exercising individual:

4.3.1 Analgesics and anti-inflammatory agents

4.3.2 Corticosteroids

4.3.3 Muscle relaxants

4.3.4 Antiresorptive agents (i.e., estrogens, calcitonin, bisphosphonates, selective estrogen receptor modulators)

4.3.5 Deposition agents (i.e., calcium and vitamin D supplements)

4.4 **Musculoskeletal Aspects of the Physical Examination.** Basic knowledge, skills, and abilities related to the physical examination of individuals with musculoskeletal diseases and disabilities.

4.4.1 Basic knowledge of and ability to understand the results of a musculoskeletal examination.

4.4.2 Basic skills in and abilities to perform range-of-motion, flexibility, muscular strength, and muscular endurance measurements.

4.4.3 Basic skills in and abilities to perform a basic posture evaluation.

4.5 **Musculoskeletal Medical and Surgical Treatments.** Basic knowledge of techniques and ability to understand key findings in reports of medical and surgical treatments used in the management of individuals with musculoskeletal diseases and disabilities.

4.5.1 Basic knowledge of techniques and ability to understand key findings in reports of spinal surgeries, including: microdiscectomy, diskectomy, spinal decompression, spinal fusion, internal fixation, and laminectomy.

4.5.2 Basic knowledge of techniques and ability to understand key findings in reports of joint-replacement surgeries.

4.5.3 Basic knowledge of techniques and ability to understand key findings in reports of surgical approaches for the treatment of ulnar neuropathies, carpal tunnel syndrome, and cubital tunnel syndrome.

4.5.4 Basic knowledge of and ability to understand key findings in reports of bone fracture setting, amputations, and joint stabilization, including taping, casting, pins, and rods.

4.5.5 Basic knowledge of techniques and ability to understand key findings in reports of ligament- and tendon-repair surgeries.

4.5.6 Basic knowledge of techniques and ability to understand key findings in reports of arthroscopic joint surgeries.

4.6 **Musculoskeletal Diagnostic Techniques.** Basic knowledge of techniques and ability to understand key findings in reports of diagnostic techniques and specific knowledge and abilities in certain diagnostic modalities currently used in the management of individuals with musculoskeletal diseases and disabilities.

4.6.1 Basic knowledge of techniques and ability to understand key findings in reports of an EMG.

4.6.2 Basic knowledge of techniques and understanding of pain assessment tools (e.g., Waddell's nonorganic physical signs in low back pain, visual analog scales, SF-36, Oswestry disability Questionnaire, anatomic pain distribution, and Beck Depression Inventory).

4.6.3 Basic knowledge of techniques and ability to understand reports of bone-density measurements.

4.6.4 Basic knowledge of techniques and ability to understand reports of MRI, CT, bone scan, or x-ray.

4.7 **Musculoskeletal Exercise/Fitness/Functional Testing.** Knowledge, skills, and abilities used in administering exercise, fitness, work simulation, and/or functional tests in individuals with musculoskeletal diseases and disabilities.

4.7.1 Knowledge of the contraindications for maximal lifting tests.

- 4.7.2 Ability to perform maximal lift tests in the following planes: floor to knuckle, knuckle to shoulder, shoulder to overhead, single arm carry, and double arm carry.
- 4.7.3 Ability to calculate the recommended weight limit (RWL) for manual material handling tasks.
- 4.7.4 Skill in assessing patient's ability to perform essential vocational functions.
- 4.7.5 Ability to administer maximal grip strength tests.
- 4.7.6 Ability to administer orthopedic and musculoskeletal exercise tests using a variety of modes and protocols.
- 4.7.7 Ability to identify probable end points for exercise testing individuals with orthopedic and musculoskeletal disease and chronic pain.
- 4.7.8 Ability to perform immediate postexercise procedures and various approaches to cooldown following orthopedic and musculoskeletal exercise testing.
- 4.7.9 Ability to record, organize, and perform necessary calculations of exercise test data for summary presentation.
- 4.7.10 Ability to administer balance tests.

4.8 **Musculoskeletal Exercise Prescription and Programming.** Knowledge, skills, and abilities in prescribing and supervising exercise programs for individuals with musculoskeletal diseases and disabilities.

- 4.8.1 Ability to select appropriate exercise equipment and/or exercise activities for individuals with musculoskeletal injuries or disabilities.
- 4.8.2 Skill in developing frequency, intensity, and duration of exercise in supervised programs.
- 4.8.3 Ability to teach and maximize compliance with independent exercise programs.
- 4.8.4 Knowledge of concepts related to industrial or occupational rehabilitation, which includes work hardening, work conditioning, work fitness, and job coaching.

4.9 **Musculoskeletal Education and Counseling.** Knowledge, skills, and abilities in conducting education programs and counseling individuals with musculoskeletal disease and disabilities. (See Core Education and Counseling.)

4.10 **Musculoskeletal Emergency Procedures.** Basic knowledge, skills, and abilities to respond with appropriate emergency procedures for use prior to, during, or after administration of an exercise test or therapeutic exercise sessions for individuals with musculoskeletal diseases and disabilities. (See Core Emergency Procedures.)

4.11 **Musculoskeletal Quality Assurance, Outcome Assessment, and Discharge Planning.** Knowledge, skills, and abilities in quality assurance, outcome assessment, and discharge planning for exercise programs for individuals with musculoskeletal diseases and disabilities. (See Core Quality Assurance, Outcome Assessment, and Discharge Planning.)

4.12 **Musculoskeletal Administration of Testing and Rehabilitation Programs.** Knowledge, skills, and abilities used in the management of rehabilitation programs and exercise testing laboratories in the areas of musculoskeletal rehabilitation. (See Core Administration of Testing and Rehabilitation Programs.)

5.0 NEUROMUSCULAR PRACE AREA

5.1 **Pathophysiology of Neuromuscular Diseases.** Basic knowledge of the epidemiology and pathophysiology of neuromuscular diseases, *including:* stroke and head injury, spinal cord injury, multiple sclerosis, Parkinson's disease, cerebral palsy, post-polio, Guillain-Barre, muscular dystrophy, and peripheral neuropathy and chronic neurogenic pain.

- 5.1.1 Basic knowledge of the epidemiology of the above conditions.
- 5.1.2 Basic knowledge of the difference between disease classifications: congenital, acquired, traumatic, progressive, and relapsing.
- 5.1.3 Basic knowledge of the comorbidities associated with each condition.
- 5.1.4 Basic knowledge of dysesthesia and paresthesia as it relates to reflex sympathetic dystrophy
- 5.1.5 Basic knowledge of symptoms and signs of neurologic emergencies, e.g., seizures, autonomic hyperreflexia.
- 5.1.6 Basic knowledge of the difference between sensory loss versus one-sided neglect.
- 5.1.7 Basic knowledge of motor (i.e., flaccidity, spasticity, weakness, dyskinesias, bradykinesia, athetoid movements) and sensory (i.e., dysesthesias, paresthesia) disturbances of patients with the above conditions.

5.2 **Clinical Exercise Physiology Applied to Neuromuscular Diseases.** Basic knowledge of the clinical applications of exercise physiology to individuals with neuromuscular diseases and disabilities.

- 5.2.1 Basic knowledge of and ability to identify the affect of fatigue on the above conditions.
- 5.2.2 Basic knowledge of factors that increase the energy cost of locomotion.
- 5.2.3 Basic knowledge of factors that reduce and increase muscular spasticity in the above conditions.
- 5.2.4 Basic knowledge of the stretch response in patients with spasticity.
- 5.2.5 Basic knowledge of interference of heterotopic bone formation with exercise in paralyzed patients.
- 5.2.6 Basic knowledge of and ability to prevent or reduce contractures in individuals with the above conditions.

5.2.7 Basic knowledge of the effects of chronic exercise on osteopenia in paralyzed individuals.

5.2.8 Basic knowledge of neurogenic bladder and orthostasis in paralyzed patients.

5.2.9 Ability to recognize pulmonary limitations in the above conditions.

5.2.10 Basic knowledge of the effects of hydration and bladder control programs.

5.2.11 Basic knowledge of temperature regulation (internal and external) in individuals with the above conditions, especially spinal cord injury and multiple sclerosis.

5.2.12 Basic knowledge and ability to differentiate between peripheral and central pain.

5.2.13 Basic knowledge of and ability to describe the patterns of weakness in each of the above conditions.

5.2.14 Basic knowledge of gait and postural deviations.

5.2.15 Basic knowledge of the biomechanical effects of orthotic devices (bracing devices) on the function of the patients with the above conditions.

5.2.16 Ability to describe uses of functional electrical stimulation (FES) with spinal cord injury.

5.2.17 Basic knowledge of the phenomenon of tenodesis for gripping in spinal cord injury.

5.3 **Neuromuscular Pharmacology.** Basic knowledge of the drug classifications used in the treatment of individuals with neuromuscular diseases, including the purposes, indications, major side effects, and the effects, if any, on the exercising individual:

5.3.1 Anticoagulants

5.3.2 Analgesics

5.3.3 Anticonvulsants

5.3.4 Anti-inflammatories

5.3.5 Antispasmodics & anticholinergics

5.3.6 Migraine preparations

5.3.7 Muscle relaxants

5.3.8 Neurolytic agents (used in nerve and motor point blocks)

5.3.9 Parkinson's drugs

5.3.10 Psychotropics

5.4 **Neuromuscular Aspects of the Physical Examination.** Basic knowledge, skills, and abilities related to the neuromuscular physical examination of individuals with neuromuscular diseases and disabilities.

5.4.1 Ability to understand the report of the muscle strength exam in each of the above conditions.

5.4.2 Ability to understand the classification of muscle stretch reflexes (deep tendon reflexes) in the above conditions.

5.4.3 Ability to understand the terminology used in describing abnormal sensation.

5.4.4 Skills and abilities to identify spasticity, increased and decreased muscle tone, tremor, weakness, and sensory loss.

5.5 **Neuromuscular Medical and Surgical Treatments.** Basic knowledge of techniques and the ability to understand key findings in reports of various medical and surgical treatments used in the management of individuals with neuromuscular diseases.

5.5.1 Ability to understand key findings in medical reports describing a spinal fusion.

5.5.2 Ability to understand key findings in reports of brain surgery for aneurysm clipping and tumor removal.

5.5.3 Ability to understand key findings in reports of nerve and motor point blocks with phenol or Botox (botulinum toxin) for spasticity.

5.5.4 Basic knowledge of the purposes of epidural catheterization of the spine and sympathetic blocks. Skill to recognize the results of tendon-release procedures.

5.6 **Neuromuscular Diagnostic Techniques.** Basic knowledge of the techniques and ability to understand the key findings in reports of diagnostic techniques used in the management of individuals with neuromuscular diseases and disabilities.

5.6.1 Ability to understand key findings in reports of needle electromyography and nerve conduction studies.

5.6.2 Ability to understand key findings in reports of x-rays after spinal cord injury.

5.6.3 Ability to understand key findings in reports of scans for a brain hemorrhage in a stroke.

5.6.4 Ability to understand key findings in reports of angiograms and MRIs for cerebral aneurysms.

5.6.5 Ability to understand key findings in reports of Doppler studies and angiograms for peripheral vascular disease and carotid artery stenosis.

5.6.6 Ability to understand key findings in reports of lumbar spinal fluid tap for infections and multiple sclerosis.

5.6.7 Ability to understand key findings in reports of cognitive/neuropsychological testing.

5.6.8 Electromyography. Basic knowledge, skills, and abilities in clinical assessment of neuromuscular disease using surface electromyography (EMG).

5.6.8.1 Ability to understand the percent of maximum contraction using EMG.

5.6.8.2 Ability to understand motor unit recruitment patterns using EMG.

5.6.8.3 Ability to understand muscle fatigue or motor facilitation with the EMG.

5.6.8.4 Ability to understand the basic principles of biofeedback utilizing surface EMG.

5.7 **Neuromuscular Exercise/Fitness/Functional Testing.** Basic knowledge, skills, and abilities used in administering exercise, fitness, work simulation, and/or functional tests for individuals with neuromuscular diseases.

5.7.1 Basic knowledge of the functional limits and benefits of assistive devices (e.g., wheelchairs, crutches, canes) for daily activities.

5.7.2 Basic knowledge of the limitations placed on exercise testing methods by orthotic devices.

5.7.3 Basic knowledge of the relative effort of using these assistive devices in comparison to the effort of walking.

5.7.4 Ability to use the results of self-selected speed of ambulation with and without the use of an assistive device to determine patient function in a community setting (e.g., shopping, commuting).

5.7.5 Ability to determine performance capabilities of self-care, household duties, yard work, recreation for fitness, and occupational simulation skills.

5.7.6 Basic knowledge of the precautions and contraindications (absolute and relative) for exercise testing of the above conditions.

5.7.7 Ability to identify specialized equipment and adaptations for metabolic testing in the above conditions.

5.7.8 Basic knowledge of differences in test protocol and procedures in the above conditions.

5.7.9 Ability to modify test protocols and procedures for patients with neuromuscular limitations, including tests involving treadmill, cycle and arm ergometry, and with assistive devices.

5.8 **Neuromuscular Exercise Prescription and Programming.** Basic knowledge, skills, and abilities in prescribing and supervising exercise programs for individuals with neuromuscular diseases and disabilities. (Also see Core Exercise Prescription and Programming)

5.8.1 Ability to develop exercise prescriptions for the above conditions.

5.8.2 Ability to instruct an individual with neuromuscular disease in techniques for performing physical activities safely and effectively in an unsupervised setting.

5.8.3 Ability to supervise a small group exercise session for individuals with neuromuscular diseases and/or disabilities.

5.8.4 Knowledge of environmental (temperature, humidity) controls during exercise in patients with the above conditions.

5.9 **Neuromuscular Education and Counseling.** Basic knowledge, skills, and abilities in conducting education programs and counseling individuals with neuromuscular disease and disorders. (See Core Education and Counseling.)

5.10 **Neuromuscular Emergency Procedures.** Basic knowledge, skills, and abilities to respond with appropriate emergency procedures for use prior to, during, or after administration of an exercise test or therapeutic exercise sessions for individuals with neuromuscular diseases and disabilities. (See Core Emergency Procedures.

5.11 **Quality Assurance, Outcome Assessment, and Discharge Planning for Neuromuscular Programming.** Basic knowledge, skills, and abilities in quality assurance, outcome assessment, and discharge planning for programs for individuals with neuromuscular diseases and disabilities. (See Core Quality Assurance, Outcome Assessment, and Discharge Planning.)

5.12 **Administration of Neuromuscular Testing and Rehabilitation Programs.** Basic knowledge, skills, and abilities used in the management of rehabilitation programs and exercise testing laboratories in the areas of neuromuscular rehabilitation. (See Core Administration of Testing and Rehabilitation Programs.)

6.0 NEOPLASTIC, IMMUNOLOGIC, AND HEMATOLOGIC (NIH) DISORDERS PRACE AREA

6.1 **Pathophysiology of NIH Disorders.** Basic knowledge of the epidemiology and pathophysiology of NIH disorders, *including:* cancer, anemia, acquired immunodeficiency syndrome (AIDS), and chronic fatigue syndrome (CFS).

6.1.1 Knowledge of the etiology, epidemiology, and pathophysiology of cancer, specifically models of carcinogenesis, risk factors and signs/symptoms for major cancer sites (lung, colon and rectum, breast, prostate, and skin), cancer primary prevention guidelines, and recommended screening procedures (secondary prevention guidelines).

6.1.2 Knowledge of the etiology, epidemiology, and pathophysiology of anemia, specifically underlying disorders that affect red blood cell formation or lifespan, iron-deficiency stages and identification according to changes in blood indices, and dietary or medical factors related to anemia formation.

6.1.3 Knowledge of the etiology, epidemiology, and pathophysiology of acquired immunodeficiency syndrome (AIDS), specifically risk factors associated with infection from the human immunodeficiency virus (HIV), the stages of HIV disease and the specific signs and symptoms associated with each stage, and immune system and opportunistic infection criteria used by the Centers for Disease Control and Prevention (CDC) to define the acquired immunodeficiency syndrome.

6.1.4 Knowledge of the basic components of the immune system and how it responds to a pathogenic challenge.

6.1.5 Knowledge of the etiology, epidemiology, and pathophysiology of chronic fatigue syndrome (CFS), specifically potential immunologic, inflammatory, or neuroendocrine changes that may cause CFS, risk factors and signs/symptoms associated with CFS, and the criteria used by the CDC to define CFS.

6.2 **Clinical Exercise Physiology Applied to NIH Disorders.** Basic knowledge of the clinical applications of exercise physiology in individuals with NIH disorders.

6.2.1 Knowledge of the effect that cancer therapy (e.g., surgery, radiation, chemotherapy) may have on functional capacity and cardiopulmonary response to exercise and ability to engage in specific musculoskeletal movements.

6.2.2 Knowledge of the influence of anemia, iron deficiency, and sickle-cell anemia on functional capacity and cardiopulmonary responses to exercise.

6.2.3 Knowledge of how HIV disease influences acute cardiopulmonary and neuroendocrine responses to exercise.

6.2.4 Knowledge of how the immune system responds to acute and chronic exercise.

6.2.5 Knowledge of how CFS affects acute cardiovascular, pulmonary, and muscular responses to exercise.

6.2.6 Knowledge of the immediate and long-term influence of cancer therapy on cardiopulmonary and musculoskeletal responses to exercise training.

6.2.7 Knowledge of the potential adaptations to exercise training in individuals with different types of anemia.

6.2.8 Knowledge of immune, cardiopulmonary, and musculoskeletal responses to exercise training in HIV patients.

6.2.9 Knowledge of potential changes in symptomatology and aerobic capacity following periods of exercise training in CFS patients.

6.2.10 Knowledge of the nutritional and fluid considerations of individuals with NIH disorders engaging in exercise training.

6.3 **NIH Disorder Pharmacology.** Basic knowledge of the drug classifications commonly used in the treatment of patients with NIH disorders, including the purposes, indications, major side effects, and the effects, if any, on the exercising individual.

6.3.1 Cancer medications, including those used in antimetabolite, antitubulin, alkylator, anthracycline, and platinum salt chemotherapy, and those used in hormonal therapy. Anemia medications, including iron, folic acid, and vitamin B-12, and those used to prevent sickling, including hydroxyurea and butyrate.

6.3.2 Medications used in the treatment of HIV disease, including antiretroviral drugs included in highly active antiretroviral therapy (HAART).

6.3.3 Medications used in the treatment of CFS, including antidepressants, anti-inflammatory drugs, and immunologic therapy.

6.4 **NIH Disorder Physical Examination.** Basic knowledge, skills, and abilities related to the physical examination for individuals with NIH disorders.

6.4.1 Basic knowledge of and ability to understand the results of a physical examination on a patient with cancer, anemia, sickle-cell anemia, HIV disease, and CFS.

6.4.2 Basic knowledge of the signs and symptoms associated with NIH disorders.

6.5 **NIH Disorder Medical and Surgical Treatments.** Basic knowledge of techniques and understanding of key findings in reports of medical and surgical treatments used in the management of individuals with NIH disorders.

6.5.1 Basic knowledge of techniques and ability to understand key findings in reports of basic types of cancer treatment techniques, including radiation, systemic therapy, and surgery.

6.5.2 Basic knowledge of techniques and ability to understand key findings in reports of results of tests used to control and treat anemia, including nutrient supplementation, management of gastrointestinal bleeding, and transfusion.

6.5.3 Basic knowledge of techniques and ability to understand key findings in reports of results of tests used to manage HIV disease, including medications, nutritional therapy, psychological interventions, and treatment of opportunistic infections and cancers.

6.5.4 Basic knowledge of CFS management, including medications and interventions varied to meet predominant symptoms.

6.6 **NIH Disorder Diagnostic Techniques.** Basic knowledge of techniques ability to understand key findings in reports of assessment techniques used on patients with NIH disorders.

6.6.1 Basic knowledge of criteria used to assess iron deficiency and anemia.

6.6.2 Basic knowledge of techniques and ability to understand key findings of lab reports of tests for complete blood count (CBC) and other clinical laboratory reports and determine iron-deficiency and sickle-cell anemia.

6.6.3 Basic knowledge of techniques and ability to understand the screening guidelines for cancer.

6.6.4 Basic knowledge of techniques and ability to understand lab reports of leukocyte and lymphocyte subset blood counts from clinical laboratory reports, and note normal and abnormal values, especially for T helper cell counts ($CD3^+$, CD4) in patients with HIV disease.

6.6.5 Ability to determine whether an individual has CFS using CDC criteria (major symptom and physical criteria).

6.7 **NIH Disorder Exercise/Fitness/Functional Testing.** Knowledge, skills, and abilities in conducting exercise, fitness, work simulation, and/or functional tests for individuals with NIH disorders.

6.7.1 Knowledge of the indications and contraindications (absolute and relative) for graded exercise testing in patients with cancer, anemia, HIV disease, and CFS.

6.7.2 Knowledge of the probable effects of NIH disorders on exercise performance, functional capacity, and safety.

6.7.3 Knowledge of the use of Universal Precautions in the exercise testing of individuals with HIV disease.

6.8 **NIH Exercise Prescription and Programming.** Knowledge, skills, and abilities in prescribing and supervising exercise programs for individuals with NIH disorders.

6.8.1 Ability to develop exercise prescriptions for individuals with NIH disorders that are safe (e.g., avoidance of high-intensity exercise and dehydration in persons with sickle-cell disease).

6.8.2 Ability to supervise exercise programs for an individual or group with an NIH disorder.

6.8.3 Ability to instruct individuals with NIH disorders in techniques for performing physical activities safely and effectively in an unsupervised exercise setting.

6.9 **NIH Disorder Education and Counseling.** Knowledge, skills, and abilities in conducting education programs and counseling individuals with NIH disorders. (See Core Education and Counseling.)

6.10 **NIH Disorder Emergency Procedures.** Basic knowledge, skills, and abilities to respond with appropriate emergency procedures for use prior to, during, or after administration of an exercise test or therapeutic exercise sessions for individuals with NIH disorders. (See Core Emergency Procedures.)

6.11 **NIH Disorder Quality Assurance, Outcome Assessment, and Discharge Planning.** Knowledge, skills, and abilities in quality assurance, outcome assessment, and discharge planning for programs for individuals with NIH disorders. (See Core Quality Assurance, Outcome Assessment, and Discharge Planning.)

6.12 **NIH Disorder Administration of Testing and Rehabilitation Programs.** Knowledge, skills, and abilities used in the management of rehabilitation programs and exercise testing laboratories in the areas of NIH Disorders. (See Core Administration of Testing and Rehabilitation Programs.)

Clinical Exercise Physiology Knowledge, Skills, and Abilities Writing Groups

William Jay Gillespie, EdD, FACSM, Editor
Chair, Clinical Exercise Physiology Exam Sub-Committee
Associate Professor and Chair
Department of Cardiopulmonary and Exercise Sciences
Bouve College of Health Sciences
Northeastern University
Boston, MA
Clinical Physiologist
Beth Israel Deaconess Medical Center
Boston, MA

Cardiovascular Practice Area

William Jay Gillespie,
Practice Area Coordinator

William G. Herbert, PhD, FACSM
Chair, Clinical Exercise Physiology Practice Board
Professor and Director, Laboratory for Health & Exercise Science
Department of Human Nutrition, Foods, and Exercise
Virginia Tech
Blacksburg, VA

Jeffrey L. Roitman, EdD, FACSM
Director, Cardiac Rehabilitation
Baptist Medical Center and Research Medical Center
Kansas City, MO

Ernest Gervino, ScD, FACSM
Director of Clinical Physiology, Cardiovascular Division
Beth Israel Deaconess Medical Center
Assistant Professor of Medicine
Harvard Medical School
Boston, MA

Joseph R. Libonati, PhD
Assistant Professor and Director
Kinetics Research Laboratory
Temple University
Philadelphia, PA

Jeffrey Ocel, PhD
Clinical Physiologist, Cardiovascular Division
Beth Israel Deaconess Medical Center
Boston, MA

Nancy O'Hare, ScD, FACSM
Clinical Physiologist, Cardiovascular Division
Beth Israel Deaconess Medical Center
Boston, MA

Pulmonary Practice Area

Reed H. Humphrey, PhD, PT, FACSM, FAACVPR,
Practice Area Coordinator
Assistant Professor, Departments of Physical Therapy & Physical Medicine and Rehabilitation
Virginia Commonwealth University/Medical College of Virginia Health Sciences
Richmond, VA

Brian W. Carlin, MD
Medical Director, Pulmonary Rehabilitation
Allegheny General Hospital
Pittsburgh, PA

Dianne V. Jewell, MS, PT, CCS, FAACVPR
Physical Therapy Clinical Education Coordinator
Sheltering Arms Rehabilitation Hospital
Richmond, VA

Metabolic Practice Area

Patricia Painter, PhD, FACSM
Practice Area Coordinator
Transplant Rehabilitation Director
University of California at San Francisco
San Francisco, CA

Susan Carey, MS
Staff Research Assistant—Renal Exercise Demonstration Project
Department of Physiologic Nursing
University of California at San Francisco
San Francisco, CA

J. Larry Durstine, PhD, FACSM
Associate Professor
Department of Exercise Science
University of South Carolina
Columbia, SC

Joanne Krasnoff, MS
Staff Research Assistant—Diet and Exercise following Liver Transplant
Department of Physiologic Nursing
University of California at San Francisco
San Francisco, CA

David Miller, MS
Transplant Exercise Physiologist
Department of Rehabilitation Services
University of California at San Francisco
San Francisco, CA

David Nieman, DrPH, FACSM
Professor of Health and Exercise Science
Appalachian State University
Boone, NC

Janet P. Wallace, PhD, FACSM
Associate Professor
Department of Kinesiology
Indiana University
Bloomington, IN

Musculoskeletal Practice Area

Carol A. Harnett, MS,
Practice Area Coordinator
Director, Wellness and Ability Management
Hartford Life
Simsbury, CT

Sherry A. Barkley, MS
HPER Instructor
Augustana College
Sioux Falls, SD

Robert W. Boyce, PhD, FACSM
Charlotte, NC

Ron Bybee, PhD, PT
University of Texas, El Paso
El Paso, TX

Fredrick S. Daniels, MS
CPTE Health Group, Inc.
Nashua, NH

Thomas E. Dreisinger, PhD, FACSM
Preventive Care, Inc.
Jefferson City, MO

Dale Moss, MS
Abbott-Northwestern Hospital
Fridley, MN

Neuromuscular Practice Area

Terry L. Nicola, MD, MS,
Practice Area Coordinator
Director, Sports Medicine Rehabilitation, and Assistant Professor
Department of Rehabilitation Medicine and Restorative Sciences
University of Illinois Medical Center
Chicago, IL

Cheryl Dudeck, MS
Coordinator, Clinical Exercise Physiology Program
Department of Rehabilitation Medicine and Restorative Sciences
University of Illinois Medical Center
Chicago, IL

James Rimmer, PhD
Research Program Director
Institute of Disability and Human Development
University of Illinois Medical Center
Chicago, IL

Neoplastic, Immunologic, and Hematologic Practice Area

David C. Nieman, DrPH, FACSM,
Practice Area Coordinator
Professor of Health and Exercise Science
Appalachian State University
Boone, NC

Ron Deitrick, PhD, FACSM
Program Director, Cardiac Rehabilitation
Clinical Coordinator, Spinal Cord Injury Research Center
West LA VA Medical Center, Physical Medicine and Rehab (117)
Los Angeles, CA

E. Randy Eichner, MD, FACSM
Professor of Medicine
Health Sciences Center
Oklahoma University
Oklahoma City, OK

Roy Shephard, PhD
Professor Emeritus of Applied Physiology
Physical Education and Health
University of Toronto, Toronto, Canada
Visiting Scientist at DCIEM
Resident Scholar in Health Studies at Brock University
St. Catharine's, ON, Canada

Index